HANDBOOK ON WOMEN AND AGING

Edited by
Jean M. Coyle

Greenwood Press
Westport, Connecticut • London

Library of Congress Cataloging-in-Publication Data

Handbook on women and aging / edited by Jean M. Coyle.
    p. cm.
   Includes bibliographical references and index.
   ISBN 0-313-28857-7 (alk. paper)
   1. Middle aged women—United States. 2. Aged women—United
States. I. Coyle, Jean M.
   HQ1059.5.U5H36   1997
   305.24'4—dc20   96–32414

British Library Cataloguing in Publication Data is available.

Library of Congress Catalog Card Number: 96–32414
ISBN: 0-313-28857-7

First published in 1997

Greenwood Press, 88 Post Road West, Westport, CT 06881
An imprint of Greenwood Publishing Group, Inc.

Printed in the United States of America

The paper used in this book complies with the
Permanent Paper Standard issued by the National
Information Standards Organization (Z39.48–1984).

10 9 8 7 6 5 4 3 2 1

Copyright Acknowledgments

The author and publisher gratefully acknowledge permission to reproduce the following copyrighted material:

Elisa Facio. Chapter 5 of *Understanding Older Chicanas* by Elisa Facio, copyright ©
1996 by Sage Publications, Inc. Reprinted by permission of Sage Publications.

Dedicated
to the memory
of my mother, Bertha Jeanette Lay Coyle,
my grandmother, Anna Maria Euler Lay,
and gerontologist Mildred M. Seltzer

Contents

PART I:
Historical and Theoretical Perspectives

PART II:
Economic Issues

PART III:
Health, Psychological, and Living Issues

PART IV:
Racial, Ethnic, and Demographic Issues

PART V:
Relationships

Preface

This reference book is designed to provide an extensive discussion of diverse topics with regard to midlife and older women. The intent in each chapter is to discuss the state of knowledge and the most current research on that topic. A wide variety of subjects reflecting many areas of the lives of midlife and older women has been selected for this volume. The major subjects covered herein include the old-old, work, rural older women, images in art, sexism and ageism, friendship, health, sex-role stereotypes, the social construction of older women, reminiscence, retirement, spirituality, voluntarism, models of lifespan psychological change, American Indians, Asian Americans, black Americans, Chicanas, suicide, economics, caregiving daughters, family relationships, historical images, singlehood, life satisfaction, widowhood, living arrangements, and fathers, daughters, and caregiving.

Many topics significant to midlife and older women are included in this volume, and there are others that might have been, or that might be included in a succeeding publication. The attempt in this book was to present an extremely varied collection of chapters focusing on issues most affecting midlife and older women. Some topics are more theoretical, while others emphasize more pragmatic concerns. Together, these chapters offer the reader an eclectic collection of information on women's issues.

Acknowledgments

I want to express my thanks to George Butler, Associate Editor, Acquisitions, at Greenwood Press, who conceived the idea of this book and invited me to develop it. I appreciate very much the support and encouragement of the previous editor, Mim Vasan, Senior Acquisitions Editor, before her retirement. Special thanks to Charles Eberline for his extremely careful copyediting and to Lynn Zelem, Production Editor, for her extensive and conscientious work in finalizing the manuscript.

I especially want to thank all the chapter authors who have shared their respective areas of expertise within this publication. They have provided insightful contributions. I would also like to thank Jan Davidson and other staff members at the American Association of Retired Persons Resource Center, Washington, D.C., and staff members at the Library of Congress, Washington, D.C., for their assistance.

Introduction

JEAN M. COYLE

Women live longer than men—an irrefutable fact. "Women form a substantial majority of the North American population over 50 and increasingly more of a majority with each succeeding age decade" (Turner & Troll, 1994, p. 2). However, lack of empirical data on women as they age has "perpetuated societal myths. . . . Preconceived notions and myths are slow to change, even in the face of an emerging body of research with women as the investigators" (Jacobson, 1995, p. 3). The focus in this book is on presenting a diverse and eclectic collection of topics related to these midlife and older women. The emphasis is on women and their concerns.

When this author was writing her dissertation on women's attitudes toward retirement in 1976, she found many articles on retirement that did not even identify the gender of the subjects. There was a presumption that only males worked and only males retired—an exaggeration of the facts, to be sure, but, nonetheless, the reality was that subjects' genders were not always specified. Even in 1996 there remain numerous unanswered questions about the lives of midlife and older women, especially how future cohorts of women will deal with their concerns—indeed, what their concerns will be. Within this volume, chapter authors—well-known experts in their areas of focus—present a review of research and knowledge of their subjects and raise questions for future research.

Erdman Palmore begins with a discussion of the effects of sexism and ageism on women. Palmore considers the "double standard of aging." Continuing this discussion, Susan Sherman looks at age and gender stereotypes, reporting research that failed to give strong evidence of a double standard. Sherman indicates that there is congruence of some negative themes across the various areas reviewed.

Historian Carole Haber examines the findings of recent historical studies about old women. Haber reveals the "distinctive past" of older women, which challenges traditional notions of being old in America. Images of aging women through time are described by Mary Grizzard, who presents a wide range of images of middle-aged and older women as depicted in diverse art forms. Also considering historical views of women, Elizabeth Markson describes the social construction of older women throughout history. Markson discusses the ambivalent attitudes toward older women.

The "Economic Issues" part of this book looks at economic status, work, and retirement. Economist Rose Rubin presents a thorough description of the economic status of older women. Rubin covers employment, income, wealth, and expenditures. The differentiation of financial situations based on gender is clearly stated.

John Rife focuses on middle-aged and older women's participation in the work force, raising the question of what we know about the employment and unemployment of these women. Rife delineates the changing labor force, income as a primary reason for women entering the labor force, women being disadvantaged in the labor market, the negative impact of unemployment, and the need for additional research.

Just as work has become increasingly important in the lives of more American women, so, too, has the retirement period of their lives. Frances Carp identifies the financial problem for retired women as a key element in their lives, often resulting from lower wages during working years and, thus, lower pensions in retirement. The need for more research specifically on women and retirement is apparent.

Diverse topics are presented in "Health, Psychological, and Living Issues." Diana Torrez provides a discussion of health characteristics of older women, particularly differentiating by race and ethnicity. Torrez considers life expectancy and mortality, specific health conditions, such as diabetes and hypertension, effects of income on health status, limitations of activities, and use of health care services. Recognizing the vast differences among older women, Torrez concludes, is the starting point to developing effective health policy.

Jan Sinnott offers an approach to capturing the "richness and complexity in the development of mature women." Sinnott discusses ways of modelling women's development as they age. She concludes by recommending a synthesis of several models.

B. Jan McCulloch explores the factor structure of life satisfaction among older women. McCulloch questions what the factor structure of life satisfaction is for separate cohorts of older women and whether a single life-satisfaction factor structure has been confirmed across cohorts of older women. The consistency found in the performance of the life-satisfaction index among older women has increased confidence that the scale found a similar interpretation across cohort groups.

Using a qualitative approach, Debra McDonald and Eileen Curl explore elderly women's perceptions of reminiscence. Reminiscence as a therapy and as a potentially beneficial intervention technique is examined.

Nancy Osgood and Marjorie Malkin examine age and gender differences in suicide and discuss major factors related to suicidal behavior in women. Older women have been neglected in research on suicide. The authors predict a significant rise in the rate of completed suicide among women 65 and over.

America's oldest women, those 85 and over, are survivors, as assessed by Sally Bould and Charles Longino, rather than victims, as they are often portrayed. In spite of higher degrees of disability among old-old women, Bould and Longino cite "the preponderance of women at the top of the population pyramid [as] ipso facto proof of their biological and psychological strength." The authors indicate that there is an "aura of survivorship" among these women, along with a sense of "aloneness" and a sense of "singularity."

Barbara Payne-Stancil views women's search for the meaning of their lives as reflected in their involvement in religious activities and practices. Payne-Stancil reports that women are more religious than men at every age. Even when religious activities decline with age, they decline less for women, and religion becomes more important to them. Payne-Stancil also considers the "baby-boomer" woman's religiosity and spiritual journey and adds her own spiritual autobiographical postscript.

While the stereotypical image of the volunteer is as an upper- or middle-class, white homemaker, Winifred Dowling reports that a number of studies show that older women are only slightly more likely to volunteer than older men and that, in general, older people are less likely to volunteer than younger age groups. Dowling predicts significant changes in the participation of older women as volunteers, with an expected increase among both the young-old and the old-old.

Frances Carp reports significant sex differences in living arrangements, with a trend toward desiring to live independently. Many older women live alone because they have no alternative, but they tend to be economically deprived, to have chronic and multiple health problems and inadequate health care, to be socially isolated, and to suffer lives of very poor quality. Carp predicts a large increase in the number of elderly women living alone in the next century.

Middle-aged and older women in four major racial and ethnic groups in the United States are the focus of "Racial, Ethnic, and Demographic Issues." Penny Ralston leads off with a review of research on midlife and older black women. Ralston examines the sociohistorical context of contemporary midlife and older black women, the roles of black women in their families, communities, and work, health behaviors, and foci for future research.

Robert John, Patrice Blanchard, and Catherine Hennessy address the lives of American Indian women elders—lives that they report are hidden because so little has been written about aging and American Indian women and because most existing information is difficult to find. The authors consider demographic characteristics, status and roles, and contributions of aging American Indian women.

Darlene Yee presents a review of the limited literature available on the aging of Asian-American women. Yee discusses the factors complicating research on Asian Americans, including the ethnic diversity of the groupings of Asian-American women.

Elisa Facio focuses on women of Mexican descent residing in the United States, one of a number of Hispanic groups that include Cuban Americans, Puerto Ricans, Mexican Americans, Central Americans, and other Spanish speakers, as the Census Bureau identifies them. The majority of research conducted on older ''Hispanic'' women has been on Mexican Americans, who comprise 14 million of the 23 million people in the United States who are categorized as Hispanic. Generalizations from this research on one Hispanic group cannot be made to all Hispanic groups. Facio examines the social construction of womanhood for older Chicanas as caregivers and as cultural teachers.

Rural older women are profiled by Vira Kivett, who reports that these women generally have been treated as an independent variable, rather than as a major unit of analysis. Kivett looks at physical well-being, psychological well-being, social characteristics, economic well-being, housing, supports, and needs. She predicts that future rural older women will become more heterogeneous, greater self-advocates, more powerful politically, and more economically independent.

Jean Pearson Scott begins ''Relationships'' by painting a portrait of family relationships for midlife and older women in a time of dramatic demographic and technological changes. Scott recommends more research grounded in theory, as well as broader representation in samples of social class, race/ethnicity, and region.

The ever-single older woman, comprising only about 5% of the population, is the focus of Richard Newtson and Pat Keith's chapter. Perhaps because marriage is considered normative behavior, those individuals who remain unmarried throughout the life course are often neglected by researchers. The majority of research suggests that ever-single aged women may be better off (e.g., more friends, better health) than the widowed, divorced, or separated. This chapter offers an extremely thorough, and rare, description of this subgroup of older women.

Using an integrative conceptual framework, Rebecca Adams examines friendships among older adult women. She looks at number, homogeneity, density, and solidarity. Adams suggests new studies comparing women and men across stages of the life course, separating out age, period, and cohort effects, distinguishing between the sociological and psychological effects of age and gender, and identifying sources of variation in friendship patterns, such as social class and ethnicity.

Widowhood, which affects almost half of all older women, is the topic of Julia Bradsher's chapter. Gender appears to be a differentiator in the widowhood experience. American society provides a unique historical, social, and cultural context for widowhood.

In her discussion of women as caregivers for the elderly, Sally Bould argues that the emotional bond between elderly mothers and their middle-aged daughters motivates the caregiving by the daughters. Bould presents an explanation of the radical change in familial caretaking between the 1910s and the 1980s and provides evidence of the elder care being provided by middle-aged daughters.

Bertram Cohler considers the relationship between older fathers and their adult daughters, on which topic the knowledge is quite limited. The daughter is the most visible caregiver. Cohler recommends systematic study of the middle-aged-daughter/older-father relationship from both social and psychoanalytic perspectives.

This volume presents a wide range of topics—although, certainly, not every possible subject that might be addressed. The authors have reviewed the most pertinent research on their topics and have posed useful questions for further research. It is evident that there has developed, especially within the past decade, a growing body of knowledge about midlife and older women. Significant research gaps remain in many areas, offering current and future researchers new challenges and opportunities.

REFERENCES

Jacobson, J. (1995). *Midlife women.* Boston: Jones & Bartlett.
Turner, B., & Troll, L. (Eds.). (1994). *Women growing older: Psychological perspectives.* Thousand Oaks, CA: Sage Publications.

Part I

Historical and Theoretical Perspectives

One

Sexism and Ageism

ERDMAN B. PALMORE

Aging in our society progressively destroys a woman but is less profoundly wounding for a man. (Sontag, 1972)

What are sexism and ageism? What happens when sexism is combined with ageism? Is sexism worse in old age? Is ageism worse against older women? In other words, do older women suffer from "double jeopardy" or a "double standard of aging"? Which has stronger effects: ageism or sexism? What are the sources of sexism in old age, and how can it be reduced? These are the basic questions for this chapter, but before we can begin to answer them, we need to clarify some concepts.

CONCEPTS

The terms *ageism* and *sexism* were coined about the same time (1969 and 1970, respectively), but sexism has become more widely used than ageism. Almost everyone has heard of sexism. Until recently, few people had heard of ageism. Now, however, there are four books on the subject (Barrow & Smith, 1979; Levin & Levin, 1980; Palmore, 1990; Bytheway, 1995), as well as numerous articles.

Both concepts refer to prejudice or discrimination against a category of people: sexism is usually directed against women, and ageism is usually directed against the aged. However, sometimes sexism is directed against men (by some extreme feminists), and ageism is sometimes directed against younger people ("positive ageism," Palmore, 1990).

Prejudice is a negative attitude toward a category of people that is inaccurate and resistant to change. Discrimination is an inappropriate treatment of a category of people, usually based on prejudice.

Sexism and ageism combine in all possible ways: a few areas show neither one, more areas are affected by one but not the other, but most areas are affected by both. Figure 1.1 is a "decision-tree" diagram for sorting out these various combinations of ageism and sexism. There may be some areas with neither ageism nor sexism (box 1), although it is hard to think of any area completely free of such prejudice.

In some areas there is sexism with little or no ageism (box 2). For example, it is generally believed that women of any age should not marry men younger than themselves, but it is all right for men to marry women younger than themselves. This is a main reason why there are over five times as many widows as widowers over 65.

On the other hand, in some areas there is ageism but little or no sexism (box 3). For example, many people believe that most old people are feeble or senile, regardless of gender. The fact is that the majority of people over 65 are neither feeble nor senile.

In most areas both ageism and sexism combine to intensify the problems of older women (box 4). For example, women of all ages tend to have lower incomes than men (sexism), but older women also tend to have even lower incomes than younger women (ageism). This situation is often called "double jeopardy" because of the combined effects (box 5).

Sontag (1972) coined the term "double standard of aging." This refers to the combination of sexism and ageism that multiplies the effects of both, more than would be expected on the basis of simply adding the two effects (box 6). For example, being physically attractive is more important in most women's lives than in men's (sexism); and there is a common belief that older persons are generally not as attractive as young people (ageism). However, women's grey hair, wrinkles, bulges, and stooped bodies receive harsher judgment than those of men. For many women, aging means a "humiliating process of gradual sexual disqualification" (Sontag, 1972), while many men enjoy more romantic success later in life because they have more status, money, and power than they had earlier. As a result, being a "spinster" or "old maid" is considered a pitiful status, while being an older bachelor is not so bad. Notice that there is no male equivalent of "old maid."

It may be objected that many older women do not mind this "sexual disqualification" and adjust to it by renouncing all interest in sexual activities or by becoming lesbians. This is true, but beside the point. The point is that sexism combined with ageism tends to enforce this "sexual disqualification" whether or not the woman likes it.

PAST OR PRESENT SEXISM?

Another complication is whether the inferior status of older women is due to present sexism against older women or to a lifetime of past sexism. Let us

Figure 1.1
Decision Tree for Ageism and Sexism

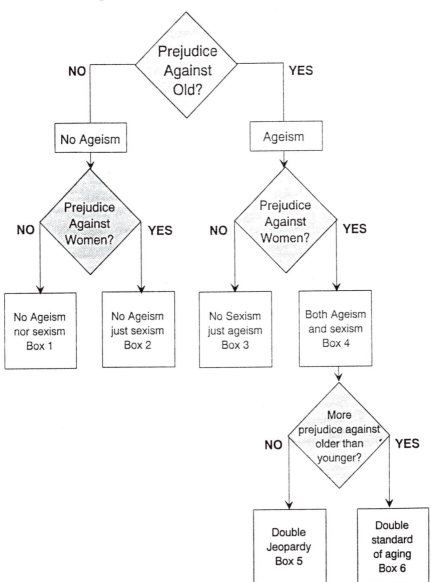

examine some of the major differences between older women and men to see the extent to which they are caused by past or present sexism.

One basic difference that underlies many of the other differences is the fact that three-fourths of men over 65 are living with their spouse, while only a minority of older women are so fortunate (42%; Treas, 1995). This is due to a combination of past and present sexism and the greater longevity of women. Women on average marry men four years older than themselves (past sexism). Older widows find fewer men eligible for remarriage because of the prohibition of marrying younger men (present sexism). The greater longevity of women (despite sexism) creates many more widows than widowers.

This difference in marital status underlies several of the other differences between men and women. Partly because more women are widowed, they are more likely to live alone, be less active sexually, be isolated, be in poverty, need home care, and be institutionalized.

Or consider the well-known income differential between men and women. The median income of women over 65 is about 57% of men's (U.S. Senate, 1990). This is partly related to more women being widowed (which in turn is due to past and present sexism, as described earlier) and partly to present discrimination against older women in employment, but is mainly due to past sexism in the form of employment discrimination, interrupted careers, and lower rates of employment. The gap between median incomes of all women and men (women's is 40% less than men's) is slightly larger in old age (43%), but this could be mainly a ''cohort effect'' because earlier generations of women did not have as much lifetime employment to produce pensions and savings for old age.

Similarly, the higher rates of mental illness among older women are probably due to a combination of past and present sexism. Actually, we do not know why women of all ages have higher rates of mental illness than men in most studies (Palmore, 1984). The higher rates for women may be due to some genetic difference in susceptibility between women and men, or to the methods of identifying cases of mental illness (women are usually more willing to admit psychiatric symptoms), or to the stresses produced by past and present sexism, or to a combination of all these explanations. It should be noted that the overall rates are higher for women despite the fact that men have more brain syndromes from alcoholism and syphilis.

DOES OLD AGE INCREASE OR DECREASE SEXISM?

A related question is whether sexism increases with age, stays the same, or decreases. The answer is that any one of these may occur, depending on the area. The ''double standard of aging'' in regard to sexuality (described earlier) is a good example of increasing sexism.

Another example is the increasing difference between women and men in the proportion in poverty. Among adults under age 65, the proportion in poverty is about 5% higher among women (14%) than among men (9%); but this proportion is about 8% higher among older women (18%) than among men (10%; U.S. Bureau of the Census, 1982, U.S. Senate, 1990). This increase is partly caused by the increasing rate of widowhood among women, but it may also be caused by increasing discrimination in employment that prevents poor older women from supplementing their income with adequate earnings.

Some forms of sexism appear to diminish in old age. For example, the gap in self-esteem appears to decline from late middle age onward (Turner, 1987). Regardless of age, women in our culture tend to have lower self-esteem and more self-criticism than do men. However, several studies have found that the gender difference in self-criticism was less among persons over age 55. What could account for this decrease? It may be a cohort difference, since these studies were cross-sectional rather than longitudinal. However, there seems to be no theoretical reason to expect such a cohort effect. A more likely explanation is that because "feminine" traits are generally rated as socially undesirable by both women and men, if "femininity" declines and "masculinity" increases as women grow older, self-concept would improve. Thus the decrease in self-criticism among women with age is not because of decreasing sexism (as reflected in the negative ratings of "feminine" traits), but because gender-role differences tend to decline with age (as reflected in less "feminism" among older women). There is considerable evidence that as men retire and women are freed from traditional child-rearing duties, there is a growing convergence of gender roles and traits in old age.

For example, several cross-sectional studies have found that self-concepts are less stereotypically sex typed in older men and women than in middle-aged and young adults (Turner, 1987). Older men come to view themselves as more nurturant, tender minded, and dependent, while older women describe themselves as more assertive, managerial, and autonomous. It is noteworthy that these differences were more related to stage of life than to chronological age. In other words, many older women find themselves freed from the traditional feminine roles and become free to "be yourself," to do what they want, when and how they want. This increases their morale and decreases their self-criticism.

Another example of decreasing sexism in old age is the fact that the differences between men and women in access to health care tend to decline. Older women have more access to good health care because they are covered by Medicare, whereas many younger women have little or no health insurance. Lack of health insurance among younger women is caused by their lower rates of employment at jobs that provide health insurance. This, in turn, is partly caused by discrimination against women in employment.

COHORT DIFFERENCES

As mentioned earlier, the question of increasing or decreasing sexism is complicated by the possibilities of cohort (generational) differences in the gaps between men and women. It is well known that among younger cohorts there are decreasing differences between women and men in educational attainment, occupational achievement, legal rights, sexual activity, marital status, physical fitness, smoking, drinking, driving, recreation, and other aspects of lifestyle. Because of these shrinking gaps, some of the differences between women and men in the present older generation may be expected to decline as newer cohorts move into the category of old age. Thus what may now appear to be increasing sexism in old age may turn out to be mainly caused by cohort differences.

SEXISM, AGEISM, AND RACISM

Which is worst in old age: sexism, ageism, or racism? There have been few attempts to answer this question quantitatively. Atchley (1991) analyzed how education, race, and gender simultaneously affect earnings of full-time workers aged 55 to 64 within various occupations. He concluded that while lower education and being black were disadvantages within most occupations, the greatest disadvantage was being a woman. For example, women in the most advantaged categories—white, college-educated women—consistently had median incomes lower than men in the most disadvantaged categories—black men who had not completed high school in jobs such as crafts and clerical work (p. 311).

Palmore and Manton (1973) analyzed the race, sex, and age inequalities shown by the U.S. census statistics and found that the relative importance of these inequalities depended on which indicator was being used. Age inequality was greater than race and sex inequality in the number of years of education completed and in the number of weeks worked. In other words, there was more discrepancy between the aged and nonaged in their education and weeks worked than there was between the whites and nonwhites and between men and women.

On the other hand, in the area of occupation, age inequality was less than racial and sex inequality. Age inequality was also less than sex inequality in the area of income. Of course, these inequalities are influenced by other factors than ageism, sexism, and racism, but at present it is difficult to control for the other factors (such as personal choice, education, and so on).

SOURCES OF AGEISM AND SEXISM

There are many sources of ageism: individual, social, and cultural (Palmore, 1990). The individual sources include authoritarian personalities, frustration and aggression, selective perception, rationalization, and death anxiety. The social sources include modernization, competition, obsolescence, segregation, and self-fulfilling prophecies. The cultural sources include the process of blaming the victim, differing value orientations, language, humor, songs, art, literature, television, and cultural lag.

There are probably just as many sources of sexism that have been documented and analyzed elsewhere (see, for example, Friedan, 1963). However, in this section we will discuss only a few sources of sexism that seem to increase in old age: humor, songs, language, and television.

Humor

Negative jokes about women of all ages are common. However, jokes about old women seem to be relatively more frequent and more negative than those about younger women (Palmore, 1971, 1990). In analyzing 264 jokes about older people, it was found that those dealing with old women were much more likely to be negative (77%) than those dealing with old men (51%). Furthermore, most of the jokes about age concealment attributed it to women ("It's terrible to grow old alone—my wife hasn't had a birthday in six years"). One of the largest categories of jokes was about old maids, and there were no equivalent jokes about old bachelors.

As any student of racism or sexism knows, negative humor is one of the most common and effective ways to perpetuate negative stereotypes about a minority group. One reason negative humor about a group is so common and effective is that it is passed off as "just a joke" or "harmless humor." In fact, negative humor is rarely harmless and is especially insidious because its viciousness is masked by its overt "funniness."

Thus the age-concealment jokes reinforce the stereotype that all older women are ashamed of their age, while older men are not. It may well be that somewhat more old women are ashamed of their age than are old men (because of the "double standard of aging"), but that is beside the point. Similarly, the status of old maid is generally considered more negative than that of old bachelor, but that too is beside the point. The point is that such negative humor reinforces prejudice against older women.

Songs

Negative songs about old age are another source of ageism in our culture. Cohen and Kruschwitz (1990) have collected and analyzed over 400 pieces of sheet music about old age in America. They found that a substantial majority present a negative view of aging and old age. In an analysis of sexism in these songs, Cohen (1993) concluded that old women are more likely to be viewed positively than negatively, but in songs dealing with negative physical aspects of aging, women are more likely than men to be mentioned. This is further evidence of the "double standard of aging" in which physical decline is seen as worse in women than in men.

Language

One of the most subtle but pervasive influences of culture on our attitudes is our language: the words we use to identify or describe a person or group; the derivations, definitions, and connotations of the words; their synonyms and antonyms; and the context in which they are used. Our language often supports ageism in all of these ways (Palmore, 1990).

In addition, two analyses of words for elders have found that many of them also reflect sexism. Covey (1988) found that terms for old women have a much longer history of negative connotations than those for old men, because women not only faced a long history of ageism, but also sexism and religious persecution (as in witch hunts).

Similarly, Nuessel (1982) found that many contemporary terms for the aged are doubly offensive because they reflect both ageism and sexism (anile, beldame, biddy, crone, grimalkin, hag, little old lady, old maid, old bag, old bat, old battle ax, spinster, witch). There are also a few ageist terms for old men (codger, coot, geezer), but the ageist vocabulary for women is "more derisive because it represents them as thoroughly repugnant and disgusting" (p. 274). Also, there are many more ageist terms for women (14) than for men (7).

Television

Television is the most important mass medium in the United States (and in most of the rest of the world). There are several ways in which television supports ageism (Palmore, 1990), and this is particularly true about ageism against women. There is clearly a sexist bias among the elders that are portrayed. Only 10% of the people on television over 65 are female (Davis & Davis, 1985), and those few tend to be portrayed negatively (Gerbner, Grass, Signorielli, & Morgan, 1980). Older women tend to be comic or eccentric figures and are likely to be treated disrespectfully. In contrast, older men are given increased sexual attractiveness as they age, often based on their increased assets and social power.

However, there are some recent exceptions to the negative image of older women, as in "Murder She Wrote" and in some recent soap operas where they are often seen as official and informal advisors (Elliott, 1984). Nevertheless, older women in the "soaps" are still more often seen as the nurturer, the adoring attendant, or the nag than in other roles.

SEXISM AND CRIME

There are very few old criminals and even fewer old female criminals. Arrest and incarceration rates for men over 65 are about one-tenth those of younger men, and older women are arrested and imprisoned even more rarely (Palmore, 1990). Part of the reason for this appears to be "positive ageism" (prejudice in favor of elders) and "reverse sexism" (discrimination in favor of women). Chaneles (1987), a criminologist, asserted: "I believe the facts [about criminality among elders] are obscured by a double standard of law enforcement toward older men and women. Except for the most serious crimes, such as murder, police and prosecutors are inclined to overlook offenses by the elderly, especially by women. They often don't make arrests, or if they do, the charges are dismissed'' (p. 49).

Similarly, despite the stereotype of the frequently victimized "little old lady," elders are victimized less often than others, and older women are victimized even less than older men (Schick, 1986). The criminal victimization rate for those over 65 is less than half that of persons aged 12 to 64 in all categories of crime except purse snatching/pocket picking; and the victimization rate for older women is less than half that of older men. The victimization rate in elder abuse for women is also half that of men, but women are more likely to be physically abused (Atchley, 1991). Rape, of course, is mostly a crime against women; but rape of older women is quite rare (less than two per year per 100,000 women 65 or older). Less than 2% of all rapes involve women over 65 (Schick, 1986).

There are a number of reasons for these low rates of victimization. Elders, and especially older women, are more fearful of crime, are more cautious, and avoid dangerous situations and areas. Elders, and especially older women, tend to stay home more and therefore discourage burglary and avoid crime on the streets. Elders, and especially older women, are less likely to provoke violent crimes by aggressive behavior. The stereotype that elders, and especially older women, tend to be poor and have little worth stealing may make them less attractive targets for property crimes.

There is one type of crime that appears to victimize elders and especially older women more often: fraud and medical quackery. Such crimes are probably encouraged by the stereotype that older people, and especially older women, are more gullible, ignorant about medical science, and desperate to try any possible cure for their disease. Thus, except for crimes of fraud and quackery, the general area of crime and victimization is one area in which ageism and sexism appear to work in favor of older women.

REDUCTION OF SEXISM AND AGEISM

How can this malevolent combination of sexism and ageism be combatted? In general, most of the strategies that have been successful in reducing racism and sexism in general could be used to reduce the combination of sexism and ageism. Individuals can take the following actions to reduce prejudice and discrimination against older women:

1. Inform yourself so you have the facts to combat the misconceptions and stereotypes.

2. Examine your own attitudes and actions and try to eliminate those that reflect sexism and ageism.

3. Inform your relatives, friends, and colleagues about the facts, especially when some prejudice is expressed or implied.

4. Do not tell ageist or sexist jokes and refuse to laugh when you hear one. (Try converting the joke to an age- and sex-neutral joke by not specifying age or sex.)

5. Do not use derogatory terms like "old maid."

6. Do not use ageist or sexist language such as equating old age and old women with dependency, deterioration, and weakness.

7. Point out to others when they are using ageist or sexist language.

8. Refuse to go along with discrimination against older women.

9. Write letters to editors of newspapers and magazines pointing out and protesting ageism and sexism in current events.

10. Write letters to local officials, state and federal representatives, and executives pointing out and protesting ageism and sexism in government.

11. Boycott products of companies that use ageist and sexist advertisements or discriminate against older women in employment.

12. Join groups that oppose ageism and sexism: "Don't agonize, organize!" (See the list of such organizations in Palmore, 1990.)

13. Support and vote for political candidates who oppose ageism and sexism.

14. Support legislation to reduce ageism and sexism.

CONCLUSION

There is some scattered evidence that both ageism and sexism are declining trends in our society; but the question of whether the combination of sexism and ageism against older women is declining has hardly been touched. Until that is researched we won't really know whether (and if so, in which areas) older women have "come a long way."

REFERENCES

Atchley, R. (1991). *Social forces and aging*. Belmont, CA: Wadsworth.
Barrow, G., & Smith, P. (1979). *Aging, ageism, and society*. St. Paul, MN: West Publishing Company.
Bytheway, B. (1995). *Ageism*. Bristol, PA.: Open University Press.
Chaneles, S. (1987, October). Growing old behind bars. *Psychology Today*, p. 48.
Cohen, E. (1993, January 18). Personal letter.
Cohen, E., & Kruschwitz, A. (1990). Old age in America represented in nineteenth and twentieth century popular sheet music. *Gerontologist, 30*, 345.
Covey, H. (1988). Historical terminology used to represent older people. *Gerontologist, 28*, 291.
Davis, R., & Davis, J. (1985). *TV's image of the elderly*. Lexington, MA: Lexington Books.
Elliott, J. (1984). The daytime television drama portrayal of older adults. *Gerontologist, 24*, 628.
Friedan, B. (1963). *The feminine mystique*. New York: Norton.
Gerbner, G., Grass, L., Signorielli, N., & Morgan, M. (1980). Aging with television. *Journal of Communication, 30*, 2.

Levin, J., & Levin, W. (1980). *Ageism: Prejudice and discrimination against the elderly.* Belmont, CA: Wadsworth.

Nuessel, F. (1982). The language of ageism. *Gerontologist, 22,* 273.

Palmore, E. (1971). Attitudes toward aging as shown by humor. *Gerontologist, 11,* 181.

———. (1984). The mentally ill. In E. Palmore (Ed.), *Handbook on the aged in the United States.* Westport, CT: Greenwood Press.

———. (1990). *Ageism: Negative and positive.* New York: Springer.

Palmore, E., & Manton, K. (1973). Ageism compared to racism and sexism. *Journal of Gerontology, 28,* 363–369.

Schick, F. (Ed.) (1986). *Statistical handbook on aging Americans.* Phoenix, AZ: Oryx Press.

Sontag, S. (1972). The double standard of aging. *Saturday Review, 55* (39), 29–38.

Treas, J. (1995). Older Americans in the 1990s and beyond. *Population Bulletin, 50* (2). Washington, DC: Population Reference Bureau.

Turner, B. (1987). Self-concepts: sex differences. In G. Maddox (Ed.) *Encyclopedia of aging.* New York: Springer.

U.S. Bureau of the Census (1982). *Money income and poverty status of families and persons in the U.S.: 1982.* Current Population Reports, Series P-60, No. 140. Washington, DC: U.S. Government Printing Office.

U.S. Senate, Special Committee on Aging. (1990). *Aging America.* Washington, DC: U.S. Government Printing Office.

Two

Images of Middle-aged and Older Women: Historical, Cultural, and Personal

SUSAN R. SHERMAN

Through the centuries unflattering descriptions have been attributed to middle-aged or older women: vicious mother-in-law, old-maid schoolmarm, crone, hag, and harridan (Formanek, 1990). While there is extensive literature on the topic of images of older women, much of it is nonempirical, and much continues to be polemical. The bulk of the research literature on images of older women of the past decade falls into three areas: historical, cultural (primarily television and film), and personal (attributions of ''old'' and of attractiveness). Before a review of these three areas, descriptions of controlled experimental research will be presented.

EXPERIMENTAL STUDIES ON AGE-GENDER STEREOTYPES

Over a decade ago I noted that research on age stereotypes largely omitted any gender differentiation, while research on gender stereotypes largely ignored older women. The situation has not changed substantially. In fact, it has been claimed (e.g., Macdonald, 1989) that scholars in women's studies have tended to ignore, stereotype, or exploit older women. The authors of each of the following experimental studies have pointed to these twin omissions (gender from age-stereotype studies, and age from gender-stereotype studies). The omissions are important because of the claims of gender-role convergence or reversal in later life (e.g., Gutmann, 1985), and because of the claim of a double standard of aging (e.g., Sontag, 1972; Secunda, 1984), such that society is more permissive of aging in men than in women.

My own research, studying age and gender stereotypes together, failed to give strong evidence of a double standard (Sherman, 1985). Over 500 students were asked to rate middle-aged or old man, woman, or person on a set of adjective pairs incorporating items from typical aging and gender research. A significant main effect of target age was found on nearly all items, but contrary to prediction, the main effect of sex of target was very limited. Out of 33 pairs, the only differences were that men were rated as more powerful, and women were rated as more warm and emotional. Contrary to prediction, middle-aged and older women were not rated as less sexual than their male counterparts. Although there was a larger decline from middle age to old age in being rated as sexual for women than for men, most of the adjective pairs did not show an age-by-gender interaction.

In a study with 138 students aged 19 to 30, and with 54 participants of senior centers aged 56 to 88, rating 12 drawings of young, middle-aged, and old persons, Wernick and Manaster (1984) found that both age groups rated young faces as more attractive than old faces. The authors suggested, however, that the need for ego integrity led older raters to perceive a smaller age difference between old and young stimulus faces, as well as to judge a smaller age difference on attractiveness. Most noteworthy, both men and women of both age groups rated female faces as more attractive than male faces. (It must be assumed that this was true for all ages of stimulus picture, as the authors did not state otherwise.) Again, it seems that experimental data do not support "conventional wisdom."

In similar fashion to Sherman's (1985) research, Turner (1987) used a sex-role-stereotype questionnaire and varied age (late 20s, late 40s, late 60s) and gender (male, female, adult). This was administered to marriage and family therapists, who "viewed people in their late 60s as less assertive, self-confident and self-directed than they viewed people in their late 40s, but . . . did not distinguish between old men and old women" (p. 552). Representing perhaps the only experimental study of age and gender stereotypes to include variation of target race, Turner and Turner (1991, 1994), using psychologists and students as subjects, found a main effect of target age and a main effect of target gender in ratings on a scale of communion and a scale of agency. There were some differences in results between the psychologists and the students, but for the most part, women were rated as higher on communion and lower on agency than were men, and older persons were rated as higher on communion and lower on agency than were middle-aged or younger persons. The researchers did not find any consistent age-by-gender interactions, although there were some interactions by race. Stereotypes did not differ substantially by age of subject. Beliefs were influenced to some extent by the perceived social role of the target (e.g., full-time homemaker, retiree, full-time worker), and when the role was controlled, some of the differences disappeared. Turner and Turner's study was noteworthy for its theoretical basis, that is, the linkages with trait theory, social role theory, and social cognition theory as they affect gender/age stereotypes. Much of the other research on either age or gender stereotypes focuses only on content.

In an experimental study using free-response descriptions and rating scales that college students and older community residents were to apply to 35- and 65-year-old men and women, Kite, Deaux, and Miele (1991) failed to find support for a double standard of aging on negative stereotype items. Limited support was found on physical descriptions: 35-year-old females were rated higher on feminine physical characteristics than were 65-year-old females, but no difference was found for males. Even the differences were mixed, demonstrating the importance of using a multidimensional conception of the target: older women were seen as both more wrinkled and more involved in the community, as compared to older men. There were strong age-of-target effects and little sex-of-target effects on the free-response descriptions. Gender-role reversals (women becoming more agentic or men becoming more communal with age) that had been hypothesized were not found. Also contrary to expectation, both men and women were rated as declining on masculine characteristics with age, whereas women were not judged as declining in femininity with age.

Considering, then, the limited experimental research that has simultaneously varied age and gender and has tested both older and younger groups (the latter usually students), we find, for the most part, strong and consistent age effects and some gender effects (although one was opposite to prediction). However, there appeared to be a lack of consistent support for gender-role convergence with age, or for a double standard of aging. It is encouraging to note that the more recent research has expanded the dimensions to which the rater is to respond. However, it must be recognized that experimental research has limitations of its own. Although we recognize diversity among the elderly, our research paradigms frequently ask respondents to answer for ''the elderly''—a category far too broad (Cook, 1992). We turn now to a review of the images of middle-aged and older women encompassing a wider range of methodologies. It must be noted that it was difficult in much of the literature considered for this chapter to separate middle-aged from older women, so much of the review will not distinguish. When age is mentioned in an article, it will be reported.

HISTORICAL IMAGES OF OLDER WOMEN

''Historically, older men have had a different social image from old women. Older men were characterized (dualistically) by artists as fools, religious leaders, wise, feeble, venerable, esteemed, contemplating, lustful, and honored. Older women—whose images are less common in Western art—were shown as helpers, feeble, evil, pious, and grandmotherly'' (Covey, 1991, p. 174).

There is a problem in defining ''old'' historically. ''Old'' needs to be seen as a relative term, and we cannot be sure if writers are talking about those who would be considered old even today, or about a larger group who were old in their own society. In Covey's (1991) historical review, for example, old age was described as beginning as early as 40 by Erasmus and Shakespeare; still, it could be a relative position that is significant. Most important, it has been noted (e.g., Covey, 1989a, 1989b, 1991) that old age has been defined earlier for women than men, partly because of the specific association for women with menopause and the end of procreation.

The historical picture of older women in literature and art has been reported as mixed (e.g., Grambs, 1989). Plato regarded aging women as wise, both spiritually and sexually (Banner, 1992), whereas others have pointed to the depiction of irrationality (Maxwell, 1990) or childishness (similar to older men) of older women (Covey, 1992–93). Banner traced the contrasting themes of the wise woman and the witch in Europe from medieval times to the eighteenth century. It appeared that to be perceived as sexual could be dangerous, so it was better to be perceived as spiritual. After the eighteenth century, "as sexuality was contained within marriage, the new female villain became not the older woman . . . but the unmarried woman" (Banner, 1992, pp. 235–236).

Some authors reviewed noted positive images such as benevolent, nurturant, powerful, free, and respected for "knowledge of rituals and herbal lore" (Grambs, 1989, p. 196). In fact, these words were formerly used as honorific titles: "Virago—a strong, experienced and wise older woman; Crone—a woman who passes on prudence and foresight and is revered by younger women; or even Witch, an older woman who becomes the tribal healer, herbalist, sexual instructor and counselor" (Hot Flash, 1992, p. 1). Furthermore, it should be noted that when older women were viewed negatively, older men were likely to be perceived negatively as well.

Banner (1992) analyzed age-disparate relationships of aging women with younger men (much less common than the reverse); Elizabeth I of England and Catherine the Great of Russia—powerful, self-aware, and wise—were perhaps the most favorable examples. Banner reported on mistresses of kings who were perceived as sensual in later years, and also noted that Benjamin Franklin recommended cross-age relationships: older women were seen as more interesting, both conversationally and sexually, and more anxious to please.

The sexuality of older women has been a problematic theme, however, across the centuries. Covey (1989b, 1991) indicated that throughout most of Western history since the Middle Ages, sexuality for older people of both genders was considered inappropriate, immoral, disgusting, unhealthy, and perverse. This was partly because sexuality for people of any age was considered sinful except for procreation. When behaviors contradicted the norms, sanctions, for example, public ridicule, were applied to deviants. In describing a review of nineteenth-century views of older women, Rodeheaver and Stohs (1991) found the theme of fading and decline, slackening and wrinkling; with age, beauty is transformed to disgust and horror.

For men, sexuality in old age was humorous, impossible, a temptation, and self-deceptive, but, with a younger partner, a source of social status; for women, sexuality was evil, controlling, deceiving, seductive, sinister, predatory, and witchlike (Covey, 1989b, 1991). Maxwell's (1990) analysis of a wide range of fictional characters demonstrated that middle-aged women—explicitly or implicitly menopausal—were described as sexually voracious. She included Chaucer's Wife of Bath and the Prioress, "preoccupied with gratifying their carnal appetites" (p. 258), and Shakespeare's Gertrude, who was overcome by lust. The connection between menopause and attribution of insanity can be traced back to Galen, who believed that the blood vessels of postmenopausal women are rigid and cannot discharge accumulated blood periodically. The congested blood therefore goes to the brain, causing insanity. This was a common belief until the 1920s (Formanek, 1990).

Witches were earlier thought of as being of any age and even could be seen (less frequently) as men; however, in the sixteenth and seventeenth centuries the label of witch became attached predominantly to older women (Covey, 1991), resulting in thousands of deaths in the seventeenth and early eighteenth centuries (Grambs, 1989). Witches served as community scapegoats, and the label of witch may have discharged the community from responsibility for poor, older, dependent women (Covey, 1991).

Older women seem to have been viewed both as excessively powerful and as powerless. In legends of ancient Greece, as well as the Roman republic and empire, powerful goddesses could be old (Banner, 1992)—not necessarily chronologically old as we now think of old age, but old enough to have adult children. But power can be punished; Lady Macbeth's "rampant lust for power openly violates prescribed gender roles, thus plunging her into unqualified madness" (Maxwell, 1990, p. 261).

The related theme of economics has also been problematic for older women, particularly older widows (Covey, 1991). An analysis of the work of the Victorian artist Hubert Herkomer (McLerran, 1993) illustrated the view of the times that the aged (men and women) were considered "as able-bodied and capable of their own financial support as anyone else" (p. 770), were redeemed by work, and were forced to live in conditions of squalor when they could not support themselves. Because their usual trades were displaced by mechanization of the garment industry, and because of their longer life expectancy, aged women were the most common occupants of workhouses for the poor (McLerran, 1993).

POPULAR CULTURE AND THE MEDIA

We turn now from historical images to seeing how they are replicated in contemporary popular culture. Most of the research on popular culture's views of older women comes from analyses of television portrayals, where, because of limited time, stereotypes are common (Davis & Davis, 1985). In general, some reviewers have noted that the aged of either gender are disadvantaged on television, and others have noted that women of any age are disadvantaged. However, it has then been indicated that older women are particularly disadvantaged. "Men tend to have interesting and productive roles in the drama of life much longer than do women. . . . [Women] tend to disappear after age 30, except in soap operas, where their numbers diminish after age 50" (Davis &

Davis, 1985, p. 47). The research indicates that "mature women . . . are . . . underrepresented, undervalued, and undersexed" (Gerbner, 1993, p. 12).

Turning first to representation, research has analyzed TV shows watched by older persons themselves, as well as shows watched by a variety of ages. Gerbner (1993), for example, analyzed 19,642 speaking parts on 1,371 TV shows on major cable and other networks covering a period from 1982 to 1992. These included prime-time shows, Saturday-morning shows, daytime serials, game shows, and local and national news. With respect to frequency, the literature reviewed was unanimous in concluding that older (or middle-aged) women were underrepresented on TV. Some comparisons were with younger women; others were with older men (e.g., Vernon, Williams, Phillips, & Wilson, 1990), who are also underrepresented (Gerbner, 1993), but not to the same extent as older women. Richard H. Davis (1987) found that of those on TV older than 65, 90% were males.

Older or middle-aged women were less likely to be underrepresented on daytime TV than on prime-time shows (R. H. Davis, 1987; Davis & Davis, 1985; Grambs, 1989). I would suggest that perhaps women—daytime viewers—can tolerate older women better than can men—prime-time viewers. Although Grambs (1989) reported that there were more older women than older men on soaps, each was shown in traditional roles (nurturer and worker). When women are considered too old for drama, they may be used in commercials (Davis & Davis, 1985), although here, too, it has been found that older men—even with graying temples—are more likely to be used in commercials than are older women. Furthermore, the latter are likely to be selling remedies for arthritis, digestion, and dentures or to be giving advice about cooking or cleaning (Davis & Davis, 1985; Grambs, 1989). Gerbner (1993) found that older women were less likely to be used as newscasters or subjects of news reports than were older men. Older-appearing male anchors appear authoritative; females are thought not to be (Lakoff & Scherr, 1984).

With regard to the measurement of value, older women on television are shown as secondary to men; men are smarter, and women are silly, nurturant, marginal, passive, or unsuccessful (Davis & Davis, 1985; Grambs, 1989; Hubbs-Tait, 1989). "The female . . . is usually 10 years younger than the lead male, and becomes increasingly unimportant to the plot as she ages. Her role becomes one of adoring attendant upon the 'rocking chair sage' " (Davis & Davis, 1985, p. 46). Grambs noted that when a woman was shown as intelligent ("Murder She Wrote"), she was nevertheless shown as deferent. An even more negative image found was that of witch, villain, or eccentric (R. H. Davis, 1987; Gerbner, 1993; Grambs, 1989). For example, on children's shows older women were more likely to be shown as villains than were either older men or younger women.

Most studies indicated that older women were not portrayed as sexual or romantic (Bell, 1992; D. M. Davis, 1990; Gerbner, 1993) and frequently were depicted as the old maid (Davis & Davis, 1985). Sexuality "is an important absence in the lives of most elderly television characters, and especially in the lives of elderly women'' (Bell, 1992, p. 309). Women are shown as losing sexual attractiveness as they age, while males are portrayed as increasingly sexually attractive, especially because of increasing attributions of power for men (R. H. Davis, 1987; Davis & Davis, 1985).

Richard H. Davis (1987) found evidence that early middle-aged women are seen as economically powerful and sexually attractive, but women older than that are seen as nurturing. When middle-aged or older women are shown as sexy, glamorous, and rich, they are also shown as "scheming, malicious, and manipulative" (Grambs, 1989, p. 20). As in historical images, to be sexy is threatening; it is more favorable to be unglamorous and ineffectual.

It is claimed that two universes are depicted on TV. One is a female universe where women dominate and might be seen as commanding and powerful, but no men are involved. The other is "a male universe of older men where there are women but not older women. . . . when men appear with women, the old stereotypes of male prominence and dominance still operate. . . . prime-time television doesn't seem to know how (or wish) to handle a continuing intimate relationship between two elderly people of the opposite sex'' (Bell, 1992, p. 310).

Finally, some of the television reviews emphasized the risks involved when unrealistic expectations are aroused. In a survey of network entertainment programs portraying women over 50, conducted in the spring of 1986, Steenland (n.d.) found images as powerful, creative, appealing, attractive, romantic, sexual, wise, respected, healthy, and affluent, in contrast to earlier decades. However, she contrasted the earlier distortions of older women as negative or invisible with the current distortions: more glamorous, less diverse, faced with fewer problems than older women in reality. Bell (1992) found little on family relationships in shows with older (male or female) characters.

Davis and Davis (1985) concluded that TV stereotyping has serious negative implications for aging women and men. Both are encouraged to deny the realities of aging and are being set up for disappointment. Additionally, men will be unable to support aging in their mates. "The realities of the aging process are still taboo on TV today. Not only are aging's negative social and economic consequences for women ignored, but the realities of the physical changes people experience as they age are invisible. . . . today's older women on TV are merely yesterday's ingenues portrayed by older actresses'' (Steenland, n.d., p. 21). Steenland contended that this is just as unrealistic. She advocated portraying older women with more reality and diversity. "Older women are finally visible on the screen. . . . Television's next challenge is to bring aging out of the closet. Reality must infiltrate the screen so that older female characters exhibit some of the scars and wisdom of five or six decades worth of living'' (Steenland, n.d., p. 24).

As another reflection of cultural norms, two recent studies have analyzed the place of older women in films. In similar fashion to the results reported in the

TV analyses, Markson and Taylor noted that there is a scarcity of older women in films, and when they do appear, they generally have been portrayed negatively, for example, as "viragos, poor old things, or minor characters" (1993, p. 158). In a historical analysis of ages of male and female Academy Award nominees and winners, Markson and Taylor found that only about one-quarter of all Best Actress winners were 40 or older, whereas about two-thirds of all Best Actors were that old. On the other hand, the low percentages of winners 60 and over were the same for men and women (8% of all winning actors and 9% of all winning actresses). In a related analysis of the Best and Supporting Actor and Actress winners since 1927, Levy (1990) found that the modal age for male Best Actor was middle aged and for male Supporting Actor was elderly (over 65), whereas for both Best and Supporting Actresses, the modal age was young (under 35). "Leading ladies have been young and beautiful, but leading men have been middle-aged and, preferably, but not necessarily, handsome" (Levy, 1990, p. 60). This means, then, that until the late 1970s, middle-aged actresses had the choice of retiring at the peak of their career or accepting less important character roles (Levy, 1990).

Levy claimed that the roles express the ideological views of powerful white, middle-class men. Markson and Taylor found that "among actresses 60 and over, roles in which women have a career or are working are rare" (1993, p. 168). When women do have a career, they are portrayed as having unhappy family relationships. "Those factors contributing to female malaise in later life, such as poverty and lack of economic opportunity, as well as societal devaluation, are generally ignored as are the strengths of experience, agency, and communion with one another" (Markson & Taylor, 1993, p. 168). Levy (1990) pointed to films in which older actresses portray the fading older actress (over age 40) in the midst of losing looks, love, and even her mind and perhaps having a drinking or drug problem—all the while being supplanted by the new young actress. Although Levy (1990) found that "of the last ten winning roles [for Best Actress] three were middle-aged, and two . . . old" (p. 71), Markson and Taylor (1993) did not interpret their data as showing a trend toward nominating older women from the 1920s through the 1980s.

The conclusion from most of the media studies is that older women are seen as powerless. If older women can be rated positively only as they gain power, does this mean that they will still "lose" because they will then be marked as "witches" or as villains? Before leaving the review of popular culture, it should be noted that in contrast to most analyses of television and films, Kehl (1988) found the following images of older women in twentieth-century fiction and poetry: independent, rejecting superficiality of youth, courageous, strong-willed, passionate, and open to change. Kehl concluded that literature has the possibility of providing more realistic understanding of aging females. Also, in a study of popular sheet music—lyrics and cover pictures—covering the years 1830 through 1980, Cohen and Kruschwitz (1990) found that the spousal relationship in old age, usually from the husband's perspective, was portrayed favorably.

However, for the most part, the research on cultural images, especially in popular culture, shows rather negative images of middle-aged and older women.

PERSONAL IMAGES OF OLDER WOMEN: ATTRIBUTIONS OF AGING AND ATTRACTIVENESS BY OTHERS AND SELF

Turning from historical and cultural to personal images, four related areas of literature were found: perceptions by others that women age sooner than men, women's own age identity, differential attributions of attractiveness by others, and older women's self-esteem. The perception of women "aging sooner than men . . . has had a long tradition in Western thought" (Covey, 1991, p. 39) and is cited repeatedly. "A man can have a reasonably lined face, and pepper-and-salt—or even white—hair, and still seem youthful, if he looks active and vital" (Lakoff & Scherr, 1984). Rodeheaver and Stohs (1991) claimed that when men are motivated to change their appearance, it is due to fear of being perceived as less powerful rather than as less youthful. After reviewing a large body of research on interpersonal attraction and age, Webb, Delaney, and Young (1989) raised an empirical question as to whether older women are expected more than older men to retain unrealistic youthful appearances. In a recent national opinion survey of persons 55 and older, men were consistently defined as becoming old later than were women—between 60 and 64 versus between 55 and 59 (Seccombe & Ishii-Kuntz, 1991). This is hardly as large a difference as much literature, including Sontag (1972), would suggest.

In an analysis of themes in humor, Palmore (1987 and this book) indicated that a common theme for older women is age concealment. Using a mail questionnaire in a cross-sectional study, Montepare and Lachman (1989) found that the discrepancy between chronological age and subjective age identity increased in old age more for women than it did for men; Rodeheaver and Stohs (1991) suggested that this is functional for adaptation and life satisfaction, due to sociocultural images of the older woman. Montepare and Lachman found, however, that for older women, younger age identity was associated with lower life satisfaction.

One of the negative images of menopause, Dan and Bernhard (1989) claimed, is that of being unattractive. In a retrospective chapter in 1989, Troll concluded that not much had changed regarding stereotypes and the double standard of aging in the twenty years since she had organized a conference on older women: "In spite of . . . portraits of charming women aged fifty, the important part of being considered a beautiful . . . older woman is to 'look young.' Full-page pictures of Gloria Steinem and other feminist icons who are now reaching the dreaded fifty (as distinguished from the earlier dreaded age of thirty or forty) attest to their not showing any of the signs of shame: no dry skin, no sagging muscles, no sallow coloring, no wrinkles" (Troll, 1989, p. 20). Lesnoff-Caravaglia (1984) concurred: "It is all right for a woman to be chronologically old, if she looks younger than her years. It is also all right for her to be sexual and old, if her skin and body give the illusion of youth. The emphasis in cosmetic advertising is always on looking younger than you are'' (p. 15).

Lakoff and Scherr (1984) suggested that with increasing age, there is an inevitable loss of the power that beauty brings, and one never knows for sure when this power will disappear. This is particularly difficult for women who have been accustomed to the power of being beautiful (Grambs, 1989). ''A man need consider a face-lift only if the signs of age and wear in his face become too apparent: pouches and jowls, not mere lines. . . . Even if a man's appearance of ageing diminishes his value in the world of work, his social desirability is not necessarily compromised: a man remains attractive to women until a much greater age than a woman to men'' (Lakoff & Scherr, 1984, p. 148). Interestingly, however, the men they interviewed said that they did not necessarily prefer younger women and were not bothered by wrinkles; they preferred women their own age, ''as long as they were in good shape'' (Lakoff & Scherr, 1984, p. 239).

A decline in ratings of attractiveness of older women can be important to the extent that physical attractiveness generalizes to attributions of other characteristics such as intelligence. Being perceived as competent can then, in a self-fulfilling prophecy, lead to increased competence (Pierson, 1987). In the extreme, negative self-feelings can lead women to have cosmetic surgery that may be dangerous or at best have a temporary effect. Lakoff and Scherr claimed that the '' 'ugliness' of ageing for women is . . . an outgrowth of our fears of lack of polarization between the sexes: a woman should be untouched and innocent, distinguishing her clearly from a man, who should not'' (1984, p. 171). The various cosmetic surgeries to keep women from looking old are also, Lakoff and Scherr asserted, to keep them from looking like men.

However, empirical research on older women's self-attributions is mixed. In interviews with 10 women in their 60s, 70s, and 80s, Furstenberg (1989) found that some women employed changes in their physical appearance as part of their aging self-concept. She suggested that the resulting self-rejection reflects society's emphasis on ''youthful appearance as the criterion for feminine attractiveness and the disqualification of women as sexual 'candidates' at much younger ages than men'' (p. 271). Similarly, in a convenience sample of 505 highly educated women whose mean age was 47, Mansfield and Voda (1993) found both ''image'' and biological issues to be cited as the most worrisome changes about menopause (either anticipated or current). With respect to psychosocial worries, 12% worried about loss of attractiveness, 9% about getting older, and 18% about increased moodiness.

On the other hand, in a questionnaire study with 30 younger and 30 older respondents, matched for health, depression, and education, although older respondents reported more concern with external physical appearance than did younger respondents, and women reported more concern than did men, there were no age-by-gender interactions. Therefore, it was suggested that women's sensitivities to these issues are developed early and continue into later life, even above the increased sensitivity in later life experienced by both genders (Ross et al., 1989).

Finally, White (1988) provided empirical data questioning the belief that middle-aged women are more sensitive to signs of aging than are men, and that women's aging is more important than men's. In telephone interviews she asked a national probability sample of 1,500 married men and women, aged 20 to 60, to comment on decline over the past three years in several body systems. She found that women reported somewhat more decline in areas in which they may actually undergo earlier decline—eyesight, energy, skin, and shape; and men reported somewhat more decline in those systems in which they actually undergo more decline—hearing and hair condition. By the 50s, men's and women's reports regarding changes in body shape were the same (about 35%), although in the 40s, nearly 40% of the women responded affirmatively, while only about 30% of the men did so. Furthermore, the pace of decline was parallel for all systems. White contended that her research calls into question the "double standard of aging," as she found that both men and women were more self-critical regarding decline than were their spouses about them, that is, husbands perceived less decline in their wives than women in general did for themselves. White also found no overall age-gender interaction on perceived decline.

CONCLUSION

We have now reviewed recent literature on historical, cultural, and personal images of middle-aged and older women, covering a wide range of methodologies. Some of these included experimental attitude measurement, analyses of art and historical texts, content analyses of television and films, and interview and mail surveys. Several conclusions will be stated, gaps in research indicated, and further research suggested.

While research on the media found the most consistently negative images, there is congruence of some negative themes across the various areas reviewed. These include judgment of women as old earlier than men, and images of older women as not sexual and not valued. Nevertheless, positive images were found as well, such as nurturant and benevolent. Contradictory images abound: wise or silly, respected or irrational, powerless or powerful. The empirical research reviewed in each section of this chapter presents a fairly complex picture.

It is difficult to distinguish between middle-aged and old in research reports. A minority of the literature refers specifically to the middle-aged; for the most part, however, the discussion is of older women, although the age of "older" can be quite varied. In discussions of historical images of older women, it is unclear whether the work refers to relatively "older" or to what in contemporary society would be considered "old." It is also not always clear whether the literature describing images of older women is comparing them to older men or to younger women (rarely is there a comparison between older women and middle-aged women). Further, critics seem to be saying both that distinctions are not made between older women and older men when they should be, and that when distinctions are made, they disadvantage women in the same ways that younger women are disadvantaged.

Much of the literature fails to distinguish between beliefs and behaviors, that is, between "stereotypes" and "discrimination" (and between seemingly discriminatory beliefs and ignorance) (Cook, 1992). There is an abundance of descriptive research showing the images of older women to which the population is exposed, whether historically or contemporaneously, but a lack of research showing whether or how this matters. There has been more research on the content of the images than on the audience. If the images matter, is it because of the message they give older persons themselves, or the message that is portrayed to younger people? We need to look at the effects of the stereotypes for older persons, for younger persons, and for all those in between.

It is important to note a distinction between self-image and image of others. As with stereotypes of the aged in general, middle-aged (or older) women may hold negative stereotypes about middle age for other persons, but not apply them to themselves. Likewise, one's self-image and the image others hold are not necessarily identical. Grambs (1989) and others have suggested that the negative stereotypes in TV and film pressure women in our culture to attempt to look younger. However, while younger persons or men may subscribe to negative stereotypes, the middle-aged or older woman may still have a positive self-image. More research is needed before we can assume a connection between stereotypes (held by self or others) and one's self-perception.

More research is needed to study the process by which various attributes are used in making judgments of older women, such as age itself, physical appearance, or competence. For example, does physical appearance become most salient when it is presented without other information? Perhaps, as much research would suggest, it is less salient after other characteristics (e.g., competence) are known. To what extent does knowing the women's age then influence attractiveness, which then influences judgment of other attributes? More research is needed on the components of attractiveness (Webb et al., 1989).

Grambs (1989) suggested that present and earlier cohorts of older women had to apologize for career achievements; newer cohorts, she claimed, should be different and gain self-esteem from achievement; therefore, age and age-related appearance may be less relevant. This is an empirical question, and we can ask how images will change as the "baby-boom" cohort, having been influenced by the women's movement, advances into old age. Will the unprecedented size of this older cohort influence images of older women? Finally, will the images of older women (and men) change as society continues to recognize broader ranges and increased flexibility of life stages for education, marriage, child rearing, leisure, and career?

REFERENCES

Banner, Lois W. (1992). *In full flower: Aging women, power, and sexuality: A history.* New York: Knopf, distributed by Random House.

Bell, John. (1992). In search of a discourse on aging: The elderly on television. *Gerontologist, 32,* 305–311.

Cohen, Elias S., & Kruschwitz, Anna L. (1990). Old age in America represented in nineteenth and twentieth century popular sheet music. *Gerontologist, 30,* 345–354.

Cook, Fay L. (1992). Ageism: Rhetoric and reality. *Gerontologist, 32,* 292–293.

Covey, Herbert C. (1989a). Old age portrayed by the ages-of-life models from the Middle Ages to the sixteenth century. *Gerontologist, 29,* 692–698.

———. (1989b). Perceptions and attitudes toward sexuality of the elderly during the Middle Ages. *Gerontologist, 29,* 93–100.

———. (1991). *Images of older people in Western art and society.* New York: Praeger.

———. (1992–93). A return to infancy: Old age and the second childhood in history. *International Journal of Aging and Human Development, 36,* 81–90.

Dan, Alice U., & Bernhard, Linda A. (1989). Menopause and other health issues for midlife women. In Ski Hunter & Martin Sundel (Eds.), *Midlife myths: Issues, findings, and practice implications.* Newbury Park, CA: Sage.

Davis, Donald M. (1990). Portrayals of women in prime-time network television: Some demographic characteristics. *Sex Roles, 23,* 325–332.

Davis, Richard H. (1987). Images of aging in the media. In George Maddox (Ed.), *The encyclopedia of aging* (pp. 343–344). New York: Springer.

Davis, Richard H., & Davis, James A. (1985). *TV's image of the elderly: A practical guide for change.* Lexington, MA: Lexington Books.

Foner, Nancy. (1989). Older women in nonindustrial cultures: Consequences of power and privilege. In Lois Grau (Ed., in collaboration with Ida Susser), *Women in the later years: Health, social, and cultural perspectives* (pp. 227–237). New York: Haworth. Published also as *Women and Health, 14*(3/4).

Formanek, Ruth. (Ed.). (1990). *The meanings of menopause: Historical, medical, and clinical perspectives.* Hillsdale, NJ: Analytic Press.

Furstenberg, Anne-Linda. (1989). Older people's age self-concept. *Social Casework, 70,* 269–275.

Gerbner, George. (1993, June). *Women and minorities on television: A study in casting and fate.* A report to the Screen Actors Guild and the American Federation of Radio and Television Artists. The Annenberg School for Communication. University of Pennsylvania, mimeo, 26 pp.

Grambs, Jean D. (1989). *Women over forty: Visions and realities* (rev. ed.). New York: Springer.

Grau, Lois. (Ed., in collaboration with Ida Susser). (1989). *Women in the later years: Health, social, and cultural perspectives.* New York: Haworth. Published also as *Women and Health, 14*(3/4).

Gutmann, David L. (1985). The parental imperative revisited. In J. A. Meacham (Ed.), *Family and individual development.* Basel: Karger.

Heisel, Marsel A. (1989). Older women in developing countries. In Lois Grau (Ed., in collaboration with Ida Susser), *Women in the later years: Health, social, and cultural perspectives* (pp. 253–272). New York: Haworth. Published also in *Women and Health, 14*(3/4).

Hot Flash. editorial (1992, Summer). *11*(3), 1.

Hubbs-Tait, Laura. (1989). Coping patterns of aging women: A developmental perspective. In J. Dianne Garner & Susan O. Mercer (Eds.), *Women as they age: Challenge, opportunity, and triumph* (pp. 95–122). New York: Haworth. Published simultaneously in the *Journal of Women and Aging, 1*(1/2/3).

Hummert, Mary Lee. (1990). Multiple stereotypes of elderly and young adults: A comparison of structure and evaluations. *Psychology and Aging, 5,* 182–193.

Kehl, D. G. (1988). The distaff and the staff: Stereotypes and archetypes of the older woman in representative modern literature. *International Journal of Aging and Human Development, 26,* 1–12.

Kite, Mary E., Deaux, Kay, & Miele, Margaret. (1991). Stereotypes of young and old: Does age outweigh gender? *Psychology and Aging, 6,* 19–27.

Lakoff, Robin Tolmach, & Scherr, Raquel L. (1984). *Face value: The politics of beauty.* Boston: Routledge & Kegan Paul.

Lesnoff-Caravaglia, Gari. (1984). Double stigmata: Female and old. In Gari Lesnoff-Caravaglia (Ed.), *The world of the older woman: Conflicts and resolutions* (pp. 11–20). New York: Human Sciences Press.

Levy, Emanuel. (1990). Stage, sex, and suffering: Images of women in American films. *Empirical Studies of the Arts, 8,* 53–76.

Macdonald, Barbara. (1989). Outside the sisterhood: Ageism in women's studies. *Women's Studies Quarterly, 17*(1–2), 6–11.

McLerran, Jennifer. (1993). Saved by the hand that is not stretched out: The aged poor in Hubert von Herkomer's *Eventide: A Scene in the Westminster Union. Gerontologist, 33,* 762–771.

Mansfield, Phyllis K., & Voda, Ann M. (1993). From Edith Bunker to the 6:00 news: How and what midlife women learn about menopause. *Women and Therapy, 14,* 89–104.

Markson, Elizabeth W., & Taylor, Carol A. (1993). Real versus reel world: Older women and the Academy Awards. *Women and Therapy, 14,* 157–172.

Maxwell, Marilyn. (1990). Portraits of menopausal women in selected works of English and American literature. In Ruth Formanek (Ed.), *The meanings of menopause: Historical, medical, and clinical perspectives* (pp. 255–280). Hillsdale, NJ: Analytic Press.

Montepare, Joann M., & Lachman, Margie E. (1989). "You're only as old as you feel": Self-perceptions of age, fears of aging, and life satisfaction from adolescence to old age. *Psychology and Aging, 4,* 73–78.

Palmore, Erdman B. (1987). Humor. In George Maddox (Ed.), *The encyclopedia of aging* (pp. 341–342). New York: Springer.

Pierson, June S. (1987). *Beauty and aging women.* Unpublished manuscript, State University of New York at Albany.

Rodeheaver, Dean. (1987). When old age became a social problem, women were left behind. *Gerontologist, 27,* 741–746.

Rodeheaver, Dean, & Stohs, Joanne. (1991). The adaptive misperception of age in older women: Sociocultural images and psychological mechanisms of control. *Educational Gerontology, 17,* 141–156.

Ross, Michael J., Tait, Raymond C., Grossberg, George T., Handal, Paul J., Brandeberry,

Linda, & Nakra, Raj. (1989). Age differences in body consciousness. *Journal of Gerontology: Psychological Sciences, 44*, P23–P24.

Seccombe, Karen, & Ishii-Kuntz, Masako. (1991). Perceptions of problems associated with aging: Comparisons among four older age cohorts. *Gerontologist, 31*, 527–533.

Secunda, Victoria. (1984). *By youth possessed: The denial of age in America.* Indianapolis: Bobbs-Merrill.

Sherman, Susan R. (1985). Sex role stereotypes of middle and old age. *Journal of Social Service Research, 8*, 23–35.

Sontag, Susan. (1972). The double standard of aging. *Saturday Review, 55*(39), 29–38.

Steenland, Sally. (n.d.). *Prime time women: An analysis of older women on entertainment television.* Washington, DC: National Commission on Working Women.

Troll, Lillian E. (1984). The psycho-social problems of older women. In Gari Lesnoff-Caravaglia (Ed.), *The world of the older woman: Conflicts and resolutions* (pp. 21–35). New York: Human Sciences Press.

———. (1989). Issues in the study of older women: 1970 to 1985. In A. Regula Herzog, Karen C. Holden, & Mildred M. Seltzer (Eds.), *Health and economic status of older women* (pp. 17–23). Amityville, NY: Baywood.

Turner, Barbara F. (1987). Psychotherapy: Age and sex stereotypes. In George Maddox (Ed.), *The encyclopedia of aging* (pp. 551–552). New York: Springer.

Turner, Barbara F., & Turner, Castellano B. (1991). Bem Sex-role Inventory stereotypes for men and women varying in age and race among *National Register* psychologists. *Psychological Reports, 69*, 931–944.

———. (1994). Social cognition and gender stereotypes for women varying in age and race. In Barbara F. Turner & Lillian E. Troll (Eds.), *Women growing older: Psychological perspectives* (pp. 94–139). Thousand Oaks, CA: Sage.

Vernon, JoEtta A., Williams, Jr., J. Allen, Phillips, Terri, and Wilson, Janet (1990). Media stereotyping: A comparison of the way elderly women and men are portrayed on prime-time television. *Journal of Women and Aging, 2*(4), 55–68.

Webb, Lynne, Delaney, Judith Jopling, & Young, Lorraine R. (1989). Age, interpersonal attraction, and social interaction: A review and assessment. *Research on Aging, 11*(1), 107–123.

Wernick, Mark, & Manaster, Guy J. (1984). Age and the perception of age and attractiveness. *Gerontologist, 24*, 408–414.

White, Lynn K. (1988). Gender differences in awareness of aging among married adults ages 20 to 60. *Sociological Quarterly, 29*, 487–502.

Three

Witches, Widows, Wives, and Workers: The Historiography of Elderly Women in America

CAROLE HABER

In 1985, in an article in *Social Science History*, Marjorie Chary Feinson posed the question "Where are the women in the history of aging?" (Feinson, 1985). At the time, the study of the history of the elderly in the United States was not even a decade old. These early histories, as Feinson noted, often ignored elderly women as they discussed the experiences of old men. Generally examining cultural paradigms enunciated by aging "authorities," the studies repeated the language and assumptions of earlier generations of experts who had focused on the declining status of the old. Initially exploring questions of rank and power, they spoke largely in masculine terms (Achenbaum, 1978; Fischer, 1977; Haber, 1983).

Although these histories did not always agree about the course or interpretation of male-centered old age, they generally concurred that most elderly men were treated with honor in colonial America. Religious admonitions cautioned the young to respect the old, while landownership and continued activity assured them power and control. By the late nineteenth century, however, cultural paradigms had radically changed. Gray hair and stooped backs were no longer seen as signs of wisdom but as symbols of obsolescence. Increasingly, old men found themselves labeled too outdated to contribute to the fast-moving industrial world and too debilitated to compete with the young (Cole, 1992). Yet, as one recent study has shown, the impact of industrialization on old men was not entirely detrimental. With industrial growth, the elderly tended to make significant financial gains. In terms of homeownership, savings, and retirement, early twentieth-century aged men generally maintained greater economic well-being than their counterparts from earlier centuries (Haber & Gratton, 1994).

But what of old women? Did their history parallel that of men, or did their gender bring new issues and realities into their lives? In many of the early histories, old women seemed little more than an appendage of the elderly man and his offspring, or a passing exception to the supposedly strong correlation between great age and power (Fischer, 1977). To a great degree, though, they were simply left shrouded in an unknown past.

In the ten years since Feinson's article, however, numerous monographs and articles have begun to uncover these invisible aged women. In so doing, they have discovered that the history of old age often appears radically different from the elderly woman's perspective (Gratton & Haber, 1993). Unlike her male counterpart, the aged woman rarely found that retirement from the work force marked a major turning point in her adult life, nor did farm ownership and inheritance guarantee her continued high status. The course of old-age history itself seems far more complex and varied when viewed through her eyes and experiences.

By focusing on the American experience, this chapter will look at the findings of recent historical studies about old women. As we shall see, old age for women often differed profoundly from both the ideals and realities of men's senescence. In each period of America's past, gender had profound implications. In terms of status, wealth, family, and work, elderly women were not simply an "exception" to the history of men's old age but possessed a distinctive past that challenged conventional notions about what it meant to be old in America.

OLD WOMEN IN EARLY AMERICA

Power, for aging men in colonial America and the early United States, often rested on continued activity and possession of valued resources. Largely remaining heads of household until their deaths, they assured their continued respect through wealth and landownership. As historians have shown, the young had little choice but to honor aged men who still controlled their livelihood or their future status. Through inheritance, aging men were able to dictate the behavior of the young as well as secure their own place in the community (Greven, 1970; Demos, 1978).

Aging women, however, found their experience to be quite different. According to Terri Premo (1990), the status of an elderly woman was won not by land or inheritance but through thriving relationships with family and friends. "Successful aging" depended on an aged woman's ability to "enjoy the rewards of family, friendship, and moral sustenance" (Premo, 1990, p. 25). While ambivalent about the physical limitations of growing old, she discovered that the qualities associated with old age—benevolence, dignity, humility, and serenity—were traits that brought increased stature to her final days. As an aging wife, the elderly woman generally defined her sphere through her role as the spouse of the household head. Part of the family enterprise, she realized that while her work diminished, it rarely ceased; maternal duties simply blended across generations. Having experienced little disruption in her life course, she remained reliant on her husband and family for her status and security.

As a result, widowhood marked the most dramatic change in the life of an elderly woman and her place in both the family and the community. With the death of her husband, a woman lost her position as the wife of the household head. As all possessions were legally his, she was dependent upon the allocations of his will. According to law, women received at least one-third of their husbands' estate—the traditional "dowager's third." While some wills lacked specificity about these provisions, most clearly spelled out the widow's allotted possessions. The provisions of wills often consigned the aged woman to a room in the house, equipped with appropriate furniture, and even granted her control of particular livestock (Shammas, Salmon, & Dahlin, 1987; Chelfant, 1955). Although these stipulations guaranteed that she would not be poverty-stricken, the explicit terms marked a dramatic change in her status. Her place in the house was now limited to a single room; the provisions allotted to her satisfied only her basic needs. The younger generation—usually a son—took over the role as the head of household, promising to support and respect his aging mother (Haber, 1983). Once widowed, she faced little chance of remarrying and regaining her role as spouse of the household head. In seventeenth-century Massachusetts only about 10 percent of all widows remarried; in early nineteenth-century Pennsylvania the figure rose to only about 20 percent (Keyssar, 1974; Wilson, 1992). While the very richest widows were often able to arrange a new union, the great majority lived out their lives according to the terms of their husbands' wills.

Some widows, however, had neither a dowager's third or a family on which to depend. In colonial America, as in the early republic, impoverished widows filled the rolls of church charities and community relief. They were the chief recipients of a town's outdoor relief in the form of rent, food, clothing, or wood. According to Priscilla Clement (1985), in Philadelphia in 1814 and 1815, 86 percent of outdoor pensioners were women, and about 38 percent of these women were widows. In Newburyport, Massachusetts, Susan Grigg estimated that in the early nineteenth century about 80 percent of the women receiving outdoor relief were widows, a figure mirrored in antebellum Charleston, South Carolina, as well (Grigg, 1984; Haber & Gratton, 1986). In such urban centers these poverty-stricken females attracted the attention of religious and community leaders. Cotton Mather, the most prominent Puritan minister, noted the large number of impoverished widows who resided in mid-eighteenth-century Boston. "A State of Widowhood," he lamented, "is a state of affliction" (Mather, cited by Keyssar, 1974, p. 99). He admonished his congregations to recognize the women's needy old age and treat them with compassion and relief. As part of a community's "deserving poor," they were worthy recipients of the city's benevolence.

Although the tenuous plight of the impoverished widow was perhaps understandable, far wealthier widows in colonial America were not automatically assured of authority or even of a peaceful old age. While receiving a large inheritance guaranteed a man power and control, it could have radically different consequences for an aging woman. Although it increased the likelihood that she could negotiate an advantageous marriage, it did not bring her authority or power. As Carol Karlsen (1987) has shown, women who were bequeathed size-able property but lacked a male heir or guardian were often feared and despised by the community. If they chose not to remarry, their very existence challenged the patriarchal structure of society.

Karlsen found, in fact, that in seventeenth-century New England such women comprised a high percentage of individuals accused and convicted of witchcraft. No individual more personified the difficulties faced by the rich widow than Katherine Harrison of Wethersfield, Connecticut. Widowed in the 1650s and left with the largest estate in the town, she encountered the wrath of the community when she chose to remain unmarried and attempted to manage her property alone. Her neighbors damaged her fences, maimed and destroyed her livestock, and finally accused her of being a witch and fortune-teller. Katherine Harrison escaped further persecution only by signing her estate over to male guardians and fleeing Connecticut entirely (Karlsen, 1987).

Not every independent or active widow faced the harsh treatment of Harrison. Elderly wives and widows certainly demonstrated great capacity and initiative at their occupations; they ran taverns, operated shops, worked as seamstresses, and even managed large estates. Generally, however, they justified their roles in terms significantly different from those used by men. In contrast to their male counterparts, they worked not to define their place in society through prominent careers but essentially for domestic reasons: they labored in order to provide for the needs of their families (Wilson, 1992). Those who did not support their industry in terms of domesticity were likely to encounter social scrutiny and reprisals. In male-dominated fields, according to Premo, "they risked censure and unhappiness, both of which might appear increasingly inappropriate and undesirable" as they aged (Premo, 1990, p. 25). Old women who dressed, acted, or spoke in a manner inappropriate to their advanced years and domestic state received condemnation from both minister and magistrate. In the early nine-teenth century Theodore Parker exclaimed from the pulpit:

Now she is an old woman of fashion, wearing still the garments of her earlier prime, which short and scanty as they were, are yet a world too wide for shrunken age to fill. . . . In youth a worm; in womanhood a butterfly; in old age, your wings all tatted, your plumage rent, a 'fingered moth'—old, shriveled, sick, perching on nothing, perishing into dust, the laughter of the witty; the scorn of the thoughtless; only the pity of the wise and good. (Parker, cited by Cole, 1992, p. 195)

Aging women were best accepted in occupations that did not challenge male authority. As seamstresses, boardinghouse keepers, and midwives, they appeared to remain within the female sphere of maternity and domesticity. Nonetheless, especially as midwives, elderly women were able to exert considerable influence in the community. Laurel Thatcher Ulrich's (1990) study of aging midwife Mar-tha Ballard clearly demonstrated the resourcefulness and activity of an aging woman in the new republic. But even a woman such as Martha Ballard was not without her constraints. With the entrance of male physicians into obstetrics, Ballard found herself and her role challenged and eventually replaced by a "professional" doctor.

Moreover, while Ballard demonstrated great resourcefulness and autonomy, even she encountered real limitations to her independence. Although she wished to live alone when her husband was in jail, her son and daughter-in-law quickly moved into "their father's house" unannounced. "Ballard," wrote Ulrich, "became a lodger in her own house, taking one room as her own, giving over the rest to her son's family" (Ulrich, 1990, p. 281). Other elderly women discovered that they too were unable to remain single household heads. In the early nineteenth century Massachusetts matron Hannah Carter Smith wrote to her daughter explaining her desire to live alone. "It is important," she stated, "that I have a house of my own on moderate terms even if there are inconveniences." In time, however, and with great reluctance, she gave up her home and assumed a new and clearly more dependent position in the family of her offspring (Smith, cited by Premo, 1990, p. 36). Although aging men generally maintained both their position as household heads and their professional identities until disability or death, there were clear restrictions to the autonomy of aging women.

In colonial and early America, therefore, the values and attitudes toward elderly women differed profoundly from those toward men. Power and authority rested with aged men who controlled wealth and possessions. The promise of inheritance served to insure the continued respect of offspring. For women, however, such factors often had detrimental effects: continued activity outside the familial sphere brought scrutiny and, at times, even condemnation; landownership could place them in social jeopardy. As wives they relied upon the status of their husbands; as widows they became dependents in their own homes. The respect and authority that they commanded came not from wealth or possessions but from domestic qualities and benevolence.

WOMEN'S OLD AGE IN THE NINETEENTH CENTURY

While not all historians agree with David Hackett Fischer (1977), who argued that a dramatic change occurred in attitudes toward old age in the early nineteenth century, his model has little bearing on the lives of old women (Premo, 1990). Although the experiences of these women did differ somewhat from those of their earlier counterparts, they did not find themselves suddenly portrayed as enduring meaningless existences. As images of old men became feminized and debased, the line between old men and women began to vanish (Cole, 1992; Haber, 1983). No longer portrayed as authoritarian or controlling, old men, like their female counterparts, were applauded for their humility, dignity, and serenity; their active involvement with the world was presumed to be at an end. Thus, while old men in the nineteenth century lived to see themselves often portrayed in sharply different terms from their colonial forerunners, women continued to construct their lives around their families and to depict their interests as domestic concerns.

Yet old women often found themselves immersed in a wider variety of family patterns than in previous eras. In the seventeenth and eighteenth centuries late age of marriage, long periods of childbirth, and high adult mortality served to limit the number of women who lived to see all their children grown and married. The great majority experienced most of their adult lives as wives and mothers, residing in two-generational households. Beginning in the mid-nineteenth century, however, declines in mortality, both for infants and for women at childbirth, meant that a larger proportion of women survived to old age and outlived their husbands. At the same time, earlier ages for both marriage and childbirth increased the probability that three generations of family members would be alive simultaneously. These wide-scale demographic changes then served to broaden the possible combinations of family patterns. Old women lived as spouses of the household head, as dependents in a household of their children and grandchildren, and as heads of their own homes.

The historiography of this varied nineteenth-century family structure has been extensive: numerous scholars have investigated the household structure of elderly men and women in the nineteenth century (for example, Chudacoff & Hareven, 1978, 1979; Hareven, 1976, 1982, 1983; Korbin, 1976; Ruggles, 1987, 1994; Smith, 1979, 1986). Of greatest importance, according to Howard Chudacoff and Tamara Hareven, is the fact that these elderly families rarely experienced dramatic transitions in demographic or social cycles. Households did not dissolve, nor did the elderly live numerous years apart from kin in "empty-nest" households. Rather, until the twentieth century, families continued to be the center of social and economic support. Old women rarely lived alone, separated from their immediate kin. Before the creation of state pensions and the rise in real income and savings, families remained the most important support of the elderly. In order to sustain kin, they shared resources, savings, and space. For elderly married men, this kinship arrangement assured that the great majority remained heads of their own homes, even as their earnings decreased with age. As long as the elderly man remained alive, the great majority of elderly women retained the status of spouse of the household head.

In the nineteenth century this household looked remarkably different from the common pattern a century later. Despite their advancing age, married couples often shared the household with an unmarried adult child or children who contributed significantly to the household income and fulfilled essential family responsibilities. According to Steven Ruggles (1994), in 1880, 72.8 percent of white elderly married couples and 61.2 percent of nonwhite elderly couples lived with at least one of their own children. Entering the work force at relatively earlier ages, or completing vital tasks on the farm, these children participated in the creation of a family fund. Although aging women were generally not considered part of the wage work force, their contribution to the familial economic arrangement was essential. By remaining within the home and fulfilling domestic tasks, they allowed their maturing children to enter the labor force. Moreover, their labor added significantly to the family income. They cooked, canned, preserved, sewed, worked gardens, operated dairies, and sold their produce to stores. As nurses and midwives, they maintained the health of the family; as teachers of growing daughters, they passed their knowledge on to the next generation. Although by the end of the nineteenth century, as Nancy Folbre (1991) has argued, they were often labeled "unproductive," throughout much of the era they were recognized as a vital part of the family economy.

While most married elderly couples retained their position as household head, as the result of ill health or financial need, some were forced to cede their roles within the family to the younger generation. Yet such transfers of power and status were not made easily. Historians such as Mary Ryan and Emily Abel have related tales of family strife in which the elderly individuals came to assume a dependent role within the family circle (Ryan, 1981; Abel, 1992). According to Ryan, for example, in mid-nineteenth-century Utica, New York, Julia and Bildad Merrill allowed their son and daughter-in-law to enter their home and become the heads of household. Before long, however, conflict between the generations emerged. Both mother and daughter-in-law claimed command over the servants and preeminence with the children. Ultimately, their dispute led to an outbreak of violence between the two women and an attempt by their church to find peace within the household. Not surprisingly, then, households that contained two complete generations of married couples in which the couple of the younger generation was listed as head of household were relatively rare. Most aging married couples managed to retain their roles as spouses and heads.

Elderly women who became widows, however, often experienced a wider variety in living arrangements. Unlike men, such women could not assume that they would live much as they had earlier; they often found their status and responsibilities radically altered. As Carole Haber and Brian Gratton have shown, ability to maintain their independence often depended on their location and income. Upon the deaths of their husbands, old farm women were likely to become dependents in the homes of their sons (Haber & Gratton, 1994; Smith, 1986). Despite those who attempted to manage property (and the small minority who succeeded), most found the rigors of farm life too demanding. Other elderly women left the farm for the city and small town. As a result, by the late nineteenth century fewer aged women than men lived in farm households. Thus, while farm ownership in the late nineteenth century tended to guarantee continued status for elderly men, for a sizeable percentage of elderly women it had a far different meaning.

In contrast, widows in cities, and especially in small villages, were more likely to remain heads of their own homes. According to Carole Shammas et al. (1987), these women often benefited from changing inheritance patterns. In the eighteenth century elderly farmers often held on to their land until death, assuring themselves of enduring power, or deeded the land to their children while continuing to guarantee themselves the support of their children. Upon their deaths, their elderly widows simply received a room in the house or provisions for their care. In the late nineteenth century, however, aging farmers with valuable property began to sell or rent their land, utilizing the funds to support themselves and their wives. Many moved into villages where the "nest egg" amassed from the sale of land guaranteed their independence. Thus in rural nonfarm settings at the turn of the twentieth century, more than two-thirds of all village women aged 60 and over were listed by census takers as either married to the household head (36 percent) or heads themselves (32 percent). Even widowhood did not necessarily lead to dependence. In the village 56 percent of widows were able to retain their authority as household heads, in contrast to 24 percent on the farm.

In urban areas, as well, women found job opportunities that supported their independence. As schoolteachers, domestics, seamstresses, and boardinghouse keepers, their paid employment, while often mirroring their domestic concerns, allowed them a degree of financial independence. As John Modell and Tamara Hareven (1978) have noted, women in their 40s, 50s, and 60s often became boardinghouse keepers as a means of keeping their own homes, rather than becoming dependent on kin.

The experience of elderly women was shaped as well by race and ethnicity. In a study of Buffalo in 1855, Laurence Glasco (1977) found that 16 percent of all native-born women headed their own homes, in contrast to 20 percent of German women and 25 percent of Irish women. African-American women also experienced old age in distinctive ways. In antebellum America few slaves had the privilege of retirement. Despite several historians' portrayal of the respect awarded to aged slaves, and especially aged women (Genovese, 1974; Jones, 1985), elderly female slaves continued to work and were often separated from their families, their diminished capabilities recognized in their selling price as "quarter hands." After the Civil War, elderly black women were three times more likely to be in the work force than their white counterparts. Far more apt to be living apart from their own children, they labored to provide for their old age (Rieff, Dahlin, & Smith, 1983).

Not surprisingly, black older women filled the outdoor-relief rosters of many large cities. In communities that provided almshouse shelter, they were often placed in areas reserved for the insane. White elderly women, as well, were hardly strangers to poverty in the nineteenth century. In every large city aged females, both black and white, filled the rolls of both outdoor pensioners and almshouse pensioners. Relief officials generally expected these women to be "worthy" recipients of relief. In contrast to men, their gender underscored the need for benevolence (Haber & Gratton, 1986).

Nineteenth-century old-age homes also targeted elderly women as appropriate recipients of care. Distinguishing between the laboring poor who were likely to be served by almshouses and those of a "better class," they directed their care toward widows and single women who had once been self-sufficient but experienced impoverishment as they advanced in age (Haber, 1983). Thus in the nineteenth century, while old men tended to be the dominant residents of alms-houses, old women made up the majority of residents of private asylums. Although in the late nineteenth century newly founded institutions opened their doors to couples and elderly men, they generally still housed women whose impoverished state could easily be linked to widowhood or the misfortunes of age (Haber, 1983; Gratton, 1986).

WOMEN'S OLD AGE IN THE TWENTIETH CENTURY

The economic growth tied to industrialization had a significant impact upon the lives of women. As increasing numbers of middle-class married women were able to live with their husbands apart from any children, single-generational households became more common. By the second decade of the twentieth century, a considerable proportion of middle-class children and their elders established separate residences. Between 1900 and 1940 the proportion of women who lived as dependents in their children's home declined from 34 to 23 percent. At the same time, a growing proportion of working-class families were now able to support their elderly mothers and save them from the shame of relying on charity (Haber & Gratton, 1994; Ruggles, 1987).

Nonetheless, single women and those whose children could offer little support continued to fill the ranks of the impoverished. With the Great Depression, their numbers clearly multiplied. As savings evaporated and homes were lost, women, like men, found themselves without any of the traditional means of support.

The perception that this group was growing and becoming increasingly impoverished served as a central justification for the establishment of state welfare. Tales and stark photographs of once-middle-class women forced into the almshouse served pension advocates well. Moreover, a report by the Social Security Board's Bureau of Research and Statistics listed all women married to men over 65 as dependents and burdens. Here, above all, was a group that demanded to be saved from the "misery of the asylum."

Not surprisingly, perhaps, the allocation of Social Security has had a profound effect upon the lives of women. Provisions in the measure restricted any relief being given to inmates of public asylums; as a result, almshouses shut their doors as private "nursing homes" and boardinghouses expanded. Most important, Social Security dramatically changed women's residence patterns. Although the trend toward separate households began before the depression (and was relatively strong among prosperous women living in small towns and villages), the economic crisis reversed the pattern. Families were forced back into complex arrangements in order to share resources and space. With the establishment of a guaranteed income, however, the tendency toward solitary living became the norm. In 1940, 58 percent of elderly women who did not reside with their husbands dwelled with kin; by 1970 only 29 percent shared homes with their relatives. As Daniel Scott Smith (1979, 1986), Steven Ruggles (1987, 1994),

Frances Korbin (1978), and Tim Heaton and Caroline Hoppe (1987) have found, the independent household marks a new chapter in the lives of old women.

While historians have agreed upon this new departure for elderly women, they have not concurred about the historical forces causing it. Some, such as Daniel Scott Smith, see this transformation as a sign of cultural change: where once elderly individuals were supported by families, they now are left to survive on their own. In his view, the culture of family support no longer dictates the living patterns of the old (Smith, 1979, 1986). Others, such as Haber and Gratton, argue that the pattern represents the fulfillment of a household structure long desired by the elderly, but economically available only to the wealthy or those with sufficient savings. Repeatedly, throughout the eighteenth, nineteenth, and early twentieth centuries women, like their middle-aged children, expressed their desire to live in their own homes, apart from the tensions and demands of the three-generational household (Premo, 1990; "Old Age Intestate," 1931; "I Am the Mother-in-Law," 1937). Only with Social Security and the assumption of guaranteed support has this ideal become a national reality.

Attitudes toward elderly women also have markedly changed. Previously, aged women were viewed as asexual beings, grandmothers dispensing child-rearing advice along with knitting and baking. Magazine advertisements of the early twentieth century made this image quite clear: with white hair in a bun, and confined to a rocking chair, the aged woman spoke to a time long past. She stood now only for repose and contemplation (Cole, 1992). By the late twentieth century, however, such an image found little support. Her sexuality discovered by the Kinsey Report, as well as Masters and Johnson, the old woman became portrayed by magazines such as *Lear's* as active, knowledgeable, and involved.

Clearly, the existences of elderly women have differed from those in the past. Changing economic conditions and social mores have transformed the lives and images of older women. Yet today, as in the past, older women experience no single reality, nor does a single interpretation define their existences. While many women have profited from changing social and economic conditions, single, unattached aged women still rank among the most impoverished of all Americans; other still-married elderly women and those with significant inheritances continue to live prosperous lives. Their relationships to friends, family, and work vary considerably. This diversity underscores the need for additional studies into the history of elderly women. As we have seen, their histories are not those of men, nor are they necessarily unified simply by the nature of their advanced age. In their past, instead, is revealed the complex nature of women's old age in America.

REFERENCES

Abel, Emily. (1992). Parental dependence and filial responsibility in the nineteenth century. *Gerontologist, 32*(4), 519–536.

Achenbaum, W. Andrew. (1978). *Old age in the new land*. Baltimore: Johns Hopkins University Press.

Chalfant, Ella. (1955). *A goodly heritage*. Pittsburgh: University of Pittsburgh Press.

Chudacoff, Howard, & Hareven, Tamara. (1978). Family transition in old age. In Tamara Hareven (Ed.), *Transitions*. New York: Academic Press.

———. (1979). Family dissolution: Life course transitions in old age. *Journal of Family History, 4*(1), 217–243.

Clement, Priscilla. (1985). *Welfare and the poor in the nineteenth-century city*. Rutherford, NJ: Fairleigh Dickinson University Press.

Cole, Thomas. (1992). *The journey of life*. New York: Cambridge University Press.

Demos, John. (1978). Old age in New England. In Michael Gordon (Ed.), *The American family in social-historical perspective* (2nd ed., pp. 220–256). New York: St. Martin's Press.

Feinson, Marjorie Chary. (1985). Where are the women in the history of aging? *Social Science History, 9*(4), 429–452.

Fischer, David Hackett. (1977). *Growing old in America*. New York: Oxford University Press.

Folbre, Nancy. (1991). The unproductive housewife. *Signs, 16*(3), 463–485.

Genovese, Eugene. (1974). *Roll, Jordan, roll*. New York: Pantheon Books.

Glasco, Laurence. (1977). The life cycles and household structure of American groups: Irish, German, and native-born whites in Buffalo, New York, 1955. In Tamara Hareven (Ed.), *Family and kin in urban communities*. New York: New Viewpoints.

Gratton, Brian. (1986). *Urban elders*. Philadelphia: Temple University Press.

Gratton, Brian, & Haber, Carole. (1993). In Search of "intimacy at a distance": Family history from the perspective of elderly women. *Journal of Aging Studies, 7*(2), 183–194.

Greven, Philip J., Jr. (1970). *Four generations*. Ithaca, NY: Cornell University Press.

Grigg, Susan. (1984). *The dependent poor of Newburyport*. Ann Arbor: University of Michigan Research Press.

Haber, Carole. (1983). *Beyond sixty-five*. New York: Cambridge University Press.

Haber, Carole, & Gratton, Brian. (1986). "Old age public welfare and race: The case of Charleston, South Carolina, 1800–1949." *Journal of Social History, 21*(2), 263–279.

———. (1994). *Old age and the search for security*. Bloomington: Indiana University Press.

Hareven, Tamara. (1976). "The last stage." *Daedalus, 105*(4), 110–125.

———. (1982). *Family time and industrial time*. Cambridge: Cambridge University Press.

———. (1986). Life course transitions and kin assistance. In David D. Van Tassel and Peter N. Stearns (Eds.), *Old age in a bureaucratic society*. Westport, CT: Greenwood Press.

Heaton, Tim, & Hoppe, Caroline. (1987). Widowed and married: Comparative change in living arrangements, 1900 and 1980. *Social Science History, 11*(3).

I am the mother-in-law in the home. (1937, November). *Reader's Digest* 11–13.

Jones, Jacqueline. (1985). *Labor of love, labor of sorrow*. New York: Basic Books.

Karlsen, Carol F. (1987). *The devil in the shape of a woman*. New York: Norton.

Keyssar, Alexander. (1974). Widowhood in eighteenth-century Massachusetts: A problem in the history of the family. *Perspectives in American History, 8,* 83–119.

Korbin, Frances. (1976). The fall in household size and the rise of the primary individual in the United States. In Michael Gordon (Ed.), *The American family in social-historical perspective* (2nd ed.). New York: St. Martin's Press.

Modell, John, & Hareven, Tamara. (1978). Urbanization and the malleable household. In Michael Gordon (Ed.), *The American family in social-historical perspective* (2nd ed.). New York: St. Martin's Press.

Old age intestate. (1931, May). *Harper's Magazine* 712–715.

Premo, Terri. (1990). *Winter friends: Women growing old in the new republic, 1785–1835.* Urbana: University of Illinois Press.

Rieff, Janice, Dahlin, Michel, & Smith, Daniel Scott. (1983). Rural push and urban pull: Work and family experiences of older black women in Southern cities, 1880–1900. *Journal of Social History, 16,* 39–48.

Ruggles, Steven. (1987). *Prolonged connections: The rise of the extended family in nineteenth-century England and America.* Madison: University of Wisconsin Press.

―――. (1994). The transformation of American family structure. *American Historical Review, 99*(1).

Ryan, Mary. (1981). *Cradle of the middle class.* New York: Cambridge University Press.

Shammas, Carole, Salmon, Marylynn, & Dahlin, Michel. (1987). *Inheritance in America.* New Brunswick, NJ: Rutgers University Press.

Smith, Daniel Scott. (1979). Life course, norms, and the family system of older Americans in 1900. *Journal of Family History, 4*(2).

―――. (1986). Accounting for change in families of the elderly in the United States, 1900–present. In David D. Van Tassel & Peter N. Stearns (Eds.), *Old age in a bureaucratic society.* Westport, CT: Greenwood Press.

Ulrich, Laurel Thatcher. (1990). *A midwife's tale: The life of Martha Ballard based on her diary, 1785–1812.* New York: Random House.

Wilson, Lisa. (1992). *Life after death: widows in Pennsylvania, 1750–1850.* Philadelphia: Temple University Press.

Four

Images of Aging Women through the Ages

MARY GRIZZARD

Every society and every epoch bears a specific relation to the world of art. While texts, records, and inscriptions may form the basis for the historian's knowledge of a place and time, images offer additional confirmation of knowledge obtained through other means. Art, much like literature, however, is selective and interpretive, but in its selectivity it is quite revealing about attitudes toward certain categories of life. We all know that there have been old people present throughout history, although in a smaller percentage of the overall population than today, for life expectancy was shorter. Therefore, we also know that there were middle-aged and old women as well, but they were represented less often than men of all ages. The strange thing is that while there are indeed many images of older women, and at times the characteristics of aging are easy to recognize, many times the images are so abstract or idealized in their youth that we have to know that these persons were, in fact, old at the time they were represented. A youthful appearance is often given, for example, to a monarch or a religious person whom we know to have been depicted late in life. This is rather like some people who continue to submit what appears to be a high-school photograph to professional journals throughout a lifetime.

Although there are a great many more representations of young women and more of men of any age in art, there are more of older women in art than one would perhaps think at first. There are also more women artists throughout history than have been traditionally reported, but a review of their work finds no more representations of older women in their art than in works of art by men artists.

When we look back into prehistory and ancient history, we see that there were many goddesses. Although goddesses are interesting phenomena, they have to be eliminated for the most part from our survey because they are by definition immortal and do not age. Of course, some exceptions come to mind, such as the Cumaean Sibyl, in Greek mythology, who escaped Apollo's amorous attentions, but was punished by becoming immortal without the usual accompanying eternal youth. There are too many other examples for us to deal with the exceptional, however.

The earliest known image of a middle-aged female dates from about 26,000 B.C. It is a small, carved ivory head, found at Dolní Vestonice in present-day Slovakia.[1] The features are so individual that they appear to be a portrait. Her nose has a small bump on the end, and her forehead and mouth are sharply angled to the left. A burial of an approximately 40-year-old woman was found nearby, with a skull bearing congenital malformations resembling those of the carving. The figurine would appear to be a portrait of this unusual individual, who was buried in the traditional fashion for that period, facing west, with adornments and implements of a sacred nature placed around her. Red ochre was sprinkled over her, and two mammoth shoulder blades were placed on top of her. At her side was the tail of a fox, and in her right hand were the animal's teeth.

The most common type of female representation in the prehistoric period is the so-called mother or earth-goddess figure, but there is no suggestion that the Dolní Vestonice figure might belong to this broader category. It is not even known for certain if such "earth goddesses" as the well-known Venus of Willendorf[2] are really fertility figures, or if they might have been associated with puberty rituals or other beliefs. In any case, the Dolní Vestonice image may have been that of a powerful, even revered person. That it was associated with a nearby burial of an older female bearing a very similar deformation of the skull suggests circumstantially that it is a portrait of that individual. We know nothing else about her, but the existence of a portrait gives one reason to believe that there was respect of some kind for this middle-aged person—some 28,000 years ago.

Though wall paintings have survived in Western Europe from the Mycenean time (ca. 1500–1200 B.C.) (and no images of older women survive), so much has been destroyed of later Greek painting that we have to generalize on the basis of vase paintings and descriptions. In classical Greece (fifth century B.C.) we see older women represented in some of the rituals in which they participated. Mothers used to partake in one of the phases of the wedding ritual: the bride's departure from home. In the British Museum there is a Greek vase on which a wedding departure is depicted. The vase dates from about 430 B.C., and is a pyxis, or cylindrical terra-cotta container. On the surface, wrapping around the curve of the vase, is a wedding couple riding in a chariot. A woman, perhaps the bride's mother, is seen in the doorway of the house they are leaving. She must be middle-aged by ancient Greek standards (with the then-shorter lifespans) to have a daughter of marriageable age. She is, nonetheless, depicted as a woman of indeterminate age, with long hair and an erect posture, standing with one hand across her chest to hold the door open as she watches her daughter leave.

There may be more emotion in that scene than is first apparent if we realize that brides had no choice whom they married. It conforms to reality, then, that the mother stands in the doorway and has little part to play in the ritual as a whole. However, in another vase[3] she is shown arranging the garments of the bride as she steps away from the door, and it is known that the mother of the bride was also allowed to carry a torch in the wedding procession. However, the bride's mother was not a major part of the entire marriage ritual, which included its arrangement, dowry payment, procession, and banquet.

In Greek funeral rituals women were apparently those who were given closest access to mourn the body of the deceased. In the Louvre Museum is a pinax, a terra-cotta plaque dated about 500 B.C., once fixed to the tomb. On this plaque the deceased is a beardless adult man lying on a bed. Several women surrounding him express their grief by tearing at their hair. A quiet woman touches the head of the deceased, and the inscription identifies her as *meter*, or mother. Facing the mother at the head of the bed is *thethe*, a grandmother.

In Greek paintings there is some age differentiation among males, who are beardless, bearded, bald, or white haired, indicating some degree of age; however, women are generally portrayed as ageless, with only minor nuances, if any, to indicate an advanced stage in life. One exceptional classical Greek red-figure cup (skyphos) is by the painter identified by stylistic grouping under the name Pistoxenos Painter. The cup is from about 470 B.C. and is from Cerveteri, north of Rome.[4] On the cup the young hero Herakles goes unwillingly to school (he later killed his teacher), followed by an old Thracian woman. She is in profile, appears to be toothless, and has wrinkles by her mouth and shoulder-length white hair. Her posture is stooped, and she leans on a walking stick with one hand and carries a lyre (a small, stringed instrument) with her other hand. With the evidence at hand, it is impossible to say who this woman is, but she may represent the force of responsibility, given the circumstances of Herakles' attitude toward formal education. The depiction is honest and does not appear to be comic or disrespectful, as representations of identifiably aged women tend to be in classical Greece.

Also in fifth century B.C. classical Greece small clay figurines were used as religious offerings—in the house, the grave, or the sanctuary. They were intended to solicit divine protection to the person offering the figurine. Success might be provided, for example, to actors on the Greek stage by a representation of actors wearing costumes and masks. One such clay duo of actors shows one dressed as an old woman and one as a bearded man. While the man has the usual actor's costume of padded tunic, phallus, and tights, the old woman (in reality a man dressed as a woman) has a sagging paunch beneath her garment and tugs at her drooping jowls. That some kind of comedy was intended is apparent by these caricatures. In the last surviving plays by Aristophanes, wicked humor is derived by making fun of elderly women. This clay group dates from the fourth century B.C. and is in the Wagner Museum in Würzburg, Germany.[5]

It says much about the ideas in Greek art as well as a certain bias in Greek society that most surviving depictions of recognizably older women are either comic or pitiable. A famous example from the Hellenistic period (ca. second century B.C.) is a sculpture of an old drunk woman grasping a wine flask with both hands. Another well-known Hellenistic statue from about the second century B.C. depicts a tired old woman carrying a basket of vegetables.[6] She is bent forward, her mouth open, with her garment sagging in front to reveal one breast. The effect is that of loneliness, for it seems that she has no one to help her with a chore that appears to have exhausted her so much. Apart from this visual evidence there is not much in the written record to indicate what the Greek attitude toward the elderly might have been. It is known that there was respect for older men, for some political positions were set aside for them,[7] and elderly women were given the important role of midwife. Nonetheless, the visual evidence as well as several of the sardonic remarks about the elderly in general that appear in Greek literature do not give a very positive outlook. Aristotle, in the *Rhetoric*, delivered a scathing description of the elderly, and the public speaker Thrasymachos of Chalkedon, active in the last half of the fifth century B.C., was said to have delivered to the Athenian Assembly a statement that, in effect, he wished he had lived in Athens a long time ago, when *neoteroi* (younger men) were obliged to be silent, and when *presbyteroi* (elderly people) guided the citizenry.[8]

Romans apparently treated their elderly citizens better than their Greek predecessors. Old age was considered a qualification for public office, for old men were viewed to have the necessary *gravitas* (seriousness). The very word *senator* derives from *senex*, the Latin word for old man. Accordingly, the elderly were cared for, accompanied in the streets, and stood up for when they entered the room.

Cicero's first wife, Terentia, lived to be 103, and his *De senectute* (On old age) expressed a kind of cheerful philosophical acceptance of aging. Therefore, respect for old age is what we find in Roman medals, mosaics, paintings, and especially portrait sculpture. Several of these Roman portrait busts are in the National and the Capitoline museums in Rome, and in all cases the individual represented exhibits all the incidental aspects that identify that person as an individual, including all the folds and wrinkles. This indicates respect for the appearance of aging, with no need to give a youthful or idealized appearance.

One especially dignified example of a Roman portrait of an elderly woman is a marble head from the 2nd century A.D., in the Museu Arqueologic Nacional de Tarragona, in Spain. Her gaze is serious; she is the very picture of Roman *gravitas*. Mouth, brow, cheeks, and eyes all show the natural softening of age. Elderly Roman women were expected to stay in their households and to be able to spin and weave cloth. Those who were upper class could also head literary salons and influence politics through their families. Although remarriage was possible for widows and divorcées, epitaphs praised women who died having known only one husband (*univira*). There is every evidence that their dignified portraits reflect the esteem in which they were held within the family.

Though older women owned businesses in the Middle Ages and Renaissance, they were more likely to be represented in art due to their role in religion or as a member of the aristocracy. Within the church, European women could lead a life outside marriage and the family. There were communities of religious women where they could develop their intellectual and spiritual capacities. Senior women could become nuns and abbesses and assume great responsibilities among the nuns of the order. Literacy among nuns meant the ability to understand Latin and to study the texts of the early church and antiquity. Accordingly, with their prominence and family wealth, abbesses would often become patrons of beautifully illustrated religious texts, and in these we see portraits of the donor-abbess.

In medieval central Europe Abbess Hildegard of Bingen (1098–1179), founder of the convent of Rupertsberg, Germany, was a writer and a visionary. When she was 40, she began to write down her thoughts and experiences, and she continued nearly until her death at age 78. She wrote books of religious inspiration, science texts, allegorical works, and songs. Popes and emperors accepted her scientific treatises, and she was widely regarded as a prophet and a sage.

One of her texts was *Scivias* (Know the ways of the Lord), consisting of thirty-five of her visions relating to the history of salvation. The text begins "And behold! In my forty-third year I had a heavenly vision." The first illustration in the text shows her at this age with a monk in a monastery. Two small rooms with red domes flank the center space, and in the large central room Hildegard sits while writing on a wax tablet as a vision descends in a great flash of light from above her head. The elderly, bald, white-bearded monk looks directly into her face as he leans in from one of the smaller domed rooms at the side.[9]

Mysticism such as Abbess Hildegard's clearly continued to be a path to holiness that had been open equally to women and men since the early Christian period. Some of the mystics, such as the Spaniard St. Teresa of Ávila (1515–82), became especially honored and influential. She came from a wealthy merchant family of Toledo, Spain. Orphaned at age 14, she entered the care of Augustinian nuns at age 16 and six years later chose a career as a nun in the Carmelite order. In the Carmelite convent at Ávila she first experienced a mystical vision at the age of 39. She continued to experience visions throughout her life and was consulted by church leaders and royalty alike. There is a very lifelike, realistic portrait of her at the age of 61 (1576) by Fray Juan de la Miseria. It is a half-length figure of St. Teresa in the robes of the Carmelite order, her hands joined in prayer as she gazes at a dove symbolizing the Holy Spirit. A banderole (scroll with lettering) curls above her head with the prayer in Latin: "Have mercy, Lord; I sing in eternity." The overall tone of the painting is one of great seriousness and respect for her actual appearance at age 61, with a long aquiline nose, a small mouth, large folds under her eyes, and sagging cheeks. She must have felt free to allow herself to be represented with accurate signs of aging. Further inscriptions on the painting give the artist, her name, and the date.[10]

Just as often, we see portraits of elderly aristocratic donor women in texts, panel and wall paintings, and mosaics. A famous medieval example of an elderly aristocratic donor is the mosaic portrait of the Byzantine Empress Theodora (sixth century) in San Vitale, Ravenna. Information about her early career largely comes from the *Secret History* by Procopius, a Byzantine historian. The account is often a rather scandalous court chronicle, but nonetheless it describes Theodora as an actress and prostitute before her marriage (522) to Justinian I. On Justinian's accession in 527, he made her joint ruler, sharing his authority with her. She is known to have been quite assertive and is credited with saving the Byzantine throne during a major upheaval, the Nika riot (532). This donor portrait on the chancel wall in San Vitale shows her standing in a palace door-way with her court retinue beside her. Justinian and his courtiers face her on the opposite wall. Although the representations are quite flat and are surrounded by heavy dark lines, these are clearly portraits of the monarchs in their later years. This portrait was completed just before she died, and the lines around her eyes definitely sag downwards along the lower lid. Forceful and assertive is certainly the impression given by her straight posture and open, steady gaze toward the viewer.

One of the most famous donor portraits in the Renaissance is in the fresco of the Trinity by Masaccio (1425), in Sta. Maria Novella, in Florence. The painting is celebrated for its understanding of geometrically constructed space and creates a quite convincing illusion of a deeply barrel-vaulted unity receding into the wall. On the equally convincing ledge that is painted to appear as if it is in front of the barrel-vaulted space are a kneeling husband and wife, who were donors of the piece. These are the Lenzi, a wealthy merchant family. Both husband and wife are represented with considerable honesty as an aged couple who gaze toward the vision of God, the Holy Spirit, and the crucified Christ. This wall painting was meant as a pious donation, as a continual prayer on behalf of the donors above their tomb in the church.

Likewise, in the same wall painting in Florence, we see the Virgin Mary as an aged woman at the time of her son's death. As always in such representations, she is to the right of the crucified Christ, and St. John is to the left. Although it is true that Mary would be at least middle aged at the time of her grown son's death, artists vary whether they represent her as older by the time of his cru-cifixion. Likewise, the Italian Renaissance artist Francesco della Cossa shows a decidedly old Mary with John below the crucified Christ (ca. 1470–75), as does also the German Renaissance artist Matthias Grünewald in his panel painting *The Small Crucifixion* (ca. 1520).[11] Oddly enough, although there are several elderly saints who come to mind, such as St. Anne, Mary's mother, and Eliz-abeth, John the Baptist's mother, they are usually depicted as ageless females, even though in both of their cases conception was considered a miracle, for they were both well beyond the usual age of motherhood.

Occasionally medieval and Renaissance paintings depict an elderly woman as part of a larger narrative scene. One such painting is by the fifteenth-century late medieval Spanish artist Bernardo Martorell. It is a panel of Christ and the woman from Canaan, an episode from Matthew 15:22–28, in which a woman asks Christ to cure her daughter who is possessed by a demon. The setting resembles the medieval streets of Barcelona near the Cathedral. The Canaanite kneels before the assembled group of Jesus and his disciples. Behind a barred window in the closest building is the possessed daughter, with her hands clenched and her head thrown back as a demon is expelled from her mouth. From this scene alone it can be said that Martorell observed attitudes and expressions very carefully. Not only is the woman from Canaan a convincing profile of an elderly woman with many wrinkles and folds, but the figure of her daughter is an accurate representation of an epileptic in a position of seizure. Until the nineteenth century, it must be remembered, epilepsy was considered a ''demoniacal infection.'' The evident aged quality of the mother's face as she beseeches Christ for a miracle makes the painting all the more moving.[12]

Among the types of medieval and Renaissance portraits of elderly women, there were many donor portraits, as previously mentioned; there were also others simply recording the appearance of the individual. Queen Isabella of Spain (1451–1504) is very frankly and realistically represented in a portrait in the Madrid Instituto de la Historia by an anonymous Hispano-Flemish artist. She is shown in a three-quarter view to midchest. Fitting all the descriptions of the sober, plain dress of the Spanish court, she wears a black dress with a high-necked, pleated white insert and a matching simple white cloth cap. The large golden cross around her neck recalls her fame as the ''Catholic monarch'' who participated with her husband Ferdinand in the conquest of Islamic Granada. Her heavily lidded eyes, solemn gaze, and the considerable fleshiness of her cheeks and double chin indicate that she was definitely an aged woman in this portrait. If she looks very wise, it could be because by this time she could look back to having sent Columbus on his voyage to discover the New World, and also to having achieved the conquest of Granada, all in the same year (1492).

It should be emphasized, however, that most aristocratic portraits were by no means as faithful to the age and appearance of the person as was that of Isabella of Spain. Certainly an example of a sharply idealized portrait is one of Mary Tudor, Philip II of Spain's second wife. It is from around 1554 and is by the Flemish artist Antonís Mor. Mary's delicate, smooth skin, lack of wrinkles, and even her slenderness and dark hair color are misleading, in complete disagreement with the fact that she was middle aged, some eleven years older than Philip, and was described by contemporaries as a fat redhead with no eyebrows and a deep voice. It should be remembered, however, that as the Catholic queen of England, the daughter of Henry VIII and Catherine of Aragon, hers was a marriage of property and power. As was the custom in such arranged alliances, this portrait may well have been one that was sent to Philip as a representation of his prospective bride. They were married for only four years before her death in 1548, but during that time England was drawn into the existing war between Spain and France, with the main results being the loss of Calais and the increasing hostility of the English people. Philip even left her in London while he led a victory over the French. Even though the idealized youthful portrait may have been part of the scheme to get her married to Philip, the marriage was not judged to be happy, either for her or for England. So much for the wisdom of attempting to hide the truth of old age!

For the most part, the baroque and rococo periods (seventeenth–eighteenth centuries) abound with sensuous, nubile young women in theatrical settings. As we recall, in the Renaissance period even the much-adored St. Teresa had a right to be represented honestly as an older woman, since her visions did not begin until she was 39 years old. Nonetheless, one of the most famous baroque sculptures, *The Ecstasy of St. Theresa* (1645–52), by Giovanni Bellini, in the Cornaro Chapel, Sta. Maria della Vittoria, Rome, represents her as a very young woman. She is semireclining, her mouth is open, and her eyes are closed, as a smiling young angel positions an arrow above her. No one has missed the erotic implications of this piece, and one has to consider how strange it is, given her real age when her visions began, and the esteem in which she was held as a religious leader.

Nonetheless, there are some outstanding baroque representations of older women, and some of the best examples tend to cluster among the northern countries, especially in the Dutch school. The Netherlands, the seven provinces centered on the economically dominant province of Holland (including Amsterdam), enjoyed a period of great prosperity in the early seventeenth century. One of the effects of prosperity was to gain independence from Spain. The purchasers of paintings were from the great Dutch urban merchant class, and a considerable percentage of the artisan class as well. Paintings on religious, historical, and mythological subjects abounded, as did landscapes and portraits.

Rembrandt van Rijn worked in Amsterdam, then a boomtown of sorts for a thriving continental and maritime trade. His *Tobit and Anna* (1626) in the Amsterdam Rijksmuseum depicts a kind of homey realism consistent with the middle-class prosperity of Amsterdam. In a middle-class interior, complete with wooden shelves, basket, and hanging garlic, the elderly, blind Tobit clasps his hands as he raises his face toward the window light. His decidedly elderly wife Anna leans toward him as he looks toward the window. According to the story, this represents either the miracle of having his sight restored or his vision of the restoration of Jerusalem. His son Tobias, under the guidance of Raphael, had cured his father's blindness. Since the story inculcates ideas of benevolence, chastity, and prayer, it was a great favorite for paintings in baroque drawing rooms. While the story is from the Old Testament, placed in the Apocrypha after Nehemiah in the Western canon, the setting is modeled on a typical middle-class milieu, a factor that would have been comfortingly familiar to the stable, prosperous merchants and artisans of Holland. Dutch interiors of this type abound, often with a biblical theme or with a general moralizing tone of civic and family stability. In such themes realistically represented elderly women often play a part to emphasize the strong values of hearth and home.

In the second half of the eighteenth century in England, Evangelicalism emerged, a reform movement within the Anglican church. Its best-known protagonists, Hannah More and William Wilberforce, appealed to the English middle and upper classes to reform personal morality, focusing on sin, guilt, and redemption. An internal support system was encouraged, already started by the Puritans, of keeping diaries and journals, with daily Bible readings and family prayer. In these beliefs women were thought to be especially important in providing a sound and stable domestic setting. Therefore, exemplary paintings of intergenerational family devotions became common in the second half of the eighteenth century in England. A painting by Samuel Dutler called *Family Prayers* (1864), in St. John's College, Cambridge, illustrates the spirit of family Evangelicalism. It shows all the women, including two elderly, white-haired family members in simple white bonnets and high-necked dresses, as they listen pensively to the devotionals read by a bald, middle-aged male seated at a table. Family stability and faithfulness to family duty are signaled by the very presence of the elderly women among the family seated in the quiet drawing room. Although it is not a large or richly furnished room, a sense of prosperity is suggested by a fancy clock and oil landscape paintings on the wall. Another message brought through these paintings undoubtedly is that hard work and sound morality bring a comfortable life.

Another of these same kinds of home gatherings of family worship, featuring the reassuring presence of elderly, well-cared-for women, is entitled *Presbyterian Catechizing*, by John Philipp. This eighteenth-century painting, in the National Gallery of Scotland in Edinburgh, is centered on an elderly man reading devotions from a text. Surrounding him in a middle-class interior with a grandfather clock and a large wooden cabinet are some two dozen family members of all ages, from infancy to some very stooped, wizened old women. Respect, care, and affection for elderly women are certainly clearly communicated in the many English eighteenth-century paintings of this type.

Although not specifically inspired by English Evangelicalism, many English late eighteenth- and nineteenth-century paintings strove to portray a generalized sense of a happy family gathering. These were commissioned as family portraits and tended to center on some remembered activity where all the family would have been present. These occasions included birthday celebrations, christenings, after-dinner concerts at the parlor piano, and the like. A family portrait of this type is the mid-nineteenth-century painting by William Powell Frith called *Many Happy Returns of the Day*, in which a child's birthday is celebrated while the family sits at the dining-room table.[13] An elderly man and woman in the scene are presumably the child's grandparents. The joys of home with an accompanying reasonable sense of longevity and economic well-being were earnestly wished-for ideals in late eighteenth-century and nineteenth-century England and America, and this allowed for a very honest representation of elderly members of the family.

In the early years of America's history, through the late eighteenth century, female life centered on private duties of the home. Through the few records, letters, embroideries, and portraits, we can evaluate women's life only a little beyond a kind of idealized model. We know through colonial newspapers that there were eighteenth-century female blacksmiths, tanners, shoemakers, gunsmiths, printers, teachers, and shopkeepers. Many of these were middle-aged widows who continued the business of their husbands. In embroidery and portraiture alike there is a theme of the steady wife who helps assume the responsibilities of her husband. An eighteenth-century needlework chairseat in the Winterthur Museum in Delaware shows a decidedly older woman walking with her husband in the pasture. The inscription says, "With half-pin' gown, unbuckled shoe, I haste to milk my lowing cow." Paired portraits with the husband were also common, and a representative example is one of the elderly, double-chinned Catherine and John Moffat of Portsmouth, around 1745. They are shown as "yokefellows," and her lace cap and book further connote a kind of family propriety.[14]

Many of the same artists who produced domestic subjects began to paint other aspects of the urban middle-class milieu, with a special fondness for the latest in omnibuses, railway stations, and street scenes. This was a wave of mid-nineteenth-century realism that produced paintings for large international exhibitions or "salons." The interior of a new form of urban transportation gave the English artist William Maw Egley the opportunity to paint a variety of social types in *Omnibus Life in London* (1859).[15] Here, men, women, and children are seated together in the small space of the omnibus coach. In the foreground is the distinctive and unforgettable profile of a well-dressed elderly woman who leans forward slightly to protect an elaborately wrapped hatbox and to cradle a collapsed, large, black umbrella between her knees. Since she does not appear to be with anyone, she serves as a reminder that there were indeed single working women who elected to live alone and often did so with a degree of comfort.

Solitude was the result of deliberate choice or a decision to favor career over family. Nurses, postal workers, and schoolteachers often chose to remain unmarried out of a desire for financial and personal independence. Widowhood would usually leave a woman in the care of close relatives. A French census in 1851 revealed that about a third of women over 50 were single, and of those some 12 percent had never married. The single older woman, whether widowed or never married, became a frequent subject in the never-ending search for interesting character studies in late nineteenth- and early twentieth-century academic paintings, produced for the salons, or official state exhibitions.

Several very strong paintings of elderly women illustrate this trend. One is by Henri-Georges Bréard and is entitled *The Newspaper* (1914). Three elderly women sit together in a simple, spare room as one of them reads aloud from a newspaper. In an English painting by Richard Miller, *Spinsters* (1904), two elderly women enjoy a cup of tea together in a comfortable small salon.

Probably the painting that first comes to mind when one thinks of representations of elderly women is the famous *Arrangement in Grey and Black No. 1: The Artist's Mother* (1872), by James Abbott McNeill Whistler. The strange title indicates Whistler's ideas of looking at a painting mainly in terms of simplified shapes and monochromatic color schemes. Nonetheless, for all his interest in the abstractions of carefully modulated pure forms, this portrait is wonderfully expressive of character. It is probably the most serene representation of widowhood by an American artist.

In effect, the tone set by Whistler's portrait of his mother is one continued by many twentieth-century artists of all nationalities, who have expressed their love and respect for their mothers through dignified paintings, sculptures, photographs, and films that captured their real appearance as elderly women. Although the styles may vary and include any number of stylizations and abstractions, the portraits of artists' mothers are by and large much more moving, tender, and observant of the individual than any other subject in their work. Indeed, this is a theme that comes closest to consistency in modern art. Although a disrespect for women is also a subtheme in modern art, these are almost always younger women, and indeed disrespect often goes into misogyny as women are represented as monsters and sexual beasts. This subtheme of misogyny in modern art is another subject, however, and since it scarcely touches on our topic of elderly women, it will not be addressed here, except to note that in general, there is a remarkably more positive attitude toward aged women.

As is clear from this survey, art only reflects the ideas of the time and place where it is created. Perhaps surprisingly, the most negative view of elderly women was seen in the images of ancient Greece. Through early school days, Americans have a rather rosy view of Greece as the cradle of democracy. However, it seems that with respect to its older women, life left much to be desired. As we have observed, as the position of older women improves in society, so does their image as it is represented in art. Art is, after all, just another component of the evidence of how we think and feel as a people.

NOTES

1. The Dolní Vestonice data are from B. Klíma, *Dolní Vestonica* (Prague: 1963). The head, only two inches in length, is now in the National Museum of Bratislava, Slovakia.

2. The Venus of Willendorf's head is a small nub with a series of braidlike designs covering the surface. The figure is only some four inches in length and is in the Naturhistorisches Museum in Vienna.

3. Athenian red-figure pyxis, ca. 460 B.C., Louvre Museum, Paris.

4. Red-figure skyphos by the Pistoxenos Painter, ca. 470 B.C., from Cervetri, in the Schwerin Museum.

5. Clay group dressed as an old woman and old man, ca. fourth century B.C., Martin con Wagner Museum, Würzburg.

6. Hellenistic sculpture (ca. 2nd century B.C.) of an old woman carrying a market basket.

7. In Sparta, the chief decisions were taken by a body called the Gerousia, a council of *gerontes* (old men). Athens was apparently less generous in its allotment of political power to the elderly, having specifically done so only in the winter of 413 B.C., immediately after a disastrous expedition to Sicily. See Garland (1990).

8. This timely observation by the rhetorician Thrasymachos of Chalkedon is recorded in H. Diels, *Die Fragmente der Vorsokratiker*, 5th ed., 2 vols. (Berlin: 1935), vol. 11, p. 85.

9. Hildegard of Bingen, *Scivias*, 2nd half of the 12th century, Formerly in the Hessische Landesbibliothek, Wiesbaden. Destroyed in World War II.

10. Fray Juan de la Miseria, *Sta. Teresa of Ávila* (1576), Carmelite Convent, Seville, Spain.

11. Francesco della Cossa, *Crucifixion with Mary and John* (ca. 1470–75); and Matthias Grünewald, *The Small Crucifixion* (ca. 1520), the National Gallery, Washington, D.C.

12. Bernardo Martorell, *Christ and the Woman from Canaan*, predella panel in the *Transfiguration* altarpiece (ca. 1445–48), Barcelona.

13. William Powell Frith, *Many Happy Returns of the Day*, mid-nineteenth century, Harrogate Art Gallery, England.

14. Catherine and John Moffat's portraits (ca. 1745) are in the Currier Gallery, Portsmouth, New Hampshire.

15. William Maw Egley, *Omnibus Life in London* (1859), in the Tate Gallery, London.

REFERENCES

Garland, R. *The Greek way of life*. (Ithaca: 1990).
Perrot, Michelle. (Ed.) *A history of private life* (Vol. 4). London: 1990.

Five

Sagacious, Sinful, or Superfluous? The Social Construction of Older Women

ELIZABETH W. MARKSON

There is an old Arab saying that when each child is born, it is surrounded by one hundred angels. For every year a male lives, an angel is added; for every year a female lives, an angel dies. Even today in contemporary American society, sexism and ageism form a deadly duo for many older women. Consider, for example, the many mother-in-law jokes but the paucity of father-in-law jokes, fairy tales with wicked old women but few evil old men, Halloween portrayals of old witches but no elderly warlocks, and the numerous cosmetics promising restoration to a "more youthful" appearance for women with "mature" skin. Although the seasoning, power, and wealth associated with aging may be aphrodisiac qualities for males, current ideals of female beauty require youthful, unwrinkled faces and lithe figures of adolescence or early adulthood. Physical youth is more central to a woman's social identity, social regard, and self-esteem than to a man's. It is true that today's older women suffer from an incurable malady: angel deficiency disease?[1] If so, how did this view of the older woman come about?

Although aging is a biological event that begins at birth and ends at death, it is the social construction of the older woman that is of concern here. Today, in Western industrialized society, age is associated with a particular number plus specific behaviors and social roles. The significance of age as a number is relatively new; in northern Europe, for example, it was not until the mid-sixteenth century that numerical age had any social significance. Indeed, few people knew how old they were (Cole, 1992). In other societies where life expectancy at birth is short and physical conditions are hard, a person may be defined as an "elder" in what we consider midlife: age 40 or 45. At any point in the lifespan, age simultaneously denotes not only a number and an assortment of physiological states but a set of social constructs, defined by the norms specific to a given society at a particular point in history.

HISTORICAL VIEWS OF THE OLDER WOMAN

"Western dualistic thought has characteristically bifurcated women as either sexual or spiritual . . . perceptions applied to aging women, as well. . . . aging women [are personified] as both 'fair' and 'foul', as figures of wisdom, of desire, or of danger," commented historian Lois Banner (1992, p. 60) in her analysis of older women through the centuries. In the past females were believed to possess magical properties, as menstruation and the lengthy human gestation period for human birth were poorly understood until the nineteenth century. These uniquely female processes were regarded as signs of fearsome supernatural powers. Magic, prophecy, healing, fertility, birth, and death were the provinces of women. For many societies, the archetype of the female has also been "Mother Death": life given by the great mother also brings seeds of death. In India Kali was the Hindu tripartite goddess of creation, preservation, and destruction. In Norse mythology Freya was goddess of both love and death—a common association in many religions. Females were often feared, as the Chinese description of female genitalia as "gateways to immortality" and "executioners of men" clearly says. Similarly, in traditional Maori religion with a belief in a literal, born-again reincarnation, the vagina was viewed as a "house for the dead"—a place where ghosts seeking a rebirth lurk (Walker, 1988).

In many societies it was particularly the older woman who was viewed as having mystical qualities. For example, according to Scottish mythology, powerful old crones, such as Black Annis and the Cailleach Bheur, who were believed to live in remote rural areas, were personifications of winter who, with the coming of spring, were transformed into young females. In ancient Greece priestesses were selected from among postmenopausal women, and only women over 60 could serve as paid ritual mourners at funerals (Banner, 1992). The word "hag," from the Greek "hagia," meaning holy one, was once a compliment, stressing the old woman's magical qualities (Walker, 1988). By the Middle Ages hag was a pejorative term for witch. How did this transformation come about? The answer lies both in forms of social organization and in their cultural definitions of older women.

In the nineteenth century Friedrich Engels, examining the evolution of gender stratification and the family, proposed that early families began as a form of "primitive communism," in which gender equality predominated. Sexual egalitarianism characteristic of primitive communism changed as forms of economic organization transformed: first into matriarchy, then, with the institution of private property, into patriarchy and its resulting subjugation of women (Engels, 1884/1972). Although subsequent anthropologists, historians, and other scholars have attempted to identify purely matriarchal societies throughout the ages, evidence for matriarchy now or in the past remains slim. Purely patriarchal societies have abounded, but available data suggest instead that matrilineal descent and matrilocal residence, existing both in past and some present societies, have been erroneously designated as indications of matriarchal power. Nor is there either evidence of a "golden age" in which elders were revered because of their age or a simple relationship between preindustrial societies and a particular image of aging.[2] The position of elders—and of females of all ages—would appear to depend rather on their ability to control, exchange, and retain goods and resources, including food, weapons, money, property, or knowledge.

ANCIENT VIEWS OF THE OLDER WOMAN

Both ancient Greece and Rome were highly stratified along social class and gender lines as patrilineal, patrilocal, and patriarchal societies. Both societies also recognized distinct periods of the life course. Yet whether young or old, females were technically under the control of father, husband, or son throughout their lives.

In Greece distinct terminology was used to designate four stages of life for both genders. Males and females alike initially were classed as *pais* or child, and old age broadly as *geras*. After puberty, however, terminology clearly distinguished gender differences in life stages. Culturally defined as governed by mental irrationality and destabilizing sex drives, females were defined primarily in sexual and reproductive terms. For example, a young, sexually mature woman was a *kore* or, if still a virgin, a *parthenos*; the mature wife-woman *gyne*; and the elderly woman *graia*. In contrast, the mature man was at *akme*, or the prime of life, and the elderly man *geron* or *presbys*. Women entered old age with the onset of menopause, as their value for sexual or reproductive purposes had ended. For men the transition into old age was more social and generational than physical, occurring usually around age 60 when a son married at the age of 30 (most often to a female half his age), and the father relinquished control of the family household (Falkner & de Luce, 1992).

Although a woman became "old" much earlier than a man, old age for either gender was abhorrent. Greek society was obsessed with youth and beauty—a fixation not unlike our own today—and regarded the elderly as dried up and ugly. Despite the repugnance for old age, many elite men lived long and productive lives. Euripides died at age 79, having just completed the *Bacchae*, and Socrates at age 70. According to most accounts, aging women had a more difficult time. Not surprisingly, given the cultural emphasis on females as sex objects, older women were often represented as deviating from the feminine and domestic virtues. In comedy aging females were portrayed as feisty, argumentative, sexually aggressive, and alcoholic; even when they were heroines in tragedy, as in the plays of Euripides, they were depicted as capable of enormous hatred and vengeance (Falkner & de Luce, 1992).

Life may have been easier, however, for older women than for younger ones. Having lost their value as "feminine," the older women were no longer subject to tight male control. Athenian widows, unlike their younger counterparts, could travel through the city as midwives, participate in religious festivals, and, as mentioned earlier, act as professional mourners (Bremmer, 1987). In Athens fourteen aging women were the priestesses of Dionysus, and the woman chosen as the priestess at Delphi, the Greeks' major oracular site, had to be postmenopausal. To honor older women's contributions to society by giving birth, Athenian sons were required by law to support their mothers in old age (Banner, 1992). Central to the position of older women in Athenian culture, some analysts have suggested, was constant male apprehension about the force of the woman as mother, her parthenogenic potency, and rampant sexuality (DuBois, 1988).

Among the Romans, too, females of all ages were defined by their sexuality and role in the family. Menstruation usually began at age 14, but a female could legally marry at age 12; a male could marry at age 14 and become head of his own family if the *pater familias*—his father or the eldest living male from whom descent was traced—was not alive. The *pater familias* held great power over all family members, including the right of life and death over his children; under Roman law, only he was recognized as able to act in a legal capacity. Older Roman males enjoyed greater respect than did their Greek counterparts. "Youth ought to obey and old age rule," said Plutarch, attempting to settle the question of whether old men should withdraw from public life (Falkner & de Luce, 1992). Nevertheless, Rome was not a gerontocracy as such but rather had a well-defined system of seniority. For example, at age 42, a male could enter the consulship, at 50 be exempt from military service, and at 60 be excused from being a senator (Falkner & de Luce, 1992).

Whether young or old, females were expected to live under perpetual guardianship (*perpetua tutela*) with a male controlling goods and resources. For a woman, both old age and "retirement" were linked to reproductive function and came with menopause (believed to occur between the ages of 40 and 50). The impact of becoming an "older woman" varied; if her value lay primarily in being a mother, a woman was less protected because she was no longer fertile. Conversely, menopause might bring her greater freedom because she could no longer bear children; limiting sexual access to her was no longer necessary. A mother might play a decisive role in arranging or ending her children's marriages, in providing advice, and in other family relationships. In later life the most impressive old women were described within the context of familial relationships, but they were also viewed by some as repulsive, especially if they had both money and power (Falkner & de Luce, 1992). As in other societies, the witch, a popular figure in Roman literature, was both old and female. For example, Horace focused on an older woman as a witch who, without legitimate power or influence, relied on magic to attain her ends (Falkner & de Luce, 1992). Ovid's *Amores* depicted an older woman, Dipsas, as both a drunkard and a witch whose alleged powers included reversing the flow of water, changing the weather, and transforming herself into a bird at night (Banner, 1992).

Paradoxically, there were also old wise women. For example, the Sibyls, ten old women believed to live throughout the Mediterranean, were prophets whose presumed predictions were collected in the Sibylline Books, eventually Rome's most sacred text. Roman portraits of the older woman—alternately depicted as wise, drunken, sexually insatiable, and demonic—highlight the fear that older women, freed from menstruation and the dangers and responsibilities of childbearing, would use their wisdom to control both men and other women (Banner, 1992).

In Judeo-Christian tradition females of all ages have been even more suspect. According to Genesis, Eve was, through her temptation of Adam, the bringer of death to humanity. Not only was the female responsible for original sin, but she exemplified salaciousness, insatiability, and enticement. Although in the Gnostic gospels Sophia was the mother of the god creator and, with God the Father and Son, formed a trinity different from the official Christian trinity (Father, Son, and Holy Ghost), these alternate accounts of the life of Christ and Christian doctrine were excluded from the Bible approved by councils of bishops during the fourth century A.D. (Pagels, 1979). The dominant view of women according to the early Christian church was summarized by Tertullian in the third century as "the devil's gateway . . . the first deserter of the divine law" (Tertullian, De cultu feminarum [On female dress], quoted in J. Smith, 1992, p. 76). The author of Ecclesiasticus affirmed this perspective: "All wickedness is but little to the wickedness of a woman" (Ecclesiasticus 25:19, quoted in J. Smith, 1992). Another theologian, the ninth-century monk Odo of Cluny, declared, "To embrace a woman is to embrace a sack of manure" (quoted in J. Smith, 1992, p. 76). To the thirteenth-century Christian theologian St. Thomas Aquinas, a mother's body was mere soil in which the father planted a seed. Female children were defective males, conceived only because the father was weak, sick, or in a state of sin (J. Smith, 1992).

Female value resided only in fertility and motherhood. Once past childbearing age, a woman ceased to represent fecundity. Her sexual attractiveness was nil. In medieval and Renaissance literature the postmenopausal woman was sometimes heavily sexualized, but most often, like Chaucer's Wife of Bath or the nurse in Romeo and Juliet, she was confined to the role of go-between in the mating game, either as romantic intermediary or sexual procurer, and was dangerous to social harmony in either role (Banner, 1992). Her redeeming worth was skill in caring for others in birth, illness, and death. Most villages had many older "medwyfs" [sic]—literally, "wise women"—who eased pain in childbirth and illness. Prelates of the church viewed these women with a jaundiced eye as possessors of forbidden knowledge that went against the will of God as punishment for Eve's sin: secrets of abortion, contraception, and alleviation of suffering in birth. By the fourteenth century the church declared war on female healers. Although no university admitted females to study medicine, any woman who cured sickness without studying medicine at a university—from which all women were barred—was a witch, a restriction not applied to men (Ehrenreich & English, 1982). Although both good and bad witches have a long and distinguished history in myth, the designation of the witch as a servant of satanic power dominated. As Banner (1992) observed: "From definitions of aging women as sexualized creatures and as go-betweens dangerous to social harmony, it was only one step to accusing them of being witches, individuals who bound themselves diabolically to the devil through an infernal sexual pact" (p. 189).

Although the Inquisition began as an effort to consolidate the power of the church by stamping out heresies such as the Catharan dissenters in southern France, its leaders soon sought other victims. Aging women were prime candidates for the inquisitors. According to the major witchcraft manual, *Malleus Maleficarum*, females were not only "of a different nature from men . . . [and] more carnal than a man" (Kramer & Sprenger, 1971, pp. 116–117), but as witches were known to "collect male organs in great numbers, as many as twenty or thirty members together, and put them in a bird's nest" (Kramer & Sprenger, 1971, p. 268). Their unbridled sexuality and unattractiveness led them to consort with the devil. Belief in their latent uncontrollable sexuality meant that suspicion of witchcraft "fell on every old woman with a wrinkled face" (Fraser, 1984, p. 113). Available data show that the median age of suspected witches was between 55 and 65 (Banner, 1992)—hardly young or even middle aged in an era when the average life expectancy at birth was around 30.

Menopause was closely linked to witchcraft. Because the link between menstruation and production of an ovum was not understood until the mid-nineteenth century, most physicians believed that menstruation was a purging of evil humors that might otherwise encourage doubly shameful conduct by the weaker, less rational sex. According to one seventeenth-century doctor: "When seed and menstrual blood are retained in women besides [beyond] the intent of nature, they putrefie [*sic*] and are corrupted, and attain a malignant and venomous quality" (Crawford, "Menstruation in seventeenth-century England," p. 55, quoted in Banner, 1992, p. 192).

Scapegoating older women as witches not only reflected the growing misogyny of the sixteenth and seventeenth centuries—when official witch hunting throughout Europe was at its height—but provided a way to eliminate the poor who were too old or too feeble to work. Older women as targets were financially profitable as well. Well-off widows' property was impounded before trial. Loss of property could also occur after death, for witches could also be tried posthumously—and their property confiscated—up to three generations afterwards. As many as two million women, primarily older, widowed, feeble, or poor, were executed in Europe. In seventeenth-century Puritan Massachusetts, those most likely to be killed for witchcraft were older women, usually single, widowed, or poor, who had a reputation for annoying their neighbors (Demos, 1982).

Scholars paid little attention to older women for many centuries except for their depraved sexuality and potential for evil. Given their alleged inferiority and their lesser likelihood of reaching old age due to higher adult mortality rates associated with childbirth, it is hardly surprising that little study centered on older women (Laslett, 1977). Until the seventeenth century, whenever scholars, writers, artists, or others wrote or depicted the ages of life, women were either subsumed under the heading of "man" or ignored. During the seventeenth century, with the advent of a market society and the dwindling of feudalism, the concept of ages and stages of life emerged in both literature and art (Cole, 1992). Although women had been shrouded by medieval Christian beliefs that the female body was the devil's hopyard, by the seventeenth century "Neoplatonic views of the body as a pathway to divine love legitimated the notion that a beautiful body reflected a beautiful soul. . . . beauty became a kind of vocation or sacred duty for women" (Cole, 1992, p. 26). This new regard for women's lives concentrated on their daily lives and duties to preserve a decorous family, a task for which aging women paid a high price, as they were frequently depicted as ugly and physically disabled.

Among the Puritans, too, belief in females as deficient beings remained. Spotlighting the patriarchal social organization characteristic of Puritan culture was the belief that a woman's relationship to God must always be negotiated through her husband, who was God's representative to her (Cole, 1992). Although historians such as Fischer (1977) have argued that a firmly established (and male) gerontocracy existed in colonial America, other historians (Demos, 1978; D. S. Smith, 1978) have noted that any high status enjoyed by the elderly resulted from their control of resources. Economic power outweighed chronological age (Haber, 1983) and even gender (Cole, 1992). However, impoverished older women—and men—dependent upon the good will of their relatives and the community, did not enjoy high status (Haber & Gratton, 1993).

NINETEENTH-CENTURY VIEWS OF THE OLDER WOMAN

During the nineteenth century, according to Cole (1992), a distinct antipathy toward old age arose with the development of middle-class culture: "Victorian moralists split the last stage of life into two apparently separate, controllable parts: the 'good' old age of virtue, health, self reliance, natural death, and salvation; and the 'bad' old age of sin, disease, dependency, premature death, and damnation . . . [setting up] a historical dynamic in which popular perceptions would swing from one pole to the other" (Cole, 1992, pp. 161–162). By 1851, according to one female commentator, being anything but young was unfashionable and un-American (Kirkland, 1851, "Growing old gracefully," cited in Cole, 1992, p. 148). Victorian morality also redefined the older woman as a maternal figure. The aging woman as go-between began to disappear in both literature and reality, and women became the architects of family life, or, if unmarried or widowed, asexual eccentrics. The stereotype of the "single woman"—an ugly, scowling woman who waited on others—emerged: "Unmarried aging women bore the brunt of what was, in effect, a reallocated misogyny" (Banner, 1992, p. 252).

Also, in the nineteenth century, with the development of science and scientific medicine, physicians became increasingly interested both in old age and the female reproductive system as pathological processes. Physicians introduced the idea of *climacteric illness*, characterized by deterioration of mental and physical vigor presaging death and an onset in women between the ages of 45 and 55 and among men aged 50–75 (Haber, 1983). Some physicians believed that menopause was part of climacteric illness; others claimed that menopause was merely a harbinger of the disease. In either case, most acknowledged that the disease was less severe among women, for their periodicity cushioned their decline into old age (Haber, 1983). As Oliver Wendell Holmes, noting the rigid gender-based division of labor, commented: "Women find it easier than men to grow old in a becoming way. . . . With old men it is different. . . . They have no pretty little manual occupations. The old man . . . does not know what to do with his fingers" (Holmes, 1891, pp. 292–293, cited in Cole, 1992, p. 150).

At the same time, an opposing theme in medicine stressed the instability of the menopausal female, echoing the age-old dual beliefs about the female aging experience. Upper- and middle-class women of all ages, who were expected to be idle and weak, got little exercise, and were constrained by corsets, were a ready market for physicians, many of whom believed that there was a direct connection between the uterus and the brain.[3] Not only did doctors perform hysterectomies in an attempt to cure "hysteria," but they also held that aging women were adversely influenced by menopause. As early as 1865, "involutional melancholia" and "climacteric insanity" were terms used to describe postmenopausal women (Banner, 1992). By 1896 psychiatrist Emile Kraepelin catalogued "involutional melancholia" as a disorder that "sets in principally, or perhaps exclusively, at the beginning of old age in men and in women from the period of menopause onwards. . . . About one third of women make a complete recovery" (Kraepelin, 1896; cited in Greer, 1991, p. 79). Kraepelin observed, however, that emotional dullness was likely to remain, judgment and memory were likely to deteriorate, and the course of the disease was tedious. The medicalization of menopause was profitable to the emerging field of gynecology, and special diagnostic categories, including "old maid's insanity," were used to describe menopause.

A countervailing force to the vilification of the postmenopausal woman stemmed from the women's movement of the late nineteenth and early twentieth centuries. Feminists such as Susan B. Anthony, Elizabeth Cady Stanton, and Frances Willard were active until well into their 60s. Moreover, medical views began to change as doctors discovered that menstruation was not a purging of "toxic humors" but was connected to production of an ovum. Inasmuch as postmenopausal women did not menstruate and presumably did not lose vital energy through a monthly flow, some medical observers believed that women were increasing their vitality. As Elizabeth Cady Stanton described it, her "vital forces," formerly centered in her reproductive organs, were "flowing" to her brain (Banner, 1992, p. 282). Nonetheless, by the end of the nineteenth century, chronological age began to be defined by social reformers and physicians alike as a social problem, directly linked to poverty and ill health: "At around 50, his [the worker's] abilities began to falter.... His strength and flexibility—as well as his salary—all declined with age'' (Haber, 1983, pp. 43–44). The connection between dependent old age and almshouse residency was clear: "Generations grew up with 'a reverence for God, the hope of heaven, and the fear of the poorhouse' " (Haber & Gratton, 1993, p. 122).

TWENTIETH-CENTURY VIEWS ON OLDER WOMEN

At the outset of the twentieth century, the positive view of older women expressed by Stanton was not supported by the cult of youth popular in the United States. Physician William Osler commented on the comparative uselessness of men (but did not mention women) over the age of 40. The worthlessness of the old was repeated by another physician, I. L. Nascher (who coined the term "geriatrics"): "We realize that for all practical purposes the lives of the aged are useless, that they are often a burden to themselves, their family, and the community at large'' (I. L. Nascher, *Geriatrics*, 1909, cited in Cole, 1992, p. 202). Nascher also expounded on personality changes with aging, saying that gender differences disappear in later life. Such inherent male personality traits as nobility, virility, and bravery and female characteristics such as nurturance, domesticity, and passivity blended into one homogeneous genderless personality: an old person (Haber, 1983). Paralleling the increased medicalization of old age was the expansion of American business and advertising from the 1890s on. Health, cosmetic, and pharmaceutical industries, emphasizing youth, health, and slimness, developed products—from corn flakes to tonics to face creams—to ensure youthful appearances. Not surprisingly, women were especially targeted as consumers.

The Persistence of "Female Equals Psychopathology" (and Old Age Makes It Worse)

The developing field of psychoanalysis also labeled females of all ages as distinctly flawed and menopause as a significant event, defining women as "aging," most often in unflattering terms. Freud's model of feminine identity echoed the views of Judeo-Christian theologians: women have weaker superegos than men and a corrupt sense of social justice because of penis envy (Freud, 1961b). Freud also had scant interest in older people of either gender and made it clear in the early days of psychoanalysis that, due to the amount of material to be covered and increasing inflexibility of the personality associated with aging, analysis was inappropriate for those aged 50 or older. For Freud, women as young as 30 were unfit analysands because of their psychic rigidity and unchangeableness; men at the same age remained youthful and pliable (Freud, 1961a).

Menopause remained inextricably tied to later-life psychopathology. The old belief that postmenopausal women were likely to be troubled by a strong sexual drive and sexual aggressiveness was repeated at the outset of the twentieth century by sexologist Havelock Ellis, who remarked on "old maid's insanity," a condition to which older unmarried women, career women, and lesbians were especially inclined (Ellis, 1905/1942). Freud, too, noted that menopause increased sexual desire in women and return of adolescent issues and the Oedipus complex. As late as the 1940s, psychoanalyst Helene Deutsch (1945), herself 60, viewed menopause as a woman's partial death. A listing of the hazards confronted by menopausal women includes reappearance of Oedipal feelings, "sublimated homosexuality of puberty," "rape" and "prostitution" fantasies, and sexual acting out. Deutsch narrated a case of a grandmother arrested in the park for soliciting men and another of a menopausal 50-year-old woman who fantasized about a female friend who "tenderly initiated adolescent boys into the mysteries of sensual love" (p. 468).

Aging women have been of little interest to subsequent psychoanalysts. As Tallmer noted in 1989: "The common expression, the 'empty nest' syndrome, reflects the current psychoanalytic emphasis on the association between aging and loss. Psychological changes in late adulthood are generally explained as reactions to loss, and, ultimately, to the most basic fear of death" (p. 231). Given how much psychopathology was attributed to women at midlife and in old age, it is not surprising that theories of normal adult development have most often relied upon a male model.

While Erikson (1968) proposed progressive epigenetic stages leading one to become a more complex, integrated self with age, his observations, discussions, and examples were based largely on upper-middle-class men, as were those of Levinson (1977). For Erikson, as for Freud, biology was destiny and determined personality. To the extent that they received attention, females, due to their inner space (i.e., the uterus waiting to be filled), were quiet, protective, and equipped with psychological abilities to care for others. The male was the criterion for adult development. Moreover, the last stage of personality development—ego integrity versus despair—covers at least one-third of one's life—a very long time to remain static in one life stage.

Challenges to Views of Female Experiences through the Life Course

Feminist psychologists have challenged the assumptions made by the Freudians about the nature of female experience. As Karen Horney (1967) remarked: "Like all sciences and all valuations, the psychology of women has hitherto been considered only from the point of view of men. . . . The psychology of women . . . actually represents a deposit of the desires and disappointments of men" (p. 56). Although they pay little attention to midlife and old age, Jean Baker Miller (1986) and other recent feminist theorists have proposed that women's desire for affiliation is key throughout their lives. While Erikson's model of adult development assumes that identity precedes intimacy and generativity, for women these two stages are fused. Females know themselves through their relationships with others, but because valued behavior is built on male models, affiliative feminine activity is largely unrecognized and perceived as passivity. Cooperation, giving, and participation in the development of others are not in direct, open pursuit of masculine goals. Females, although tacitly labeled as inferior beings, are more able to use their feelings of vulnerability and dependency to create a sense of internal worth. It is not penis envy that is the key to the feminine psyche but fear of the ability to be "like a man"—strong, self-sufficient, and competent—that creates problems for her.

Recent contributions to role theory complement formulations of adult developmental psychology and differentiate male versus female patterns of behavior in later life. In their work on disengagement based on the Kansas City Studies of Adult Life, Cumming and Henry (1961) gave a structural-functionalist interpretation to gender differences in aging described by Oliver Wendell Holmes. They proposed that women's passage through the life course is smoother than that of men, for their roles retain an essential sameness from girlhood to death—that of homemaker, kinkeeper, and nurturer. Aging men, in contrast, confront critical changes. When their instrumental roles as breadwinners are lost through retirement, males lack the sources of reward upon which they have relied most of their adult lives.

More recent analyses of subsequent cohorts and gender roles have emphasized discontinuity rather than sameness as characteristic of women's lives. Required to adjust to many role shifts—entry into the labor force, childbearing and child care, changes in husband's job, empty nest, career reentry, widowhood, and so on—a woman is more likely than a man to be flexible and to be able to cope with life changes (Kline, 1975; Lopata, 1971). She is also more likely to have same-gender friends upon whom she can depend for social support. Harking back to Nascher's view that gender-related personality characteristics change with the aging process, Gutmann proposed a different twist. His work has shown that personality apparently changes in both men and women as they age; women become more aggressive while men become more nurturant and affiliative—a transformation that seems to hold true cross-culturally (Gutmann, 1987).

Why do negative stereotypes about middle and old age in women's lives persist despite contrary empirical evidence? Neither menopause, the empty nest, nor old age in themselves correlate to decrease in well-being or to depression, although these events may be exacerbated by other negative life experiences such as poverty or poor health. The answer seems to lie in the still-persistent belief that a woman's essence lies in her youthfulness—itself a symbol of her potential to procreate. Yet, at least theoretically, once women are free of child-care responsibilities, they are able to be stimulated by changes, to focus on their own presents and futures, and to design their own lives.

The Persistence of Ambivalence

With the reduction of adult mortality associated with childbearing, clearly there are more older women than older men. American women 65 or over now outnumber their male age peers 3:2—a dramatic increase from thirty years ago, when the ratio was 6:5. Old age is a territory pioneered and inhabited by women for longer periods, and, given present patterns of life expectancy, women will comprise most U.S. elders in the future. Yet few gerontologists or others paid attention to gender in old age until relatively recently. Both men and women were lumped together as "elderly"—implying that gender becomes irrelevant in old age—and male models of aging were defined as "normal aging." Although women undergo more exams, lab tests, and blood-pressure checks than men, they receive fewer major diagnostic or therapeutic interventions, even for gender-sensitive testing such as breast exams, Pap tests, and mammograms (Clancy & Franks, 1993). Most medical and pharmaceutical research continues to be based on males, their problems, and their issues, with little attention to women's unique problems (Culpepper, 1993).

The women's movement, too, has largely ignored older women, reflecting the ambivalence that many founders felt to old age in general and their own mothers in particular. As one older woman activist commented: "From the beginning of this wave of the women's movement . . . the message has gone out to those of us over sixty that your sisterhood does not include us. . . . You do not see us in our present lives, you do not identify with our issues, you exploit us, you patronize us, you stereotype us. Mainly you ignore us" (Macdonald, 1989, p. 6). Yet, as Reinharz (1986) noted, there are unrecognized links between feminist and gerontological theories. Just as feminists reject models of gender-based division of labor as the right and proper distribution of tasks, elder advocates rebel against models of old age emphasizing withdrawal from socially useful roles.

Older Women in the Media: The Example of Film

Throughout the twentieth century, the mass media have wielded a powerful influence on how women of all ages are perceived and how they perceive themselves. It is no accident that feminist critics have observed that women are likely to be portrayed in the media through male eyes. As Annette Kuhn remarked in her book *Women's Pictures*: "One of the major theoretical contributions of the woman's movement has been its insistence on the significance of cultural factors, in particular in the form of socially dominant representations of women and the ideological character of such representation, both in constituting the category 'woman' and in delimiting and defining what has been called the 'sex-gender system' " (Kuhn, 1982, p. 4).

During the past twenty years a dearth of roles for women in American film has been noted. According to a report by the Screen Actors Guild, women of all ages comprised only about 29 percent of roles in feature films in 1989. As

Cohen observed: "Men in film have retreated to their own clubhouse for a while, treating women with passive exclusion or active denigration" (Cohen, 1991, p. 39). Older actresses in American film have most often portrayed stereotypical viragos, sacrificing or evil mothers, "poor old things," or minor characters. At first glance, however, the films of the 1980s appeared to feature older women, for three of the ten Academy Award winners for Best Actress were aged 60 or older. Had the "graying of America," with the rapid growth of the older population, increased opportunities for older women in film—a change from the usual practice of relegating older actresses to cameo or walk-on parts? Had the emerging new psychology of women influenced cinematic depictions mirroring gender stereotypes about older women in particular? An analysis of 1,169 Academy Award nominees for Best Actor, Best Actress, Best Supporting Actress, and Best Supporting Actor from 1927 (the first year in which the Academy Awards were given) through 1990 would say no (Markson & Taylor, 1993).[4]

In April 1968 at the age of 60 when she won her second Oscar for Best Actress, Katharine Hepburn cabled Screen Actors Guild president Gregory Peck, saying, "They don't usually give these things to the old girls, you know." She may not have known how accurate she was, for Hepburn and Marie Dressler, who won in 1930–31 at the age of 62, were the only two women 60 or over to win as Best Actress in the then 40-year Academy history. Hepburn later won two more Oscars as Best Actress, accounting for half the awards made to women over the age of 60. Except Hepburn, older women nominees for Best Actress have been rare. Among nominees for the category of Best Actor or Best Actress, women, with an average age of 37 over a 63-year period, have been consistently younger than men, whose average age was 43 ($p = .0001$). Gender differences between males and females have been remarkably consistent through the decades, excepting the 1980s when three actresses—Katharine Hepburn, Jessica Tandy, and Geraldine Page—inflated the total. Even given the Hepburn-Page-Tandy effect, no significant decade trend can be found. Moreover, in an analysis spanning the Academy Awards for 63 years, only one in five of all female nominees for Best Actress was over the age of 39, compared with more than half of all men. Among those winning an Oscar, females over the age of 39 accounted for only 27% of all winners for Best Actress, whereas men in the same age range comprised 67%. It was not until the 1980s that the average age of actresses winning the award increased to almost age 45, alas not due to an increasing appreciation of the graying of America but to the Hepburn-Page-Tandy effect in three films (*On Golden Pond, Trip to Bountiful*, and *Driving Miss Daisy*).

Plus ça change, plus que c'est le même chose? In the first three years of the 1930s, three older women (Marie Dressler twice, May Robson once) were nominated for Best Actress, the difference being that the three older women nominated in the 1980s won. In the 1980s, similar to preceding decades, half the female winners were under age 38, compared with half the men, who were aged 45 or older. Even given the Hepburn-Page-Tandy effect, youth remained a powerful criterion for winning an award for women, while middle age was an equally powerful criterion for award-winning men. Once past the age of 59, however, nominations and winners dropped for both genders. The types of roles portrayed by male and female nominees for Best Actress/Actor aged 60 or over, however, varied sharply. Males nominated—but not winning—as Best Actor depicted roles as family doctor, lawyer, judge, newspaper magnate, successful mystery writer, TV reporter, Jewish Nazi hunter, con man, and jazz musician; male Oscar winners portrayed a statesman (Disraeli), U.S. marshal, TV reporter, and pool hustler. Only two men, one of whom was a former professor, were retired. In contrast, roles played by female nominees included a shopkeeper, nanny, pianist, owner of an art gallery, and twelfth-century queen; none focused primarily on their professional identities. The three roles by award-winning aging women during the 1980s were of housewives or retirees. Despite the growing proportion of midlife and older American women in the labor force, with a few notable exceptions, women's occupational involvement is invisible or minimized. Those few films in which women's careers have been salient, such as *Mildred Pierce* or *Autumn Sonata*, emphasize the negative impact of work pursuits upon family relationships. Although 15% of real-world women aged 60 and over are in the labor force, roles in which women have a career or are working are rare for actresses 60 and over.

Nor do women's relationships with one another receive much attention. Unlike men, who have entire film genres (westerns and gangster, war, and "buddy" pictures) dedicated to their relationships, even in the "women's movies" the spotlight has been almost exclusively on their relationships to men whether or not males are physically represented on the screen. Films of the 1960s and 1970s portrayed many mother-son relationships but almost no mother-daughter relationships. During the 1980s film depictions of mother-daughter relationships emphasized conflict and enmeshment, for, as Walters pointed out, "Except for the rare feminist exceptions . . . this thematic of antimonies (love/hate, bond/separate, enmeshment/autonomy) runs through almost all the cultural material on mothers and daughters in the 1980s" (Walters, 1992, p. 191). Yet, as Jean Baker Miller has pointed out, women's desire for affiliation is key to their sense of self; in American society, as in many others, females are groomed as the carriers of human communication.

In the real world women's friendships also provide a buffer throughout the life course, enabling them to cope with gender inequality, responsibilities of home and family, often dual demands of home and job, and transitions and events of later life. Only recently has Hollywood discovered portrayal of women's friendships as noteworthy to consider for Oscars with the 1991 Academy Award nominations of Geena Davis and Susan Sarandon for *Thelma and Louise* and Jessica Tandy for *Fried Green Tomatoes*. *Thelma and Louise* has often been described in the press as a "female buddy picture," underscoring the lack of a women's film genre comparable to the male "buddy picture." Both films are notable in that "older women"—Susan Sarandon at 45, Kathy

Bates at 42, and Jessica Tandy at 82—play key roles. *Fried Green Tomatoes* is doubly striking. Not only are women's affiliations with one another portrayed, but a frankly old woman (a mother figure) causes positive change in the life of a middle-aged daughter figure. Yet it is primarily through Tandy's life review rather than her current life that Bates changes. Should we infer that once a woman is explicitly old, life review is the most significant occupation left for her?

That so few women of any age are in featured roles in Hollywood films reflects the "revisionist" or backlash response to the women's movement. That *Thelma and Louise* has been widely criticized as a "male-bashing" film, although *Fatal Attraction* and a host of other films in which women are either evil or victimized have seldom been reproached as "female bashing," makes the point. Another factor contributing to the absence of women overall and older women in particular is the composition of screenwriters. A recent Writers Guild report showed that white men, predominantly under the age of 40, have written 80% of films shown in the last few years. This is a marked change, for as little as a decade or so ago, the highest wages were paid to writers in their 50s, but by 1987 the highest pay went to writers in their 30s. A "Hollywood gray list" of writers aged 40 and over severely limits opportunities for employment (Lehr, 1992). Young writers are sought to cater to the anticipated film audience; prevailing "wisdom" holds that the primary film audience is composed of 15–25-year-old males. Yet this young male audience comprises only about 8% of the total U.S. population and has a per capita discretionary income far less than that of men and women 60 and older, who constitute 17% of the population. Perhaps women of all ages are less likely to go to films when their choices may be between one of the numerous horror films or a sequel to *Terminator*. As Americans grow older and older with females predominating in older age groups, the decision makers and power brokers in Hollywood remain males, younger and younger each year.

FUTURE DIRECTIONS

Changing from one form of social organization to another is always painful, as the recent experience of Eastern Europe in its transition from communism to capitalism has shown. Caught in the midst of both backlashes against the women's movement of the 1960s and subsequent legislation expanding female options and against the civil and human rights movements, the social definition of female experience is shifting. Changes in the social construction of older women, and of females of all ages, clearly affect their lives. Many factors still define and circumscribe their options to be treated with dignity. Among older women, for example, six in ten of those aged 55 or older and in the labor force work in retail sales, administrative and clerical, and services—all areas with wages below the national average for all occupations (U.S. Department of Labor, 1989). In old age women of every marital status have lower money incomes than their male counterparts due to lower wages, inadequate pension coverage, economic dependency on men, and widowhood. The median income for all women 65 and over remains only 56% of that of old men. Old women comprise almost three-fourths of the elderly poor, and they are far more likely to receive Supplemental Security Income. Widowhood or divorce may still spell financial disaster. Most vulnerable to poverty are widows who are very old and members of minorities. Over half of elderly African-American and Latina women not living with family members have incomes below the poverty level; half of all women aged 75 or over who live alone subsist on incomes below 150% of the poverty level.[5] Unmarried, separated, widowed, or divorced older women are subjected to greater financial stress than older men, an exposure that overwhelms their ability to maintain a sense of control, in turn resulting in greater psychological stress (Keith, 1993). Low-income aging women with few economic resources to cope with aging are more likely to have circumscribed lives and more physical and psychological health problems (Murrell, Himmelfarb, & Wright, 1983; Stallones, Marx, & Garrity, 1990). The experience of being an older woman cannot be understood without taking account of the social context in which she lives. The cultural construction of old age for both men and women in postindustrial society encourages elders to internalize their own limitations and to settle for less than their actual capacities (Phillipson, 1982).

What of the future? Increasingly, poverty in the United States has become feminized, with single mothers with young children and old women among the poorest in the nation. According to current projections, by the year 2020 two out of five elderly women will be living on incomes less than $9,500 in today's dollars (U.S. House of Representatives, 1992) and primarily dependent on Social Security and Supplemental Security Income. Clearly they will not be among the ranks of WOOPies (well-off older persons) enjoying the growing elder consumer market. It seems likely that if older women were no more likely to brave financial strain than men, there would be no significant gender differences in their sense of mastery and psychological distress so often overtly or tacitly discussed in studies of gender development throughout the life course.[6] We are giving birth to new social constructions of women throughout the life course, but the gestation period is long and the rebirth is painful. Therein lies a challenge for all of us.

NOTES

1. I am indebted to Mary Kay Cordill for her accurate labeling of this condition of older women.

2. Prominent in many societies, whether Eastern, Western, or African, is the divergent image of aging based on gender. An extensive review of the social construction of female aging throughout the multiple societies making such distinctions is, however, beyond the scope of this paper. Rather, I am focusing on those societies—ancient Greece, ancient Rome, and the Judeo-Christian tradition—that I consider most influential on western past and present images of aging women.

3. *Hysteras* is the Greek word for uterus, from which the term "hysteria" is derived.

4. Of the 585 nominations for actresses and 584 for actors nominated for Academy Awards, 1927–90, 310 were for Best Actress, 309 for Best Actor, and 275 each for Best Supporting Actress and Actor. These and the following data on Academy Award winners and nominees are drawn from Markson and Taylor (1993).

5. In interpreting poverty levels, note that the federal government applies different income standards for those under age 65 and those 65+. On one's 65th birthday, a man or woman is magically considered to need less money than on the previous night at age 64.99. The formula for establishing the poverty level is based on a 1955 government survey that found that poor households spent about one-third of their income on food; those 65 and over were assumed to need less food than younger people. In 1993, the poverty index for an elderly couple was calculated at $1,000 less in annual income than that for a couple younger than 65. For individuals 65 or over, the index was $588 less per year.

6. One of my students has proposed that it is specifically the economic and sometimes physical dependence of the elderly that makes them subjects of opprobrium. If this is indeed a major cause of ageism, then the economic situation of old women in future generations is a critical factor in their vulnerability, extending beyond misogyny.

REFERENCES

Banner, Lois W. (1992). *In full flower: Aging women, power, and sexuality*. New York: Knopf.

Clancy, Carolyn M., & Franks, Peter. (1993). Physician gender bias in clinical decision making: Screening for cancer in primary care. *Medical Care, 31*(3), 213–218.

Cohen, John. (1991, June). Neomacho. *American Film*, pp. 36–39.

Cole, Thomas R. (1992). *The journey of life: A cultural history of aging in America*. New York: Cambridge University Press.

Culpepper, Emily E. (1993). Ageism, sexism, and health care: Why we need old women in power. In G. R. Winslow & J. W. Walthers (Eds.), *Facing limits: Ethics and health care for the elderly* (pp. 191–209). Boulder, CO: Westview Press.

Cumming, Elaine, & Henry, William. (1961). *Growing old*. San Francisco: Jossey-Bass.

Demos, John. (1978). Old age in early New England. In Michael Gordon (ed.), *The American family in socio-historical perspective, 2nd edition*. New York: St. Martins Press, 220–256.

Demos, John. (1982). *Entertaining Satan: Witchcraft and the culture of early New England*. New York: Oxford University Press.

Deutsch, Helene. (1945). *Psychology of women: A psychoanalytic interpretation*. New York: Grune & Stratton.

Dubois, Page. (1988). *Sowing the body: Psychoanalysis and ancient representations of women*. Chicago: University of Chicago Press.

Ehrenreich, Barbara, & English, Deirdre. (1982). *For her own good*. New York: Anchor Books.

Ellis, Havelock. (1905/1942). The sexual impulse in women. In *Studies in the psychology of sex*, vol. 1 (pp. 192–256). New York: Random House.

Engels, Friedrich. (1884/1972). *The origin of the family, private property, and the state*. New York: International Publishers.

Erikson, Erik H. (1968). *Identity, youth, and crisis*. New York: Norton.

Falkner, Thomas M., & de Luce, Judith. (1992). A view from antiquity: Greece, Rome, and elders. In Thomas R. Cole, David D. Van Tassel, & Robert Kastenbaum (Eds.), *Handbook of the humanities and aging*. New York: Springer.

Fischer, David Hackett. (1977). *Growing old in America*. New York: Oxford University Press.

Francis, Doris. (1991). Friends from the workplace. In Beth B. Hess & Elizabeth W. Markson (Eds.), *Growing old in America*. New Brunswick, NJ: Transaction Books.

Fraser, Antonia. (1984). *The weaker vessel*. New York: Knopf.

Freud, Sigmund. (1961a). Some psychical consequences of the anatomical distinction between the sexes. In J. Strachey (Ed. and Trans.), *The standard edition of the complete psychological works of Sigmund Freud* (Vol. 7). London: Hogarth Press.

Freud, Sigmund. (1961b). Types of onset of neurosis. In J. Strachey (Ed. and Trans.), *The standard edition of the complete psychological works of Sigmund Freud*. (Vol. 12). London: Hogarth Press.

Greer, Germaine. (1991). *The change: Women, aging, and the menopause*. New York: Knopf.

Gutmann, David. (1987). *Reclaimed powers: Toward a new psychology of men and women in later life*. New York: Basic Books.

Haber, Carole. (1983). *Beyond sixty-five: The dilemma of old age in America's past*. New York: Cambridge University Press.

Haber, Carole, & Gratton, Brian. (1993). *Old age and the search for security*. Bloomington: Indiana University Press.

Holmes, Oliver Wendell. (1891). *Over the teacups*. Boston: Houghton Mifflin.

Horney, Karen. (1967). *Feminine psychology*. New York: Norton.

Keith, Verna M. (1993). Gender, financial strain, and psychological distress among older adults. *Research on Aging, 15*(2), 123–147.

Kline, Chrysee. (1975). The socialization process of women. *Gerontologist, 15*(6), 486–492.

Kramer, Heinrich, & Sprenger, Johann. (1508/1971). *Malleus maleficarum: The classic study of witchcraft* (M. Summers, Trans.). London: Arrow.

Kuhn, Annette. (1982). *Women's pictures: Feminism and cinema*. London: Routledge & Kegan Paul.

Laslett, Peter. (1977). *Family life and illicit love in earlier generations*. Cambridge: Cambridge University Press.

Lehr, D. (1992, January 26). Screen writers talk about Hollywood's graylist. *Boston Globe*, pp. B-37, B-39ff.

Levinson, Daniel J., et al. (1978). *The seasons of a man's life*. New York: Knopf.

Lopata, Helena Z. (1971, Spring). Widows as a minority group. *Gerontologist* (Part 2), 67–77.

Macdonald, Barbara. (1989, Spring/Summer). Outside the sisterhood: Ageism in women's studies. *Women's Studies Quarterly, 17*(1/2), 6–11.

Markson, Elizabeth W., & Taylor, Carol A. (1993). Real versus reel world: Older women and the Academy Awards. *Women and Therapy, 14*(1/2), 157–172.

Miller, Jean Baker. (1986). *Toward a new psychology of women*. (2nd ed.). Boston: Beacon Press.

Murrell, S. A., Himmelfarb, S., & Wright, K. (1983). Prevalence of depression and its correlates in older adults. *American Journal of Epidemiology, 117,* 173–185.

National Research Council. (1988). *The aging population in the twenty-first century: Statistics for health policy.* Washington, DC: National Academy Press.

Pagels, Elaine. (1979). *The Gnostic gospels.* New York: Random House.

Phillipson, Chris. (1982). *Capitalism and the construction of old age.* London: Macmillan.

Reinharz, Shulamit. (1986). Friends or foes: Gerontological and feminist theory. *Women's Studies International Forum, 9*(5), 503–514.

Smith, Daniel Scott. (1978). Old age and the great society: A New England case study. In Stuart F. Spicker, Kathleen M. Woodward, & David D. Van Tassel (Eds.), *Aging and the elderly.* Atlantic Highlands, NJ: Humanities Press.

Smith, Joan. (1992). *Misogynies: Reflections on myth and malice.* London: Faber & Faber.

Stallones, L., Marx, M. B., & Garrity, T. F. (1990). Prevalence and correlates of depressive symptoms among older U.S. adults. *American Journal of Preventive Medicine, 6*(5), 295–303.

Tallmer, Margot. (1989). Empty-nest syndrome: Possibility or despair. In T. Bernay & D. W. Cantor (Eds.), *The psychology of today's woman: New psychoanalytic visions* (pp. 231–252). Cambridge, MA: Harvard University Press.

U.S. Department of Health and Human Services, Administration on Aging. (1991, March). *What you should know about the aging of America.* Washington, DC: Administration on Aging (xerographic copy).

U.S. Department of Labor. (1989). *Labor market problems of older workers: Report of the Secretary of Labor.* Washington, DC: U.S. Department of Labor.

U.S. House of Representatives. (1992). *Living in the shadows: Older women and the roots of poverty.* Report of the Subcommittee on Retirement Income and Employment of the Select Committee on Aging. Washington, DC: U.S. Government Printing Office.

Walker, Barbara. (1988). *The crone: Woman of age, wisdom, and power.* New York: Harper.

Walters, Suzanna D. (1992). *Lives together, worlds apart: Mothers and daughters in popular culture.* Berkeley: University of California Press.

Woods, William. (1974). *A history of the devil.* New York: Putnam.

Part II

Economic Issues

Six

The Economic Status of Older Women

ROSE M. RUBIN

The aging of the population and the sustained entry of women into the labor force are two of the most compelling societal changes of the twentieth century. These changes have influenced virtually all facets of both household and national life, including family composition, consumption patterns, the distribution of income, entitlement expenditures, and national savings. Yet very few changes in national policy have responded to these dramatic shifts. This lack of policy response may be assumed, at least in part, to persist because those most heavily affected by these changes are women, particularly older women whose economic status is becoming increasingly vulnerable. These currently elderly women who have not succeeded in affecting social policy have been referred to as "the silent majority" (Datan, 1989).

During the past quarter century the number of women 55 years old and over in the United States has increased, so that one in every ten persons now falls into this demographic category. Although substantial gains have been made in the income levels and economic status of older persons, older single women remain one of the groups most likely to be poor. Many analyses of the elderly either look at the household as a unit or disaggregate by work status (retired versus nonretired) or by age group. In contrast, to develop a clear picture of the economic status of older persons in the United States, it is necessary to analyze the economic situation for women as distinct from that for men. The important factors influencing the economic status of women tend to revolve around marital status and age cohort. Older married women are, in general, much more economically secure than their single counterparts, and younger cohorts among the elderly have different patterns than do more aged women.

In order to motivate both research on issues of older women and future policy developments affecting them, a coherent perspective on their economic status is needed by gerontology researchers, students, and policy makers. The objective of this chapter is to provide an overview and synthesis of research findings on the economic status of older women. The goal is to develop a clear picture of both the economic diversity and general fiscal vulnerability of this most rapidly growing group. The chapter contains six sections covering the demographics of older women, their employment status, income by sources, assets and savings, and expenditure patterns, followed by an overview and conclusions.

DEMOGRAPHIC CHARACTERISTICS OF OLDER WOMEN

Age Distribution

Since the turn of the century the conditional life expectancies (on reaching age 65) of women have far outstripped those of men (Hurd, 1990). In 1990 a 65-year-old woman could expect to live 19 years, or 4 years longer than a man aged 65, and this difference is forecast to continue to increase (U.S. Bureau of the Census, 1994).

The percentage of females in each cohort group over age 55 is larger than the corresponding share for males, while the reverse is the case for younger ages. There are 84 men per 100 women aged 65–69, 65 men per 100 women aged 75–79, and only 34 men per 100 women aged 85+ (U.S. Senate Special Committee on Aging, 1991). In 1990, 15 percent of women were age 65+, 7 percent were age 75+, and 2 percent were 85+, compared to 10 percent, 4 percent, and 1 percent for men in these cohorts. By the year 2050 these shares for women are projected to be 25 percent, 15 percent, and 7 percent (Taeuber & Allen, 1993), and all of these women were already born at least a decade ago. This means that most of the very old will continue to be women, and also that younger women must prepare for financing their consumption for a very extended period following retirement age.

Education

For those with less education than high school, the educational attainment of older men and women is fairly similar, as about one-fourth completed eight years or less and about 15 percent have some high school (table 6.1). But at higher levels of education the similarities decline. Almost 40 percent of older women are high-school graduates, but only 9 percent completed four or more years of college (U.S. Bureau of the Census, 1994).

Since level of educational attainment is considered to be a major determinant of employment opportunity and earnings, the underlying issue is how the return to education compares for older women and men. The differential income return to education between older men and women was much greater for those with a college degree than for high-school graduates (U.S. Bureau of the Census, 1994).

Table 6.1
Demographic Characteristics of Persons Aged 65+ by Gender, 1993

	Males	Females
Total (millions)	12.8	18.0
White (millions)	11.4	16.1
Black (millions)	1.1	1.6
% below Poverty Level	8.9%	15.7%
PERCENT DISTRIBUTION		
Marital Status		
Single	4.4%	4.4%
Married	76.8	42.2
Widowed	14.3	47.6
Divorced	4.5	5.8
Living Arrangements*		
Alone	16.0	41.0
With spouse	75.0	41.0
With other relatives	7.0	17.0
With non-relatives	3.0	2.0
Years of School Completed		
8 years or less	25.0	23.5
1-3 years of high school	14.9	16.1
4 years of high school	29.7	37.4
1-3 years of college	14.3	13.9
4 or more years of college	16.1	9.0
Labor Force Participation		
Employed	15.1	7.9
Unemployed	0.5	0.3
Not in labor force	84.4	91.8

*Numbers may not add to 100% due to rounding.
Source: U.S. Bureau of the Census. (1994). *Statistical Abstract of the United States: 1994* (114th ed.). Washington, DC: U.S. Government Printing Office.

Since a much larger share of elderly men are at least college graduates, this is one important factor that has influenced income differentials.

Household Type\Marital Status

In strong contrast to the picture for women, older men tend to be married, and relatively few live alone. While only 40 percent of older women are married, three-fourths of men aged 65 and over are married with spouse present. Perhaps surprisingly, only about 5 percent of both groups are divorced. Almost half of elderly women are widowed (including over a third of those aged 65 to 74 and two-thirds of those over age 75), while fewer than 15 percent of older men are widowed (U.S. Bureau of the Census, 1994).

These differences in marital status translate into quite distinct living arrangements for elderly men and women. Over two-fifths of older women live alone, and an additional fifth live with someone else, considerably more than twice the share of older men either living alone or with someone else (U.S. Bureau of the Census, 1994). This 20 percent of elderly women living with relatives or others poses a special problem in the measurement of poverty among the elderly. Low-income individuals may not be counted as poor if they are residing in nonpoor households, but the reason they live with others is often their lack of income. Schulz (1992) suggested that at least a third of these elderly had income below the poverty level and that most were not counted. Thus official poverty statistics of the elderly are likely to understate the case of poor older women.

One factor that is generally not acknowledged in descriptions of the household type or the living arrangements of older women is the extent to which they are raising grandchildren. At least 5 percent of the country's children under age 18 lived with grandparents in 1992, and half of these lived with a grandmother alone (Glasse, 1993).

EMPLOYMENT

Since the importance of women, including older women, to the labor market continues to grow, an understanding of the factors that influence their labor-force participation decisions is important. The retirement decision can be viewed as the converse of the participation decision. Leaving the labor force not only reduces current earnings income, it may also affect the individual's potential future income from both public and private retirement sources. Further, poverty patterns at the societal level, particularly for elderly women, may be related to prior labor-force participation decisions (Weaver, 1994).

Employment Characteristics

Only 8 percent of women over age 65 are employed, with the remainder not in the labor force, but almost twice this share of older men are labor-force participants. Marital status is a significant determinant of the likelihood of work of older women. Older divorced or single women, who are likely to have to rely on their own pensions and earnings, have a much stronger work attachment than do married women (Herz, 1988). Divorced women over age 65 are twice as likely to be in the labor force as married women the same age (U.S. Department of Labor, 1993). However, both elderly single men and women and, also, married men have reduced their labor-force participation rates by more than half since 1960, but the participation rate for older married women has slightly increased over this long term (U.S. Bureau of the Census, 1994).

Part-time work is prevalent for older women. Almost three-fifths of employed women over age 65 work part-time, with many concentrated in low-wage retail or service industries (Schulz, 1992).

Among those elderly who remain in the labor force, only a very limited share of either women or men are unemployed. This may reflect the likelihood that the elderly who become unemployed withdraw from the labor force. In fact, being unemployed is one of the most important single predictors of transition out of the labor force; for the elderly, unemployment significantly increases the probability of leaving the labor force. Thus there is some question as to whether the usual distinction between unemployment and being out of the labor force is meaningful for older workers (Peracchi & Welch, 1994). When the Bureau of Labor Statistics revised its employment survey, effective in 1994, the new estimates were found to reflect somewhat higher unemployment for women and for the elderly, so future unemployment data for older women may be expected to reveal somewhat higher rates.

There has been more variation over time in employment among the near-elderly, as participation rates of women aged 50 to 54 and 55 to 59 have increased substantially, while rates of those aged 60 to 64 have remained fairly constant (Herz, 1988; Gendell & Siegel, 1992; U.S. Department of Labor, 1993). In a somewhat different study using data from the Current Population Survey, Peracchi and Welch (1994) found that women under 60 have higher participation rates than they did 20 years ago, but that those aged 60 or over have lower participation rates. However, projections of the labor-force participation rates for older women, unlike those for men, indicate increases through 2005 for all ages except 75+, as shown in table 6.2 (Gendell & Siegel, 1992). This is not surprising, as the scant labor-force experiences of today's elderly women are not likely to be repeated among future cohorts (Herz, 1988). When currently younger women reach retirement age, they will have had much more extensive work experience than previous cohorts of women, and their participation rates are expected to increase (Peracchi & Welch, 1994).

Retirement

Since 1950 the average age of retirement for both women and men has decreased sharply, by about 6 years to the current age of 63.5. Among women, the decline was from age 68 to 63.4. However, most of this decline occurred by 1970, and it has since leveled off for both men and women (Gendell & Siegel, 1992). The major measure of entry into retirement is initial award of Social Security retirement benefits, for which the lower limit is age 62. Among those beginning Social Security benefits in 1989, about 50 percent of men and 60 percent of women received initial benefits at age 62.

Since age at retirement has generally been measured in terms of the long-run

Table 6.2
Labor-Force Participation Rates by Age Group and Gender

Age Group (years)	Males			Females		
	1990	1995*	2005*	1990	1995*	2005*
45-49	92.3	92.0	91.6	74.8	79.1	85.1
50-54	88.8	88.8	88.8	66.9	71.0	77.6
55-59	79.8	79.4	78.8	55.3	58.4	64.5
60-64	55.5	54.7	53.3	35.5	37.9	40.9
65-69	26.0	26.6	27.9	17.0	18.2	20.7
70-74	15.4	15.4	15.5	8.2	8.4	8.5
75+	7.1	7.4	7.2	2.7	2.5	2.6

*Projected rates.
Source: Gendell, M., & Siegel, J. S. (1992). Trends in retirement age by sex, 1950–2005. Monthly Labor Review, 115 (7), 22–29.

trends in labor-force participation of men, Gendell and Siegel (1992) argued that the measure should be calculated for women as well as men, because participation rates for women in different age subgroups over 55 differ from those for men. Studies of the retirement decision of single women indicate that its determinants are similar to those for men, but decisions regarding retirement are more complicated for married women (Hurd, 1990). As an example, in married-couple households where the couple self-identified as both retired, three-fourths of the women did not work in the year before the couple entered the retirement stage, indicating that these wives probably had considered themselves homemakers and had not worked outside the home in prior years (Rubin & Nieswiadomy, 1995).

Weaver (1994) has compiled a very useful literature review of the retirement decisions of older women. The important conclusions he drew are that wives are more likely to discontinue working if their husbands are retired; neither the presence of dependents in the household nor the health status of husbands is a major determinant of the work and retirement patterns of older women; wealth and unearned income influence the work and retirement decisions of unmarried women, but not those of married women; work is positively related to its financial reward for women; and married women are more likely to work if they can augment the lifetime value of their Social Security benefits. Although Weaver noted that these results have appeared consistently in the literature, he cautioned that this body of studies is limited in size and coverage and that several studies he reviewed employ older data sets.

Occupations of Older Women

The majority of older working women continue to be employed in stereotyped occupations, the traditional low-paying occupations where more than half the workers are women (Taeuber & Allen, 1993). Nearly two-thirds of women aged

55 or over are in three traditionally female job categories: sales, services, and administrative support (Herz, 1988). Women aged 65 or over are over-represented in sales and service jobs, and also in being self-employed or unpaid family workers. These job categories for older women may reflect the low rates of pension coverage in these areas. Receipt of a pension other than Social Security is an important determinant of whether women continue to work beyond normal retirement age (Herz, 1988).

INCOME AND SOURCES OF INCOME

Median income for older women was $8,189 in 1992, compared to $14,548 for men (U.S. Bureau of the Census, 1994). However, income patterns differ substantially between elderly married and single women, with those who are married consistently better off. This is reflected in the fact that 14 percent of all elderly women were in poverty in 1989, but almost a fourth of elderly women living alone were in poverty (U.S. Senate Special Committee on Aging, 1991). Whether they are retired or not, Social Security is the financial mainstay of single women once they reach eligibility age, because their pension income is low and very little income is generated from their meager level of financial assets (Rubin & Nieswiadomy, 1994).

Since "real income" reflects the purchasing power of dollar income, or money income after taking account of inflation, real income is generally viewed as a better determinant of living standards than unadjusted money income. Nieswiadomy and Rubin (1995) analyzed change in the real income of retired households from 1972 to 1987 and found that while it increased slightly during this period for couples and single males, single females experienced a 13 percent decline in real income.

There are several difficulties in the measurement of income that affect analyses of the income of elderly women. First, income is frequently reported by household unit, rather than by the individual, so that the income of spouses cannot be separated, and only the income of single persons is reported by gender. This is done, for example, in Social Security (Girad, 1994) reports such as *Income of the Population 55 or Older*. Second, it is typical in many surveys for income to be underreported, particularly income from assets. Thus income at lower levels that is predominantly from Social Security, other transfer programs, and earnings tends to be more accurately reported than higher levels of income that include more income from assets.

Four sources provide almost all of the money income of the elderly: earnings from work, Social Security benefits, other public and private pensions, and income from assets. The share of income provided by each of these sources varies by age, marital status, and sex. As can be seen in table 6.3, for those of near-retirement age (55–64), males' median income is almost two and a half times that of females; and for full-time workers, males' earnings are almost two-thirds greater than females' earnings. For those aged 65 or over, both median income

Table 6.3
Comparison of Income of the Older Population by Gender

	Males	Females
Median income (1992)		
Age 55-64	$25,271	$10,168
Age 65+	14,548	8,189
Average earnings of full-time workers (1992)		
Age 55-64	38,843	23,751
Age 65+	38,719	19,932
Pensions		
Mean lump-sum distribution (1993)	14,162	6,956
Median lump-sum distribution (1993)	5,364	2,637
Mean monthly pension income (1991)	859	481
Mean combined pension and Social Security income (1991)	1,383	958
Social Security: Average monthly retiree benefit (1993)		
All benefits	789	581
Without reduction for early retirement	902	737
With reduction for early retirement	686	522

Sources: Silverman, Celia, Anzick, Michael, Boyce, Sarah, Campbell, Sharyn, McDonnell, Ken, Reilly, Annmarie, & Snider, Sarah. (1995). *EBRI databook on employee benefits* (3rd ed.). Washington, DC: Employee Benefit Research Institute; U.S. Bureau of the Census. (1994). *Statistical Abstract of the United States: 1994* (114th ed.). Washington, DC: U.S. Government Printing Office.

and earnings are nearly twice as large for males as for females. Further, for those receiving pensions, both average lump-sum distributions and average monthly pension income are roughly twice as large for males as for females. Social Security retiree benefits are also considerably higher for males than for females, even though many women receive benefits based on their spouse's earnings record.

Earnings

While currently earned income from labor (wages and salaries) constitutes nearly three-fourths of total income in the United States, this figure is much lower for older women. Nonetheless, almost three-quarters of nonmarried women aged 62 to 64, and a third of those aged 65 or over, relied on their own earnings for at least half their total income (Herz, 1988).

In the research literature income is generally recorded by economic units (households), and earned income for married older women is not obtainable separately. However, average earnings differ significantly between older men and women. For full-time full-year workers, women over 65 earned $19,932 in 1992, about half the earnings of older men, while near-elderly (aged 55–64) women earned $23,751 (table 6.3).

Social Security

Social Security is the major income-protection program for the elderly, and it is the most important source of income for a large share of older women, particularly those at the lowest income level. The fact that the Social Security program favors traditional households is one of the underlying factors in the high incidence of poverty among single elderly women (Burkhauser, 1994). Because income from Social Security depends upon either the worker's or spouse's contributions to the system (based on earnings level and length of employment), many women who have not worked may ultimately receive larger payments than those who have been in the labor force. Currently, even working women are out of the labor force an overall average of 11.5 years, compared to 1 year for men; and since women's earnings have tended to be lower than men's, an older woman may be better off receiving payments from the contribution record of a spouse or ex-spouse (if married at least ten years) than from her own earnings record (Doup, 1992). This is why average retiree benefits for women ($581) are closer to those for men ($789) than are earnings.

Social Security poses one of the major policy issues that is likely to affect the income of widows in the future, as there is considerable question regarding the continuing viability of the spouse benefit. If Social Security ceases to be viewed as sacred in the attempts to reduce the federal budget deficit, then the current spouse benefit provision may become a target for budget cutters. In contrast, Burkhauser (1994) suggested that the spouse benefit should be raised from a two-thirds survivor benefit to three-quarters, and that survivors of two-earner families should receive the same three-quarters benefit, based on the total benefit previously paid to the couple.

Private Pensions

Women are much less likely than men to receive private pension benefits. Schulz (1992) reported that in one study only 27 percent of women were found to receive a pension (24 percent from own employment plus 3 percent from survivor benefits), which was half the pension rate for men. Average monthly pension income for those women with pensions in 1991 was $481, only 56 percent of men's average pension. These figures are approximately the same as

Table 6.4
Distribution of Income of Persons Aged 65+ by Gender, 1992

	Males	Females
$1-$2,499	2.1%	4.8%
$2,500-$4,999	4.7	16.8
$5,000-$9,999	23.6	39.8
$10,000-$14,999	21.4	17.6
$15,000-$24,999	25.9	13.4
$25,000-$49,999	16.0	6.4
$50,000-$74,999	3.3	0.8
$75,000 and over	2.9	0.4

Source: U.S. Bureau of the Census. (1994). *Statistical Abstract of the United States: 1994* (114th ed.). Washington, DC: U.S. Government Printing Office.

those found by Rubin and Nieswiadomy (1994) from the Consumer Expenditure Survey data, that retired single females receive only about half as much pension income as retired single males and less than one-third as much as retired married couples. For those women receiving lump-sum pension distributions, the average was also less than half that for men (table 6.3).

Since pension wealth declines sharply for widows upon the death of their husbands, the Retirement Equity Act of 1984 was designed to encourage the selection of pension options with survivorship rights. However, even this does not overcome the proclivity toward poverty of elderly widows. Because the correlation between economic status and pension eligibility is strongly positive, few poor widows would have been eligible for pension benefits even with survivorship rights, which are unlikely to have a large impact on widows' high poverty rates (Hurd, 1990).

Poverty and the Distribution of Income

Although the poverty status of the elderly has declined dramatically since 1970, older women remain at high risk for being impoverished. By 1993, 16 percent of women over age 65 were below the poverty level, and nearly one-third had incomes less than 150 percent of the poverty level. Women constitute about three-fourths of the elderly poor and are 76 percent more likely to be in poverty than older men (Allen, 1993b).

Table 6.4, giving the distribution of income of the elderly, reveals the income disparities between men and women, with 61 percent of women and only 30 percent of men having income below $10,000. Burkhauser and Smeeding (1994, p. 5) found that it is "this wide disparity between the economic well-being of older women and men that constitutes the most pressing unfinished business of social policy toward the aged."

While the percentages of older married men and women in poverty are the same, the shares of those in poverty are much higher for single (widowed, divorced, separated, or never-married) elderly women than for single males. Two out of three elderly persons are women, among whom two-thirds are living alone and constitute the group most likely to be in poverty (Koelln, Rubin, & Picard, 1995). Koelln, Rubin, and Picard (1995) concluded that "the income situation of older singles is very different from that of couples, with widowed females experiencing the lowest incomes of any demographic group." A widow is four times more likely to live in poverty after retirement than a married woman, with half of the widows becoming poor following their husband's death (Doup, 1992). Schwenk (1991) found that three-quarters of older women living alone have incomes below $10,000, and 60 percent of their income was from Social Security. Further, among industrialized countries this problem is considerably worse in the United States than anywhere else (Burkhauser & Smeeding, 1994). Thus being old, single, and female in the United States constituted the criteria for what Minkler and Stone (1985) termed "triple jeopardy" a decade ago, and this still applies today. Further, this situation will not be ameliorated by anything except transfer payments until the aging of a generation of women who are covered by fuller pensions and the higher levels of Social Security and savings generated by higher salaries.

In-kind Benefits

In-kind, or noncash, benefits are also important determinants of material welfare, but these are rarely included in the calculation of either income or poverty levels. Among the elderly, only 5 percent of married couples receive one or more in-kind benefits exclusive of health financing (i.e., Medicare), compared to 16 percent of single women receiving at least one in-kind benefit. The four major sources of in-kind benefits received by single older women are energy assistance (10 percent), food stamps (8 percent), public housing (6 percent), and rental assistance (3 percent) (U.S. Senate Special Committee on Aging, 1991). These noncash transfers have income-based eligibility criteria and provide important cushions for the economic welfare of those elderly who qualify.

WEALTH

Hurd (1990) concluded that "although income is practically the only measure of economic status in use, life cycle considerations suggest that, at least for the retired elderly, wealth is a better measure because it measures consumption opportunities." However, most measures of wealth, like those for income, are for households rather than individuals within the household unit, and it is not possible to separate the assets of husbands and wives.

In 1988 female householders aged 65+ reported a median net worth of $47,233, approximately two-thirds the level of that of all older households (U.S.

Senate Special Committee on Aging, 1991), but this group does not include the poorest older women living with others. A crucial finding of the selected financial assets reported by household units in the Consumer Expenditure Survey is that the asset value of single females is only about one-third that of married couples or single males. This small asset value is closely related to the relatively low after-retirement income reported by single females, who have low asset income (Rubin & Nieswiadomy, 1995).

Ownership of a house simultaneously provides an important equity asset and a stream of housing consumption services over time. Thus homeownership is an important determinant of both the wealth assets of a household and its spending on housing. Schwenk (1991) found marked differences in both homeownership and the income generated from assets among older women in different living arrangements. She noted that women living alone were less likely than others to be homeowners and also had dividend and interest income less than half the level of older married couples.

In a recent study of changes in older households from 1972 to 1987, increased shares of homeowners were found for all household types, with the largest increases for single males, followed by single females, since married couples already had 80 percent ownership in 1972. Also, the share of homeowners without a mortgage increased for the single owners, but decreased for married couples (Nieswiadomy & Rubin, 1995).

Nieswiadomy and Rubin (1995) analyzed the change over time in the financial assets and savings patterns of three retiree household groups over age 55 and noted marked declines from 1972 to 1987 in the assets of all elderly. Assets of married couples and single females declined to about half, and assets of single males declined to three-quarters of the earlier levels. In 1972 positive saving from income was 10 percent for married couples, 16 percent for single males, and 8 percent for single females. By 1987 only married couples still showed positive savings, which had declined to only 2 percent of after-tax income. Both single retired male and female households were dissaving, as their annual income was less than expenditures, and single females were spending considerably more than their income.

EXPENDITURES

Household expenditure patterns can be viewed as one of the clearest indicators of household consumption and, therefore, of living standards. In particular, spending on the necessity areas of food, housing, and health care gives an indication of how well the household is living. As with income and wealth data, expenditures are reported for the household or consuming unit and are only reported for individuals for men and women who are single and live alone.

Single females suffer the most substantial decline among elderly demographic groups in postretirement income, but this is not offset by concurrent expenditure decreases, as noted earlier. Average total expenditures of single females declined only slightly in the face of a one-quarter decrease in after-tax income, so that postretirement dissavings were as high as 15 percent of after-tax income. With assets initially one-third or less of those for other groups, single females begin dissaving in the first quarter of retirement (Rubin & Nieswiadomy, 1995).

In a comparison of expenditures by retirees from 1972 to 1987, single males spent 21 percent more than single females, and married couples spent 87 percent more than single females. Among the nonretired groups over age 50, single males spent 33 percent more than single females, and married couples spent 80 percent more than single females.

Nieswiadomy and Rubin (1995) examined expenditure patterns of retirees over age 50 by household type and over time. They found that for spending on necessities from 1972 to 1987, different patterns were seen for food and apparel than for housing. All retiree households allocated lesser budget shares to the necessity areas of food and apparel over time, but single females significantly increased housing shares.

Housing

One of the most notable aspects of the expenditure patterns of older women is the large share of spending devoted to housing. In extensive analyses of the expenditure patterns of the elderly, Nieswiadomy and Rubin (1995) and Rubin and Nieswiadomy (1994) found that housing expenditure shares remained virtually constant over time for married couples, declined for single men, and rose for single women. While single females allocated 43 percent of their budgets to housing, single males have reduced this share to under 30 percent, now comparable to that for married couples. The researchers concluded that this large housing share expended by older women is not caused primarily by spending on shelter, but by utilities and household operations. However, single females spend larger amounts on housing and all subcategories of housing than single males or married couples.

One often-overlooked factor in the housing situation for older women is their residence in mobile homes. Single women comprise almost a third of mobile-home dwellers aged 55 to 64 and over 40 percent of those aged 65 or over (Glasse, 1993).

The housing situation is beginning to reach crisis proportions for older women in the United States, particularly for those who are single. Over three-fourths of older tenants in public and subsidized housing are women. In nearly a third of cases, older female renters spend over half of their limited incomes on housing, and housing consumes an especially large share of income for older minority women (Glasse, 1993). Since single females spend a considerably greater budget share on housing, there is a need for further study on elderly female living arrangements and housing assistance programs.

Table 6.5
Health Insurance Coverage of the Near-Elderly (Aged 55–64), 1993

	Males	Females
Employer coverage	67.1%	61.3%
Other private	10.3	15.1
Total public	16.9	16.6
Uninsured	13.3	13.5

Source: Silverman, Celia, Anzick, Michael, Boyce, Sarah, Campbell, Sharyn, McDonnell, Ken, Reilly, Annmarie, & Snider, Sarah. (1995). *EBRI databook on employee benefits* (3rd ed.). Washington DC: Employee Benefit Research Institute.

Health Care

The establishment, growth, and universal coverage of the elderly by Medicare has significantly reduced their potential to suffer the risks of medical costs. About two-thirds of the elderly have Medigap or supplemental health care insurance, and since 1992 the eligibility of impoverished elderly for Medicaid coverage is assured. The elderly remain vulnerable to large medical outlays that exceed Medicare limits and to the risks of long-term care, for which few have insurance.

Although those aged 65 or over have universal health insurance coverage, the picture is much more variable for the near-elderly, as shown in table 6.5. More men aged 55 to 64 have employer health coverage than women, but it is not possible to distinguish how many have coverage through spouse's employment. Approximately the same shares of near-elderly men and women have public insurance (17%) or are uninsured (13%).

OVERVIEW AND CONCLUSIONS

When the elderly are not viewed as a homogeneous entity and the economic conditions of subgroups of the older population are examined, the diversity of their financial situations can be clarified. It becomes readily apparent that the economic status of older women differs in important ways from that of older men. Change is a notable aspect of data on the economic status of the elderly in recent decades; and for older women, economic changes have been greater than for men and have not been consistently positive.

For elderly women, age of retirement has declined, life expectancy has increased, and the likelihood of becoming widowed at some time has increased. Thus older single women are now among those most likely to be impoverished. It might appear that they have not anticipated having an increased lifespan or the financial requirements this entails over a longer period of time. However, an even more plausible explanation is that many of these women never had the resources to have planned for a very extended period of retirement. A crucial issue then becomes, what will it take to prevent this pattern from being repeated in future generations of elderly women?

Betty Friedan, the eminent feminist, has begun to emphasize economics, and particularly gender parity in income, as having highest priority. She noted that what is needed is both increased effort to integrate economic policies with social concerns and an understanding of the impact of economic policy on social outcomes (Erickson, 1994). It may be that workers, especially women, are encouraged by early-retirement features of the Social Security system to retire too soon. Further, the Social Security system discriminates against women in dual-earner families, a factor that involves increasing numbers of households.

One particular area in need of policy initiatives is affordable adequate housing. Since elderly single females spend a considerably greater budget share on housing than males, further study of living arrangements and housing assistance programs available for older women is needed (Wolf & Soldo, 1988; Rubin & Nieswiadomy, 1995).

As the population ages, larger shares will be retirees, particularly among women with their longer life expectancies. Closely related is the need for greater recognition by both businesses and workers that retirement requires planning and that women workers need to be encouraged to utilize formal retirement-planning programs where they are available. Thus availability of preretirement planning needs to be enhanced to facilitate women's financial readiness for retirement.

Several policies aimed at preventing poverty among women in old age have focused on pension reform, but pension reform, while needed, is not sufficient. In addition to reforms of both public and private pensions, the underlying issue of greater parity in the labor force must be solved. Such parity requires solutions to disrupted job tenure, achieving enhanced occupational integration, and higher returns to educational attainment. The economic status of future cohorts of older women depends upon changes in the economic status and employment situation for women in general and throughout their lifetimes.

REFERENCES

Allen, Jessie. (1993a). Caring work and gender equity in an aging society. In Jessie Allen & Alan Pifer (Eds.), *Women on the front lines: Meeting the challenge of an aging America* (pp. 221–240). Washington, DC: Urban Institute Press.

———. (1993b). The front lines. In Jessie Allen & Alan Pifer (Eds.), *Women on the front lines: Meeting the challenge of an aging America* (pp. 1–10). Washington, DC: Urban Institute Press.

Burkhauser, Richard V. (1994). Protecting the most vulnerable: A proposal to improve Social Security insurance for older women. *Gerontologist, 34*(2), 148–149.

Burkhauser, Richard V., & Smeeding, Timothy M. (1994). Social Security reform: A budget neutral approach to reducing older women's disproportionate risk of poverty. *Aging Studies Program Policy Brief, 2.* Syracuse University, Center for Policy Research.

Datan, Nancy. (1989). Aging women: The silent majority. *Women's Studies Quarterly, 17*(1–2), 12–18.

Doup, Liz. (1992, December 15). Becoming poor in old age. *Fort Worth Star-Telegram,* section D, p. 6.

Epstein, Lenore A. (1980). Some problems in measuring the economic status of the aged in the United States. In Clark Tibbitts & Wilma Donahue (Eds.), *Social and psychological aspects of aging* (pp. 232–262). New York: Arno Press.

Erickson, Kathleen. (1994). Interview with Betty Friedan: On women, ageing, and the economy. *Region, 8*(3), 12–17.

Fahs, Marianne C. (1993). Preventive medical care: Targeting elderly women in an aging society. In Jessie Allen & Alan Pifer (Eds.), *Women on the front lines: Meeting the challenge of an aging America* (pp. 105–132). Washington, DC: Urban Institute Press.

Foster, Susan E., & Brizius, Jack A. (1993). Caring too much? American women and the nation's caregiving crisis. In Jessie Allen & Alan Pifer (Eds.), *Women on the front lines: Meeting the challenge of an aging America* (pp. 47–74). Washington, DC: Urban Institute Press.

Gendell, M., & Siegel, J. S. (1992). Trends in retirement age by sex, 1950–2005. *Monthly Labor Review, 115*(7), 22–29.

Glasse, Lou. (1993). Housing crisis for older women. *Journal of Housing, 50*(4), 135–136.

Grad, Susan. (1990). Income change at retirement. *Social Security Bulletin, 53*(1), 2–10.
———. (1994). *Income of the population 55 or older, 1992.* Washington, DC: U.S. Department of Health and Human Services, Social Security Administration Office of Research and Statistics, 13–11871.

Harrison, B. (1986). Spending patterns of older persons revealed in expenditure survey. *Monthly Labor Review, 109*(10), 15–18.

Herz, Diane E. (1988). Employment characteristics of older women, 1987. *Monthly Labor Review, 111*(9), 3–12.

Holahan, Carole. (1981). Lifetime achievement patterns, retirement, and life satisfaction of gifted aged women. *Journal of Gerontology, 36*(6), 741–749.

Hurd, Michael D. (1990). Research on the elderly: Economic status, retirement, and consumption and saving. *Journal of Economic Literature, 28*, 565–637.

Jacobs, Ruth Harriet. (1993). Expanding social roles for older women. In Jessie Allen & Alan Pifer (Eds.), *Women on the front lines: Meeting the challenge of an aging America* (pp. 191–220). Washington, DC: Urban Institute Press.

Koelln, Kenneth, Rubin, Rose M., & Picard, Marion Smith. (1995). Vulnerable elderly households: Expenditures on necessities by older Americans. *Social Science Quarterly, 76*(3), 619–633.

Lamphere-Thorpe, Jo-Ann, & Blendon, Robert J. (1993). Years gained and opportunities lost: Women and healthcare in an aging America. In Jessie Allen & Alan Pifer (Eds.), *Women on the front lines: Meeting the challenge of an aging America* (pp. 75–104). Washington, DC: Urban Institute Press.

Leonard, Fran. (1982). *Older women and pensions: Catch 22.* Center for Studies in Aging Resource Center, North Texas State University.

Malveaux, Julianne. (1993). Race, poverty, and women's aging. In Jessie Allen & Alan Pifer (Eds.), *Women on the front lines: Meeting the challenge of an aging America* (pp. 167–190). Washington, DC: Urban Institute Press.

Minkler, Meredith, & Stone, Robyn. (1985). The feminization of poverty and older women. *Gerontologist, 25*(4), 351–357.

Moon, Marilyn. (1991). Consumer issues and the elderly. *Journal of Consumer Affairs, 24*(2), 235–244.

Nieswiadomy, Mike, & Rubin, Rose M. (1995). Change in expenditure patterns of retirees, 1972–1973 and 1986–1987. *Journals of Gerontology: Social Sciences, 50B*(5), S274–S290.

Peracchi, Franco, & Welch, Finis. (1994). Trends in labor force transitions of older men and women. *Journal of Labor Economics, 12*(2), 210–242.

Pifer, Alan. (1993). Meeting the challenge: Implications for policy and practice. In Jessie Allen & Alan Pifer (Eds.), *Women on the front lines: Meeting the challenge of an aging America* (pp. 241–252). Washington, DC: Urban Institute Press.

Rayman, Paula, Allshouse, Kimberly, & Allen, Jessie. (1993). Resiliency amidst inequity: Older women workers in an aging United States. In Jessie Allen & Alan Pifer (Eds.), *Women on the front lines: Meeting the challenge of an aging America* (pp. 133–166). Washington, DC: Urban Institute Press.

Rubin, Rose M., & Koelln, Kenneth. (1993a). Determinants of household out-of-pocket health expenditures. *Social Science Quarterly, 74*(4), 721–735.

———. (1993b). Out-of-pocket health expenditure differentials between elderly and nonelderly households. *Gerontologist, 33*(5), 595–602.

Rubin, Rose M., Koelln, Kenneth, & Speas, Roger. (1995). Out-of-pocket health expenditures by elderly households: Change over the 1980s. *Journals of Gerontology: Social Sciences, 50B*(5), S291–S300.

Rubin, Rose M., & Nieswiadomy, Mike. (1994). Expenditure patterns of retired and nonretired persons. *Monthly Labor Review, 117*(4), 10–21.

———. (1995). Economic adjustments of households on entry into retirement. *Journal of Applied Gerontology, 14*(4), 481–496.

Schulz, James H. (1992). *The Economics of Aging* (5th ed.). New York: Auburn House.

Schwenk, Frankie N. (1991). Women 65 years or older: A comparison of economic well-being by living arrangement. *Family Economics Review, 4*(3), 2–8.

———. (1993). Changes in the economic status of America's elderly population during the last 50 years. *Family Economics Review, 6*(1), 18–27.

Silverman, Celia, Anzick, Michael, Boyce, Sarah, Campbell, Sharyn, McDonnell, Ken, Reilly, Annmarie, & Snider, Sarah. (1995). *EBRI databook on employee benefits* (3rd ed.). Washington, DC: Employee Benefit Research Institute.

Sinicropi, Anthony V. (1983). Economic security and income maintenance. In Woodrow W. Morris, Iva M. Bader, & Sara C. Wolfson (Eds.), *Hoffman's daily needs and interests of older people* (pp. 53–65). Springfield, IL: Charles C. Thomas.

Taeuber, Cynthia M., & Allen, Jessie. (1993). Women in our aging society: The demographic outlook. In Jessie Allen & Alan Pifer (Eds.), *Women on the front lines: Meeting the challenge of an aging America* (pp. 11–46). Washington, DC: Urban Institute Press.

U.S. Bureau of the Census. (1994). *Statistical abstract of the United States: 1994* (114th ed.). Washington, DC.

U.S. Department of Labor, Bureau of Labor Statistics. (1993). *Employment in perspective: Women in the labor force.* Washington, DC: U.S. Government Printing Office.

U.S. Senate Special Committee on Aging, the American Association of Retired Persons, the Federal Council on the Aging, and the U.S. Administration on Aging. (1991). *Aging America: Trends and projections* (1991 ed.). Washington, DC: U.S. Department of Health and Human Services.

Walsh, Roberta W., & Kolodinsky, Jane. (1992). Prices, income, and the economic status of older, single women: Implications for health care and housing policies. *Forum for Social Economics, 22*(1), 48–59.

Weaver, David A. (1994). The work and retirement decisions of older women: A literature review. *Social Security Bulletin, 57*(1), 3–24.

Wolf, D. A., & Soldo, B. J. (1988). Household composition choices of older unmarried women. *Demography, 25*, 387–403.

Seven

Middle-aged and Older Women in the Work Force

JOHN C. RIFE

> I didn't go to work outside the home until six years ago and I was pretty apprehensive about it. But it has been really good for me. I have a different view of myself now. . . . I am more than just a mom and a wife.

> For me, my job was important for more reasons than income. It gave me a sense of achievement outside the home. Losing my job has been very hard, especially since I have had such trouble finding another good one.

These two statements demonstrate that work has different meanings for each of us. Employment can provide opportunities for personal growth, socialization, prestige, and economic sufficiency. Involuntary unemployment can result in increased stress, feelings of depression and anxiety, and financial dependence upon family and government resources.

The topics of employment and unemployment have received significant attention since the 1930s when, during the Great Depression, researchers began examining the psychological effects of long-term joblessness (Zawadski & Lazarsfeld, 1935). However, most of these studies have focused only on young and middle-aged men. The study of middle-aged and older women's employment experiences has not received significant research attention (Coyle, 1989). This gap in our knowledge has left the academic and policy-making communities with little information on the specific labor-market needs, aspirations, and experiences of middle-aged and older women. In addition, little is known about women's adjustment to unemployment and how their adjustment may differ from that of men (Donovan, Jaffe, & Pirie, 1987). As noted by authors such as Barrow (1986) and Blau (1985), additional research on middle-aged and older women in the work force is needed.

The current state of research on women and employment lags far behind their rates of participation in the labor force. Middle-aged women between the ages of 45 and 64 have steadily increased their presence in the work force. Whereas only 33 percent of women aged 45 to 64 were in the labor force in 1950, that number increased to 58 percent in 1990 and is projected to increase to approximately 65 percent by the year 2000 (U.S. Bureau of the Census, 1965; U.S. Department of Labor, 1985, 1990).

Unlike older men, whose participation in the labor force has declined over the past thirty years (Palmore, 1985), the participation of women aged 65 or over has remained relatively stable during this century. In 1900, 8.3 percent of these older women were in the labor force. In 1989 the percentage was 8.4 percent (Manheimer, 1994).

Although there are increasing numbers of women in the labor force, relatively little research, when compared with that on men, has been completed on their career aspirations, labor-market problems, and occupational patterns. Therefore, this chapter will address the following question: What do we know about the employment and unemployment experiences of middle-aged and older women? To answer this question, this chapter will examine and discuss recent research that has been completed on middle-aged and older women's employment and unemployment experiences. The following topical areas are included:

- Women in the labor force
- Employment and social functioning
- Discrimination in the workplace
- Unemployment and underemployment
- Job-search assistance

After the review of research in these five areas, a summary of major findings and conclusions concerning the employment experiences of middle-aged and older women will be presented.

WOMEN IN THE LABOR FORCE

Over twenty years ago, Kreps (1972) reviewed the literature on the participation of women in the labor force. While few research studies had been completed at that time, it was clear that women were becoming a significant portion of the labor force. Since that time, authors such as Rix (1990), Rosenthal (1990), Ruhm (1996), and Sandell (1987) have noted that the percentage of middle-aged women between 45 and 64 in the work force has steadily increased during the past forty years. In reflecting on this trend, Marshall (1983) and Manheimer (1994) have noted that the increased labor-force participation of women has direct implications for the social and economic status of older women in the future. This fact has also been recognized by groups such as the Roundtable on

Older Women in the Work Force (n.d.), which has met to discuss the subject of older women in the work force. This group has noted the important role that older women play in the labor market.

To fully understand the influence of middle-aged and older women in our work force, it is first important to define several terms. Women and men are defined as participants in the labor force by the U.S. Department of Labor if they are working, or unemployed but looking for work. Although government definitions differ, many experts define middle-aged workers as those between ages 45 and 64.[1] Older workers include persons aged 65 or over (Rix, 1990).

Labor-force participation among men has steadily declined since World War II (Manheimer, 1994; Ruhm, 1996). The availability of employer-paid pensions and Social Security benefits at age 62 are two significant factors that help to explain the decline in labor-market participation among middle-aged and older men (Schick & Schick, 1994). For women, however, the rate of labor-force participation is different. Since the 1940s the labor-market participation of women has increased dramatically. Factors such as World War II, during which many women went to work to support the war effort, and changes in gender roles and expectations have contributed to the increase of middle-aged and older women in the work force. In a study of labor-force participation, DeViney and O'Rand (1988) examined gender-cohort succession and retirement among older women and men from 1951 to 1984. Trends in occupational changes and retirement policies were examined to discuss how the job-force participation and retirement of older workers has changed over time. The authors noted that changes in the economy have produced more participation by women and reformed retirement policies have lessened male participation.

During the past twenty years this trend toward increased labor-force participation among middle-aged and older women has continued. In 1972, 44 percent of all women were in the labor force; in 1992 this percentage had increased to 58 percent (U.S. Department of Labor, 1992). For women aged 45 to 64, almost 59 percent were in the labor force in 1990, compared to only 49 percent in 1970 (U.S. Department of Labor, 1985, 1990).

While research has failed to keep pace with this increase of women in the work force, several recent publications underscore the growing interest in older women and work. Allen and Pifer (1993) explored common issues of aged women. Portions of this work are devoted to the subject of older women and employment. There is a discussion of new job opportunities for women, common occupations of women, discrimination, equity in pay, and projections for the future. Arendell and Estes (1991) examined work-related issues that affect older women. Inequalities in home and work roles were discussed, including discrimination in the workplace. Suggestions to lessen the discrimination faced by women were presented in the areas of Social Security, housing, and health. Further illustrating the growing interest in women and employment issues, Coyle (1989), in her annotated bibliography on women and aging, identified over twenty book, book-chapter, and serial references on the subject of older women and employment.

Several research studies have also been completed that examine the labor-force characteristics of middle-aged and older women, including patterns of job entry, reentry, and retention. Herz (1988) examined recent employment trends, changing work-life patterns, and occupational segregation between men and women in the work force. She also discussed the effects of race, education level, job opportunities, employment sector, and marital status upon labor-force participation. Herz noted that women with higher levels of education are more likely to work. Differences in earnings were reported to be impacted by marital status, with married women less likely to continue employment. Herz also found that the working experience of women prior to age 55 affects their labor-force participation as older workers.

In a study of 607 married couples on the topic of retirement and gender differences, Henretta, O'Rand, and Chan (1993) found that there were differences in retirement patterns depending upon the wife's employment during child rearing. Women who were employed showed little difference in relation to men. However, women who stayed at home during child rearing had a tendency to retire at a slower pace than men.

Shaw (1985) also examined the labor-force status and characteristics of older women who work. This author presented profiles of older women in terms of their characteristics, work experience, education, occupations, and earnings. Topics such as equal opportunity, age discrimination, and comparable worth were also highlighted. In a related publication Shaw (1983) examined the working lives of middle-aged women based on ten years of interviews. Drawn from the National Longitudinal Survey of the Work Experience of Mature Women, these data describe the characteristics and occupational trends among a nationally representative sample of 4,000 women aged 30 to 44. As in other recent research, Shaw highlighted the increased growth of middle-aged women in the work force.

Two recent studies have examined the retirement and employment patterns of older African Americans. Jackson and Gibson (1985) found that many African Americans work in old age because of low retirement benefits. They suggested that older African-American workers are more comfortable financially, but less satisfied with their personal life than African-American retirees.

Richardson and Kilty (1992) used a sample of 234 African-American professionals to measure their retirement and employment patterns. Workers with a strong commitment to work, those with limited financial investments, and those who relied on coworkers for social interaction continued working longer. Implications include assisting older African-American workers in making the transition between full-time employment and retirement. The authors noted that more research is needed on the employment experiences of older African-American adults.

During a time when many men have retired earlier than those in previous decades, why are women remaining in the labor force longer? Certainly such factors as greater employment opportunities for women, increased levels of education among women, and the personal job satisfaction experienced by many women have some influence on this trend. However, Manheimer (1994) asserted that the primary factor has been financial need. A related article by Iams (1986) supported Manheimer's assertion. This research examined the postretirement employment of a group of retired women. Data were collected through the 1982 Social Security Administration's New Beneficiary Survey. Subjects examined included pensions, health, additional income, and longest-held-job characteristics. The presence of a pension largely determined whether or not a woman worked after she began receiving Social Security benefits. The author noted that many women who do not receive a pension continue working to add to their low incomes. Regarding labor-force reentry among U.S. homemakers in midlife, Moen, Downey, and Bolger (1990) examined variables that influence homemakers to reenter the work force. Of all the variables studied, only age, marital dissolution, and education affected reentry to the job market considerably. Women in middle age who experienced divorce (often referred to as displaced homemakers) were likely to enter or reenter the labor force for income purposes.

Women are more likely than men to work in part-time positions (Rix, 1990). Bolnick (1987) examined the advantages of part-time work for older women who have served as secretaries. The author discussed a changing pattern among older secretaries who are of retirement age but who wish to continue working. Many times they are able to continue employment through part-time or temporary assignments, frequently at their previous job. Advantages for employees and employers were discussed in this article. In addition, this article included an evaluation of the effects of Social Security and taxes on earnings. In a related book Kahne (1985) also discussed the value and importance of part-time work for older workers. Part-time work provides both income and important social and psychological benefits for older workers.

In an article on gender differences in orientation toward retirement, Hatch (1992) reported findings from a study that surveyed the attitudes and orientation toward retirement of previously married female and male older workers and never-married older workers. Previously married women, due to poor financial states during retirement years, were found to be less likely to feel that older workers should retire. Previously married men identified themselves as being retirees more than the women. Women and men who were never married showed little variance in their attitudes toward retirement. However, the women were found to have a more positive outlook on life and their personal well-being than the men.

With men retiring earlier and the percentage of middle-aged women between 45 and 64 in the labor force continuing to increase, the subject of women and employment is very important. The work force in the United States is becoming more diverse, and middle-aged women are a significant part of this growing diversity. Additional research is needed to more fully document the characteristics and trends of middle-aged and older women who continue working. This trend of women in the work force has important implications for research, government labor policies, and employers.

EMPLOYMENT AND SOCIAL FUNCTIONING

With the increase of middle-aged and older women in the work force, some research has been published that addresses the relationship between their labor-force participation and social-psychological, and economic functioning. However, in comparison to similar research on men, the number and breadth of these studies are really quite meager. Coyle (1989) noted this trend in her examination of research on women and aging. This section summarizes what is known about the relationship between social-psychological and economic functioning and the labor-force activity of middle-aged and older women.

Social-Psychological Functioning

Prior research has shown that paid employment provides women with feelings of self-worth, empowerment, and self-control (Ferree, 1976; Rubin, 1981). Employment also appears to be related to the life satisfaction experienced by working women. Riddick (1985) examined the topic of life satisfaction for older female homemakers. This study used a representative sample of the population of women to determine levels of life satisfaction. The sample consisted of 403 homemakers, 698 retirees, and 119 older workers. Employment status was found to impact the level of life satisfaction of older women. Older employed women had a greater level of life satisfaction than those who were homemakers or had already retired. Income and health problems affected the life satisfaction of all three cohorts.

In a related study Henry (1991) examined the relationship of life satisfaction with patterns of past employment and homemaking responsibility for older women. This study focused on a group of older women in Brooklyn, New York. Their past patterns of employment and homemaking experiences were compared with their current level of life satisfaction. Results of the study suggested that past employment and homemaking do not significantly affect life satisfaction. Variables such as perceived health and financial well-being were found to be more related to life satisfaction.

These two studies by Riddick and Henry suggest that while current employment does seem to be related to perceptions of life satisfaction among older women, past employment does not. One possible explanation for this is that many older women tend to take on new roles, such as volunteering, following retirement. One study has examined this issue. Stephan (1991) reported results from a study conducted to assess the volunteer activity of retired older women. The author presented two views in regard to the relationship between volunteering and employment. One view suggested that retired women volunteer in order to gain employment opportunities, whereas the other view proposed that they volunteer as a substitute for employment. Results from the study provided support for the latter view, although the data also supported the notion that volunteering can lead to employment for some older women.

McNeely (1989) examined the topics of gender, job satisfaction, earnings, and other characteristics of human service workers during and after midlife. This study examined the level of job satisfaction experienced by public welfare workers during and after midlife. The study also examined the status of women in the workplace in terms of job status and earnings. The findings suggested that females with levels of education, occupational status, and number of years on the job similar to those of their male counterparts are often employed in lower-status and lower-paying jobs. However, they also often report higher job satisfaction than their male counterparts.

Two studies have examined the relationship between labor-force activity and social support experienced by older women. Depner and Ingersoll (1982) examined the relationship between labor-force status and social support. In their study the authors found that the social support of a retired woman is related to age, gender, and participation in the labor force in later life. Another study has shown that paid work can mediate the effects of spousal death on an older woman's health. In a study by Aber (1992), 157 widows (aged 55–75) were sampled to determine the relationship between paid work, health, and independence during widowhood. Results suggested that paid work during married life may assist in health protection in widowhood. Positive results from paid work in widowhood may include greater recognition of personal abilities, improved stress management, and increased self-confidence.

Economic Functioning

Olson (1990) discussed the need for ensuring the economic security of aging women. The author noted that despite the fact that 58 percent of the elderly are women, 71 percent of the poor elderly are women. Women are increasing their labor-force participation; however, they face unequal employment opportunities due to such factors as gender discrimination that can result in extended periods of unemployment and wage disparities when compared with men. In a related publication Rayman (1990) also examined the subject of inequality experienced by older women workers and suggested that this inequality in the labor force has an adverse effect on women's economic well-being.

In another study Estes, Gerard, and Clarke (1984) also examined the topic of women and the economics of aging. These authors asserted that social and economic problems encountered by women early in life tend to result in the disparities found between men and women in old age. In an article on the relationship between poverty, retirement, and widowhood, Holden, Burkhauser, and Feaster (1988) discussed the chance of older persons falling into poverty after retirement. Results of this study showed that a fall into poverty by those who were not poor before a husband retired is closely related to the event of retirement and the death of a retired husband. The authors noted that when a husband dies, a woman is often vulnerable to becoming impoverished. Age discrimination also impacts on the economic status of middle-aged and older women. This topic is discussed in the next section.

DISCRIMINATION IN THE WORKPLACE

Age discrimination is a significant obstacle for many older women who are seeking employment (Rosenthal, 1990). Nationally, the Age Discrimination in Employment Act (ADEA) is intended to protect workers aged 40 or over from discriminatory practices at work. Provisions in this legislation cover hiring, compensation, working conditions, promotions, employee training, termination, and retirement. Over the past decade the number of age-discrimination charges filed with the Equal Employment Opportunity Commission (EEOC) has grown dramatically. In 1980, 11,397 charges of age-related discrimination were filed with the EEOC. In 1987 the number of annual charges had grown to 24,110 (American Association of Retired Persons, 1993). While this increase is of concern, age discrimination against older workers is not new. For example, Hushbeck (1989) noted that age discrimination can be documented as affecting older workers in the late nineteenth century following the Civil War.

Nuccio (1989) noted that the double standard of aging defines women as old at an earlier age than men and that this has led to speculation that discrimination in employment may be a problem for women at ages younger than 40, the age established by Congress as the lower limit for age-discrimination protection. Weiss (1984) presented information on issues concerning job discrimination and older women. Legal issues and remedies were explained. This publication will be useful to people interested in understanding the issues of employment discrimination, age, and legal remedies for older women. More recently, this same author (Weiss, 1989) has written a handbook on litigating age- and sex-discrimination cases. This reference will be useful to those persons who are interested in exploring whether or not to file an age-discrimination case.

Other authors have discussed the subject of age discrimination upon middle-aged and older workers. Achenbaum (1991) examined the historical context of the Age Discrimination in Employment Act. The author discussed ADEA as a combination of two pieces of legislation and noted the resemblance of the antidiscriminatory section to Title VII of the Civil Rights Act of 1964.

The American Association of Retired Persons (1987) outlined provisions of the ADEA, who is covered, discrimination remedies, and issues in filing a lawsuit. This guide is helpful for persons interested in knowing more about the ADEA and those considering filing a lawsuit. Hushbeck (1989) explored discrimination against older workers beginning during the American Revolution and continuing through industrialization. The effects of big business on older workers during industrialization were discussed. Issues such as economic instability, unemployment, and technological change were also examined. Chapters on organizational and institutional impediments to older workers and public and private-sector responses to the plight of older workers were included.

Wanner and McDonald (1983) also examined the effects of discrimination upon older workers, including women. They noted that the decline in older workers' wages is a form of discrimination if the older worker's productivity has remained the same. Some possible reasons given for this decline include that older workers may be forced to take new jobs at lower wages or may be fearful of not finding alternative employment and accept lower wages. Other authors have discussed legal provisions for guarding against age discrimination (Fretz & Dudovitz, 1987), the effects of age discrimination (Borgatta, 1991; Dreyer, 1992; Hassell & Perrewe, 1993), criteria for age-discrimination suits, including overqualification (Levine, 1993), common mistakes made by employers related to age discrimination (Perry, 1992), and special issues for women and the disabled (Quirk, 1991).

UNEMPLOYMENT AND UNDEREMPLOYMENT

With the increase of women in the labor force and the impacts of age and gender discrimination, the problem of unemployment for middle-aged and older women has become an important concern. During the 1980s the unemployment rate for older women exceeded the rate for men. Older women, as compared to men, are particularly vulnerable during periods of unemployment. Recent research has shown that older women are more likely to experience severe emotional and financial difficulties when faced with extended unemployment. Older women are often unemployed for longer periods than older men and may have less orderly and less extensive work histories (Rife, Toomey, & First, 1989).

The special obstacles faced by older women in the workplace are reflected in statistics about poverty in the United States. Women possess less economic resources than men and are disproportionately represented among the unemployed and poor. Many women are members of the "working poor"—those who often work one or more jobs but whose wages fail to provide a decent standard of living above the poverty level. The jobs held by many women are characterized by low pay and status. For example, women held 62 percent of all service industry jobs in 1986, and their annual average earnings were only 64.3 percent of what men were earning (Harrington, 1987).

While the rate of unemployment for older workers over age 50 may be lower than that for other age groups, those who experience unemployment are often subject to more serious consequences (Atchley, 1985). Older workers, and especially older women, are more likely to remain unemployed for longer periods of time than are other age groups. Often, these periods of unemployment extend beyond the length of their unemployment benefits (U.S. Department of Labor, 1989).

Although unemployment and underemployment are problems for many middle-aged and older women, few studies have examined the effects of joblessness on women. While research is now beginning to correct this bias, we lack a complete understanding of how women may differ from men in their adjustment to unemployment.

Two recent international studies have documented some differences between men and women when they become jobless. Shamir (1985) and Davies and Esseveld (1985) found that women may substitute housework, child care, and other family-type responsibilities for prior employment roles. The authors of both studies suggested that this identification of multiple roles may buffer some of the negative impact of unemployment, especially when the women are not financially pressed. They also suggested that women value their nonwork activities more than men, and so the loss of work is not as significant to their total self-concept. However, Davies and Esseveld noted that women report that housework does not fully compensate for the loss of a social role provided by employment.

Regarding the impact of unemployment on the mental health of women, Briar (1978), in a study of industrial unemployment affecting 52 women and men during the 1970–72 recession, reported that most of her unemployed participants displayed feelings of worthlessness from their job losses. Donovan, Jaffe, and Pirie (1987, p. 302), in a study of 61 unemployed women, found that the loss of income from joblessness was "the most devastating experience" for women, but that other effects, such as a loss of self-esteem, increased family strain, and loss of workplace social supports, also had an adverse impact. Castro, Romero, and Cervantes (1987) studied Latino women following the closing of a tuna plant. Interviewed eighteen months after the closing, these women were still experiencing stress. Brenner and Levi (1987) followed unemployed women over two years and compared them to women who were employed. These authors documented a lower degree of well-being and higher levels of depression in the unemployed women.

The relationship between involuntary unemployment and serious mental health problems has been further documented by Robins et al. (1984). These authors asserted that working women who become impoverished by unemployment are at a high risk of experiencing serious mental health problems. The authors noted that while rates of mental health problems do not seem to differ by gender, women are more likely to suffer from such disorders as depression and anxiety, while men manifest their distress through the abuse of substances.

While it is commonly thought that the support provided by friends and relatives may mediate the stress and depression often experienced by unemployed persons, some research is emerging that qualifies this assumption for middle-aged and older women. This research indicates that friends and relatives can actually contribute to the stress and anxiety experienced by unemployed women. Ratcliff and Bogdan (1988) reported that while some unemployed middle-aged women suffer from a lack of caring friends and relatives, it seems more typical that a woman may be surrounded by "caring" others who actually undermine the importance of the work activity that she values as important. Rife (1995) has also found this to occur in his study of middle-aged and older unemployed women over the age of 50.

Finally, the seriousness of income loss by unemployed women is underscored by the fact that many women are the sole or primary wage earners of their families. Even when a family has multiple wage earners, women's wages contribute 33.6 percent of white family income and 52.7 percent of black family income (Abramovitz, 1984). Further, Manheimer (1994) noted that most women who work do so out of economic necessity rather than for personal fulfillment. Accordingly, the loss of income by women is a serious threat to their economic independence.

JOB-SEARCH ASSISTANCE

Given the challenges faced by middle-aged and older women who are searching for employment, a number of publications are available that attempt to assist them during the job search. Many of these offer suggestions and advice on such job-search tasks as completing applications, developing a resume, and participating in interviews. For example, Azibo and Unumb (1980) identified techniques for finding and securing employment. Specific focus was placed on planning to overcome labor-market problems faced by single, divorced, separated, widowed, and married homemakers. Brody (1983), in a book on midlife career changes, also examined job-search strategies for middle-aged women. Fredericks (1981) outlined several steps that are important to a woman's job search: self-assessment, goal setting, resume development, and job-search and interview techniques.

Allen and Gorkin (1985), in their book *Finding the Right Job at Midlife*, provided tips on job seeking for middle-aged and older workers. The authors focused on such topics as identifying skills, resumes, applications, and career planning. In a book with a similar purpose and theme Anthony and Roe (1991) provided the over-40 job seeker with an easy-to-follow self-assessment tool in order to prepare for the job search. This book discusses the importance of individual skills and strengths and provides suggestions for overcoming obstacles and barriers to employment. The book is divided into three parts: examining yourself as a potential employee, how to market yourself and locate employment opportunities, and detailed information on how to interview successfully.

Birsner (1987) also offered tips and suggestions for the female job seeker. The author included material on writing resumes and letters and discussed such topics as the emotional stages of unemployment, time management, image, finances, and leisure activities during the job search. The National Center for Women and Retirement Research (n.d.) has published a workbook that will be of interest to middle-aged and older women. Topics include assertiveness, support systems, a healthy work environment, coping with stress, and work after retirement.

Using personal case studies, Berman (1980) examined issues related to older women reentering the work force and offered advice for job searching, training, and accepting a job. Sources of information on educational programs, financial aid, and career counseling were also provided. The case studies are realistic and will be of interest to women considering reentering the work force. Crawley and Dancy (1984) also provided useful tips and suggestions for the older worker seeking employment. They presented sample resumes, application forms, and cover letters, as well as possible questions the older worker may face during an interview. In a similar publication, Harty (1991) also provided advice for the older job seeker. Topics covered include ideas for improved self-assessment, job discovery, polish and preparation, and examining the interview process. Morgan (1987) has produced an informative and useful job-seeking manual for the older worker. The author identified obstacles that older workers must confront and offered helpful advice while also assisting the older worker to identify strengths that can be used to obtain employment. The book helps to build the self-confidence of the older worker and is practical in the tips and advice offered.

Three publications examine ways of increasing the job-placement success of middle-aged and older women. An article by Rife (1992) described a group practice strategy used to assist older women in finding employment. This author has found that group counseling can be an effective technique for increasing the job-search self-efficacy of older female workers. In a book on building public/ private coalitions for promoting older women's employment opportunities, the Older Women's League (1987) identified effective strategies for increasing opportunities for the employment of older women. The book also discussed advantages and potential problem areas when building coalitions. In a publication on program resources, Miller (1989) examined employment and training services for middle-aged displaced homemakers who are entering the labor force.

In two books that address self-employment opportunities for the middle-aged and older worker, the authors provided suggestions on starting a business. Myers and Anderson (1984) provided exercises on job-search planning, identifying skills, and examining career interests. Special attention was given to starting businesses and using transferable skills. Case studies of successful older entrepreneurs and a listing of profitable businesses and franchises were provided. Selden (1989) also discussed going into business for oneself. The author helped readers to assess their interest in self-employment, identified entrepreneurial characteristics, and addressed myths about self-employment. Information was also presented on organizing the business, the business plan, start-up financing, and record keeping. This is a helpful book for those who are considering self-employment.

Finally, Stark (1983) offered advice to the middle-aged and older woman seeking to reenter the work force. This book includes information on career options, goal setting, job-search strategies, interviewing, and balancing home and work. Exercises on decision making at each stage of the job search are provided. Resume writing is also discussed. This is a useful source for the older female job searcher.

SUMMARY OF RESEARCH FINDINGS

The purpose of this chapter has been to present recent research findings on women, aging, and work. This research, while in many ways incomplete and exploratory in nature, nonetheless indicates that middle-aged and older women are a significant segment of our work force and that their characteristics and needs often differ from those of men. Research on work and middle-aged and older women is best characterized by several principle themes:

Theme One: Our Labor Force Is Changing

During the twentieth century the percentage of middle-aged and older women in the labor market has increased steadily. Since World War II this trend has continued even while men have been retiring at earlier ages. Middle-aged and older women are more likely to reenter the labor market, and they will remain in the labor force longer than men. However, once they are hired, occupational segregation of women in low-wage, service-sector jobs often results in wage disparities between women and men. Women are also more likely to be part-time workers than are men.

Theme Two: Income Is the Primary Reason Women Enter the Labor Force

Middle-aged and older women enter the labor market or continue working for many reasons: self-definition and esteem, social support, a sense of belonging, and a sense of fulfillment. Work is related to life satisfaction for many women. However, the primary reason that middle-aged and older women work is to obtain income to support themselves and their families. Caring for children, families, and even ill parents often means that women are more likely than men to move in and out of the labor force. This movement has an impact on wages and often results in wage disparities.

Theme Three: Women Are Often Disadvantaged in the Labor Market

Middle-aged female workers are more likely to work in low-wage, low-benefit positions than are their male counterparts. Middle-aged and older women are also less likely to qualify for pensions because they have been employed for shorter periods, are in positions that do not provide pensions, or qualify for pensions that provide inadequate retirement incomes. While Title VII of the Civil Rights Act and the Age Discrimination in Employment Act bar gender and age discrimination in the workplace, middle-aged and older women are likely to experience discrimination at some point during their work-force participation.

Theme Four: Unemployment Has a Negative Impact

Middle-aged and older women are often employed in low-pay, high-turnover positions that result in frequent layoffs. Older workers are more likely to remain unemployed beyond the length of unemployment benefits than are other age groups. Because of the double impact of both age and gender discrimination, middle-aged and older women are particularly vulnerable. Often, extended unemployment results in affective disorders such as depression and anxiety. It can also have serious economic consequences.

Theme Five: Additional Research Is Needed

Inadequate attention has been paid to the experiences and needs of middle-aged and older female workers by both the academic and policy-making communities. Most research on employment and older workers has focused only on men. The small body of research on women and employment that exists lacks coherence and consistency. It is often based on small unrepresentative samples, is exploratory or descriptive in nature, and lacks a theoretical basis for inquiry. Few studies are longitudinal. Even fewer replications have been completed. Studies that examine differences among women based on marital status, education, ethnicity, family and economic characteristics, and type of occupations are also lacking. The present state of research on work and middle-aged and older women is best described as immature.

Current research is needed in five topical areas: (1) labor-force characteristics of middle-aged and older women, (2) the impact of age discrimination upon job seeking, (3) the long-term effects of unemployment, (4) effective strategies for assisting women to find and secure employment, and (5) current older-worker social and economic policies in the United States such as Social Security and early-retirement incentive programs. Research designs that are longitudinal and lead to both theory and policy development are also needed. As well, research that is inclusive and examines differences among women based on age, ethnicity, marital status, educational level, and type of occupation is also important.

CONCLUSION

The percentage of middle-aged and older persons in the United States will continue to increase dramatically during the next thirty years. The future status of middle-aged and older female workers will be influenced by social, economic, and legislative factors. With legislated changes in the Social Security program, which will prevent retirees from drawing full benefits until age 67 or perhaps later, more women may need to work for extended periods. In addition, most analysts predict that the labor-force participation of women will continue to gradually increase well into the next century. Additional research will be needed to better understand the impact of these trends on our work force, on our families, and on middle-aged and older women themselves.

NOTE

1. Government definitions of "older workers" vary according to legislative program and type of service. For example, under the Age Discrimination in Employment Act (ADEA), workers are defined as "old" and eligible for protection from age discrimination at age 40. At age 55, workers are defined as "older" and are eligible for employment assistance services under Title V of the Older Americans Act. Currently, workers are eligible for early Social Security benefits at age 62.

REFERENCES

Aber, Cynthia. (1992). Spousal death, a threat to women's health: Paid work as a "resistance resource." *Image: The Journal of Nursing Scholarship, 24*(2), 95–99.

Abramovitz, Mimi. (1984). Blaming women for unemployment: Refuting a myth. *Social Casework, 65*, 547–553.

Achenbaum, W. Andrew. (1991). Putting ADEA into historical context. *Research on Aging, 13*(4), 463.

Allen, Jeffrey, & Gorkin, Jess. (1985). *Finding the right job at midlife*. New York: Simon & Schuster.

Allen, Jessie, & Pifer, Alan. (1993). *Women on the front lines: Meeting the challenge of an aging America*. Washington, DC: Urban Institute Press.

American Association of Retired Persons. (1987). *The Age Discrimination in Employment Act Guarantees you certain rights. Here's how . . .* Washington, DC: Author.

———. (1993). Federal and state age discrimination charges increase 112 percent, 1980–1990. *Working Age, 9*(1), 5.

Anthony, Rebecca, & Roe, Gerald. (1991). *Over 40 and looking for work? A guide for the unemployed, underemployed, and unhappily employed*. Holbrook, MA: Bob Adams.

Arendell, Terry, & Estes, Carroll. (1991). Older women in the post-Reagan era. *International Journal of Health Services, 21*(1), 59–73.

Atchley, Robert. (1985). *Social forces and aging* (4th ed.). Belmont, CA: Wadsworth.

Azibo, Moni, & Unumb, Therese. (1980). *The mature women's back-to-work book*. Chicago: Contemporary Books.

Barrow, Georgia. (1986). *Aging, the individual, and society* (4th ed.). St. Paul, MN: West Publishing Company.

Berman, Eleanor. (1980). *Re-entering: Successful back-to-work strategies for women seeking a fresh start*. New York: Crown.

Birsner, E. Patricia. (1987). *The 40+ job-hunting guide*. New York: Arco.

Blau, Zena. (1985). *Current perspectives on aging and the life cycle: Work, retirement, and social policy*. Greenwich, CT: JAI Press.

Bolnick, Rae. (1987). Unretired secretaries. *Secretary, 47*(9), 19–21.

Borgatta, Edgar. (1991). Age discrimination issues. *Research on Aging, 13*(4), 476–484.
Brenner, Sten, & Levi, Lennart. (1987). Long-term unemployment among women in Sweden. *Social Science and Medicine, 25*(2), 153–161.
Briar, Katharine. (1978). *The effect of long-term unemployment on workers and their families.* San Francisco: R & E Research Associates.
Brody, Jean. (1983). *Mid-life careers.* Philadelphia, PA: Westminster, John Knox.
Castro, Felipe, Romero, Gloria, & Cervantes, Richard. (1987). Long-term stress among Latino women after a plant closure. *Sociology and Social Research, 71*(2), 85–88.
Coyle, Jean. (1989). *Women and aging: A selected, annotated bibliography.* Westport, CT: Greenwood Press.
Crawley, Brenda, & Dancy, Joseph. (1984). *Mature/older job seeker's guide.* Washington, DC: National Council on the Aging.
Davies, Karen, & Esseveld, Johanna. (1989). Factory women, redundancy, and the search for work: Toward a reconceptualization of employment and unemployment. *The Sociological Review, 37*, 219–252.
Depner, Charlene, & Ingersoll, B. (1982). Employment status and social support: The experience of the mature woman. In M. Szinovacz (Ed.), *Women's retirement: Policy implications of recent research.* Beverly Hills, CA: Sage Publications.
DeViney, Stanley, & O'Rand, Angela. (1988). Gender-cohort succession and retirement among older men and women, 1951 to 1984. *Sociological Quarterly, 29*(4), 525–540.
Donovan, Roberta, Jaffe, Nina, & Pirie, Valerie. (1987, July–August). Unemployment among low-income women: An exploratory study. *Social Work,* pp. 301–305.
Dreyer, R. S. (1992, January). Too old for what? *Supervision, 53,* pp. 16–17.
Estes, Carroll, Gerard, Lenore, & Clarke, Adele. (1984). Women and the economics of aging. *International Journal of Health Services, 14*(1), 55–68.
Ferree, Myra. (1976). Working class jobs: Housework and paid work as sources of satisfaction. *Social Problems, 23,* 431–441.
Fredericks, Susan. (1981). *How grandma got a job—In the business jungle.* Great Neck, NY: Todd & Honeywell.
Fretz, Burton, & Dudovitz, Neal. (1987). *The law of age discrimination: A reference manual.* Chicago: National Clearinghouse for Legal Services.
Garner, J. Dianne, & Mercer, Susan. (Eds.). (1989). *Women as they age: Challenge, opportunity, and triumph.* New York: Haworth Press.
Harrington, Michael. (1987). *Who are the poor?: A profile of the changing faces of poverty in the United States in 1987.* Washington, DC: Justice for All National Office.
Harty, Karen. (1991). *50 and starting over: Career strategies for success.* Hollywood, CA: Newcastle.
Hassell, Barbara, & Perrewe, Pamela. (1993). An examination of the relationship between older workers' perceptions of age discrimination and employee psychological states. *Journal of Managerial Issues, 5*(1), 109–120.
Hatch, Laurie. (1992). Gender differences in orientation toward retirement from paid labor. *Gender and Society, 6*(1), 66–85.
Henretta, John, O'Rand, Angela, & Chan, Christopher. (1993). Gender differences in employment after spouse's retirement. *Research on Aging, 15*(2), 148–169.
Henry, Mary. (1991). The relationship of life satisfaction to patterns of past employment

and homemaking responsibility for older women. *Journal of Women and Aging,* *3*(1), 5–21.

Herz, Diane. (1988, September). Employment characteristics of older women, 1987. *Monthly Labor Review, 111,* pp. 3–12.

Holden, Karen, Burkhauser, Richard, & Feaster, Daniel. (1988). The timing of falls into poverty after retirement and widowhood. *Demography, 25*(3), 405–414.

Hushbeck, Judith. (1989). *Old and obsolete: Age discrimination and the American worker, 1860–1920.* New York: Garland Publishing.

Iams, Howard. (1986). Employment of retired-worker women. *Social Security Bulletin, 49*(3), 5–13.

Jackson, James, & Gibson, Rose. (1985). Work and retirement among the black elderly. *Current Perspectives on Aging and the Life Cycle, 1,* 193–222.

Kahne, Hilda. (1985). *Reconceiving part-time work: New perspectives for older workers and women.* Totowa, NJ: Rowman & Allanheld.

Kreps, Juanita. (1972). Sex in the marketplace: American women at work. In M. Purvine (Ed.), *Manpower and employment: A source book for social workers* (pp. 151– 161). New York: Council on Social Work Education.

Levine, Marvin. (1993). Age discrimination in employment: The over qualified older worker. *Labor Law Journal, 44*(7), 440–444.

McNeely, R. L. (1989). Gender, job satisfaction, earnings, and other characteristics of human service workers during and after midlife. *Administration in Social Work, 13*(2), 99–116.

Manheimer, Ronald. (1994). *Older Americans almanac.* Detroit, MI: Gale Research.

Marshall, F. Ray. (1983). *Work and women in the 1980s: A perspective on basic trends affecting women's jobs and job opportunities.* Washington, DC: Women's Research and Education Institute.

Mercer, Susan, & Garner, J. Dianne. (1989). An international overview of aged women. *Journal Of Women and Aging, 1*(1–3), 13–45.

Miller, Jill. (1989). Displaced homemakers in the employment and training system. In S. Harlan & R. Steinberg (Eds.), *Job training for women: The promise and limits of public policies.* Philadelphia: Temple University Press.

Moen, Phyllis, Downey, Geraldine, & Bolger, Niall. (1990). Labor-force reentry among U.S. homemakers in midlife: A life-course analysis. *Gender and Society, 4*(2), 230–243.

Morgan, John. (1987). *Getting a job after 50.* Princeton, NJ: Petrocelli.

Myers, Albert, & Anderson, Christopher. (1984). *Success over sixty.* New York: Summit.

National Center for Women and Retirement Research. (n.d.). *Employment and retirement issues for women.* Southampton, NY: Long Island University.

Nuccio, Kathleen. (1989). The double standard of aging and older women's employment. *Journal of Women & Aging, 1*(1–3), 317–338.

O'Bryant, Shirley. (1991). Older widows and independent lifestyles. *International Journal of Aging and Human Development, 32*(1), 41–51.

Older Women's League. (1987). *Building public/private coalitions for older women's employment: An OWL guidebook.* Washington, DC: Author.

Olson, Paulette. (1990). Mature women and the rewards of domestic ideology. *Journal of Economic Issues, 24,* 633–643.

Palmore, Erdman. (1985). *Retirement: Causes and consequences.* New York: Springer Publishing Company.

Perry, Phillip. (1992, October 24). Don't get sued for age discrimination. *Editor and Publisher, The Fourth Estate, 125*, 24–25.

Quirk, William. (1991). *New hiring, promotion, and termination rules for the 1990's: New rules dealing with the disabled, older workers, and women*. New York: Institute for Management, Panel Publishers.

Ratcliff, Kathryn, & Bogdan, Janet. (1988). Unemployed women: When "social support" is not supportive. *Social Problems, 35*(3), 54–63.

Rayman, Paula. (1990). *Resiliency amidst inequality: Older women workers in an aging United States*. Southport, CT: Project on Women and Aging, Southport Institute for Policy Analysis.

Richardson, Virginia, & Kilty, Keith. (1992). Retirement intentions among black professionals: Implications for practice with older black adults. *Gerontologist, 32*(1), 7–16.

Riddick, Carol. (1985). Life satisfaction for older female homemakers, retirees, and workers. *Research on Aging, 7*(3), 383–393.

Rife, John. (1992). A group practice strategy for helping unemployed older women find employment. *Journal of Women and Aging, 4*(1), 25–38.

————. (1995). Older unemployed women and job search activity: The role of social support. *Journal of Women and Aging, 7*(3), 55–68.

Rife, John, Toomey, B., & First, R. (1989). Adjustment to unemployment among older women. *Affilia: The Journal of Women and Social Work, 4*(3), 65–77.

Rix, Sara. (1990). *Older workers*. Santa Barbara, CA: ABC-CLIO.

Robins, Lee, Helzer, John, Weissman, Myrna, Orvaschel, Helen, Gruenberg, Ernest, Burke, Jack, & Regier, Darrel. (1984). Lifetime prevalence of specific psychiatric disorders in three sites. *Archives of General Psychiatry, 41*, 949–958.

Rosenthal, Evelyn. (Ed.). (1990). *Women, aging, and ageism*. New York: Haworth Press.

Roundtable on Older Women in the Work Force. (n.d.). *Roundtable on older women in the work force: Proceedings and recommendations*. Washington, DC: Author.

Rubin, Lillian. (1981). *Why should women work?* Center for Research and Education for Women, University of California at Berkeley.

Ruhm, Christopher. (1996). Historical trends in the employment and labor force participation of older Americans. In William Crown (Ed.), *Handbook on employment of the elderly*. Westport, CT: Greenwood Press.

Sandell, Steven. (Ed.). (1987). *The problem isn't age*. New York: Praeger.

Schick, Frank, & Schick, Renee. (Eds.). (1994). *Statistical handbook on aging Americans*, Phoenix, AZ: Oryx Press.

Selden, Ina. (1989). *Going into business for yourself: New beginnings after 50*. Glenview, IL: Scott, Foresman.

Shamir, Boas. (1985). Sex differences in psychological adjustment to unemployment and reemployment: A question of commitment, alternatives, or finance? *Social Problems, 33*(1), 67–79.

Shaw, Lois. (Ed.). (1983). *Unplanned careers: The working lives of middle-aged women*. Lexington, MA: Lexington Books.

————. (1985). *Older women at work*. Washington, DC: Women's Research and Education Institute.

Stark, Sandra. (1983). *Returning to work: A planning book for women*. New York: McGraw-Hill.

Stephan, Paula. (1991). Relationships among market work, work aspirations, and volunteering: The case of retired women. *Nonprofit and Voluntary Sector Quarterly, 20*(2), 225–236.

U.S. Bureau of the Census. (1965). *The statistical history of the United States from colonial times to the present.* Stamford, CT: Fairfield.

U.S. Department of Labor. (1989). *Labor market problems of older workers.* Washington, DC: U.S. Government Printing Office.

———, Bureau of Labor Statistics. (1985, June). *Handbook of labor statistics.* Washington, DC: U.S. Government Printing Office.

———. (1990, January). *Employment and earnings.* Washington, DC: U.S. Government Printing Office.

———. (1992). Unpublished tables on 1991 work experience. Washington, DC: U.S. Government Printing Office.

Wanner, Richard, & McDonald, Lynn. (1983). Ageism in the labor market: Estimating earnings discrimination against older workers. *Journal of Gerontology, 38*(6), 738–744.

Weiss, Francine. (1984). *Older women and job discrimination: A primer.* Washington, DC: Older Women's League.

———. (1989). *Employment discrimination against older women: A handbook on litigating age and sex discrimination cases.* Washington, DC: Older Women's League.

Zawadski, Bohan, & Lazarsfeld, Paul. (1935). The psychological consequences of unemployment. *Journal of Social Psychology, 6*(2), 244–251.

Eight

Retirement and Women

FRANCES M. CARP

Retirement is a rather recent phenomenon in the industrial nations. Their expanding populations and increases in life expectancy brought pressure to remove older persons from the labor force in order to make room for younger ones (Sussman, 1972). Contrary to the commonly held view that the retiree struggles to adjust to a life without work, a review of the literature shows that retirement has become a normal event for most older workers in the industrialized sectors of the world (Phillipson, 1989).

However, most workers who have been studied were men. One reason is that women's entry to the labor force and consequent involvement with retirement are even more recent than societal creation of the phenomenon. Also, "The notion of retirement as a male phenomenon rests on the premise that a man's status and identity is obtained through work while a woman's social position is derived primarily through her family roles" (Erdner & Guy, 1990, p. 129).

There have been dramatic changes in women's roles in American society, particularly within the past quarter century. Women comprised 18% of the labor force in 1890, 44% in 1965, 55% in 1985, and 60% in 1990. This was accompanied and partly explained by advances in education among women. Young women who want or need to work are no longer limited to the triad: teacher, secretary, nurse. Other options are open to them. Increasingly, college women prepare for careers that have rewards intrinsic to the work, their careers are important to women pursuing them, and career women have high life satisfaction (Carp, 1992). Other women must try to find and keep any jobs that pay for the necessities of life. Work is important in the lives of increasing numbers of American women, and so, therefore, is retirement—the valedictory of a successful career or exit from work because there are no job opportunities for older women.

There is need for research on the retirement experience of female as well as male workers, and the further need for research on the relationships of retirement to employment history, types of work, and retirement attitudes—all of which may influence study outcomes within one gender group and on all of which women vary from men (Belgrave, 1989; Phillipson, 1989). Hendricks (1993) expanded on this theme, recognizing that it is egregious to assume that all men or all women have the same experiences, and that failure to recognize the roles of personal resources and of participation in the labor force perpetuates inequality. He noted that feminist scholars have added an important analytic dimension to customary research procedures by emphasizing that gender is not only an attribute but also a relationship, and that the work of feminist scholars has sensitized investigators to gender as well as racial/ethnic and social-class biases in previous work. Now we turn to substantive research on women's retirement.

FINANCIAL CONSIDERATIONS

The most consistent research finding is that retirement is financially problematic for women. Old women in all racial and ethnic groups in this country have fewer economic resources than do old men (Hatch, 1990), and old women from minority groups are the poorest (Logue, 1991; Rayman, Allshouse, & Allen, 1993). Though income drops significantly at retirement, the transition from work to retirement is no longer economically perilous for most married couples, but the transition during retirement from spouse to survivor remains financially hazardous, much more so for widows than for widowers (Burkhauser, 1990).

Writing about poverty among older women, Meyer (1990) subtitled her article "The Gendered Distribution of Retirement Income in the United States." Nuccio (1989) discussed the "double standard in our patriarchal society that values youth." In this society older women bear unusually heavy economic penalties that increase with age. Over the entire life course the "economic risks of gender roles" are apparent (Burkhauser & Duncan, 1989). The economic well-being of women is threatened more greatly than that of men by life events such as divorce or separation, death of the spouse, birth of a child, loss of proximity to other family members, disability, or loss of work due to illness. These investigators suggested that today's social safety net was designed to protect the family of the 1930s and does not meet the needs of people in today's world.

Women are penalized in wages during working years and in pensions after retirement. The poverty experienced by many working women extends to their retirement and colors their psychological, physical, and social well-being (Perkins, 1992).

Work experiences, occupation, and characteristics of industry and business build up different economic resources in retirement for men versus women and minorities (Hatch, 1990). Women are moving toward work patterns traditionally associated with men, but they are not converging with men in pay at work or in retirement benefits. This is attributed largely to women's interrupted job records (Hatch, 1990). These broken job histories result from limited opportunities, social prohibition against women having careers, husbands' pride in the role of provider, and women's allegiance to the caregiver role. Most working-class women are limited to occupations with equal (but low) wages for women and men and that often carry no retirement benefits. Women in sex-segregated jobs—where men get better assignments and pay—leave those jobs with insecure retirement incomes.

Pension-covered career positions last longer and more frequently end with permanent retirement (Ruhm, 1991). However, for many men and women, the job ends before the person is ready to retire, and retirement is followed by postcareer employment of some sort. In attempting to reenter the work force, older people are at a disadvantage compared to younger people, and older women are at an even greater disadvantage than are older men (Hardy, 1991). The disadvantage is clear even when preretirement job status and education are controlled. Thus, in addition to gender bias in educational opportunity and job status, gender per se is an additional impediment to work-force reentry. Working-class women, with histories of low-paid jobs without retirement benefits, have few financial resources for retirement and often must try to find work to supplement their incomes (Perkins, 1993). Jobs available to them are limited and pay poorly. Despite greater commitment to paid work among women approaching retirement age, work absences and intermittent careers, as well as concentration in low-pay work, leave women heavily dependent on Social Security for retirement incomes.

WHAT LIES IN THE FUTURE?

Probably this heavy dependence on Social Security benefits will persist. Rix (1993) and others have suggested that reform in the Social Security system is necessary to provide more equitable benefits by taking into consideration such factors as marital status, living arrangements, and work experiences as they are at the end of the twentieth century. Private pension programs should also be reformed. Significant reform in either seems unlikely, and longer work lives may be necessary. Considering the disadvantage of older women in labor-force reentry, their future is not rosy.

The situation is not unique to the United States. Ginn and Arber (1993) wrote of the "pension penalties" due to the "gendered division of occupational welfare" in England. Women's pension benefits are reduced if they are married, have a child, work part-time, are employed in the private sector, or have been in their jobs a short time and have low earnings. Ginn and Arber concluded that unless the state makes more generous provision for their retirement, elderly women in Great Britain will increasingly face lives of poverty. Gee and McDaniel (1991) observed that pension policies in Canada have become politicized, and that results of recent changes have had deleterious effects, among them decreased incomes for women.

Views regarding the Social Security system in the United States vary widely. This is exemplified in a review of three books on the topic (Weber, 1989). Kingston, Hirshorn, and Cornman (1986) described Social Security as well suited to the interdependent and mutually supportive society of this country and viewed arguments about the inequity of the system as illogical and divisive and as failing to take into account the contributions of women and immigrants to the Social Security fund. Other authors (Bernstein & Bernstein, 1988) labeled Social Security "the system that works" and considered it not only to be effective in assisting today's older persons in their retirement but also as financially solvent well into the next century. The third book (Longman, 1987) concluded that cultural values that allocate resources to the old will result in "baby boomers" not receiving full Social Security benefits, so that they are "born to pay" unless changes are made.

Kingston et al. (1986) argued that despite criticisms of Social Security as fraught with intergenerational inequalities for the future, "baby boomers" will benefit from the system as it was designed. They will receive a smaller rate of return than previous and current cohorts of recipients, but the rate they receive will be reasonable in terms of what they will have invested. According to these authors, the retirement problems of "baby boomers" will lie rather in health care costs, the financing of Medicare, and the budget deficit. They perceived the real problems in Social Security to be inadequacy of benefits to working women and to divorced beneficiaries and displaced homemakers. (Women predominate in both the divorced and the displaced homemaker categories.) Thus there is lack of agreement among experts regarding intergenerational equity in Social Security benefits, particularly for the approximately eight million persons born from about 1946 to about 1965, a large population cohort that is approaching retirement age.

Demographic changes will continue to have important implications not only for the Social Security program, but also for other issues that impact the well-being of retired women. Age-distribution shifts in the population and changes in labor-force participation are drastically altering the dependency ratio: the proportion of the population in the labor force relative to the proportion not in it. The number of workers is declining in comparison to the number of those who have not yet entered and those who have left work life. An increasing proportion of the population is economically dependent upon a decreasing proportion of workers (Friedland, 1989). This puts increasing stress on national and personal/family finances.

Moreover, the composition of the "dependent" is altering because of increased life expectancies and lower birth rates. Traditionally, most nonworkers were below the age of 18. Increasingly, those 65 and older comprise a greater proportion. In setting priorities for programs such as Social Security and health care, as well as for budgeting attention and money within families, the strain of attempting to meet the needs of both the young and the old is obvious. This is a youth-oriented society, and most members, including older women, agree that the welfare of children and young people deserves high national and family priority for the future well-being of individuals, families, and the nation. Equitable distribution between youth and elders of economic resources provided by a smaller work force is a difficult problem and may give rise to intergenerational conflict. Women, who comprise an increasing majority of the elderly population, are at particular risk when intergenerational priorities are set.

The rapidly growing proportion of older women is increasingly diverse in terms of many factors, including education, types of jobs held, and continuity of employment histories, as well as current housing and living arrangements, marital status, and social support systems. This growing diversity emphasizes the need for research that takes into account both between- and within-gender differences to provide factual bases for appropriate financial provisions for women in retirement. For both research and public action, prospects look bleak. Without radical changes, more and more older women will spend more and more years in retirement without funds adequate to meet their basic needs, let alone the needs whose satisfaction gives life meaning. Poverty affects all aspects of women's lives during retirement, which is an increasing proportion of their lifespans.

ANTICIPATIONS OF RETIREMENT

The retirement process begins long before the "gold watch day" or the final "pink slip day." People are aware that exit from the work force is inevitable, and they form preconceptions regarding their own retirements. Individuals often express contradictory feelings about leaving the world of work, and a variety of meanings are attached to it. Among men and women professionals aged 50–60, definitions of retirement ranged from social death through ambivalence to positive anticipation (Karp, 1989). Among professional and semiprofessional women aged 57–78, Skirboll & Silverman (1992) found three distinct groups: retirement anticipators, retirement resistors who were still working, and retired women still resisting retirement.

The influence of economic status is clear in the finding that previously married women, who often face bleak financial situations in retirement, are less likely than previously married men to agree that older workers should retire, and are less likely to describe themselves as retired (Hatch, 1992). Fear of retirement and negative attitudes toward retirement were observed in persons who expected to have little personal control over their lives after retirement (Fletcher & Hansson, 1991), which may reflect the economic vulnerability that is more pervasive among women and societal stereotypes that assign women dependent roles. Anticipatory attitudes toward retirement and actual retirement are both related to health status among women but not among men (Midanik, Soghikian, Ransom, & Polen, 1990). However, women's more positive reactions toward retirement in this study may not be attributable to gender alone. The study was being conducted by a major health maintenance organization (HMO), Kaiser Permanente Medical Care Program, and respondents were members of this HMO, which provides prepaid health care. Women's more positive reactions toward retirement in this study may stem from their lesser job satisfaction (at lower-level jobs) in a situation that is unusually secure with regard to continuing health care, a major budget item for older persons and especially older women.

Identification with the job is important: Women with stronger work identities have more negative attitudes toward retirement (Erdner & Guy, 1990). Because work is a significant factor in personal identity for increasing numbers of women, and because women are moving into higher-level jobs, this has important implications for their attitudes toward retirement in the future.

PREPARATION FOR RETIREMENT

Getting ready for retirement by learning what it will be like and what can be done ahead of time to improve retirement life through classes, reading, radio, and television makes for an easier transition into retirement and a more satisfactory life during retirement for women and men, rural and urban (Dorfman, 1989). Women exacerbate their situation by failing to take part in this "anticipatory adaptation." Women are inferior to men in amount of financial planning, adequacy of planning, and attendance at retirement workshops (Richardson, 1990).

Finances are the major focus of most retirement-preparation programs, because incomes typically drop significantly at retirement. Though financial resources are likely to be especially poor for women, they do not try to obtain information about retirement benefits or learn budgeting strategies. Women are much more likely than men to go into retirement overvaluing the pensions they will receive (Ghilarducci, 1990). Whether this is a "head in the sand" reaction of denial related to aversion against exposure to unpleasant informational programs, or whether it results from such nonexposure, it has unfortunate consequences for women. Insufficient retirement income is disadvantage enough; allowing it to hit one unexpectedly after one has retired is truly double jeopardy, greatly increasing the difficulties of adjustment to the new stage of life and putting women at further disadvantage.

Perkins (1992) attributed the gender difference in retirement preparation to women's traditional societal roles, which emphasize dependence and passivity. Married women do not participate in retirement-preparation seminars available at work, but rely on their husbands to prepare for retirement (Slowik, 1991). Women approaching retirement following the dissolution of long-term marriages, newly without a husband on whom to rely, do not act to acquire financial-planning skills (Hayes & Anderson, 1993). Too often, money matters have been the domain of the husband, so that these women are left in ignorance regarding such matters and are especially in need of instruction. Without it, their well-being in retirement is severely jeopardized, even with relatively good incomes. Perkins (1992) attributed women's aversion against facing up to the realities of retirement not only to the prevailing myth among women that they will be taken care of in old age, but also to their fear of growing old in this youth-oriented society that allows men—but not women—to grow "more distinguished-looking" with age. Cultural stereotypes that affect women throughout their lives seem to underly their reactions to impending retirement.

RETIREMENT AS AN EVENT: TIMING AND REASONS

There are gender differences in leaving the world of work. Women are more likely to retire before age 62, never to have married or to have divorced and not remarried, and to report good health, as well as to have lower retirement incomes (Waltz, Craft, & Blum, 1991). The decision to stop working has different causal factors for women than for men, and for married women than for women without husbands. As a result of greater longevity and earlier retirement ages, marriage is the context within which most retirements take place, but this is true for fewer women (about two-thirds) than men (nearly 90%) (Atchley, 1992). Men are more likely to leave for work-related reasons; women are more likely to leave for family reasons, and married women are often pressured into joining their husbands in retirement before they want to quit working (Szinovacz, 1991). A woman who worked during child-rearing years is likely to retire earlier, especially following her husband's retirement, while women who were not employed during child-rearing years retire more slowly than do men (Henretta, O'Rand, & Chan, 1993).

Retirement is more likely for both African-American and Euro-American women—whether married or not—when a household member needs assistance. In both ethnic/racial groups, unmarried women are more likely than married women to leave work in order to provide such care, even if leaving work results not only in loss of present income but also in lower or no benefits when they come to retirement age. (Hatch & Thompson, 1992).

ADJUSTMENT TO RETIREMENT

Women retirees are vulnerable in making this transition not only because of poor economic resources and failure to acquire information and make an "anticipatory adjustment" to retirement, but also because of the lack of research into women's retirement and the fact that generalizations from findings on studies of men are not justified. In addition to greater gender-related economic jeopardy, which entails also greater insecurity in regard to health care, women must deal with all of the psychological effects of retirement that affect men. Responses to retirement have been shown to depend upon occupational status, age, and percentage of income that is retained (Richardson & Kilty, 1991). Women who worked at jobs with low occupational status are the most vulnerable to adjustment problems. Loss of the work role often results in poor self-image, feelings of uselessness, loneliness, anomie, and isolation (Perkins, 1992).

After reviewing the literature, Phillipson (1989) was sanguine about people's adaptation to retirement. However, older persons have the highest suicide rate of any age group, and they are more determined to die. They are less likely than younger persons to communicate or even hint at their suicidal intentions to others (and thus avoid possible intervention). Fewer of their attempts are just "pleas for attention." They use methods that are more difficult for others to detect ahead of time and that are more sure to succeed in achieving death (e.g., gunshots) (de Leo & Ormskerk, 1991). Suicidal tendencies differ for men and women at different ages or life stages, and this difference seems to be affected by other factors that are often associated with retirement, such as relocation, loss of social support, or bereavement, and by other consequences of unsuccessful adjustment to retirement, such as feelings of hopelessness and alcohol abuse.

In relation to retirement, women experience a larger number of more severe stressors ("life events") than do men, which may explain the gender difference, since "life events" are cumulative in producing stress. In a study of cohabiting spouses/partners of suicide victims, most (82%) surviving partners considered life events as the precipitating stresses. Interpersonal losses or conflicts (death, separation, discord), loss of home (eviction), and personal physical illness were among the more commonly mentioned (Heikkinen, Aro, & Lonnqvist, 1992).

Wives who do not work outside the home are affected by the retirements of their husbands. Prior to that date, thoughts of each partner may turn to expectations regarding changes in activities retirement may bring. Vinick and Ekerdt (1992) studied such couples in regard to anticipations prior to the husband's retirement and reports of experience a year after retirement. A major finding was the likelihood of disagreement in preretirement expectations between spouses, and therefore the "obvious desirability" for couples to share expectations with each other, because lack of consensus may be detrimental to adjustment to the new state.

The popular belief that retirement precipitates a crisis in most marriages was not upheld by the data (Vinick & Ekerdt, 1989). There was no change in hostile verbal exchanges or in physical spousal abuse. However, wives of recently retired men often complained about their husbands' intrusion into "their" domain at home. There may be some truth in the old adage "I married him for better or for worse—but not for lunch." No difference in marital conflict or violence was found in comparisons of retired men and women with their working counterparts (Bachman & Pillemer, 1991).

Studies of adjustment to retirement that included women as well as men are summarized by Richardson and Kilty (1991). Among both professional and nonprofessional women, in comparisons of retirees to those still at work, retirees have lower morale, lower psychological well-being, greater dissatisfaction with life, and more frequent self-reports of poor health. Loss of work often results in poor self-image, feelings of uselessness, loneliness, anomie, and isolation. Sociability increases after retirement, but women feel deprived of the social contacts that were available through work. Professional women have more difficulties than nonprofessional women in adjusting to retirement, and, unlike men, high job satisfaction prior to retirement on the part of women resulted in poorer adjustment to it. On the other hand, and not surprisingly, retired women with higher incomes have higher morale than do retired women with low incomes. Compared to homemakers, women retirees show higher morale, visit friends more often, and feel less lonely. In their own study comparing gender differences in adjustment to retirement, Richardson and Kilty found that women who had worked at low-status jobs were the most vulnerable to problems in adjusting to retirement.

Retired women were interviewed about their commitment to work versus family responsibilities during their working years (Rotman, 1989). There was no difference in work commitment attributable to degree of family responsibility, and Rotman concluded that women need not be categorized in one role or the other, but that they can be involved satisfactorily in both family and work. A study by Adelman (1993) suggested that both may be better than either one alone. Women aged 60 or older were asked to describe themselves as retired only, homemakers only, or both retired and homemakers. Single-role women (retired only and homemaker only) did not differ in well-being, but women who described themselves as "both retired and homemaker" had higher self-esteem and lower depression scores than did single-role women. This should be encouraging news to the increasing numbers of women who are, either by choice or by necessity, both working outside the home and being homemakers.

Hanson and Wapner (1994) found that mandatory retirement can be experienced in four ways: transition to old age, new beginning, continuation, and imposed disruption. Overwhelmingly, women described the experience as continuation. The researchers explained this as a result of the fact that formal roles have less importance for women than for men. Women maintain lifelong "continuity amidst discontinuity" by deriving their identities from informal roles and interpersonal relationships. Loss of the work role does not disrupt women's sense of continuity, which is based elsewhere.

RETIREMENT LIVING: RETIREMENT AS A LIFE STAGE

Retirement spans many years. It is much longer than most developmental stages that have been studied (infancy, childhood, adolescence) and may come to rival the working years in duration. Soon it will not be unusual for a woman to spend a third of her life in retirement. During this long period patterns of living undergo many changes as the demands and resources of the surrounding environment of people and things alter, and as the woman undergoes physical and psychological changes. Finances tend to be an increasing problem due to greater needs for health care and pharmaceuticals as age advances, and to inflation, which diminishes the market value of fixed incomes. These financial concomitants of living in retirement must be kept in mind in considering every facet of the lives of retired women.

Patterns are many and varied, depending upon past experiences and present resources. The current cohort of retired women includes many who never married. When they were young, the choice often was either work or marry. It was common practice for elementary and high schools to refuse applications from teachers who were married. If the applicant was a young woman, job-application forms and interviews for other work such as secretarial or nursing asked about intention to marry. In retirement, what has become of the women who never married? The stereotypical "old maid" who has taught school or been a secretary or a nurse and spends her declining years as a frustrated, bitter dependent in some relative's home is a familiar literary figure, but she seems quite inappropriate to today's cohort. O'Brien (1991) studied retired women 80 or older who had opted for work and never married. Their self-concepts were positive. Most felt that they were better off than their age peers. They had satisfying relationships with family and friends. Those in advanced old age needed more support from social services than did women their age who married and had children.

In a study of both-retired marital pairs, family finances and personal health were less crucial to successful adaptation in retirement than was the spouse's adjustment to it (Haug, Belgrave, & Jones, 1992). For wives, higher education assisted adjustment, while for husbands, wives' lower education figured prominently in their own adjustment during retirement years.

Well-educated women living in a retirement community were serious users of the mass media—in their own way. They selected content for its educational value. They read "good books," listened to "good music," and watched "quality programs" on television (Chatman, 1991). Professional and managerial retirees attributed their life satisfaction to their involvement in pursuits that nurtured and helped other people and to their relationships with extensive networks with other women (Wingrove & Sleven, 1991).

Francis (1991) showed how interpersonal networks or "convoys" formed during working years can continue to provide support in retirement. The group studied was unusual in its potential for forming group identity because its members' work had involved participation in a major social experiment (public housing), and they had participated jointly in union activities and opposition to sex discrimination on the job. The generalizability of this model of a social support group being formed at work and continuing into retirement to women with different work experiences needs to be tested. Development of this "convoy" may depend heavily upon the unique work and union experience of the particular group of women.

However, the concept is attractive. Means for enabling and facilitating development of mutually supportive networks at work that continue as "convoys" in retirement should be sought. Retired women are at particular risk with regard to informal support systems. The spouse is considered to be the most important element in the informal support system, and loss of spouse to be the most stressful of "life events." Widows now spend much more time in retirement than do widowers, and this trend will continue. The divorce rate continues to climb. Many older women never married or had children, and this too may be an ongoing tendency. Families tend to be smaller, and children do not stay "down on the farm" but live highly mobile lives, often at great distances from parents. As a consequence of these trends, the kinship support system is often thin, nonexistent, or not readily available for older women. Therefore, they have a special need for informal support systems based on nonkin relationships.

Jacobs (1990) demonstrated that women in retirement have strong needs for friendships with other women. To some older women, making friends comes naturally, but it is difficult for others. Jacobs reported that some women "settle for" paid therapists or self-help groups to meet their needs for interpersonal interaction. Therapy or organized groups can be beneficial in solving problems related to friendship formation, but they are not substitutes for informal social support networks in the "real world."

A "convoy" formed during working years and viable in retirement is a promising solution. Research should identify the elements necessary to formation and continuation of such groups. Communities can provide activities that foster development of friendships and informal support systems, beginning in midlife. Older women who lack the skill can learn how to make connections with others, given proper instruction. "You can't teach an old dog new tricks" has been disproved for old people. The subtitle for Schaie and Geiwitz's (1982) chapter on learning and memory is "Old Dogs, New Tricks."

With the recent societal emphasis on voluntarism, attraction of retired women as volunteers is societally useful because there are so many of them. Voluntarism may provide an opportunity to extend the informal social support system as well as to meet the need to feel useful. Stephan (1991) tried to clarify conflicting findings that retired women involve themselves in volunteer work as a means of getting paid work versus the view that women do volunteer work because of societal constraints that force them to find substitutes for satisfactions they had received from paid work. Her findings supported the latter position, though a minority of the women she studied were seeking paid work by offering volunteer time.

Issues regarding health and retirement have created a literature much too voluminous and contradictory to review here. Health is seen as a major reason for retiring and as a common rationalization for getting out of disliked jobs; and retirement is perceived as a threat to physical and mental health, even to longevity: "If he retires, he'll be dead in six months."

A recent report from the Kaiser Permanente Health Organization study (Midanik, Soghikian, Ransom, & Tekawa, 1995) said that among persons aged 60–66, over a two-year period the only difference between those who had retired and those still working was that retirees reported less stress than they had at baseline. Self-reports on mental health and coping ability and scores on a standard test of depression showed no differences related to retirement. In regard to health habits, there were no differences in alcohol abuse or in smoking, but more retirees engaged in regular exercise at follow-up. However, data on women did not fall into these patterns. Stress reduction among the retired was not found among women, and the "no difference" between retired and working persons on the several indexes of alcohol abuse were not found: Retired women were less likely to report alcohol problems than were still-working women. The overall results may reflect in part the disproportionate sex ratio of respondents: 342 men and 253 women. This study involved an all-too-common inappropriate treatment of data. Response differences between components of any sample—such as men and women—must be tested first. Only if "no difference" is found may the data be "pooled." If there are response differences between the component groups and there are differences in the number of persons in the two, conclusions based on unjustified pooling give undue weight to the behavior of the larger group and may not adequately represent either group. All research that includes both men and women should be scrutinized for such methodological problems before its results are taken seriously.

In another study that compared male and female retirees, women were more likely than men to smoke, use seat belts, and eat foods high in fiber; while men were more likely to exercise and use alcohol excessively (Leigh & Fries, 1992–93). Apparently there are differences between retired men and women in behaviors related to health and safety. A longitudinal study could clarify whether retirement has anything to do with these differences.

HOW TO MAKE RETIREMENT BETTER FOR WOMEN: OPTIONS FOR THE FUTURE

Research

Throughout this chapter there has been emphasis on the need to conduct research relevant to women's retirement. Findings from studies of men cannot be generalized to enlighten the retirement of women until such generalizability has been demonstrated to be appropriate by replicating the studies with women. Studies that include women but use disproportionate numbers of men may be invalid and of disservice to both genders if overall tests of hypotheses are made, lumping all subjects, prior to tests of sex differences. Data may be pooled between genders only after gender differences have been demonstrated to be absent in the data.

Finances

The single greatest jeopardy confronting women in retirement is financial. Lower economic status and economic security relative to those of men are lifelong heritages, and their amelioration lies in equitable job opportunities, security, and earnings during working years as well as retirement benefits. The Social Security system is of particular importance due to the heavy dependence of women on it. The relevance of its details to the late 1990s and beyond should be analyzed in terms of today's and tomorrow's world and women's places in it. Private pension plans should be similarly updated. Perhaps only as women gain political clout will such efforts be undertaken.

Preparation for Retirement

Women are most in need of and least likely to seek out or even passively accept information about their own retirements that could enable them to make realistic plans for the inevitable. A major deterrent against taking part in retirement-preparation programs lies within women's own minds. They "leave it up to my husband" or stick their heads in the sand in hopes that it will go away or be all right. Women must take more responsibility for themselves in actively pursuing retirement-preparation programs and doing their own planning for their own lives in retirement.

Retirement preparation should begin long before the event. Many programs offered at work begin only shortly before the last day of employment and consist primarily or exclusively of explaining company policies. Income is the most problematic area, but explanation of company policy is scarcely adequate preparation, particularly at that late date. Women are far less well aware of what their retirement incomes will be than are men, and if they are married, they tend to leave "money matters" to their husbands, which leaves them helpless at widowhood. Because retirement incomes are less for women, financial planning is both more difficult and more important. If anything, women should be even better informed about the income side and better skilled in the outgo side of household financial management than men. Health is a major consideration for retired women and a major item in their budgets. Before retirement, midlife women should seek out accurate information about women's health problems, preventive measures, and health care options in their personal preparation for retirement (Saxon, 1993).

Employers, women's advocacy groups, educational institutions, and others that offer retirement-preparation programs can be instrumental in empowering women with respect to their finances, health, living arrangements, informal social support system, and other issues so that they can deal positively with these matters when they arise in the future. Retirement educators should start this process of information and empowerment before dependency sets in (Hayes, 1990; Meade & Walker, 1989). To make up for ignorance, inexperience, and resistance to preparation programs, women may require more counseling than men (Richardson, 1993).

Francis (1990) described the retirement program run by a local unit of the AFL-CIO to facilitate the retirement transition of female members. It may be a model for union-run programs and an inspiration to programs with different sponsors. Major elements of the program are provision of (1) pre- and postretirement workshops that provide factual information and encourage planning skills relevant to women's retirement and (2) a social setting in which contacts established at work can be continued in retirement.

Closure on the Working Phase of Life

In the olden days the norm among workers was a man who held the same job until he was too old to work, at which point his employer gave a party for employees, family, and friends and presented him with a gold watch. Today the norm is a man or woman who changes jobs or even has several careers. Departure from the life of work may be marked by an ''occasion'' that is (overtly or covertly) simply the last in a series of ''farewells.'' That is the ''up'' side, especially for women. Often ''retirement'' is gradual, unwilling acceptance of the fact that the last job was indeed the ''last'' job.

Thomas Robb (1991), formerly of the Presbyterian Office on Aging, pointed to the apparently universal human need for rites of passage that help the person to redefine self-understanding and appropriate community behavior as that individual moves through transition events into successive life stages, and so to improve his or her adjustment and well-being in the new phase of life. Religious institutions have such rites for baptism, confirmation, matrimony, and burial. Robb suggested that it is time for religious groups to develop a rite of passage into retirement that will recognize it as a defining life event, convey a sense of closure to the working phase of life, and facilitate adjustment to and enjoyment of retirement.

REFERENCES

Adelman, Pamela K. (1993). Psychological well-being and homemaker vs. retiree identity among older women. *Sex Roles, 29*(3–4), 195–212.

Atchley, Robert C. (1992). Retirement and marital satisfaction. In Maximiliane Szinovacz, David J. Ekerdt, & Barbara H. Vinick (Eds.), *Families and retirement* (pp. 145–158). Newbury Park, CA: Sage Publications.

Bachman, Ronet, & Pillemer, Karl A. (1991). Retirement: How does it affect marital conflict and violence? *Journal of Elder Abuse and Neglect, 3*(2), 75–88.

Belgrave, Linda L. (1989). Understanding women's retirement: Progress and pitfalls. *Generations, 12*(2), 49–52.

Bernstein, Merton C., & Bernstein, Joan B. (1988). *Social Security: The system that works.* New York: Basic Books.

Burkhauser, Richard V. (1990). How public policy increases the vulnerability of older widows. *Journal of Aging and Social Policy, 2*(3–4), 117–130.

Burkhauser, Richard V., & Duncan, Greg J. (1989). Economic risks of gender roles: Income loss and life events over the life course. *Social Science Quarterly, 70*(1), 3–23.

Carp, Frances M. (Ed.). (1992). *Lives of career women: Approaches to work, marriage, children*. New York: Plenum Press.

Chatman, Elfreda A. (1991). Channels to a larger social world: Older women staying in contact with the great society. *Library and Information Science Research, 13*(3), 281–300.

de Leo, Diego, & Ormskerk, Sylvia C. (1991). Suicide in the elderly: General characteristics. *Crisis, 12*(2), 3–17.

Dorfman, Lorraine T. (1989). Retirement preparation and retirement satisfaction in the rural elderly. *Journal of Applied Gerontology, 8*(4), 432–450.

Erdner, Ruth A., & Guy, Rebecca F. (1990). Career identification and women's attitudes toward retirement. *International Journal of Aging and Human Development, 30*(2), 129–139.

Fletcher, Wesla L., & Hansson, Robert O. (1991). Assessing the social components of retirement anxiety. *Psychology and Aging, 6*(1), 76–85.

Francis, Doris. (1990). Women workers, workplace friends, and retirement: A union model. In Christopher L. Hayes & Jane M. Deren (Eds.), *Pre-Retirement planning for women: Program design and research* (pp. 89–113). New York: Springer.

———. (1991). Friends from the workplace. In Beth B. Hess & Elizabeth W. Markson (Eds.), *Growing old in America* (4th ed.). New Brunswick, NJ: Transaction Publishers.

Friedland, Robert. (1989). Questions raised by the changing age distribution of the U.S. population. *Generations, 13*(3), 11–13.

Gee, Ellen M., & McDaniel, Susan A. (1991). Pension politics and challenges: Retirement policy implications. *Canadian Public Policy, 17*(4), 456–472.

Ghilarducci, Teresa. (1990). Pensions and the uses of ignorance by unions and firms. *Journal of Labor Research, 11*(2), 203–216.

Ginn, Jay & Arber, Sara. (1993). Pension penalties: The gendered division of occupational welfare. *Work, Employment, and Society, 7*(1), 47–70.

Hanson, Kaaren, & Wapner, Seymour. (1994). Transition to retirement: Gender differences. *International Journal of Aging and Human Development, 39*(3), 189–207.

Hardy, Melissa A. (1991). Employment after retirement: Who gets back in? *Research on Aging, 13*(3), 267–288.

Hatch, Laurie R. (1990). Gender and work at midlife and beyond. *Generations, 14*(3), 48–52.

———. (1992). Gender differences in orientation toward retirement from paid labor. *Gender and Society, 6*(1), 66–85.

Hatch, Laurie R., & Thompson, Aaron T. (1992). Family responsibilities and women's retirement. In Maximiliane Szinovacz, David J. Ekerdt, & Barbara H. Vinick (Eds.), *Families and retirement* (pp. 99–113). Newbury Park, CA: Sage Publications.

Haug, Marie R., Belgrave, Linda L., & Jones, Susan. (1992). Partners' health and retirement adaptation of women and their husbands. *Journal of Women and Aging, 4*(3), 5–29.

Hayes, Christopher L. (1990). Social and emotional issues facing midlife women: The important role of retirement planning. In Christopher L. Hayes & Jane M. Deren (Eds.), *Pre-retirement planning for women: Program design and research* (pp. 27–40). New York: Springer.

Hayes, Christopher L., & Anderson, Deborah. (1993). Psycho-social and economic adjustment of mid-life women after divorce. *Journal of Women and Aging, 4*(4), 83–99.

Heikkinen, M., Aro, H., & Lonnqvist, Jouko. (1992). The partners' views on precipitant stressors in suicide. *Acta Psychiatrica Scandinavica, 85*(5), 380–384.

Hendricks, J. (1993). Recognizing the relativity of gender in aging research. *Journal of Aging Studies, 7*(2), 111–116.

Henretta, John C., O'Rand, Angela M., & Chan, Christopher. (1993). Gender differences in employment after spouse's retirement. *Research on Aging, 15*(2), 148–169.

Jacobs, Ruth H. (1990). Friendships among old women. *Journal of Women and Aging, 2*(2), 19–32.

Karp, David A. (1989). The social construction of retirement among professionals 50–60 years old. *Gerontologist, 29*(6), 750–760.

Keddy, Barbara, Cable, Beryl, Quinn, Susan, & Melanson, Judith. (1993). Interrupted work histories: Retired women telling their stories. *Health Care for Women International, 14*(5), 437–446.

Kingston, Eric R. (1989). Don't panic: It's working: What baby boomers need to know about Social Security. *Generations, 13*(2), 15–20.

Kingston, Eric R., Hirshorn, Barbara A., & Cornman, John M. (1986). *The ties that bind: The interdependence of generations.* Cabin John, MD: Seven Locks Press.

Leigh, J. Paul, & Fries, James F. (1992–93). Associations among health habits, age, gender, and education in a sample of retirees. *Journal of Aging and Human Development, 36*(2), 139–155.

Longman, Phillip. (1987). *Born to pay: The new politics of aging in America.* Boston: Houghton Mifflin.

Logue, Barbara J. (1991). Women at risk: Predictors of financial stress for retired women workers. *Gerontologist, 31*(5), 657–665.

Meade, Kathy, & Walker, Joanna. (1989). Gender equality: Issues and challenges for retirement education. *Educational Gerontology, 15*(2), 171–185.

Meyer, M. H. (1990). Family status and poverty among old women: The gendered distribution of retirement income in the United States. *Social Problems, 37,* 551–563.

Midanik, Lorraine T., Soghikian, Krikor, Ransom, Laura J., & Polen, Michael R. (1990). Health status, retirement plans, and retirement: The Kaiser Permanente Retirement Study. *Journal of Aging and Health, 2*(4), 462–474.

Midanik, Lorraine T., Soghikian, Krikor, Ransom, Laura J., & Tekawa, Irene S. (1995). The effect of retirement on mental health and health behaviors: The Kaiser Permanente Retirement Study. *Journals of Gerontology, 50B*(1), S59–S61.

Nuccio, Kathleen E. (1989). The double standard of aging and older women's employment. *Journal of Women and Aging, 1*(1–3), 317–338.

O'Brien, Mary. (1991). Never married older women: The life experience. *Social Indicators Research, 24,* 301–315.

Perkins, Kathleen E. (1992). Psychosocial implications of women and retirement. *Social Work, 37*(6), 526–532.

———. (1993). Recycling poverty: From the workplace to retirement. *Journal of Women and Aging, 5*(1), 5–23.

Phillipson, Chris. (1989). Towards a sociology of retirement. *Reviewing Sociology, 6*(2), 3–10.

———. (1990). The sociology of retirement. In John Bond & Peter Coleman (Eds.),

Ageing in society: An introduction to social gerontology (pp. 144–160). London, England: Sage Publications.

Rayman, Paula, Allshouse, Kimberly, & Allen, Jessie. (1993). Resiliency amidst inequity: Older women workers in an aging United States. In Jessie Allen & Alan Pifer (Eds.), *Women on the front lines: Meeting the challenge of an aging America* (pp. 133–166). Washington, DC: Urban Institute Press.

Richardson, Virginia. (1990). Gender differences in retirement planning among educators: Implications for practice with older women. *Journal of Women and Aging, 2*(3), 27–40.

———. (1993). *Retirement counseling: A handbook for gerontology practitioners.* New York: Springer.

Richardson, Virginia, & Kilty, Keith M. (1991). Adjustment to retirement: Continuity *vs.* discontinuity. *International Journal of Aging and Human Development, 33*(2), 151–160.

Rix, Sara E. (1993). Women and well-being in retirement: What role for public policy? *Journal of Women and Aging, 4*(4), 37–56.

Robb, Thomas B. (1991). Liturgical rites of passage for the later years. *Journal of Religious Gerontology, 7*(3), 1–9.

Rotman, Anita. (1989). Female social workers: Career or family? *Affilia, 4*(4), 81–90.

Ruhm, Christopher J. (1991). Career employment and job stopping. *Industrial Relations, 30*(2), 193–208.

Saxon, Sue V. (1993). Pre-retirement health needs of women. *Journal of Women and Aging, 4*(4), 57–66.

Schaie, K. Warner, & Geiwitz, James. (1982). *Adult development and aging.* Boston: Little, Brown.

Skirboll, Esther & Silverman, Myrna. (1992). Women's retirement: A case study approach. *Journal of Women and Aging, 4*(1), 77–90.

Slowik, Clare M. (1991). The relationship of preretirement education and well-being of women. *Gerontology and Geriatrics Education, 11*(4), 89–104.

Stephan, Paula E. (1991). Relationships among market work, work aspirations, and volunteering: The case of retired women. *Nonprofit and Voluntary Sector Quarterly, 20*(2), 225–236.

Sussman, Marvin B. (1972). An analytic model for the sociological study of retirement. In Frances M. Carp (Ed.), *Retirement* (pp. 29–73). New York: Behavioral Publications.

Szinovacz, Maximiliane. (1991). Women and retirement. In Beth B. Hess & Elizabeth W. Markson (Eds.), *Growing Old in America* (pp. 293–303). New Brunswick, NJ: Transaction Publishers.

Vinick, Barbara H., & Ekerdt, David J. (1989). Retirement and the family. *Generations, 13*(2), 53–56.

———. (1992). Couples view retirement activities. In Maximiliane Szinovacz, David J. Ekerdt, & Barbara H. Vinick (Eds.), *Families and Retirement* (pp. 129–144). Newbury Park, CA: Sage Publications.

Waltz, Thomas, Craft, John, & Blum, Nancy. (1991). Social work faculty in retirement: A national study. *Journal of Social Work Education, 27*(1), 60–72.

Weber, George H. (1989). Three books on Social Security: A complex portrayal. *Social Thought, 15*(1), 53–56.

Wingrove, C. Ray, & Sleven, Kathleen F. (1991). A sample of professional and managerial women: Success in work and retirement. *Journal of Women and Aging, 3*(2), 95–117.

Part III

Health, Psychological, and
Living Issues

Nine

The Health of Older Women: A Diverse Experience

DIANA J. TORREZ

The older adult population is the most rapidly increasing segment of the U.S. population. Since 1900 the number of older adults (those persons 65 years of age or older) has increased over ten times (3.1 million to 33.2 million), and their percentage of the population has more than tripled (4.1% to 12.7%). This increase is projected to continue at a rate of 1.3 percent annually until 2010, and then the number of older adults is projected to increase annually by 2.8% between 2010 and 2030 (U.S. Bureau of the Census, 1995). This has resulted in concern among health care providers and policy makers, since older adults use a disproportionate amount of total health care expenditures. Although in 1987 they represented 12.3% of the population, older adults accounted for 36% of the total health care expenditure. This extensive use of services is the result of an increasing number of disabilities that often accompany the aging process (AARP, 1992).

Since, on the average, women live longer than men, the health problems of older adults, in reality, are often those of older women. Women experience a greater life expectancy than men, and, as a result, they comprise the majority of older adults. In 1994 women 65 years of age or older numbered 20 million. This represented a sex ratio of 3 women for every 2 men. These differences increased with age. Between ages 65 and 69 the ratio was only 6 to 5, but by 85 and over this ratio was 5 to 2 (U.S. Bureau of the Census, 1995). Although women live longer than men, as a result of their life-course experiences they have a greater probability of being less educated and of being poorer and sicker. Consequently, older women exhibit higher health service utilization rates than older men. Older women's health care experiences merit close examination and must be differentiated from those of men.

Health characteristics of U.S. older women also differ by race and ethnicity;

therefore, the "health of older women" cannot be presented as a homogeneous experience. If the health care issues of older women are to be effectively addressed, the heterogeneity of this group, with its significant differences in health, education, and income, must be acknowledged. Although 90% of older adults are white, the minority older adult population is increasing rapidly. It is projected that between 1990 and 2050 the African-American older population will triple and the Hispanic older population will quadruple (U.S. DHHS, 1988). Consequently, this chapter presents an analysis of older women's health with special attention to ethnic differences.

LIFE EXPECTANCY AND MORTALITY

Redford (1984) noted that women possessed a protection against certain threatening pathological conditions associated with aging that resulted in greater life expectancy for women than for men. The longevity gap between men and women has increased since 1900, and in 1992 women, on the average, lived 7 years longer than their male counterparts; their life expectancy was 79.1 years, compared with 72.3 years for men. Although women enjoy greater longevity then men, the life expectancy of minority women is on the average 5 years less than that of white women. The life expectancy of African-American women is 73.9 years, compared to 79.8 years for white women (NCHS, 1995). In addition, although older women have experienced an increase in life expectancy, this increase has not been as great for African-American women. For instance, life expectancy at 65 for white females increased 4.1 years; however, for African-American females it only increased 2.3 years (Cohen and Van Nostrand, 1995).

This life-expectancy differential is the result of significantly higher mortality rates among African Americans at nearly all ages. African Americans report a death rate that is generally one and one-half times greater than that of whites (Sullivan, 1989). During the 1960s and 1970s researchers noted that African Americans who survived to 75 years of age began to experience greater life expectancy than whites. This reversal is known as the racial mortality crossover (Wing, Manton, Stallard, Hornes, & Tryoler, 1985). However, the age level of this crossover effect has risen in recent decades, and in 1990 African Americans did not begin to experience lower mortality rates until age 85.

Although national health data on the life expectancy of Hispanics do not exist, recent studies report that Hispanics' life expectancy has been increasing in the past several decades and is now similar to that of whites. As with white older adults, the majority of older Hispanics are women (57%). Cuellar (1990) noted that Mexican-American women age sooner and die faster due to the "stress, wear, and tear" of living. Mexican-American women report a fertility rate that is one and one-half times greater than that of whites. Consequently, they are taxed by giving birth to, and raising, a larger number of children. Further, U.S. Mexican-born women in their late 40s and 50s reported a birthrate that was twice that of middle-aged white women. Since this pattern has been recognized

Table 9.1

Mortality Rates for all Causes According to Age, Sex, Race, and Hispanic Origin, 1992

(Rates per 100,000 Population)

	55-64	65-74	75-84	85+
White female	799.2	1,909.1	4,969.4	14,015.9
(Male)	1,398.5	3,287.0	7,440.9	17,956.2
Black female	1,405.4	2,796.6	5,483.0	13,264.1
(Male)	2,493.8	4,746.7	8,744.5	16,717.1
American Indian or Alaskan Native female	912.4	1,743.2	3,307.1	6,878.7
(Male)	1,384.0	2,604.0	5,239.7	9,381.3
Asian or Pacific Islander female	476.2	1,095.0	2,873.1	9,561.8
(Male)	766.8	1,962.5	4,919.7	12,628.8
Hispanic female	598.2	1,354.2	3,149.7	8,772.4
(Male)	1,061.1	2,322.3	4,924.1	10,895.4

Source: National Center for Health Statistics. (1995). *Health, United States, 1994.* Hyattsville, MD: Public Health Service.

for thirty years, it suggests that fertility patterns may be contributing to accelerated aging.

Becerra and Shaw (1984) stated that it was not surprising that members of some minorities lived shorter lives, since they lived in triple jeopardy—they were poor, old, and members of a minority group. Minority older women, therefore, live in quadruple jeopardy. These four factors—age, race/ethnicity, income and sex—are essential to an understanding of the health status and health needs of older women (Lacayo, 1980).

HEALTH STATUS

Mortality Rates

The life-expectancy gap between men and women is attributable to men's higher mortality rates throughout their lives. Among older women, as previously noted, differences in mortality are also evident. African-American women exhibit the highest mortality rates, and Asian and Pacific Islander women exhibit the lowest mortality rates (table 9.1). Asian and Pacific Islander and Hispanic older women report lower mortality rates than white women at all ages after 55 years. American Indian women experience slightly higher mortality than white women during the ages 55–64. However, after 65, they also report lower rates than white women. African American women, however, report a mortality rate that is twice that of white women until the age of 85, at which time their mortality rate is slightly lower than that of whites.

American Indian women's lower mortality rate after 65 years of age is partially attributable to their significantly higher mortality at younger ages, particularly during ages 5 to 14 and ages 24 to 44 years. The mortality rates of African-American women are notable not only because they are higher than those of white women, but because during ages 55–64 they are also higher than those of white men and during the ages of 64–74 are only slightly lower. The pattern found among the specific mortality rates for men and women mirrors those of the overall mortality rates.

Specific Mortality Rates

The leading causes of death (diseases of the heart, cancer, and cerebrovascular diseases) among older adults are the same as those found among the general population. However, differences by sex and ethnicity again exist. The specific mortality rates for older adults revealed four patterns (table 9.2):

1. Older men exhibit higher mortality rates for diseases of the heart, cerebrovascular diseases, and malignant neoplasms than older women.

2. Among older women, African Americans exhibit the highest mortality for diseases of the heart, cerebrovascular diseases, and malignant neoplasms. Asian and Pacific Islander older women exhibit the lowest rates for these diseases. White older women exhibit higher mortality rates for these causes of death than Hispanic or American Indian older women.

3. The crossover effect can be observed for African American women at age 85 for diseases of the heart and cerebrovascular diseases. At 85 their rates are lower than those of white women; however, their rates remain higher than those of the other three ethnic groups. No crossover effect is observed for malignant neoplasms.

4. Although older men exhibit higher rates for cerebrovascular diseases than older women, at age 85 a crossover effect is observed for all ethnic groups except American Indians and Native Alaskans.

These patterns demonstrate that although older women generally experience lower specific mortality rates than older men, as women enter the "very old category" (85 years and older), this gender mortality advantage may disappear. This is true for cerebrovascular mortality rates. Waldron (1980) concluded that 46% of the mortality difference between men and women was the result of heart disease. He noted that premenopausal women had a hormonal protection that decreased their risk of heart attack. However, after menopause, this protection decreased and the heart disease rate among women tripled. By age 75 the difference between the sexes for heart disease was nearly eliminated.

In addition, these patterns reveal the effect of ethnicity on health. The mor-

Table 9.2
Mortality Rates for Specific Causes of Death According to Age, Sex, Race, and
Hispanic Origin, 1990–92

(Rates per 100,000 Population)

White male

Age	Cerebrovascular Disease	Diseases of the Heart	Malignant Neoplasm
55-64	44.7	499.8	501.4
65-74	148.9	1,196.1	1,088.3
74-84	518.4	2,865.0	1,867.6
85+	1,523.3	7,416.5	2,744.7

Black male

Age	Cerebrovascular Disease	Diseases of the Heart	Malignant Neoplasm
55-64	139.5	806.0	826.5
65-74	315.5	1,597.7	1,590.0
74-84	701.4	3,042.9	2,473.6
85+	1,395.1	6,337.6	3,255.2

American Indian or
Alaskan Native male

Age	Cerebrovascular Disease	Diseases of the Heart	Malignant Neoplasm
55-64	42.9	428.2	289.4
65-74	126.7	840.6	618.8
74-84	321.4	1,831.0	1,095.2
85+	872.7	3,709.1	1,463.6

Asian or Pacific
Islander male

Age	Cerebrovascular Disease	Diseases of the Heart	Malignant Neoplasm
55-64	55.6	231.2	272.3
65-74	161.7	612.7	652.0
74-84	475.8	1,675.8	1,195.2
85+	1,359.0	4,705.1	1,879.5

Hispanic male

Age	Cerebrovascular Disease	Diseases of the Heart	Malignant Neoplasm
55-64	50.5	343.8	287.2
65-74	127.6	816.0	652.0
74-84	360.3	1,856.8	1,206.4
85+	842.9	4,479.4	1,858.1

Table 9.2 (continued)

White female

Age	Cerebrovascular Disease	Diseases of the Heart	Malignant Neoplasm
55-64	34.8	187.2	369.1
65-74	112.1	569.5	677.8
74-84	443.4	1,814.4	1,020.0
85+	1,645.7	6,446.5	1,385.2

Black female

Age	Cerebrovascular Disease	Diseases of the Heart	Malignant Neoplasm
55-64	93.7	432.6	471.2
65-74	226.4	991.2	783.3
74-84	580.0	2,210.3	1,082.4
85+	1,480.5	5,742.9	1,478.6

American Indian or Alaskan Native female

Age	Cerebrovascular Disease	Diseases of the Heart	Malignant Neoplasm
55-64	38.6	191.5	228.6
65-74	101.6	469.0	453.2
74-84	313.8	1,070.8	600.0
85+	700.0	2,704.8	804.8

Asian or Pacific Islander female

Age	Cerebrovascular Disease	Diseases of the Heart	Malignant Neoplasm
55-64	43.2	93.7	204.3
65-74	118.4	310.9	347.5
74-84	359.4	1,071.9	620.7
85+	1,361.8	4,087.3	1,054.5

Hispanic female

Age	Cerebrovascular Disease	Diseases of the Heart	Malignant Neoplasm
55-64	36.3	148.7	214.5
65-74	96.84	428.2	392.9
74-84	291.6	1,225.8	640.6
85+	912.8	4,138.7	985.4

National Center for Health Statistics, Health, United States, 1994
Hyattsville, Maryland: Public Health Service. 1995.

tality rates of older women differ significantly by ethnic group, with older African Americans exhibiting the highest specific mortality rates in all age groups. African-American older women, aged 65–74 years, generally experience mortality rates for diseases of the heart, cerebrovascular diseases, and malignant neoplasms one and one-half times greater than those of white older women. However, Hispanic women aged 65–74 years exhibit mortality rates for these three leading causes of death that are similar to those of white women in this age category. Further, after age 75, Hispanic women exhibit mortality rates that are substantially lower than those of whites. As expected from the overall mortality rate, Asian women continue to enjoy significantly lower mortality rates for specific causes of death.

The differences in the mortality rates of older women are reflective of their different life-course experiences. For instance, both Asian and African-American women's mortality rates are related to economic status throughout their lives, with African Americans reporting some of the lowest lifetime family incomes, while Asians report some of the highest family incomes. Although Hispanic women's incomes are more similar to those of African Americans than to those of whites, their mortality rates more closely resemble those of whites. The literature has come to refer to this phenomenon as "epidemiologic paradox" (Markides & Coreil, 1986). Researchers have theorized that the culture of Hispanics acts as a protective barrier against the adverse effects of poverty. The cultural elements that have often been cited are diet and family support.

Other Mortality Rates

Diabetes. Although not among the three leading causes of mortality, diabetes is an important contributor to women's morbidity and mortality rates. In 1992, among men, diabetes was the ninth or tenth leading cause of death, dependent on ethnicity. However, among white females diabetes was the seventh leading cause of death. Further, for African-American, Hispanic, and American Indian women, diabetes was the fourth leading cause of death. Among Asian women it was ranked sixth as cause of death.

Death rates from diabetes were substantially higher for African-American women in all age groups, including those in the age group 85 years and older (table 9.3). No crossover effect was evident for the African-American diabetes mortality rate.

In diabetes the single most important risk factor is obesity, and this is disproportionately found among African-American women of all ages (U.S. DHHS, 1988). During 1988–91, 49.5% of African-American women were overweight, as compared to 32.4% of white women. This percentage increases with age: 60.8% of African-American women aged 65–74 years report being overweight, compared with 36.5% of white older women (U.S. Bureau of the Census, 1995). In addition, the percentage of overweight white older women has decreased from

Table 9.3
Mortality Rates for Diabetes among Older People by Race and Sex, 1986

(Rates per 100,000 Population)

	Total	65-74 yrs	75-84 yrs	85+ yrs
White	14.8	53.5	114.3	206.2
African American	21.5	120.5	214.0	312.3
Male				
White	12.8	55.8	116.9	207.6
African American	16.5	100.8	178.2	223.9
Female				
White	16.7	51.6	112.7	205.6
African American	26.0	135.0	235.8	351.0

Source: U.S. Department of Health and Human Services. (1988). *Health status of minorities and low-income groups* (3rd ed.). Washington, DC: U.S. Government Printing Office.

1960, when it was 43.2%. In contrast, the prevalence of overweight African-American older women increased from 47.8% in 1960 (U.S. DHHS, 1988).

Among the Hispanic older population, diabetes is also a serious health concern. Mexican-American women similarly report higher percentages of overweight persons (47.9%) than whites. The 1988 National Health Interview Survey (NHIS) reported that among Hispanics 65 to 74 years of age, 13.4% were diagnosed with diabetes. This rate compares with 8.4% for the general population. Stern (1985) noted that among the Mexican-American older population socioeconomic status and diabetes are inversely related. Rosenwaike (1987) found that although Mexican-born women generally exhibit lower death rates than Mexican-born men, this is not the case for diabetes. Mexican-born women's death rate from diabetes was 32.2 per 100,000, compared with 24.7 for men.

Hypertension. Another important contributor to mortality and morbidity, particularly for African-American women, is hypertension. Cuellar (1990) noted that hypertension is a risk factor for cardiovascular morbidity and mortality and a possible etiologic factor in other illnesses in later life. Data from the Nutrition Examination Survey for 1976–80 revealed that hypertension prevalence was the highest for African-American women between the ages of 65 and 74 years (82.9%). The prevalence among African-American men (67.1%) was similar to that of white women (66.2%). The lowest prevalence of hypertension was found among white men (59.2%). A comparison of the rates of hypertension among African-American and white older adults aged 65–74 years demonstrates that African Americans experience a hypertension rate that is one and one-half times that of whites, 524.8 per 1,000 and 357.2, respectively. Similar rates are exhibited by African Americans and whites 75 years of age and older, 538.9 and 360.5, respectively.

Redford (1984) noted that there are other conditions that, although rarely identified as causes of death, result in disability and interfere with normal functioning for many older women. Among these is osteoporosis, which results in the bone fracturing with little trauma. It can, therefore, result in great pain, disability and dependency for older adults. Because it has been estimated that as many as 50% of women over 60 years of age suffer from this condition Ryan (1983) concluded that this was a major health problem for aging women. Arthritis, a similar pathological condition of the musculoskeletal system, is also far more common in women than in men. The likelihood of arthritis also increases with age. In 1991, for women between the ages of 55 and 64, the rate for arthritis was 390.6; for women between 65 and 74 years of age, it was 493.2; and for women between the ages of 74 and 85 the rate increased to 609.6 (Cohen and Van Nostrand, 1995).

Osteoporosis and arthritis are important conditions for older adults, since these conditions can cause accidents that may result in death or disability. Redford (1984) noted that falls among older adults are important contributors to injury deaths.

Analysis of Mortality Rates as Health Measures

These health data provide an objective measure of the health of older women. However, other measures, such as "self-assessed health status" (SAHS), have been used to examine the broader health issues of older adults (Redford, 1984). Previous studies have consistently reported that older women evaluate their health as poorer than older men (Fillenbaum, 1979; Verbrugge, 1976; Cantor & Mayer, 1976). However, Cohen and Van Nostrand's (1995) report, *Trends in the Health of Older Americans*, did not reveal significant differences in SAHS between the sexes (table 9.4) (Cohen and Van Nostrand, 1995).

Differences, however, were revealed among older women. Among white women, 39.3% evaluated their health as excellent or very good, and 26.7% evaluated their health as fair or poor. Among African-American women, only 23% reported their health as excellent or very good, compared with 44.9% who evaluated their health as fair or poor. The self-assessed health measures of African-American older women are consistent with the picture of poor health painted by their high mortality rates.

While the self-assessed health status data of African Americans is consistent with their objective health statistics, this cannot be said of Hispanics. Mortality data suggest that the health status of Hispanic older women is similar to that of white older women, and therefore one might expect that Hispanic SAHS data would be similar to that of whites. However, this is not the case for Hispanics. A 1989 report from the Commonwealth Fund Commission reported that Hispanic older adults self-assess the worst health of all older groups, with 54% of Hispanic older adults reporting fair or poor health. There are also striking differences among the Hispanic ethnic groups. For example, 46% of Cubans and

Table 9.4

Respondent-assessed Health Status by Age, Sex, and Race, United States, 1992

(in Percentages)

Characteristics	Respondent Assessed Health Status				
	Excel-lent	Very Good	Good	Fair	Poor
All persons	37.9	28.6	23.0	7.6	2.8
Age					
65 years and over	15.6	22.6	33.1	19.6	9.1
Sex and Age					
Male					
65 years and over	16.4	22.4	32.0	19.4	9.8
Female					
65 years and over	15.1	22.7	34.0	19.8	8.5
Race and Age					
White women					
65 years and over	15.9	23.4	34.1	19.2	7.5
African American women					
	8.0	15.0	32.1	26.1	18.8

Source: Cohen, R.A., and Van Nostrand, J.F. (1995). *Trends in the health of older Americans: United States, 1994.* National Center for Health Statistics. Vital Health Statistics 3(30).

54% of Mexican-American older adults report poor or fair health, compared to 63% of all older Puerto Rican adults.

Income is also positively associated with self-assessed health status. For the general population, 30.3% of persons with family incomes which ranged from $10,000–$19,000 reported poor or fair health as compared with 23.4% of persons with family incomes which ranged between $20,000–$34,999 and only 18.2% of persons with family incomes of more than $35,000. Similarly, those older adults with incomes above $35,000 were most likely to assess their health as excellent or good, while those with incomes below $10,000 were more likely to evaluate their health as fair or poor (table 9.5). Since minorities are disproportionately represented in the low-income categories, the majority of the Hispanic and African-American differential noted previously can in all likelihood be attributed to income differences (U.S. DHHS, 1988).

The self-assessed health status data are important because they provide a broader perspective of older adults' health than can be attained from national health statistics. However, national data are only available for whites, African Americans, and, as a result of the Commonwealth study, for Hispanics. Unfortunately, these national data do not exist for Asians and American Indians.

LIMITATIONS OF ACTIVITIES

In addition to self-assessed health status data, other important measures of women's health are "number of limitations of activities" and "utilization of

Table 9.5

Respondent-assessed Health Status by Family Income and Age, United States, 1988

(in Percentages)

Characteristics	Respondent-assessed Health Status				
	Excel- lent	Very Good	Good	Fair	Poor
Family Income and Age					
Under $10,000					
65 years and over	11.7	17.2	31.1	25.0	15.0
$10,000 - $19,000					
65 years and over	15.5	21.7	32.5	21.3	9.0
$20,000 - $34,999					
65 years and over	18.2	23.5	34.9	17.0	6.4
$35,000 or more					
65 years and over	25.1	25.8	30.9	11.9	6.3

Source: U.S. Department of Health and Human Services. (1988). *Health status of minorities and low-income groups* (3rd ed.). Washington, DC: U.S. Government Printing Office.

health services.'' The national data on limitations of activities are again limited to whites and African Americans. This information is important because these limitations may be the result of past health problems that were not adequately addressed, current chronic health problems, and/or lack of access to adequate health services. It is evident from the data (table 9.6) that African-American older women are twice as likely to experience personal care activity limitation as white women. It is also interesting to note that although white older women experience more activity limitations than white men, they fare better than African-American older men. It was noted earlier that African-American older men do have higher rates of specific mortalities than white older women. This fact is reflected in the data on limitations of activities.

The number of persons with limitations of activities also increases with age. Those persons who are over 85 years of age are twice as likely to experience limitations of personal and routine care activities as those persons aged 70 years or over. Although the data do not provide gender breakdowns for African Americans over 85 years of age, it is clear that by the age of 85 only one-third of African Americans report no limitations, as compared to one-half of whites. Since the women significantly outnumber men by the age of 85, it is women who experience the most limitations of activities and, therefore, are dependent on others for assistance in performing everyday activities (Cohen and Van Nostrand, 1995).

Table 9.6
Persons 70 Years and Older in Selected Types of Activities as a Result of Chronic
Conditions, by Race, Sex, and Age, 1993

(in Percentages)

Type of Limitation	White Male	White Female	Black Male	Black Female
70 years and over				
Personal care activities	6.7	8.6	10.7	15.6
Routine care activities	8.8	14.2	10.9	18.1
Other activities	22.9	16.9	23.6	15.4
Not limited	61.6	60.3	54.8	50.9
	White Male	White Female	Black Both Sexes	
85 years and over				
Personal care activities	13.9	20.1	37.1	
Routine care activities	18.4	24.6	18.4	
Other activities	17.8	13.6	9.3	
Not limited	49.9	41.7	35.2	

Note: Personal care activities include eating, bathing, dressing, and getting around at home. Routine
care activities include doing everyday household chores, doing necessary business, shopping, or
getting around for other purposes. They exclude persons who need help of others with personal
care activities. Other activities exclude those persons who need help of others with personal or
routine care activities.

Source: Cohen, R.A., and Van Nostrand, J.F. (1995). *Trends in the health of older Americans:
United States, 1994.* National Center for Health Statistics. Vital Health Statistics 3(30).

UTILIZATION OF HEALTH CARE SERVICES

Health Insurance

Prior to examining the utilization of health care services by older adults, it is
necessary to examine health insurance coverage, since this is the single most
important factor in utilization of health care. Although the majority of older
adults are covered by Medicare, nonwhite older adults are more likely not to be
insured by Medicare. Also, whites are nearly twice as likely to supplement
Medicare with private insurance. Supplemental insurance assists with out-of-
pocket costs not covered by Medicare.

In 1989, 96% of all older Americans received Medicare, with or without
private insurance or Medicaid. Slightly less than 17% of all older adults received
Medicare only. Although there was little difference in the health coverage of

Table 9.7

Health Coverage for Persons Sixty-Five and Over According to Type of Coverage and Selected Characteristics, 1989

(in Percentages)

Characteristic	Medicare and Private Insurance	Medicare and Medicaid	Medicaid Only
Total	73.5	5.7	16.8
Age			
65 - 74 years	74.2	5.0	15.5
75 years and older	72.3	6.8	19.0
Sex			
Male	73.9	4.0	17.2
Female	73.4	6.8	16.4
Race			
White	77.3	4.5	14.7
African American	39.3	16.5	37.9
Income			
Less than $14,000	64.8	11.4	21.5
$14,000 - $24,999	81.2	2.6	13.4
$25,000 - $34,999	80.0	2.4	12.5
$35,000 - $49,999	80.3	1.9	10.2
$50,000 or more	76.5	1.1	12.6

Source: National Center for Health Statistics. (1993). *Health, United States and health people 2000 review 1992.* Hyattsville, MD: Public Health Service.

men and women, there were significant differences among white and African-American older adults (table 9.7). The majority of white older adults supplemented Medicare with private insurance (77.3%). However, only 39.3% of African Americans supplemented Medicare with private insurance. Instead, 16.5% supplemented Medicare with Medicaid, and 37.9% had Medicaid insurance only. This difference can be explained by the effect income has on the ability to supplement Medicare with private insurance. Since African-American older adults have lower incomes than whites, they are less likely to be able to afford to supplement Medicare. The significantly higher Medicaid coverage of African Americans again attests to the African-American/white income differential in old age, when the poverty rate for African Americans continues to be three times that of white older adults.

A study by the Commonwealth Fund (1989) reported that 28% of older Hispanics have Medicare only and no supplemental insurance, while 33% of older Hispanics have Medicare and Medicaid. This is again the result of a poverty level among Hispanic older adults that is twice that of white older adults. Although these ethnic differences are not available by gender, since in all ethnic groups women outlive men, it can be deduced that nonwhite women are less likely to be covered by Medicare or private insurance. They are more likely to have Medicaid as their sole source of insurance. This is significant since the inability to supplement Medicare with private insurance results in increased out-of-pocket costs. This is a financial difficulty for nonwhite older adults who have low incomes. In addition, the fact that many nonwhite older adults supplement Medicare with Medicaid or have only Medicaid insurance is significant since Medicaid is not always accepted by all physicians or hospitals.

Health Care Utilization

Physician contact is generally accepted as a measure of health care utilization, since most medical care occurs in physicians' offices. Although health status is an important predictor of physician contact, physician contact is also affected by insurance coverage, ambulatory sites, and physicians' practice patterns (U.S. DHHS, 1988). Older women and men between ages of 65 and 74 have approximately the same number of physician contacts, 9.3 and 10.4. Although 1990 data revealed that the place of contact for women was more likely to be in the physician's office than for men, 61.6% and 57.6%, respectively, this was no longer the case by 1993, when for 56.7% of men and 56.5% of women, the place of contact was the physician's office. However, men are still more likely than women to come into contact with physicians in hospitals, 14.6% and 12.6%, respectively (NCHS, 1995). This suggests that regardless of health status, men wait longer to contact the physician, and as a result of the delay, their health status may have worsened.

African-American older adults also report more physician contacts than whites, 11.5 and 9.7, respectively. Whereas whites are more likely to contact physicians in their offices (58.4%), less than half (48.2%) of African Americans report this pattern. Instead, African Americans report twice as many physician contacts in hospitals (24.3%) as whites (12.3%). A Commonwealth Fund Study (1989) also reported that Hispanic older adults had more annual physician contacts than whites. This, in all likelihood, is a reflection of Hispanic and African-American older adults' poorer health relative to whites. Since both Hispanics and African Americans are more likely to contact physicians in hospitals, this may indicate that they wait until their health problem is of a serious nature before seeking treatment.

Women over 65 years of age have lower rates of hospital utilization than men. Their discharge rate is 321.5 per 1,000, compared with 368.0 for older men. This may be attributable to their rates of physician contacts (NCHS, 1995). Older women may seek treatment for health problems earlier than men, thereby decreasing the risk of hospitalization. Data from the National Hospital Discharge Survey (1986) reveal that although African-American older men and white older men have similar hospital utilization (discharge rates 357.3 per 1,000 and 363.3, respectively), older white women were found to be higher utilizers of hospitals than minority older women, 316.1 per 1,000 and 304.2, respectively. This may be the result of minority women's lower rate of health insurance coverage. Minority women may be reluctant to be hospitalized if they do not have adequate health insurance to cover the costs.

These data, however, indicate that the average length of stay is longer for minority older adults than whites. The average length of stay for white older men is 8.2 days, compared with 9.4 days for older minority men. The same pattern emerges for older women, with white older women reporting 8.7 days as average length of stay. Minority older women report an average length of hospital stay of 10.1 days. This measure is important because the average length of stay is considered to be an indicator of the severity of the illness. This measure, therefore, indicates that minority older adults experience poorer health than do white older women.

CONCLUSIONS

As the number of older adults increases, it is necessary to develop health policy that will effectively address their needs. Demographers have projected that by 2030, 22% of the population will be 65 years of age or older (U.S. DHHS, 1988). Past gerontological literature has emphasized the need for a comprehensive understanding of older women's needs, since they comprise the majority of the older population. However, this chapter has demonstrated that in order to acquire a comprehensive understanding of older women's health needs, it is necessary to acknowledge the heterogeneity of this group. It is evident that older women's aging experience is affected by ethnicity, and this is particularly true with regard to health. The health characteristics of women in their later years are to a significant degree the outcome of their socioeconomic status throughout the life course.

The poverty rate does rise with age among the elderly. For instance, in 1992, 11% of those between the ages of 65 and 74 lived in poverty, compared with 16% of those persons over 75 years. In addition to age, however, sex and ethnicity increase the risk of living in poverty. For instance, older women experience a higher prevalence of poverty than men, 16.0% and 9.0%, respectively. Older adults who are members of minority groups exhibit higher rates of poverty. The rate for African American older adults is 33%, compared with 22% for Hispanics and 11% for whites. Consequently, older women who are members of minority groups are at greatest risk of living in poverty (U.S. Bureau of the Census, 1995).

Examination of the median income of the older population reveals similar patterns. Older women report lower incomes than men, and nonwhite older persons report lower incomes than whites. Consequently, the lowest incomes are reported by minority older women (table 9.8).

The economic inequalities observed in the larger society are mirrored in the health characteristics of older adults. Women's lower socioeconomic status rel-

Table 9.8

Median Income of Persons Age 65 and Older by Age, Race and Hispanic Origin, 1987

Age	White	African American	Hispanic
Male			
65-plus	$12,398	$7,167	$6,803
65-69	14,504	8,328	8,704
70-plus	11,336	6,658	6,183
Female			
65-plus	7,055	4,494	*
65-69	7,171	4,640	*
70-plus	7,027	4,436	*

*Unavailable.

Source: U.S. Department of Health and Human Services. (1988). Health status of minorities and low-income groups (3rd ed.). Washington, DC: U.S. Government Printing Office.

ative to men is reflected in their health outcomes. Although women exhibit longer life expectancies than men, they report more disabilities than men. Similarly, among women, nonwhites generally report lower incomes and worse health outcomes. African Americans report shorter life expectancies, higher specific mortality rates, poor self-assessed health, and lower health coverage than white women. Hispanic older women although reporting similar objective mortality measures to white older women, have poorer self-reported health and a higher rate of disability. The socioeconomic status of women throughout their life course is important because it determines what health resources are available to them in addressing their health problems.

In conclusion, if the health of older women is to be addressed, it must be understood in its broadest context. The effect of gender and ethnicity on health must be better understood. Effective health policy for older women must begin by acknowledging and integrating the vast differences that exist among older women. However, further research regarding factors that influence women's health is needed. The contradiction between the low mortality rates and high morbidity rates of women needs to be further examined. Redford (1984) noted that if effective and efficient health policy for older adults is to be developed, the interaction between the biological, behavioral, and social factors that impact health must be better understood. She concluded that it is time to integrate all these factors and change the current disease orientation and the medical treatment focus. Although Redford made this recommendation over a decade ago, little has changed. The U.S. health programs for older adults continue to have a medical focus. Given the fact that this has proven to be a costly path, it is again important to emphasize that in addition to increasing life expectancy, as a society, we must also be focused on improving the quality of older adults' lives.

REFERENCES

American Association of Retired Persons. (1993). *A Profile of older Americans*. Washington, DC: Administration on Aging.

Becerra, Rosina, & Shaw, David. (1984). *The Hispanic elderly: A research reference guide*. New York: Academic Press.

Cantor, M., & Mayer, M. (1976). Health and the inner city elderly. *Gerontologist, 16*(1), 17–25.

Cohen, R. A., and Van Nostrand, J. F. (1995). *Trends in the health of older Americans: United States, 1994*. National Center for Health Statistics. Vital Health Statistics *3*(30).

Commonwealth Fund Commission on Elderly People Living Alone. (1989, September). *Poverty and poor health among elderly Hispanic Americans*. New York: The Commonwealth Fund.

Cuellar, Jose. (1990). Hispanic aging: Geriatric education curriculum development for selected health professionals. In *Minority Aging* (pp. 365–414). DHHS Publication No. HRS-P-DV-90-4. Washington, DC: United States Department of Health and Human Services.

Fillenbaum, G. G. (1979). Social context and self-assessments of health among the elderly. *Journal of Health and Social Behavior, 20*, 45–51.

Hanis, Craig, Ferrell, R. E., Barton, Sara, et al. (1983). Diabetes among Mexican Americans in Starr County, Texas. *American Journal of Epidemiology, 118*, 659–672.

Hanis, Craig, Ferrell, R. E. & Schull, William. (1985). Hypertension and sources of blood pressure variability among Mexican Americans in Starr County, Texas. *International Journal of Epidemiology, 14*(2), 231–238.

Lacayo, Carmela. (1980). *A national study to assess the service needs of the Hispanic elderly*. Los Angeles: Asociacion Nacional por Personas Mayores.

Markides, K., & Coreil, Jeannine. (1986). The health of Hispanics in the Southwestern United States: An epidemiologic paradox. *Public Health Reports, 101*(3), 254–265.

Morrison, B. (1984). Physical health and the minority aged. In R. L. McNeely & John Colen & R. L. McNeely (Eds.), *Aging in Minority Groups* (pp. 161–173). Beverly Hills, CA: Sage Publications.

Mueller, W. H., Joos, Sandra, Hanis, Craig, Zavaleta, A. N., Eichner, J., & Schull, William. (1984). The diabetes alert study: Growth, fatness, and fat patterning, adolescence through adulthood in Mexican Americans. *American Journal of Physical Anthropology, 64*(4), 389–399.

National Center for Health Statistics. (1993) *Health, United States and Health People 2000 Review 1992*. Hyattsville, MD: Public Health Service.

National Center for Health Statistics. (1995). *Health, United States, 1994*. Hyattsville, MD: Public Health Service.

Redford, Linda J. (1984). The health of older women. *Convergence in Aging: A Publication of the Mid-America Congress on Aging, 2*, 16–36.

Rosenwaike, Ira. (1987). Mortality differentials among persons born in Cuba, Mexico, and Puerto Rico residing in the United States, 1979–81. *American Journal of Public Health, 77*(5), 603–606.

Ryan, K. J. (1983). Estrogen replacement therapy. In R. Cape, R. Coe, & I. Rossman (Eds.), *Fundamentals of Geriatric Medicine*. New York: Raven Press.

Stern, M. P. (1985). Diabetes in Hispanic Americans. In *Diabetes in America*. NIH Publication Number 85–1468. Washington, DC: U.S. Government Printing Office.

Sullivan, L. W. (1989, July). Keynote remarks presented at the American Association of Retired Persons' Minority Initiative Conference, Washington, DC.

U.S. Bureau of the Census. (1995, May). *Sixty-five plus in the United States*. Statistical Brief. U.S. Department of Commerce.

U.S. Department of Health and Human Services. (1988). *Health status of minorities and low-income groups* (3rd ed.). Washington, DC: U.S. Government Printing Office.

Verbrugge, L. (1976). Females and illness: Recent trends in sex differences in the United States. *Journal of Health and Social Behavior, 17*, 387–403.

Waldron, I. (1980). Sex differences in longevity. In S. G. Haynes & M. Feinleib (Eds.), *Second conference on the epidemiology of aging*. Washington, DC: U.S. Department of Health and Human Services.

Wing, S., Manton, K. G., Stallard, E., Hornes, C. G., & Tryoler, H. A. (1985). The black/white mortality crossover: Investigations in a community based study. *Journal of Gerontology, 40*, 78–84.

Ten

Developmental Models of Midlife and Aging in Women: Metaphors for Transcendence and for Individuality in Community

JAN D. SINNOTT

Mature and aging women in this historical time voice experiences of their development over time that are complex, are unique, and transcend traditional polarities. Models of women's development in the second half of life often seem to have been the products of minds viewing behavior through specific, rather limited cultural and epistemological lenses. Typically a "standard," lifespan, male-focused, developmental model is simply applied to women (the nonstandard case). Then "women's problems" are noted as exceptions to the standard. Reproductive biology often is regarded as the most interesting factor driving the system, although the differences or problems that social roles impose on women may be noted. The problem of research distortions created by our lenses is certainly not unique to studies of mature women (e.g., Bem, 1993; Kuhn, 1962). Women and men in standard textbooks of development are fragmented creatures described by researchers using their favorite tools. The resulting picture shows models, but more theories or general trends than models, of progressively larger individual differences, greater accumulated losses, and the possible growth of wisdom and concern for others beyond the self. Of course, my brief description of developmental research does not do any of it justice, especially my own work, but I want to make the point that we are not doing a good-enough job in capturing the richness and complexity in the development of mature women. Part of the problem is that our typical models are not equal to the task.

More recent models in psychology and other sciences could be used to obtain a broader and more complex perspective. These newer approaches to theorizing reflect the transformations in thought and technology that have been radically changing the way we look at many aspects of life, including behavior. These transformations include, for example, the feminist movement, concerns about ecology and sustainable economies, and the population explosion. To theorize within these types of transformations, one needs to think in the newer terms of multivariate process models such as general systems theory (Buckley, 1968; Ford, 1987; Miller, 1978; Bertalanfy, 1968) or self-constructing systems (described by Waldrop, 1992).

Neither the old nor the new set of lenses (models) is the "best" way to view women's maturity and aging. Using both sets of lenses can provide us with a more complex and useful picture. Using both also allows us to examine a larger variety of issues with a broader range of tools. We can hear both the individual chords and the melody of women's mature lives. One of the major motivating factors for mature adults is the desire to give life meaning by going beyond the self and identifying with a larger whole. Models used to study mature women must conceptually incorporate those self-transcendent and communal qualities while describing increasing individuality, all within cohort and time-related changes.

In this chapter I shall discuss the newer and older ways of modelling women's development during the second half of life. I shall speak as a psychologist, but as one aware that this topic demands an interdisciplinary approach. Along with descriptions of the older and newer models will be a discussion of some theories and issues that might be addressed using these models. Next, I will mention some methods available to do research within these models, as well as potential methods that could be constructed to take advantage of the newer models and topics. This review will close with a description of one synthesis of newer and older models in addressing a specific research problem, and a discussion of the ways in which that synthesis of several models, rather than use of a single model, could enrich our research questions and research methods.

HISTORICAL CHANGES AND OUR CHOICE OF RESEARCH MODELS

Women have always been influenced by a huge number of inner and outer forces, but especially by the views cultures hold of them and by their ability to bear children. With apologies to Freud, both biology and culture have been destiny. While ancient cultures or those of some indigenous peoples may have been structured around valued feminine roles and world views (e.g., see Eisler's *The Chalice and the Blade* [1987] or Underwood's *The Walking People* [1993]), the recent millennium in Western and Eastern cultures has valued hierarchies of power, male dominance, heterosexism, polarization of roles and groups, specialization, competition, and biological (or other) determinism. Culture, as a quasi-living system (Ford, 1987; Miller, 1978), was a strong force favoring these stances at this point in human evolution. The individual, not the community, was favored, and material aspects of the here and now, not transcendent values and goals, were emphasized. In many ways, in general systems theory terms, it was an "adolescent" culture.

But now a conjunction of circumstances has turned many of these Western industrial cultural forces on their heads. The older view of woman as sexual property, as victim, as a vessel for the child, has been challenged. Although at earlier times the older view could be justified in part by the imperatives of a historical period (e.g., underpopulation) and the imperatives of a culture (e.g., the rules of religious tradition), the justifications have been crumbling fast since the old rules no longer worked well. We, as a middle-aged culture, have a new interest in transcendent values and community. Perhaps we even have a new-found need to balance individualism and individual transcendence.

While the older view of women has been crumbling, its implications and constraints on models of middle age and old age in women have still been very strong since models generally lag behind cultural change. Globally, women's status still depends on their husbands' status and mainly increases only when they bear many children. Thus a study of the mature or older woman (who is less often chosen as a partner and who cannot bear children) largely has remained a biologically focused study about biological losses to which women must adjust. If traditional cultures worldwide still hold that a woman's main role is to nurture children, our studies of her roles or her generativity in midlife automatically take place in the context of family, not in the context of work or in the larger world. Since the research that is then produced using the older view of women gives the message that women develop through family roles, that research itself reinforces the original limiting lenses. Limited models tend to lead to additional limited models that suit the past. They do not fit the times of transformation in which we are living and doing research.

In recent decades, especially in "developed" countries such as the United States, the world has swiftly changed, and so have the roles and identities of many mature women. For example, a woman's lifespan has lengthened dramatically, even beyond that of her male companions, so that mature and older women make up the bulk of the mature adult population. It is harder for mature and older women to continue to acquiesce to "dominant" males when those males are harder to find and become weaker and sicker faster than the women do.

Changing a model is hard. A scientist at the National Institutes of Health who shall be nameless, and who had a hard time dealing with these worldwide changes, once tried to save the old model at all costs. He suggested during a conference discussion period that we might alleviate this model "problem" by getting women to sicken and die at the same rate as men. While his particular idea was not enacted, the older models have been quite durable, perhaps because few have taken the time to analyze their assumptions.

But hanging on to old models will not be easy either. Many of a woman's years (more than half in "developed" countries) are spent without the need to bear or care for children, so the old-fashioned childbearing/nurturing role is not a sustainable one for women. The ecology of roles is being seriously damaged. World population is soaring to a frightening degree, to the point where having many offspring is not a blessing and birth control is often chosen. Many women also now have more employment choices open to them; older models will not do justice to their decisions in maturity. Now the mature woman is almost compelled to create her own future in response to a world situation never before encountered in the history of our species.

SOME HISTORICALLY RECENT SOLUTIONS: NEW MODELS

We have some new abstract modelling possibilities to help us. New physics theories (see summaries in Capra, 1975; Sinnott, 1981; Wolf, 1981), general systems theory (Miller, 1978; Sinnott, 1986, 1993b, 1994b), theories of self-regulating systems (Jantsch, 1980; Kelly, 1994; Waldrop, 1992), and Eastern philosophical approaches (e.g., Capra, 1975; Zukav, 1979) are becoming more accessible and are opening new ways to conceptualize dynamic psychological processes over long periods of time. Where the older Western philosophies emphasized a small number of polarized concrete roles that might be exchanged, the newer approaches emphasize the continuum of roles and the process of ongoing change and transformation. Humanist (e.g., Bolen, 1984; Maslow, 1968), transpersonal (e.g., Anderson & Hopkins, 1991), and existential (e.g., Frankl, 1963) psychology have arrived. They provide models of human behavior and development that can accommodate individuality, community, and transcendence.

A difficulty in dealing with these changes centers on identity. If we keep transforming, and if we model mature women as transforming, how can we "be" what we "are"? What are our lives about when the old rules and identity labels disappear? How can we convey the meaning of our lives to others who are using different labels or lenses? In the past we, as women, could perhaps take comfort that no matter what existential confusion we found ourselves in, we could at least see ourselves as mothers. Can we stand facing the limits of our lifetime with the uncertainty that comes of variable, nonbiological roles? In the new model for middle-aged and old women's identity, women move from a labeled role through an identity core with many manifestations to an "identity" defined as a characteristic way of relating to, or being with, or dancing with others, as we move through life, to a final version of identity that goes beyond the self without loss of the self. This new sort of identity can carry the kinds of boundaries within which the mature woman in today's world can construct her complex identity (Gergen, 1991). Identity continuity need not be a problem in new models.

CHARACTERISTICS OF OLD AND NEW MODELS

In this section we will discuss the abstract dimensions of models used for most of the currently available research on middle-aged and older women. Here we define a "model" broadly, in an Aristotelian way, as a brief description of the form and nature of a behavioral event or process. The abstract form of the model, as well as the issues usually addressed by it, will be examined in later sections devoted to models used in the past and models more appropriate for today. Notice that the definition of model in itself constitutes a model; other definitions of model could be used. We are always limited by our models, but without any model our discourse lacks structure. There is never a lens-free awareness, but being conscious of one's lenses helps.

All models may differ along several dimensions: whether they attempt to give descriptive versus inferential information; how detailed they are; their genesis and historical period of origin; whether they are based on single-factor or multifactorial antecedent conditions; whether they are mechanistic, organismic, or constructionist; whether they are analog or digital; the degree to which they are nested in explicit theory; the type of issue to which they are applied; the degree to which they are developmental and lifespan; the degree to which they are assumed to be generalizable to most humans; the degree to which the model is nomothetic (seeking information on average behavior) versus idiographic (seeking information on changes within a single self who is also a reference point at any one time for other states of the self); the complexity of their view of women; the degree to which the assumptions inherent in the model are made conscious; whether they permit respondents a sense of meaning; whether data within them can be abstract or narrative-quality data; whether they permit qualitative or quantitative analyses; and whether the model is based on Newtonian science versus new physics science (see Sinnott, 1981), chaos and complexity theory, and systems theory. Of course, there could be many more characteristics.

Because of global change, the most useful models for future work appear to be those that give both descriptive and inferential information; contain meaningful detail; give analog information; are constructionist; are at least potentially multifactorial (e.g., biopsychosocial); are nested in theory; can be applied to a wide range of issues and types of women; are developmental and lifespan; are both nomothetic and idiographic, thereby allowing for summaries and for individual differences; describe a complex view of women, as opposed to a simplistic view such as "women as 'other' "; make assumptions conscious; permit meaning and narrative; permit both qualitative and quantitative analyses; and are based on new physics sciences and systems theory. Of course, no single model of middle age and aging in women is likely to have all these ideal features, but the most useful models at least have the potential for including many of these features.

To get a sense of these features of models, let us examine as an example the characteristics of a very simplistic older model, but one still widely held in our culture: "Most behavior of women in middle age and old age is determined by their going through menopause." This model is used to give both descriptive and inferential information, but its intent is to make inferences about the causes of behavior (i.e., menopause). Descriptive information about women's behavior in midlife may be generated in response to this model, but that information is at least implicitly tied to the notion of biological causality. Detail is lacking in the model as it is stated here; we do not see speculations about a causal path, for example. The genesis of this model is quite ancient, smacking of primitive wisdom and taboos. The model focuses on a single cause, a biological one in this case, ignoring, for example, the social/interpersonal dimensions. It sounds like a cross between a mechanistic effect and an organismic unfolding, given that surgically induced menopause would be thought to lead to the same conclusions in behavior that naturally occurring menopause would. The model's tone is digital; a woman is either menopausal or not, with all perimenopausal changes lumped into the position of "menopausal" (although it is known that changes in female hormone production are very gradual). The model is nested in specific biological theories about lifespan changes in the reproductive system, but in general and very vague psychosexual and physiological psychology theories about this event. This model has been applied, rightly or wrongly, to a very wide variety of behaviors and issues. The model is developmental and lifespan only in the sense that it applies to a biologically developmental event, menopause. The model has been generalized to all women. The model has been used in both nomothetic and idiographic ways, but tends to be used to describe a norm or average behavior most of the time. The view of women that seems to be held in this model is simplistic. Assumptions are not made conscious in the model. The only meaning for women that finds a home in this model is a reproductive meaning for life, in which a woman's story is her childbearing and body story. Either qualitative or quantitative data could be generated by this model, and it is based on Newtonian science.

Now imagine the kinds of scientific questions that could be asked if even one parameter of this model changed: for example, causality could be changed from single-factor causes to multifactorial causes. A researcher could creatively vary many of the less-than-optimal model parameters mentioned previously to enrich research on women, while leaving the more optimal parameters alone. Awareness of the model's parameters allows a researcher to be conscious of its strengths and weaknesses to address a given research question.

ISSUES USUALLY ADDRESSED BY OLDER MODELS

We will examine the model assumptions of three areas of research (in addition to the "menopause is at the root of it all" view mentioned earlier) that have been classic ways to describe the behavior of middle-aged and older women: Erikson's psychosocial developmental theory; androgyny and other sex-role research; and intimate-relationship research. Model assumptions usually are unconscious in all of these research areas. Our purpose in bringing model assumptions to consciousness in these selected areas is to call attention to the fact that the models can be expanded and modified from their initial interesting, but limited, forms. This could benefit research on women and aging, even in those research areas where much already has been done.

Erikson's Theory

Within Erikson's theory (Erikson, 1950), as applied to women, the essential conflicts that might first occur in midlife and old age involve generativity (versus stagnation) and integrity (versus despair). A woman becoming aware of her shortening lifespan can choose to develop by becoming a creator of something that will be larger than her individual life and that will go on after she personally dies. She might mentor children, create a business, or write a book, identifying with the larger community of humanity rather than simply with her own body and life. The opposite choice (stagnation) is to try to hold the line against change and aging, defending rather than creating. In old age the Eriksonian conflict may be between integrity, which is shown by the woman's weaving her life story into a coherent story, or by despair (the alternative choice) that her life is meaningless and has no coherent story in the face of approaching death. Erikson's way of looking at a portion of women's lives has been experienced as very meaningful to women and to men in general in spite of its derivation from the experiences of Western industrial men.

Erikson's model yields both descriptive and inferential data, but it is not particularly detailed, and it does emerge from the study of men's lives, specifically in Western capitalist nations in the twentieth century. Multifactorial conditions are assumed, if not tested, and the model is somewhat constructionist but also heavily organismic. Behavior in this model is analog; one might be more or less generative, not absolutely either/or. The theory is not explicit but speaks in a general way about general trends. It is usually applied specifically to family or work relationships and issues of disengagement and dying, but it does flow from a developmental viewpoint. The theory is generally assumed to apply to most human beings. Researchers in this tradition seem to use the model to study average behavior, while clinicians use it to describe changes in individual behavior over time. This is assumed to be a complex view of women, but it usually is applied in a simplistic way. This theory permits meaning to exist within the woman and does permit both qualitative and quantitative analyses, at least as it is usually applied. It is largely based on Newtonian logic. This theory and model, then, is best for painting a broad picture of a woman's life within a traditional context, explaining why the traditional woman does what she does and arguing from logic rather than from data.

Sex Roles

The second approach we will focus on, seen in the theories of sex roles and androgyny (e.g., Bem, 1993; Carter, 1987; Sinnott, 1981, 1986, 1987, 1993a), attempts to describe in both pictures and numbers how behavior is connected to sex roles (the stereotypic gender-related role behavior of men and women) that change developmentally over time. (For a survey of this area, see Susan Sherman's chapter in this volume.) The theory in its current manifestation suggests that roles are first polarized into male and female roles, which then either are reversed or are combined into a complex role, then ultimately transcended to the point that sex roles matter relatively little to the individual or to the construction of the individual's identity.

Looking at the underlying model behind these sex-role theories, we see that some information related to them is descriptive, but much less is inferential, despite the existence of several standard measurement tools. Although gender roles have existed for millennia, this area of study is contemporary with Freudian psychology, social learning theory, the feminist movement, and awareness of the rapidly changing American experience. While sex-role theory was originally a rather simple enterprise, we currently find more and more associated variables and context effects (Bem, 1993). Organismic models (e.g., Freud) have been challenged by mechanistic ones (e.g., Bandura) and later by constructionist ones (e.g., Kohlberg). Most approaches have been digital, labeling respondents in a polarized way, rather than analog ("to what degree am I masculine or feminine?"). Sex-role studies are nested in explicit theory; they are usually applied to clinical, personality, and developmental issues, such as adaptivity. Sex-role theory has been assumed to be generalizable to all humans. Investigators seek information about average behavior and generally are not very complex in their view of women. This work does not usually allow respondents to achieve a narrative quality for their responses and does not ask questions about the meaning of sex roles in women's lives. Quantitative analyses are the norm. The model uses Newtonian logic. This set of theories, then, rests on models that are good for both specific detailed investigations and painting the broader picture, but still are essentially intrapersonal and uncritically accepting of arguments about women's traditional place and behavior as defined by society. They do not address the transcendent meanings mature and older women try to bring to their role-related experiences. There is no room in the model for these meanings.

Intimate Relationships

A third popular approach to research on mature women is a series of studies focused on women as contexted within relationships. (For a survey of work in this research area, see chapters by Rebecca Adams and Bertram Cohler, among others, in this volume.) The relationships might be marital or family or empty-nest or grandparent ones, or simply may involve the woman's desire for many aspects of life to have a relational structure or purpose, a link to other persons or truths (e.g., Gilligan, 1982; Josselson, 1992).

These models tend to give descriptive data and vary greatly in the amount of detail they provide. These are largely twentieth-century models, fueled by the feminist movement, clinical experiences, and postmodernism. They are generally based on multifactorial antecedent conditions and are constructionist. They are analog models, usually loosely nested in specific theory, and are applied to lifespan-developmental clinical, personality, family, marital, or moral issues.

There are usually only weak attempts to generalize to all humans; nomothetic hopes are usually fulfilled by idiographic methods and case studies. The views of women in this area of research are complex, and some of the models theoretically permit intention, community, transcendence, and meaning to exist within personal narratives to some degree. Qualitative analyses are much more common than quantitative ones. These relational models usually use portions of general systems theory as well as a Newtonian scientific logic. These models of women in relationship (to others or to some bigger picture) have space to capture more of the complexity of women's own experiences in midlife and aging and seem to be less bound by the traditional views of women's place and roles.

Again, notice that the purpose of consciously specifying the model underlying these four major long-term strains of research is to examine the possibilities that more complex work will follow. When we see what the model's limits have been, we can spend less time refining research and having empirical fights in areas where the underlying model does not serve our needs and spend more time recasting the research questions based on a more complex model that captures additional salient research interests. For example, the research question "Should women take replacement hormones to control their erratic behavior during menopause?" reinforces the status quo politically loaded model of women as erratic biological creatures at the mercy of their bodies, however the data come out. Expanding the model from nomothetic to idiographic enriches the question, leads to better medical care, and circumvents the political agenda: "What changes in an individual woman's behavior might usefully lead to discussion of the pros and cons of replacement hormone use during menopause?" With conscious assumptions, the choice becomes ours as researchers.

NEWER MODELS AND ISSUES

Here is a brief listing of some newer multidisciplinary research models that, by virtue of both their content and their underlying assumptions, are built on more complex models. These areas might be used as a stimulus for some important research on women in midlife and aging. The references cited, which represent only a small sample of pertinent references, will permit the reader to learn more about the approach than can be articulated in this short chapter.

- Chaos theory and complexity theory (properties of self-organizing systems) (Cavanaugh & McGuire, 1994; Devaney, 1989; Gleick, 1987; Goldstein, 1994; Jantsch, 1980; Kelly, 1994; Waldrop, 1992)
- General systems theory (properties of human and cultural living systems) (Bertalanfy, 1968; Ford, 1987; Miller, 1978; Sinnott, 1989b, 1989c, 1993b, 1994a, 1994b)
- Eastern philosophy (Capra, 1975; Zukav, 1979)
- The "new" physics (relativity theory, quantum theory) (Capra, 1975; Herbert, 1986; Pagels, 1982; Prigogine & Stengers, 1984; Sinnott, 1981, 1989b, 1989c, 1993b, 1994a, 1994b; Wolf, 1981; Zukav, 1979)

- Environmental psychology (Demick & Nazarro, 1994; Gore, 1992)
- Theory of psychological archetypes (Bolen, 1984; Campbell, 1972; Campbell & Moyers, 1988; Jung, 1982)
- Humanistic psychology (Maslow, 1968; Rogers, 1961)
- Transpersonal psychology (Anderson & Hopkins, 1991; Sinnott, 1994a; Weibust & Thomas, 1994)
- Existential psychology (Frankl, 1963; May, 1969; Yalom, 1980)
- Mind/body (mutually influencing one another) studies (Epstein, 1989; Locke & Colligan, 1986; Sheikh & Sheikh, 1989)
- Postformal reasoning (cognitive development of the mature individual in society; its effects on relationships and organizations; and so on) (Commons, Richards, & Armon, 1984; Sinnott, 1989a, 1992, 1995; Sinnott & Cavanaugh, 1991)
- Creation of community (Underwood, 1993; Whitmyer, 1993)
- "New" biology, cooperative evolution (Augros & Stanciu, 1987; Maturana & Varela, 1988)
- Lifetime learning, plasticity (Berg, Klaczynski, Calderone, & Strough, 1994; Denney, 1994; Sinnott, 1994b; Sinnott & Johnson, 1996)
- Learning through intense or long-term relationships (Hogue, Bross, & Efran, 1994; Meacham & Boyd, 1994; Sinnott, 1984, 1994b)
- Search for personal meaning and spirituality (Keen, 1994; Moore, 1992; Sinnott, 1994a; Weibust & Thomas, 1994)
- Nonpolarized roles or descriptors (Bem, 1993)
- Individuals as creators of their own experience (Feinstein & Krippner, 1988; Sinnott, 1984)

Recall for a moment the dimensions of models presented earlier in this chapter, for example, that "a model might provide descriptive versus inferential information." The eighteen areas I have just mentioned can generally produce research possessing both dimensions discussed, both descriptive and inferential data produced in this case, because they are more complex models. Most of the eighteen areas naturally generate studies that are both single factor and multifactorial; they naturally generate mechanistic and organismic and constructionist studies. Each of the eighteen areas represents a complex idea of person in society evolving over time. Each is abstract enough to transcend the trap of considering just one historical period or just one detailed operational definition as the whole truth. Each provides information that can be analyzed as nomothetic or idiographic information, mathematical models and narrative analyses. On the whole, they are more representative of the complexity of the transcendent person in community over time than most simpler models.

Let us examine the eighteen areas a bit more fully, in the context of research and theory on intimate relationships. Many of the eighteen areas (including general systems theory, new physics, and postformal thought) make some use of common principles. Several are listed here. We can keep our discussion short enough for the boundaries of this chapter by looking at these similar underlying principles. What research questions can we address using that newer model? What might using it tell us, over and above what research questions using a simpler model would tell us?

The common principles I just mentioned are the following: Change can occur in a system only if the system includes disorder, potential, and unstructuredness; systems coconstruct their reality with other systems; systems that survive have porous boundaries; systems go through predictable "life stages" as they lose potential and gain more structure; change occurs when systems interact; and systems strive for continuity. Notice the dynamic nature of all these process-oriented statements of principles.

In the context of intimate relationships we see at once that research based on these common principles that underlie several of the models I am offering for consideration demands that we think of change over time in a biopsychosocial and historical context. The mature woman is a "changing over time" respondent who cannot be conceptualized in static, polarized terms. In line with the first statement, she cannot "become" unless there is some chaos or unstructured part of her life that she as a system can make into something new. The process must be "messy" to work at all; without relational space or emptiness, relationships cannot develop. Among other things, to study relationships within this principle means to study within a relational ecology. It means that women can become aware of their power residing in "loss." Research using this principle might include a long-term study of individual differences in women's patterns of taking relationships apart to make room for a shift in connections.

Systems also coconstruct reality with other systems. In relational terms, we each decide what our relationship is, and out of a commitment to that belief we go on to make it reality. But neither of us can create the relationship alone. Consider what the studies of long-term marital or intimate-partner satisfaction obtain when they get ratings of satisfaction. If you and I cocreate the intimate partnership we know, our satisfaction may be linked mainly to our cocreated reality being supported, and to little else. Our awareness of this partnership-making process depends on a cognitive development that realizes that our relational reality must be a cocreated one that we can influence, but not alone. Interesting research questions here could include the development of awareness over time, and its effect on the behavior of the couple, given the social context in which they live. It could include the effect of changes in the developmental trajectory of one partner on the development of the other partner, as seen close up in Newtonian space on a day-to-day basis, and as seen from a distance in the new physics nonlocal space of the couple's lifetime.

Systems that survive have porous boundaries, that is, they let information come in and out. We find it difficult to ask what women consider (not necessarily choose), what information they process, and what the constraints are on that information processing as they make relational choices. Research in this area might find ways to enhance the processing of more information by the woman or by the living system of society in ways that are compatible with each other. If the woman or the society is too rigid (nonporous) in its boundaries in respect to the other, no amount of information will be the "right" amount for an exchange to take place. Researchers might study this process, thinking of it in systems terms.

Systems have life stages going from total potential in a young system to total rigidity in a dead system. The effect of any societal or behavioral intervention will depend on the "age" of the system receiving it. The quality of interaction between two person systems will partly depend on their mutual "age" compatibility. What do we know about the effects of having a relationship of two "older" versus two "younger" versus two "dissimilar-age" systems? What does this do to social supports?

Change occurs when systems interact. We have too little data on the styles of interaction among intimates in multigenerational families. We know too little about how breakdowns occur in family interactions or in the interactions affected by memory loss or Alzheimer's disease. How much can a system bear before it breaks down entirely? Who are the "invulnerable" women who get the most even from impoverished interactions with their intimates? We might learn from them.

Systems strive for continuity. We know that this is true on a personal level. But are we studying the effects of social systems striving for continuity? When models of research on mature women are slow to become more complex, will we be able to offer our social living system what it needs to feel its continuity, in spite of changes, and therefore not resist our attempts to change it? At what point is the system in "ready state," available for change? Perhaps it is time to study living-system change. These are just a few examples of ways our research questions might become broader if we think in new model terms in one research area, that of intimate relationships. Of course, the many methods associated with the eighteen areas and new models should be explored within each model.

SUMMARY

Mature and aging women speak of their great diversity of complex patterns of development of person in society over time, development often motivated by a need to transcend individualism, simple identities, and traditional and polarized descriptions of life and themselves. This chapter suggests that at the current historical time many traditional models are too limited to find all the richness in mature women's behavior as they live within global conditions of rapid change. Researchers studying mature women might make a special effort to analyze the assumptions of research models in light of model characteristics mentioned here and to consider some of the eighteen models (such as chaotic systems, postformal thought, new physics, or transpersonal psychology) listed here. The joint power of traditional and nontraditional models may enhance research on mature women since, used together, the models are metaphors for the life experiences voiced by mature and aging women.

REFERENCES

Anderson, S., & Hopkins, P. (1991). *The feminine face of god.* New York: Bantam.

Augros, R., & Stanciu, G. (1987). *The new biology.* Boston: New Science Library.

Bem, S. (1993). *The Lenses of gender: Transforming the debate on sexual inequality.* New Haven, CT: Yale University Press.

Berg, C., Klaczynski, P., Calderone, K., & Strough, J. (1994). Adult age differences in cognitive strategies: Adaptive or deficient? In J. Sinnott (Ed.), *Interdisciplinary handbook of adult lifespan learning* (pp. 371–388). Westport, CT: Greenwood Press.

Bertalanfy, L. von. (1968). *General system theory.* New York: Braziller.

Bolen, J. (1984). *Goddesses in everywoman: A new psychology of women.* San Francisco: Harper & Row.

Buckley, W. (Ed.). (1968). *Modern systems research for the behavioral scientist: A sourcebook.* Chicago: Aldine.

Campbell, J. (1972). *Myths to live by.* New York: Bantam.

Campbell, J., & Moyers, B. (1988). *The power of myth.* New York: Doubleday.

Capra, F. (1975). *The tao of physics.* New York: Bantam.

Carter, D. (Ed.). (1987). *Current conceptions of sex roles and sex typing.* New York: Praeger.

Cavanaugh, J., & McGuire, L. (1994). Chaos theory as a framework for understanding adult learning. In J. Sinnott (Ed.), *Interdisciplinary handbook of adult lifespan learning* (pp. 3–21). Westport, CT: Greenwood Press.

Commons, M., Richards, F., & Armon, C. (Eds.). (1984). *Beyond formal operations.* New York: Praeger.

Demick, J., & Nazarro, N. (1994). Adult learning environments: Perspectives from environmental psychology. In J. Sinnott (Ed.), *Interdisciplinary handbook of adult lifespan learning* (pp. 137–158). Westport, CT: Greenwood Press.

Denney, N. (1994). The effects of training on basic cognitive processes: What do they tell us about the models of lifespan cognitive development? In J. Sinnott (Ed.), *Interdisciplinary handbook of adult lifespan learning* (pp. 408–425). Westport, CT: Greenwood Press.

Devaney, R. (1989). *An introduction to chaotic dynamical systems.* Redwood City, CA: Addison-Wesley.

Eisler, R. (1987). *The chalice and the blade: Our history, our future.* San Francisco: Harper Collins.

Epstein, G. (1989). *Healing visualizations.* New York: Bantam.

Erikson, E. (1950). *Childhood and society.* New York: Norton.

Feinstein, D., & Krippner, S. (1988). *Personal mythology: The psychology of your evolving self.* Los Angeles: Tarcher.

Ford, D. (1987). *Humans as self-constructing living systems: A developmental perspective on behavior and personality.* Hillsdale, NJ: Erlbaum.

Frankl, V. (1963). *Man's search for meaning.* Boston: Beacon Press.

Gergen, K. (1991). *The saturated self.* New York: Basic Books.

Gilligan, C. (1982). *In a different voice: Psychological theory and women's development.* Cambridge, MA: Harvard University Press.

Gleick, J. (1987). *Chaos: Making a new science.* New York: Viking.

Goldstein, J. (1994). *The unshackled organization.* Portland, OR: Productivity Press.

Gore, A. (1992). *Earth in the balance.* Boston: Houghton Mifflin.

Herbert, N. (1986). *Quantum reality.* Garden City, NY: Doubleday.

Hogue, A., Bross, L., & Efran, J. (1994). Learning in psychotherapy: A Batesonian perspective. In J. Sinnott (Ed.), *Interdisciplinary handbook of adult lifespan learning* (pp. 186–202). Westport, CT: Greenwood Press.

Jantsch, E. (1980). *The self-organizing universe.* New York: Pergamon Press.

Josselson, R. (1992). *The space between us.* San Francisco: Jossey-Bass.

Jung, C. (1982). *Complete works.* London: Routledge & Kegan Paul.

Keen, S. (1994). *Hymns to an unknown god: Awakening the spirit in everyday life.* New York: Bantam.

Kelly, K. (1994). *Out of control: The rise of neo-biological civilization.* Reading, MA: Addison-Wesley.

Kuhn, T. (1962). *The structure of scientific revolutions.* Chicago: University of Chicago Press.

Locke, S., & Colligan, D. (1986). *The healer within: The new medicine of mind and body.* New York: Dutton.

Maslow, A. (1968). *Toward a psychology of being.* New York: Van Nostrand Reinhold.

Maturana, H., & Varela, F. (1988). *The tree of knowledge.* New York: New Science Library.

May, R. (1969). *Love and will.* New York: Norton.

Meacham, J., & Boyd, C. (1994). Expanding the circle of caring: From local to global. In J. Sinnott (Ed.), *Interdisciplinary handbook of adult lifespan learning* (pp. 61–73). Westport, CT: Greenwood Press.

Miller, J. (1978). *Living systems.* New York: McGraw-Hill.

Moore, T. (1992). *Care of the soul.* New York: Harper Collins.

Pagels, H. (1982). *The cosmic code: Quantum physics as the language of nature.* New York: Simon & Schuster.

Prigogine, I., & Stengers, I. (1984). *Order out of chaos.* New York: Bantam.

Rogers, C. (1961). *On becoming a person.* Boston: Houghton Mifflin.

Sheikh, A., & Sheikh, K. (1989). *Eastern and Western approaches to healing: Ancient wisdom and modern knowledge.* New York: Wiley.

Sinnott, J. (1981). The theory of relativity: A metatheory for development? *Human Development, 24,* 293–311.

———. (1984). Postformal reasoning: The relativistic stage. In M. Commons, F. Richards, & C. Armon (Eds.), *Beyond formal operations* (pp. 298–325). New York: Praeger.

———. (1986). *Sex roles and aging: Theory and research from a systems perspective.* New York: Karger.

———. (1987). Sex roles in adulthood and the aging years. In D. Carter (Ed.), *Current conceptions of sex roles and sex typing* (pp. 155–177). New York: Praeger.

———. (1989a). Adult differences in the use of postformal operations. In M. Commons, J. Sinnott, F. Richards, & C. Armon (Eds.), *Adult development: Comparison and applications of developmental models* (pp. 239–278). New York: Praeger.

———. (1989b). Changing the known, knowing the changing: General systems theory paradigms as ways to study complex change and complex thought. In D. Kramer & M. Bopp (Eds.), *Transformation in clinical and developmental psychology* (pp. 51–69). New York: Springer-Verlag.

———. (1989c). General systems theory: A rationale for the study of everyday memory. In L. Poon, D. Rubin, & B. Wilson (Eds.), *Everyday cognition in adulthood and old age* (pp. 59–72). New Rochelle, NY: Cambridge University Press.

———. (1992). The use of complex thought in resolving intragroup conflicts: A means to conscious development in the workplace. In J. Demick & P. Miller (Eds.), *Adult development in the workplace* (pp. 155–175). Hillsdale, NJ: Erlbaum.

———. (1993a). Sex roles. In V. S. Ramachandran (Ed.), *Encyclopedia of human behavior, 4,* (pp. 151–158). San Diego, CA: Academic Press.

———. (1993b). Teaching in a chaotic new physics world: Teaching as a dialogue with reality. In P. Kahaney, L. Perry & J. Janangelo (Eds.), *Theoretical and critical perspectives on teacher change* (pp. 91–108). Norwood, NJ: Ablex.

———. (1994a). Development and yearning: Cognitive aspects of spiritual development. *Journal of Adult Development, 1,* 91–100.

———. (Ed.). (1994b). *Interdisciplinary handbook of adult lifespan learning.* Westport, CT: Greenwood Press.

———. (1995). The development of complex reasoning: Postformal thought. In F. Blanchard-Fields & T. Hess (Eds.), *Perspectives on cognitive change in adulthood and aging.* New York: McGraw-Hill.

Sinnott, J., & Cavanaugh, J. (Eds.). (1991). *Bridging paradigms: Positive development in adulthood and cognitive aging.* New York: Praeger.

Sinnott, J., & Johnson, L. (1996). *Reinventing the university: A radical proposal for a problem focused university.* Norwood, NJ: Ablex.

Underwood, P. (1993). *The walking people.* San Anselmo, CA: A Tribe of Two Press.

Waldrop, M. (1992). *Complexity: The emerging science at the edge of order and chaos.* New York: Simon & Schuster.

Weibust, P., & Thomas, E. (1994). Learning and spirituality in adulthood. In J. Sinnott (Ed.), *Interdisciplinary handbook of adult lifespan learning* (pp. 120–134). Westport, CT: Greenwood Press.

Whitmyer, C. (Ed.). (1993). *In the company of others: Making community in the modern world.* Los Angeles: Tarcher.

Wolf, F. (1981). *Taking the quantum leap.* New York: Harper & Row.

Yalom, I. (1980). *Existential psychotherapy.* New York: Basic Books.

Zukav, G. (1979). *The dancing wu li masters.* New York: Bantam.

Eleven

Life Satisfaction and Older Women: Factor Structure Consistency across Age Cohorts

B. JAN McCULLOCH

The Life Satisfaction Index (LSI) (Neugarten, Havighurst, & Tobin, 1961) continues to be used as a measure of older adult psychological well-being. Studies using the LSI can be grouped into two major categories: (1) those examining substantive issues regarding the effects of social and environmental factors as well as physical health on well-being (e.g., Baldassare, Rosenfield, & Rook, 1984; Beckman, 1981; Kivett, 1988; McCulloch, 1990); and (2) methodological studies examining the factor structure of the LSI and its appropriateness as a measure of older adult quality of life (e.g., Adams, 1969; Hoyt & Creech, 1983; Liang, Lawrence, & Bollen, 1987; McCulloch, 1992). Methodological studies continue to underscore the importance of examining LSI factor structure among specific older adult populations. For example, contradictory results concerning the performance of the scale across aging groups have been reported. Some researchers found consistent scale performance in random samples of older adults (Liang, 1984) and among older whites and African Americans (Liang et al., 1987), while others reported variability in the performance of the LSI across populations including gender/race and income/age groups (e.g., Hoyt & Creech, 1983; McCulloch, 1992; Wilson, Elias, & Brownlee, 1985).

MEASUREMENT ISSUES REGARDING THE LSI

Two specific issues have emerged regarding the validation of the LSI as a measure of quality of life among older adults. First, inconsistencies have been

This research was partially supported by the National Institute on Aging, Grant #AG00029, and was initially begun when the author was a postdoctoral fellow at the Center for the Study of Aging and Human Development, Duke University Medical Center, Durham, North Carolina.

noted in the dimensionality of the scale. For example, the original version was hypothesized to be a multidimensional scale with five subscales: zest, resolution and fortitude, congruence, self-concept, and mood tone (Neugarten et al., 1961). Subsequent studies reported revised factor structures for the scale, with support for both four-factor (Adams, 1969) and three-factor solutions (Hoyt & Creech, 1983; Liang, 1984; Liang et al., 1987; McCulloch, 1992; Wilson et al., 1985).

A second issue concerns variability of the LSI factor structure across population subgroups. Confirmatory factor analysis techniques have been used to examine LSI structure (Hoyt & Creech, 1983; Liang, 1984; Liang et al., 1987; McCulloch, 1992; Wilson et al., 1985), with researchers hypothesizing the structure of life satisfaction with either first- or second-ordered factors (Bollen, 1989; Jöreskog & Sörbom, 1989; Marsh & Hocevar, 1985). The first-order model hypothesized that the dimensions of life satisfaction were measured by scale items and that these dimensions were correlated with one another. Hoyt and Creech (1983), for example, reported that a first-order, eight-item, three-factor model provided an acceptable fit to data from separate gender/race subgroups (older white men, older African-American men, older African-American women, and older white women). This three-factor model, however, did not fit consistently across groups, with Hoyt and Creech (1983) concluding that it could not be assumed that scale items were interpreted similarly across gender/race groups. In addition, review of LSI items loading on the three factors prompted Hoyt and Creech to rename the dimensions of life satisfaction. Dimensions were identified as satisfaction with the present (previously identified as mood tone), future orientation (previously zest for life), and satisfaction with the past (previously congruence).

Others (Wilson et al., 1985) also reported across-group differences in the factor structure of the LSI. Wilson et al. (1985) examined Hoyt and Creech's (1983) three-factor version of the LSI among four income/age retiree groups. Results showed that although the model was tenable for three of the four groups (high income/younger age, high income/older age, and low income/older age), the first-order, three-factor LSI structure did not provide an acceptable fit for low-income/younger-age retirees.

In randomly divided subsamples of national data, Liang (1984) and Liang et al. (1987) examined a second-order or hierarchical, three-factor LSI factor structure. Hierarchical operationalization provided a means of explaining the interrelationships, or covariance, among LSI factors, an explanation not possible with first-order factor analyses (Marsh & Hocevar, 1985). In these examinations, life satisfaction, the second-order latent construct, was hypothesized to account for correlations among the first-order factors of mood tone, zest for life, and congruence. Results showed that the hierarchical conceptualization of life satisfaction provided an adequate fit across all four random groups (Liang, 1984) and that the model did not differ significantly across African-American and white racial groups (Liang et al., 1987). More recently, McCulloch (1992) investigated LSI item pool, coding scheme, and factor structure discrepancies in the use of the LSI as a measure of well-being among older gender/race groups. Results showed (*a*) that coding scheme made little difference in the performance of the LSI as a measure of quality of life; (*b*) that different item pools affected the fit of LSI factor structure models across groups; and (*c*) that a three-factor, first-order LSI factor structure, as compared with a hierarchical factor structure, provided the most parsimonious fit in separate groups. These results underscored the misspecification of life satisfaction when LSI items have been summed and used as a unidimensional construct.

In summary, previous studies have provided needed information about the suitability of the LSI as a quality-of-life measure in some specific population subgroups. Although studies examining the LSI with random samples reported consistent scale performance among older adults (Liang, 1984) and among older whites and African Americans (Liang et al., 1987), studies examining life-satisfaction factor structure among other specific populations showed differences in the performance of the scale across subgroups. Differences have been noted across gender/race groups (Hoyt & Creech, 1983; McCulloch, 1992) and income/retiree groups (Wilson et al., 1985). Examination of LSI satisfaction performance among older women, however, has remained unexplored.

LIFE SATISFACTION AMONG OLDER WOMEN

An examination of the factor structure of life satisfaction among older women is needed for two reasons. First, although studies examining the life status of older women have increased over the past two decades, relatively little information is available regarding the measurement of quality of life among this specific aging population subgroup. Second, and more specifically related to the LSI as a measure of quality of life, there is the possibility that cohorts of older women interpret the individual items comprising the scale differently. If women interpret items differently, this difference may confound results reported for the relationship of environmental, social, and health factors to well-being across the whole of later life for aging women. For example, if LSI items, such as "These are the best years of my life," are interpreted differently by women in early old age as compared to women of advanced age, results concerning the relationship of physical health to well-being may be affected. Examination of the face validity of LSI items suggests that some differential interpretation might be possible. Examples of such items include "I feel old and somewhat tired" and "I feel my age, but it does not bother me"—statements that may have different meanings for a 67-year-old woman as compared to an 89-year-old woman.

The purpose of this study, therefore, was the examination of life-satisfaction factor structure across three cohorts of older women. Two research questions were investigated: (1) Was a common LSI factor structure confirmed *within* separate cohorts of aging women? (2) Was a common LSI factor structure replicated *across* cohorts of older women?

METHODS

Sample

The data used in the present study were of a subsample of older women from the 1974 Myth and Reality of Aging Survey (see Harris & Associates, 1975, for a full description of the sample). Data consisted of a nationally representative sample of 2,797 adults 65 years of age or older. It should be noted that although the survey oversampled older African Americans, the numbers of African-American and other minority women in each cohort were small. Cohort data were available for less than 100 older African-American and less than 10 older Hispanic women, a constraint that precluded the examination of cohort/race confirmatory factor analysis models in this study. The unweighted sample of older women was divided into three cohort groups with complete data: a random sample of young-old women, 65–74 years of age, $n = 327$; old women, 75–80 years of age, $n = 318$; and very old women, 81 years of age and older, $n = 294$. The original survey provided data on 1,080 women 65–74 years of age (Harris & Associates, 1975). For the purposes of the present study, however, a random sample (.33) of the total young-old women was selected to provide approximately equal sample sizes across cohort groups and thus minimize the influence of differential sample size on goodness-of-fit indicators (Bollen, 1989; Jöreskog & Sörbom, 1989).

Data used for this study were chosen for two specific reasons. First, these older women provide further information about life satisfaction with a sample that has previously been examined (e.g., Hoyt & Creech, 1983; Liang, 1984; Liang et al., 1987; McCulloch, 1992), providing a method of comparison across studies. Second, few data sets are available that meet the criteria necessary for such a study: inclusion of LSI items and sufficient numbers of very old women to allow for an examination of life-satisfaction factor structure across aging cohorts.

Statistical Methods

Confirmatory factor analysis procedures were used to examine differences in the fit of LSI models across older women's cohorts (Jöreskog & Sörbom, 1989). Models were developed to examine research objectives. First, among separate cohorts of older women, what was the factor structure of life satisfaction? Second, was a single life-satisfaction factor structure confirmed across cohorts of older women? To answer these questions, two sets of confirmatory factor analysis procedures were employed: (1) separate sets of confirmatory factor analyses were used to examine the fit of hypothesized models for each cohort group, and (2) stacked confirmatory factor models were used to examine the equality of models across cohort groups.

When confirmatory factor models were stacked, the consistency of factor structure across older women's cohorts could be examined. Examinations began with the least restrictive model, M_1, one that did not constrain any model parameters across cohorts to be equal, and continued with models constraining parameter estimates across the three groups to be equal (Bollen, 1989). Lambdas (λs), or the factor loadings of measured indicators on LSI dimensions, were constrained in the first equality constraint model, M_2. Succeeding models (M_3–M_5) constrained additional parameters in the following order: M_3: gammas (γs), or factor loadings of LSI dimensions on life satisfaction; M_4: zetas (ζs), errors in first-order equations; and M_5. M_5, with epsilons (εs) or estimates of measurement error for LSI scale items also constrained, was the most restrictive model. This final model posited a life-satisfaction factor structure with lambdas, gammas, zetas, and epsilons constrained to be equal. Models, nested in this succeedingly restrictive fashion, that continue to adequately fit data across groups provide confidence in the assumption that the same life-satisfaction factor structure is operating across groups and thus increase confidence that errors encountered when parameter estimates differ across groups have been reduced (Bollen, 1989).

In accordance with LISREL specifications (Jöreskog & Sörbom, 1989), the following symbols represented well-being components:

ξ (xis)	Second-order latent construct (life satisfaction)
γ (gammas)	Structural coefficients, direct causal links between latent second and first-order constructs
η (etas)	First-order latent constructs, dimensions of life satisfaction (present, past, and future)
ζ (zetas)	Errors in first-order latent equations
λ (lambdas)	First-order factor loadings or coefficients of indicators regressed on LSI dimensions
y's	Observed indicators or LSI items
ε (epsilons)	Error in observed indicators

Polychoric Correlation Coefficients. Prior to confirmatory factor analysis, polychoric correlation coefficients were estimated using PRELIS, a preprocessor program for LISREL (Jöreskog & Sörbom, 1989). LSI scale items were coded as dichotomous variables (McCulloch, 1992), indicating that statistical assumptions would be violated if they were analyzed as continuous variables. Polychoric correlation coefficients provided the most accurate correlations when variables were dichotomous (Babakus, Ferguson, & Jöreskog, 1987; Muthén, 1983). Resulting confirmatory factor analysis estimates, including estimates of first- and second-order factors and standard errors, were closer to their true values because covariances were estimated with polychoric correlation coefficients.

Table 11.1
Use of LSI Items in Eight- and Eleven-Variable Models

LSI Items	Eight-Variable Models	Eleven-Variable Models
Satisfaction with the Present		
Happy-As happy as when I was younger	X	X
Happier-Life could be happier than it is now	X	X
Best Yrs-These are the best years of my life	X	X
Future Orientation		
Expect-Expect some interesting and pleasant things to happen in the future	X	X
Present-Things I do are as interesting as ever		X
Feel Old-I feel old & somewhat tired		X
Boring-Most things are boring or monotonous		X
Plans-I have made plans for a month/year	X	
Satisfaction with the Past		
Satisfied-As I look back, I am well satisfied	X	X
Gotten Ex-Gotten what I expected out of life	X	X
Past OK-Would not change the past	X	X
Breaks-Gotten more breaks than most		X

Note: Items presented in abbreviated form for table. Readers are referred to Neugarten et al. (1961) for a complete citing of LSI items.

Life-Satisfaction Structure among Separate Cohorts of Older Women. In the first set of procedures, two competing life-satisfaction models were examined (table 11.1). The first model represented a first-order, three-factor, eleven-item model, a scale construction previously supported by Liang (1984) and Liang et al. (1987). The second model hypothesized a first-order, three-factor, eight-variable model, a model previously supported by Hoyt and Creech (1983), Wilson et al. (1985), and McCulloch (1992). Based on previous examinations of the LSI (McCulloch, 1992), first-order, rather than second-order, models were used in these initial comparisons. After competing eight- and eleven-variable, first-order models were compared, a final, within-group model was examined. For this model, LSI factor structure was hypothesized to be hierarchical, with a second-order life-satisfaction factor explaining the interrelationships of first-order dimensions.

Life-Satisfaction Factor Structure across Cohorts of Older Women. The second set of confirmatory factor analyses examined the equality of the second-order, eight-item factor structure across the three cohorts of older women. The purpose of this specific set of analyses was the confirmation of a single factor structure—the final model in the first set of confirmatory factor analyses—across age groups of older women, one that appropriately measures quality of life regardless of cohort group. As a basis of comparison across these groups, an initial or baseline model (M_1), with all LSI items hypothesized to represent a unidimensional life-satisfaction construct, was used to compute post hoc incremental fit indices. Incremental indices of fit included χ_{diff} (Bollen, 1989), Δ_2 (Bollen, 1989), ρ_2 (Bentler & Bonett, 1980; Tucker & Lewis, 1973), and Hoelter's Critical N (CN) (Hoelter, 1983).

RESULTS

Comparison of Eight-Variable and Eleven-Variable, First-Order LSI Factor Models

The first set of analyses, addressing the fit of hypothesized first-order models in separate older women's cohorts, provided support for an eight-variable model (table 11.2). Across all older-women cohorts, the eight-variable, first-order model provided a better fit as compared to the eleven-variable, first-order model. It should be noted that for all models, relatively good fits were achieved, with both eight- and eleven-variable models fitting most acceptably for the middle cohort of aging women, women ranging in age from 75 to 80 years. Eight-variable models, across all measures of fit, however, performed better than eleven-variable models.

After comparisons of eight- and eleven-item models, a second-order factor was examined. As noted earlier, hierarchical models provide additional information regarding the interrelationship of life-satisfaction factors because the higher-ordered construct, life satisfaction, is included to explain the covariance among LSI dimensions, or first-ordered factors (Marsh & Hocevar, 1985). The resulting model, providing the basis for the second set of analyses, showed that life satisfaction explained significant amounts of variance in first-order factors (figure 11.1). Among young-old women, for example, the factor loadings of future orientation, satisfaction with the present, and satisfaction with the past on the higher-order latent life-satisfaction construct were .72, .76, and .85, respectively. Acceptable first-order factor scores also were found among women in old (.57, .60, and .93) and very old cohorts (.69, .67, and .65), demonstrating the relationship of life satisfaction to dimensions. Goodness-of-fit indices for models in this series remained acceptable across the three cohorts of older women (table 11.2). (It should be noted that when three-factor first- and second-order models are compared in this fashion, mathematically identical assessments of the fit of models to data occur.)

Equality Constraint Models: Replicability across Older-Women Cohorts

The second set of analyses, examining the consistency of LSI factor structure across cohorts of older women, provided additional support for the eight-variable

Table 11.2
Comparisons of LSI, First-Order Factor Analysis Indicators of Fit for Older Women's
Cohorts

Indicators of Fit	Three-Factor, Eight-Variable Models	Three-Factor, Eleven-Variable Models
Young-Old Women:		
n=327		
χ^2	26.59	105.88
χ^2/df	26.59/17 = 1.56	105.88/41 = 2.58
GFI	.980	.943
AGFI	.958	.908
RMSR	.020	.034
p-value of χ^2	.06	<.001
Old Women:		
n=318		
χ^2	16.65	69.25
χ^2/df	16.65/17 = .98	69.25/41 = 1.69
GFI	.987	.962
AGFI	.973	.938
RMSR	.016	.026
p-value of χ^2	.479	.004
Very-Old Women:		
n=294		
χ^2	24.73	67.53
χ^2/df	24.73/17 = 1.45	67.53/41 = 1.65
GFI	.981	.960
AGFI	.959	.936
RMSR	.020	.026
p-value of χ^2	.101	.006

model (table 11.3). Comparison with the baseline, unidimensional model (M_1) showed that acceptable fits remained across increasingly restrictive equality constraint models. The final model in this series (M_5), the most restrictive model in the series, hypothesized that across cohorts first- and second-order factor loadings (lambdas and gammas) as well as equation and measurement errors (zetas and epsilons) were equal. This model continued to fit data acceptably, as demonstrated by both individual and incremental indices of fit.

Examination of parameter estimates for the final life-satisfaction model, M_5, showed that the eight-item LSI structure was consistent across cohorts of older women (table 11.4). Life satisfaction, as measured by the LSI, consisted of three first-order factors, satisfaction with the past, future orientation, and satisfaction

Figure 11.1
Hierarchical Eight-Item, Three-Factor LSI Factor Structure

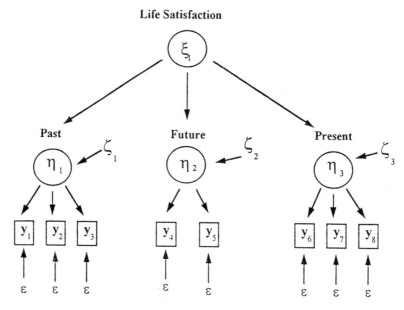

Life Satisfaction

with the present. A higher-order factor, life satisfaction, was responsible for the interrelationship of first-order factors. Standardized estimates, or factor loadings, for the observed indicators of LSI dimensions ranged from .417 to .811, with all indicators above the minimum recommended value of .40 (Liang, 1986). Additionally, correlations among LSI dimensions showed that across cohorts of older women satisfaction with the past, future orientation, and satisfaction with the present were interrelated. Correlations ranged from .407 for the correlation of satisfaction with the past and future orientation to .474 for future orientation and satisfaction with the present (table 11.4).

In summary, two sets of confirmatory factor analyses were used to address research questions. Results showed (1) that an eight-item, three-factor hierarchical factor structure was confirmed separately for each cohort of older women; and (2) that a hierarchical conceptualization of this three-factor, eight-item LSI factor structure was consistent across cohorts, a model providing the most parsimonious fit to data regardless of age grouping.

CONCLUSIONS

The purpose of this study was the examination of measurement issues related to the replicability of the LSI as a measure of quality of life across cohorts of older women. The consistency found in the performance of the LSI among older women, regardless of age group, increased confidence that the scale was inter-

Table 11.3
Comparisons of Goodness-of-Fit Indices for Eight-Variable, Second-Order Equality Constraint Models

Goodness of Fit Indicator	Unconstrained M_1	Constrained M2	Constrained M3	Constrained M_4	Constrained M_5
X^2-Square		78.23	83.44	85.62	89.46
p-value		.068	.061	.114	.407
GFI					
Young-Old Women		.979	.978	.978	.977
Old Women		.984	.982	.981	.981
Very-Old Women		.977	.976	.976	.975
RMSR					
Young-Old Women		.021	.023	.024	.025
Old Women		.018	.021	.021	.022
Very-Old Women		.025	.026	.027	.028
X^2_{diff}	240.13 * df-9	229.86 * df-1	224.65 * df-5	222.47 * df-11	218.63 * df-27
Δ_2	.934	.930	.924	.938	.989
ρ_2	.920	.932	.931	.950	.993
CN	943	957	949	1000	1146

*$p < .0001$; model a significant improvement over baseline model.

Note: X^2_{diff} reported for models M_2–M_5 was calculated as the difference between each model and a baseline model hypothesizing a one-factor model with all items loading on a single life-satisfaction factor ($X^2 = 308.09$, $df = 60$, $p < .0001$).

Table 11.4

LISREL Estimates for Eight-Variable, Three-Factor Constrained LSI Model

Parameters	Unstandardized Parameter Estimates	Standardized Parameter Estimates
Second-Order Factor Loadings		
γ_1: Satisfaction with the Present	1.000	.799
γ_2: Future Orientation	.743	.696
γ_3: Satisfaction with the Past	.586	.746
First-Order Factor Loadings		
Satisfaction with the Present		
λ_1: Happy-As happy as when I was younger	1.000	.811
λ_2: Happier-Life could be happier than it is now	.515	.417
λ_3: Best Yrs-These are the best years of my life	.686	.595
Future Orientation		
λ_4: Future-Expect some interesting and pleasant things to happen in the future	1.000	.700
λ_5: Plans-I have made plans for a month/year	.697	.489
Satisfaction with the Past		
λ_6: Satisfied-As I look back, I am well satisfied	1.000	.651
λ_7: Gotten Ex-Gotten what I expected out of life	1.190	.690
λ_8: Past OK-Would not change the past	1.016	.536
Error Variances in First-Order Equations		
ζ_1: Satisfaction with the Present	.361	
ζ_2: Future Orientation	.443	
ζ_3: Satisfaction with the Past	.515	
Correlations Between First-Order Factors		
	(2)	(3)
Present		
Future (2)	.474	
Past (3)	.440	.407

Table 11.4 (Continued)

Parameters	Unstandardized Parameter Estimates	Standardized Parameter Estimates
Measurement Error Variances in Observed Indicators		
Satisfaction with the Present		
ϵ_1: Happy-As happy as when I was younger	.218	
ϵ_2: Happier-Life could be happier than it is now	.527	
ϵ_3: Best Yrs-These are the best years of my life	.360	
Future Orientation		
ϵ_4: Future-Expect some interesting & pleasant things to happen in the future	.325	
ϵ_5: Plans-I have made plans for a month/year	.483	
Satisfaction with the Past		
ϵ_6: Satisfied-As I look back, I am well satisfied	.227	
ϵ_7: Gotten Ex-Gotten what I expected out of life	.260	
ϵ_8: Past OK-Would not change the past	.427	

Goodness-of-Fit Indicators	Young-Old Women	Old Women	Very-Old Women
Overall χ^2 for Constrained Model 89.46, $p = .407$			
GFI	.977	.981	.975
RMSR	.025	.022	.028

Note: All parameter estimates significant at or below .05.

preted similarly across cohort groups. This consistency also increases confidence in results reporting information about the relationship of environmental, social, and health factors to life satisfaction because the confounding effects of measurement inconsistency were not found across cohorts of older women. The final model, consistent across young-old, old, and very old cohorts, was a hierarchical model with the second-order construct, life satisfaction, accounting for the interrelationships among three first-order LSI dimensions (satisfaction with the past, future orientation, and satisfaction with the present).

In addition, conclusions underscored the importance of examining scale measurement properties prior to investigations of substantive issues. Results specific to the LSI as a measure of quality of life showed that three items frequently included as adequate measures of life satisfaction, although not reducing goodness-of-fit indicators to unacceptable levels, affected the overall performance of the scale. These items, "The things I do are as interesting as they ever were," "I feel old and somewhat tired," and "I have gotten more of the breaks in life than most of the people I know," contributed to an overall less parsimonious fit when compared with the eight-variable model reported by Hoyt and Creech (1983) and confirmed in subsequent studies (McCulloch, 1992; Wilson et al., 1985).

The consistency of LSI factor structure among older women was examined with data previously used to investigate the LSI as a measure of quality of life. When the results of the present study are compared with previous ones, some conclusions are possible. First, for studies that have examined specific population subgroups as compared with the random division of study populations, the eight-item version of the LSI performed more adequately than the eleven-item version. For example, the eight-item version has been confirmed among older gender/race groups (Hoyt & Creech, 1983; McCulloch, 1992), income/retiree groups (Wilson et al., 1985), and cohorts of older women. Second, comparisons suggest that even though an eight-item model has been confirmed across these specific population groups, older African-American men and women are likely to interpret the items differently as compared with white elders (Hoyt & Creech, 1983; McCulloch, 1992). As noted earlier, the limited numbers of older African-American women precluded the possibility of examining race/cohort differences in the performance of the LSI in the present study.

Caveats must be considered when interpreting these results. First, earlier analyses have reported race/gender differences in the factor structure of the LSI. It is possible that had adequate numbers of older African-American women been available for this study, cohort/race differences would have been discernible. Future methodological studies are needed with adequate numbers of older African-American men and women to examine the replicability of LSI factor structure across cohort/race/gender groups. It is likely, based on previous studies, that the LSI performs differently among whites as compared with African Americans. Additionally, data are currently unavailable regarding LSI factor structure among other minority groups, such as Hispanics or Asian Americans. Second, it must be recognized that results were obtained with archival data. It is possible that the consistent eight-variable, second-order LSI factor structure reported in this study might not be replicated with current representative samples.

It also must be recognized that the replicability of the LSI across older women's cohorts provides confidence in the consistent performance of the scale; it does not, however, address the more complex issues about validity of the scale among women across the whole of old age. Issues regarding the appropriateness of this revision of the scale continue to need examination. Does the eight-item version of the scale adequately represent quality of life? Does the eight-item version of the LSI represent a valid measure of Neugarten et al.'s (1961) original conceptualization of life satisfaction? When the eight-item version of the LSI is compared with qualitative assessments of older women's life satisfaction, does the scale continue to represent a valid operationalization of life satisfaction?

Future studies also are needed that examine issues regarding the measurement consistency of scales used to measure constructs other than life satisfaction. For example, the frequent use of burden scales (e.g., Zarit, Reever, & Bach-Peterson, 1980) and functional assessments of health (Fillenbaum, 1988) also would benefit from attention to measurement issues. Does the same factor structure for these measurement tools hold across specific population subgroups? Do cultural factors, such as differences in the definition of filial responsibility, affect the factor structure of scales measuring constructs such as caregiver burden?

In conclusion, this study has examined the performance of the LSI (Neugarten et al., 1961) as a measure of older women's quality of life. Results showed a consistent life-satisfaction factor structure with eight items measuring satisfaction with the past, future orientation, and satisfaction with the present. Findings increase confidence in the performance of the scale as a consistent measure of well-being for older women.

REFERENCES

Adams, D. L. (1969). Analysis of a life satisfaction index. *Journal of Gerontology, 24*, 470–474.

Babakus, E., Ferguson, C. E., & Jöreskog, K. G. (1987). The sensitivity of confirmatory maximum likelihood factor analysis to violations of measurement scale and distributional assumptions. *Journal of Marketing Research, 26*, 222–228.

Baldassare, M., Rosenfield, S., & Rook, K. (1984). The types of social relations predicting elderly well-being. *Research on Aging, 6*, 549–559.

Beckman, L. J. (1981). Effects of social interaction and children's relative inputs on older women's psychological well-being. *Journal of Personality and Social Psychology, 41*, 1075–1086.

Bentler, P. M., & Bonett, D. G. (1980). Significance tests and goodness of fit in the analysis of covariance structures. *Psychological Bulletin, 88*, 588–606.

Bollen, K. A. (1989). *Structural equations with latent variables.* New York: John Wiley & Sons.

Fillenbaum, G. (1988). *Multidimensional functional assessment of older adults: The Duke older Americans resources and services procedures.* Hillsdale, NJ: Lawrence Erlbaum Associates.

Harris, L., & Associates. (1975). *The myth and reality of aging in America.* Washington, DC: National Council on Aging.

Hoelter, J. W. (1983). The analysis of covariance structures: Goodness-of-fit indices. *Sociological Methods and Research, 11*, 325–344.

Hoyt, D. R., & Creech, J. C. (1983). The life satisfaction index: A methodological and theoretical critique. *Journal of Gerontology, 38*, 111–116.

Jöreskog, K. G., & Sörbom, D. (1989). *LISREL VI: Analysis of linear structural relationships by the method of maximum likelihood.* Chicago: International Education Services.

Kivett, V. R. (1988). Aging in a rural place: The elusive source of well-being. *Journal of Rural Studies, 4*, 125–132.

Liang, J. (1984). Dimensions of the life satisfaction index A: A structural formulation. *Journal of Gerontology, 39*, 613–622.

———. (1986). Self-reported physical health among aged adults. *Journal of Gerontology, 41*, 248–260.

Liang, J., Lawrence, R. H., & Bollen, K. A. (1987). Race differences in factorial structures of two measures of subjective well-being. *Journal of Gerontology, 42,* 426–428.

McCulloch, B. J. (1990). The relationship of intergenerational reciprocity to the morale of older parents: Equity and exchange theory comparisons. *Journals of Gerontology: Social Sciences, 45,* S150–S155.

———. (1992). Gender and race: An interaction affecting the replicability of well-being across groups. *Women and Health, 19,* 65–89.

Marsh, H. W., & Hocevar, D. (1985). Application of confirmatory factor analysis to the study of self-concept: First- and higher-order factor models and their invariance across groups. *Psychological Bulletin, 97,* 562–582.

Muthén, B. (1983). Latent variable structure equation modeling with categorical data. *Journal of Econometrics, 22,* 43–65.

Neugarten, B. L., Havighurst, R. J., & Tobin, S. S. (1961). The measurement of life satisfaction. *Journal of Gerontology, 16,* 134–143.

Tucker, L. R., & Lewis, C. (1973). A reliability coefficient for maximum likelihood factor analysis. *Psychometrika, 38,* 1–10.

Wilson, G. A., Elias, J. W., & Brownlee, L. J., Jr. (1985). Factor invariance and the life satisfaction index. *Journal of Gerontology, 40,* 344–346.

Zarit, S. H., Reever, K. E., & Bach-Peterson, J. (1980). Relatives of the impaired elderly: Correlates of feelings of burden. *Gerontologist, 20,* 649–655.

Twelve

Reminiscence among Older Women

DEBRA McDONALD AND EILEEN DEGES CURL

For the last three decades the concept of reminiscence has been discussed among many professional groups, as well as being the basis for scholarly research and publication by practitioners from a myriad of professions. Among professions the use of reminiscence has "taken root" and provided practitioners in sociology, anthropology, psychology, gerontology, nursing, education, occupational therapy, medicine, and pastoral care with an independent intervention that can be used in the day-to-day care of clients.

With the use of reminiscence as an interdisciplinary intervention, many questions arise in the literature regarding the status of reminiscence. Examples of these questions include the following: (1) are definitions of reminiscence consistent? (2) is reminiscence beneficial? and (3) is reminiscence a "therapy"? These questions, and others, appear with measured regularity in the literature addressing reminiscence. This chapter will address these questions, in part, and will advance a contemplative stance for those with an interest in the concept of reminiscence.

REMINISCENCE AND LIFE REVIEW: SAME OR DIFFERENT?

Haight and Burnside (1993) wrote that the terms *reminiscence* and *life review* have been used interchangeably for the last three decades, since Butler (1963) used both terms in the title of his seminal article on life review. Use of the terms reminiscence and life review has been problematic for scholars and practitioners because in some instances the terms are used to describe the same concept, while at other times the terms address distinctively different concepts. A sampling of phrases used to define reminiscence and life review are delineated in the following paragraphs.

Reminiscence

Lamme and Baars (1993) broadly defined reminiscence as "the silent or oral, purposive or spontaneous recalling of past events and experiences" (p. 298) in a person's life. Enlarging on this definition, Wong (1991) identified reminiscence as potentially "both a private and social activity" (p. 154) in which ventilation of emotions, expression of one's views, sharing of burdens, obtaining recognition, enlarging one's life experiences, and forging new friendships can occur. Wholihan (1992) used a simpler definition by describing reminiscence as the act of recalling the past. Burnside and Haight (1992) and Kovach (1991) narrowed the definition by stressing that reminiscence focuses on recalling and relating past experiences that were especially significant or memorable to the reminiscer. Similarly, Bramlett and Gueldner (1993) viewed reminiscence as "an opportunity for [people] to enjoy remembering the richness of their past experiences" (p. 69).

Other definitions of reminiscence include possible outcomes or benefits of the act of reminiscing. For example, Moore (1992) wrote of reminiscence as the mental recall of long-forgotten experiences or facts, whereby the process of telling about past experiences facilitates seeing the purpose of one's life. Haight and Burnside (1993) expanded on this idea by viewing reminiscence as a psychosocial, informal, supportive intervention, mainly using positive recall, that can decrease isolation and increase self-esteem, alertness, friendships, connectedness, and socialization. Merriam (1993b) went on to categorize the uses of reminiscence as having therapeutic, informative, and enjoyment functions.

Life Review

In Butler's 1963 seminal article on life review, the geropsychiatrist wrote:

I conceive of the life review as a naturally occurring, universal mental process characterized by the progressive return to consciousness of past experiences, and particularly, the resurgence of unresolved conflicts; simultaneously, and normally, these revived experiences and conflicts can be surveyed and re-integrated. (p. 66)

Within the literature many writers still subscribe to Butler's definition of life review (DeGenova, 1992; Farris & Gibson, 1992; Wallace, 1992; and Merriam, 1993a), but a number of diverse definitions of life review can also be found.

Magee (1993) described life review as recall and reflection upon long-forgotten incidents, during which the emotions are recaptured and the experiences are conveyed to a listener. The goal of reflection is integration of the memories into an acceptance of one's present self by critically evaluating the experiences. Burnside and Haight (1992) wrote of life review as "a retrospective survey of existence, a critical study of a life, or a second look at one's life" (p. 856). In 1993 Haight and Burnside expanded their previous work by discussing life review as a psychoanalytic, evaluative, reframing process. They further explicated life review as being a structured, empathetic, and valuing experience that may focus on pleasant or unpleasant recall. As identified by Haight and Burnside, the goal of life review is integrity, with anticipated outcomes being increased self-esteem, well-being, wisdom, life satisfaction, and peace and decreased depression.

Staudinger, Smith, and Baltes (1992) defined life review as "the construction or reconstruction, interpretation, and evaluation of an individual's life course" (p. 272). Stevens-Ratchford (1993) studied life review and reminiscence together and defined the combined concept of life-review reminiscence in this way: "Any structured or directed participation in reminiscing for therapeutic purposes, regardless of whether the person evaluates his or her past experiences" (p. 413).

Synthesis

Because the concepts of reminiscence and life review are used interchangeably in the literature, conceptual clarity between the definitions of the two terms is needed (Merriam, 1993b; Burnside, 1990; Burnside & Haight, 1992; Haight & Burnside, 1993; Kovach, 1990). To synthesize a definition of reminiscence to be used among professions, the reviewed definitions of reminiscence were combined. Advanced for consideration is a synthesized definition of reminiscence as a psychosocial intervention in which the memorable past is recalled, reflected upon, and shared with others, usually in a group setting.

By comparing this synthesized definition of reminiscence with the life-review definitions cited, one can begin to see commonalities and to delineate differences between the two concepts. Both reminiscence and life review use memory and recall. Also, both concepts have the potential to evoke pleasant or unpleasant feelings, have the potential to be used across the lifespan, may be structured or free-flowing, and are considered to be therapeutic. Differences between reminiscence and life review begin with the theory base of each concept and continue throughout the goals, the practitioner/client roles, the process, and the outcomes (Haight & Burnside, 1993).

Psychosocial theory serves as the basis for reminiscence and is congruent with the goals of reminiscence, which include increasing socialization, improving communication skills, and developing rapport with others. In contrast, life review builds on the psychoanalytic framework of Erikson's (1963) eight stages of development, with the goal being a sense of integrity related to the eighth stage. Because the goals of reminiscence and life review differ, the roles and processes used to attain the goals also differ (Haight & Burnside, 1993).

During reminiscence a practitioner uses a supportive-listener approach, while during life review a practitioner reviews with clients their perceptions of the developmental stages of life they have experienced. For negative events that occurred during stages, the practitioner uses counseling skills to reframe the events in terms acceptable to clients, thus promoting progress developmentally.

Helping clients evaluate and reframe events during the life-review process typically requires a dyadic relationship (one practitioner to one client) rather than the group-process relationship commonly used for reminiscing. Purported outcomes of the reminiscence group process include decreasing isolation, increasing alertness, and facilitating friendships and a sense of connectedness with others. Anticipated outcomes of the life-review process include less despair and more satisfaction with life due to the wisdom and peace often associated with gaining a sense of integrity (Haight & Burnside, 1993).

In this section interdisciplinary definitions of reminiscence and life review were extracted from pertinent and obtainable literature. A synthesized definition of reminiscence was advanced. In the next sections theoretical and then research perspectives about reminiscence are explored.

THEORETICAL PERSPECTIVE

Reminiscence has become a popular care option with the elderly in both the United States and the United Kingdom. This popularity has led to a growing body of reminiscence literature in various disciplines, theoretically extolling the potential benefits for participants (Middleton & Buchanan, 1993).

Wong (1991) proposed that reminiscence can be both a private and a social activity and postulated that the socialization that occurs in sharing life histories facilitates new friendships. Wong further wrote of the possibility of reminiscence groups being initiated in a variety of settings and urged readers to contemplate how reminiscence groups could be community based as part of an informal support network for seniors.

In the discipline of sociology, Lamme and Baars (1993) also stressed the importance of reminiscence as a social activity by emphasizing the influential role the social environment has upon reminiscence in elderly individuals. This emphasis is due to the fact that many of the experiences occurring across the lifespan that lead to reminiscence are organized by society. For instance, when elders are pushed to accept changes, the reflection necessary to effect change may lead older adults to think of how different their lives might have been if they were younger now. Lamme and Baars further wrote that reminiscence fosters a sense of continuity by facilitating the integration of new experiences.

In the disciplines of philosophy and pastoral care, respectively, Singer (1993) and Wendt (1992) used the literature to reminisce personally. These reminiscences committed to writing personal reflections of memorable people and places for future readers to review and contemplate.

In the discipline of nursing, Moore (1992) wrote of reminiscence relieving depressive symptoms in the elderly. Other proposed benefits of a reminiscence program include changes in awareness, alertness, enthusiasm, and spontaneity within a week of initiating a reminiscing protocol. Wholihan (1992) advanced the idea that reminiscence may be a tool for nurses to use in the care of terminally ill clients, because recalling accomplishments and good feelings is the kind of remembering frequently seen in social interactions among hospice clients, staff, and caregivers.

In review, theoretical benefits of reminiscence have been documented in the literature across several professions. Although purported benefits of reminiscence are frequently identified, empirically derived benefits are, at times, less definitive.

RESEARCH PERSPECTIVE

To examine the current empirical benefits identified in the literature, twelve available research studies exploring the concept of reminiscence were reviewed, encompassing the time period between 1990 and 1993. Research-based studies exploring life review and life histories were purposely omitted due to conceptual differences from reminiscence. Qualitative studies on reminiscence will be addressed first, to show the linkage between qualitative and quantitative studies. Following the examination of these studies, quantitative research studies will be examined.

Kovach (1991) examined the interpretations reminiscers made of personal experiences from the past. The 21 female subjects in the study were interviewed by the same interviewer for approximately 30 minutes. Content analysis techniques yielded eight reminiscent themes from the transcribed interviews. Themes generated from the findings were grouped as either validating reminiscences (i.e., positive self-appraisals, choices, positive social connections, joy, past-to-present comparisons) or lamenting reminiscences (i.e., regrets, lack of choice, difficulties). Reminiscers may have a predominance of one or more themes. Kovach encouraged researchers to identify dominant reminiscence themes and to examine their relationship to variables such as self-esteem, mood, and life satisfaction during periods of tranquillity as well as during life transitions and crises.

Newbern (1992) explored subjects' remembrances of self-care practices in the South from the turn of this century to 1945. A convenience sample of 60 subjects 65–96 years of age was drawn from nursing homes, private dwellings, senior centers, and high rises in three Southern states. An open-ended, semistructured format was used during the "mostly" audiotaped interviews. The subjects reminisced and reported on remedies, preventives, and healing methods that migrated with persons from the British Isles, Europe, and Africa. Subjects' reminiscences documented the prevalence of self-care in the interviewed group and supported the use of reminiscence to provide the context for "cold" historical facts.

Trice (1990) used a qualitative interview approach to explore elderly persons' perceptions of meaningful life experiences. Nine women and 2 men ($N = 11$) comprised the sample of independently living elders in this study. From the data, Trice extracted significant passages and formulated and validated the meanings with 4 of the participants who were involved in sharing their experiences.

By clustering themes, Trice found that the informants in the study identified feeling concern for others, feeling helpful or needed, a perception that the reminiscer's actions or activities had been useful to another, and an overall feeling of positiveness about self and helpful activities.

McDonald (1993) explored elderly women's perceptions of reminiscence using a qualitative approach. The sample consisted of 10 women, aged 65 or older, who resided in an extended-care facility. Informants were asked to attend eight reminiscence therapy sessions that occurred twice a week over four weeks. Interviews were conducted following the second and final reminiscence therapy sessions, with informants being asked to share their perceptions about reminiscence therapy and the reminiscence process.

Latent content analysis techniques were used to analyze data. From broad groupings, themes relating to thoughts, feelings, and physical sensations experienced following reminiscence therapy emerged. McDonald (1993) recommended searching for physiological measures relating to relaxation, which can be studied quantitatively, and searching for methods of exploring reminiscence as a memory-enhancement intervention.

Durham and Whittemore (1993) studied the effects of playing tapes of golden age radio upon institutionalized elders' memory recall, reactions to the memories, and participation in planned nursing-home activities. The study included 12 female nursing-home residents with a mean age of 90 years. Subjects were included in this study upon recommendation of the activity director. The residents included in the study consisted of those who were oriented, disoriented, and forgetful. One month before the study participation levels in activities were determined to be from 11 to 20 activities per week.

Researchers played golden age musical and comedy tapes on a tape player for approximately twenty minutes. The golden age musical programs were well received, as residents joined in singing, clapping, smiling, and laughing while listening to the tapes. In contrast, the golden age comedy programs were reported to evoke little response in Durham and Whittemore's (1993) study. Memory-recall response to a trivia activity was positive even in those who did not respond to the golden age tapes. One month after the study, subjects' participation levels showed a slight increase and ranged from 14 to 21 activities per week. Durham and Whittemore (1993) recommended the use of golden age musical programs as therapeutic interventions for residents in nursing homes. The researchers further recommended additional research on the use of comedy tapes with groups of mixed gender and young-old and old-old cohorts.

Franks, Hughes, Phelps, and Williams (1993) investigated the importance placed upon contact between youth and their grandparents. The population for the investigation was composed of 80 students recruited from five midwestern college campuses. The age range for participants was from 17 to 50 years, with a mean age of 22. Forty-seven participants were female and 33 were male.

Franks et al. (1993) used a qualitative design and one-to-one interviews to question participants about various aspects of their relationship with a significant elder. Data were collected and results consolidated and grouped by themes. Three key themes relating to roles played by elders, lessons learned from the relationship, and ways in which the relationship diminished common stereotypes about the elderly emerged from the data. From these findings, Franks et al. found that for the majority of those sampled, a relationship with a significant elder had a positive influence on participants' values, goals, and life choices. Franks et al. recommended that organizations (schools, churches, community) include significant elders in any activity that would normally include parents.

Past qualitative research studies have yielded data richly steeped in elderly women's perspectives about reminiscence and these women's lived experiences. The next section highlights several quantitative research studies.

Burnside's (1990) dissertation studied the effect of reminiscence on affect, fatigue, and life satisfaction in older women using the Affect Balance Scale, the Life Satisfaction Index A, and the Pearson and Byars Subjective Fatigue Checklist. The reliability and validity of all three instruments were reported as adequate.

Burnside's (1990) sample consisted of volunteers of older women ($N = 67$) who lived in apartment complexes in a metropolitan area. A quasi-experimental pretest/posttest, nonequivalent-groups design was used. Participants were divided into three reminiscence groups, which met for eight reminiscence sessions over a four-week period, and a no-treatment control group. The resulting quantitative data yielded no significant statistical improvement in fatigue, affect, or life satisfaction for those women who attended reminiscence groups. Burnside's (1990) qualitative data, however, verified that the older women in the study found reminiscing to be enjoyable. Burnside encouraged other researchers to seek out new measurements in future studies.

Bramlett and Gueldner (1993) studied reminiscent storytelling as a therapeutic modality to enhance the perception of power in well, independently living elders. The study measured changes in self-reported power (personal control) in two groups of elders by administering Barrett's Power as Knowing Participation in Change Scale, Version II (PKPCT, VII). The PKPCT, VII, is a semantic differential scale with four subscales. Construct validity and subscale reliabilities range from 0.57 to 0.84 in adult populations under the age of 60 with a greater than twelfth-grade education. In Bramlett and Gueldner's study, Pfieffer's Short Portable Mental Status Questionnaire was used as a screening tool. An investigator-developed General Information Questionnaire was also administered.

The sample consisted of 81 well, independently living elders with a mean age of 71.5 years. Subjects were recruited from church groups, community groups, and residents of subsidized apartment complexes. The sample was 81% female, with 83% either married or widowed. A pretest and posttest design was used with experimental and control groups. Subjects in the experimental group participated in a series of three one-hour reminiscence storytelling sessions conducted by the primary investigator. These sessions occurred over one week. All participants were tested with the PKPCT, VII, immediately following the third reminiscence session and again five weeks after the third reminiscence session. Subjects in the control group met only for testing using a schedule identical to that of the experimental group. No significant difference was found between the posttest scores of the reminiscence group and the control group. Thus the results of Bramlett and Gueldner's (1993) study did not confirm the value of reminiscence as a therapeutic measure. However, Bramlett and Gueldner encouraged researchers to continue designing investigations to validate the circumstances in which reminiscence has the most potential to benefit participants.

Merriam (1993b), as part of the Georgia Centenarian Study, examined how older adults use reminiscence. The sample consisted of centenarians, 80-year-olds, and 60-year-olds who were living independently and were cognitively intact. Two hundred and eighty-eight persons participated in the study. Of the participants, 70% were white, 30% were black, 67% were female, and 33% were male. The seventeen-item Uses of Reminiscence scale was utilized in Merriam's study. The scale was analyzed by means of a principal-component factor analysis followed by varimax rotation. "This procedure yielded three factors having eigenvalues greater than 1.0 that together explained 55.8% of the total variance" (p. 445). Factor 1 was labeled as "therapeutic" and consisted of the most items. Factor 2 was labeled "informative," and factor 3 was labeled as "enjoyment."

Merriam (1993b) described reminiscence as a multidimensional concept and encouraged researchers to define explicitly the type of reminiscence one is dealing with in order to link particular forms of reminiscence to desired outcomes. This type of attention to the careful conceptualization of the phenomenon may maximize the potential for reminiscence to be a viable therapeutic and educational intervention.

DeGenova (1993) studied reminiscence and other variables possibly affecting life satisfaction in later life. The study assumed that elderly people reflect on their lives in an evaluative sense. Life revision, reminiscence, and regretfulness were assessed using the researcher-designed Life Review Index (LRI). The LRI, a self-report, additive index of forty-nine questions, is divided into seven subgroups. The internal consistency (reliability) of the life-revision, reminiscence, and regretfulness subscales was reported as .84, .82, and .84, respectively. Content validity was measured by gathering opinions of elderly people and professionals in the field. Life satisfaction was measured using the Life Satisfaction Index A.

The sample consisted of 81 females and 41 males secured by random selection from a city directory. The sample had a mean age of 72.1 years. The educational mean was 12.5 years. Of the sample, 68% were married, 28% were widowed, 2% were divorced or separated, and 2% were never married.

DeGenova (1993) found that for the overall sample, social activity and health were significant predictors of life satisfaction, while reminiscence did not significantly predict life satisfaction. However, discriminant analysis of the equality of group covariance between all variables of interest revealed that there was a significant difference between those with and those without a spouse present. In the final analysis the strongest predictors of life satisfaction were health and social activity when a spouse was present, but when a spouse was absent, reminiscence was the second-highest predictor of life satisfaction. These findings suggest the possibility that when widowed, one sorts through the memories of life and finds meaning in the past. Therefore, these findings may help to explain the positive relationship between reminiscence and life satisfaction.

In 1991 McCrone studied the efficacy of resocialization (i.e., use of a sensory stimulus like a prop to facilitate reminiscence) with institutionalized, confused elderly. The Short Portable Mental Status Questionnaire was used in the study. Adequate test-retest reliability ($r = .82$) and predictive validity ($r = .92$) were documented.

Eighty nursing-home residents, drawn from three nursing homes, met for thirty minutes twice a week over a six-week time span. Resocialization, in the experimental group, was found to be significantly more effective in decreasing cognitive inaccessibility than the extra attention received by the control group. However, one month after termination of the reminiscence, the groups were tested, and McCrone (1991) found that the effect of treatment had not been maintained.

Stevens-Ratchford (1993) studied the effects of life-review reminiscence activities on depression and self-esteem in 24 residents who lived in a lifetime-care arrangement in a retirement community. Stevens-Ratchford defined life-review reminiscence activities as "the engagement of persons in past-oriented thinking and discussions after the presentation of organized visual and auditory stimuli of people, objects, and events from the past" (p. 416). Residents ranged in age from 69 to 91, with a mean age of 79.7 years. Two subjects were single, 8 were married, and 14 were widowed. Educational background ranged from high school to subjects holding graduate degrees. All subjects possessed functional hearing in a group and were free of depression as measured by the Beck Depression Inventory (BDI). The validity and reliability of the BDI with older populations were reported as relatively high. Rosenberg's Self-Esteem Survey was used to measure self-esteem. Test-retest reliability was reported as .85, and the scale's validity with other self-esteem measures ranged from $r = .56$ to $r = .83$.

Subjects were divided into male and female groups and randomly assigned to experimental and comparison groups. The experimental group participated in six two-hour sessions of life-review reminiscence activities on three consecutive Tuesdays and Wednesdays. The sessions consisted of slide-tape presentations that included classical and period music. Participants were allowed time for reflection and then were asked to write their reflections in response to the presentation. The remainder of each session was dedicated to group discussion. After four weeks the BDI and Rosenberg's Self-Esteem Survey were readministered to the experimental and comparison groups. The depression pretest mean scores were slightly higher than the depression posttest mean scores in all groups. The self-esteem posttest means were slightly higher than the means of the self-esteem pretest in all groups. However, neither the difference in depression scores nor the difference in self-esteem scores were statistically significant. Nonetheless, the experimental group's response to participation supports previous work that life-reviewing or reminiscence activities are a positive experience for older persons (Stevens-Ratchford, 1993).

In this section studies investigating the concept of reminiscence were briefly reviewed. The results of explorations and investigations into the concept of reminiscence have produced varying results. The next section will address ideas for researchers and practitioners to contemplate as the concept of reminiscence is studied in the future.

RESEARCH-BASED CONSIDERATIONS FOR STUDYING REMINISCENCE

Upon review of research findings, one is left with mixed feelings regarding the status of reminiscence research. Contemplatively questioning the meaning of the mixed results and seeking answers that will lead researchers and practitioners, across disciplines, to a more comprehensive understanding of the dimensions of reminiscence are necessary as reminiscence research continues.

As noted earlier in this chapter, the concept of reminiscence has been defined in a myriad of ways. Acceptance of a synthesized definition of reminiscence is a first step in conceptualizing whether a researcher is working with reminiscence or another related, but different, intervention.

Interdisciplinary practitioners interested in conducting research must carefully delineate goals and objectives to be achieved during future studies. Delineating the goals and objectives will assist in clearly communicating the phenomenon under study to practitioners across disciplines.

Furthermore, as the available literature is reviewed, there is a noticeable lack of standardized reminiscence protocols being studied. The length of intervention, the use of structured versus unstructured formats, and the design of studies vary widely. Replication of previous studies is lacking.

Within the literature a definite chasm exists between qualitative versus quantitative research findings. The literature supports the notion of reminiscence being an enjoyable type of intervention. Perhaps this feeling of enjoyment can be correlated with the social aspect of reminiscence, since reminiscence is usually a group activity. The enjoyment factor requires more contemplation as practitioners search for a means of qualifying and quantifying the affective aspect of reminiscence. Perhaps physiological measures can also be found that will assist in quantifying the positive aspects of reminiscence.

As research continues into the issues affecting aging women's mental health, hopefully, continued scholarly research of reminiscence will be in the forefront of topics being investigated. The value of reminiscence is still being determined, with practitioners perhaps searching for different ways of perceiving and quantifying effectiveness of the elusive concept of reminiscence.

REFERENCES

Bramlett, M. H., & Gueldner, S. H. (1993). Reminiscence: A viable option to enhance power in elders. *Clinical Nurse Specialist, 7*(2), 68–74.

Burnside, I. (1990). The effect of reminiscence groups on fatigue, affect, and life satisfaction in older women (Doctoral dissertation, University of Texas at Austin, 1990). *Dissertation Abstracts International, 51*, 4274B.

Burnside, I., & Haight, B. K. (1992). Reminiscence and life review: Analysing each concept. *Journal of Advanced Nursing, 17*, 855–862.

Butler, R. N. (1963). The life review: An interpretation of reminiscence in the aged. *Psychiatry, 26*, 65–76.

DeGenova, M. K. (1992). If you had your life to live over again: What would you do differently? *International Journal of Aging and Human Development, 34*(2), 135–143.

———. (1993). Reflections of the past: New variables affecting life satisfaction in later life. *Educational Gerontology, 19*(3), 191–201.

Durham, P. R., & Whittemore, M. P. (1993). Memory recall and participation levels in the elderly: A study of golden age radio. *Educational Gerontology, 19*(6), 569–575.

Erikson, E. H. (1963). *Childhood and society* (2nd ed.). New York: W. W. Norton.

Farris, M., & Gibson, J. W. (1992). The older woman sexually abused as a child: Untold stories and unanswered questions. *Journal of Women and Aging, 4*(3), 31–44.

Franks, L. J., Hughes, J. P., Phelps, L. H., & Williams, D. G. (1993). Intergenerational influences on midwest college students by their grandparents and significant elders. *Educational Gerontology, 19*(3), 265–271.

Haight, B. K. & Burnside, I. (1993). Reminiscence and life review: Explaining the differences. *Archives of Psychiatric Nursing, 7*(2), 91–98.

Kovach, C. R. (1990). Promise and problems in reminiscence research. *Journal of Gerontological Nursing, 16*(4), 10–14.

———. (1991). Content analysis of reminiscences of elderly women. *Research in Nursing and Health, 14*, 287–295.

Lamme, S., & Baars, J. (1993). Including social factors in the analysis of reminiscence in elderly individuals. *International Journal of Aging and Human Development, 37*(4), 297–311.

McCrone, S. H. (1991). Resocialization group treatment with the confused institutionalized elderly. *Western Journal of Nursing Research, 13*(1), 30–45.

McDonald, D. (1993). *Elderly women's perceptions of reminiscence.* Unpublished master's thesis, Fort Hays State University, Hays, KS.

Magee, J. J. (1993). Using religious paradox to facilitate life review groups with shame-driven older adults. *Pastoral Psychology, 41*(3), 159–168.

Merriam, S. B. (1993a). Butler's life review: How universal is it? *International Journal of Aging and Human Development, 37*(3), 163–175.

———. (1993b). The uses of reminiscence in older adulthood. *Educational Gerontology, 19*(5), 441–450.

Middleton, D., & Buchanan, K. (1993). Is reminiscence working? Accounting for the therapeutic benefits of reminiscence work with older people. *Journal of Aging Studies, 7*(3), 321–333.

Moore, B. G. (1992). Reminiscing therapy: A CNS intervention. *Clinical Nurse Specialist, 6*(3), 170–173.

Newbern, V. B. (1992). Sharing the memories: The value of reminiscence as a research tool. *Journal of Gerontological Nursing, 18*(5), 13–18.

Singer, M. G. (1993). Alan Donagan: Some reminiscences. *Ethics, 104*(1), 135–142.

Staudinger, U. M., Smith, J., & Baltes, P. B. (1992). Wisdom-related knowledge in a life review task: Age differences and the role of professional specialization. *Psychology and Aging, 7*(2), 271–282.

Stevens-Ratchford, R. G. (1993). The effect of life review reminiscence activities on depression and self-esteem in older adults. *American Journal of Occupational Therapy, 47*(5), 413–420.

Trice, L. B. (1990). Meaningful life experience to the elderly. *Image, 22*(4), 248–251.

Wallace, J. B. (1992). Reconsidering the life review: The social construction of talk about the past. *Gerontologist, 32*(1), 120–125.

Wendt, W. S. (1992). The way it was: Seminary reflections, 1930–1934. *Concordia Historical Institute Quarterly, 65*(2), 70–80.

Wholihan, D. (1992). The value of reminiscence in hospice care. *American Journal of Hospice and Palliative Care, 9*(2), 33–35.

Wong, P. (1991). Social support functions of group reminiscence. *Canadian Journal of Community Mental Health, 10*(2), 151–161.

Thirteen

Suicidal Behavior in Middle-aged and Older Women

NANCY J. OSGOOD AND MARJORIE J. MALKIN

Because suicide is primarily a male phenomenon, especially in the later years, suicidal behavior in women, particularly older women, has not received the attention it deserves. Many middle-aged and older women engage in self-destructive behaviors, and many die. The risk of death from suicide is particularly great for women between the ages of 45 and 54. This chapter will examine age and gender differences in suicide and attempted suicide, discuss explanations for the differences, and highlight major factors related to suicidal behavior in women.

AGE AND GENDER DIFFERENCES IN ATTEMPTED AND COMPLETED SUICIDE

Demographic Trends

The most consistent findings from research on suicidal behavior are that (1) males kill themselves more than females, and females attempt suicide more than males; and (2) older adults more often complete suicide, while younger people more often attempt suicide. Males are three to four times more likely than females to commit suicide. The highest rate of completed suicide occurs in males 65 or older, while the highest rate of attempted suicide occurs in women under age 30.

Males and females show different patterns in their rates of completed suicide. For males, suicide rates climb throughout life, reaching their highest levels in late life. For females, on the other hand, suicide rates increase slowly but steadily, peak in midlife (approximately age 45–54), and then gradually decline through late life. From 1979 through 1992, 13,686 women aged 65 or over in the United States committed suicide (Adamek & Kaplan, 1996). The suicide method chosen contributes to the lethality of the act, and the use of firearms is the most apt to lead to a fatal consequence. Adamek and Kaplan (1996) analyzed suicide rates obtained from the Compressed Mortality File (CMF), 1979–1992, from the Office of Analysis and Epidemiology, National Center for Health Statistics (NCHS), Centers for Disease Control, comparing methods of suicide as classified by ICD-9 codes for women 65 or over. They found that in 1992 firearms accounted for 38 percent of all suicides among women 65 or over, compared to 28 percent of all suicides among women 65 or over in 1979, which represents a statistically significant increase in firearm suicide among older women from 1979 to 1992. Adamek and Kaplan also demonstrated that most age groups of women showed a declining trend in firearm suicide from 1979 to 1992. Only the oldest (65 or over) and youngest (10–14) age groups of females showed significant increases in the rate of firearm suicide from 1979 to 1992. The firearm suicide rate for women under 65 declined by 33 percent, while women 65 or over experienced a 24 percent increase in the rate of suicide by firearms from 1979 to 1992. Older white women and older black women both experienced a significant increase in firearm suicide in this time period. Since 1982 firearms have become the method of choice for older female suicides. As Adamek and Kaplan pointed out, "The rising trend in suicide rates among women 65 and over and their growing use of firearms as a method of choice are cause for concern" (p. 76). For both older men and older women, suicide attempts are low compared to completed suicides. It is estimated that the ratio of attempted to completed suicide is 200 to 300:1 in the young and 4:1 in those 65 or older. Van Casteren, Van der Veken, Tafforeau, and Van Oyen (1993) recently reported on suicide and attempted suicide in Belgium from 1990 to 1991. They gathered information on suicides and suicide attempts by age and gender using data on suicides and suicide attempts collected by the Belgian sentinel network of 122 general practitioners working within a population of 134,300 inhabitants. Analyses of reported cases revealed that among people younger than 60 years of age, the incidence of attempted suicide was almost twice as high in women as in men. Beyond 59 years, the incidence rates were comparable between men and women. Suicide attempts were much more common in younger women than in older women. Older women more often completed the suicidal act.

   Middle-aged and older women also exhibit indirect life-threatening behaviors (ILTBs), which are covert, less direct forms of suicidal behavior such as self-starvation and refusal to take life-sustaining medications and follow prescribed medical regimens (Osgood, Brant, & Lipman, 1991). In a recent article in *Issues in Law and Medicine* Osgood and Eisenhandler (1994) discussed "acquiescent suicide" as a particularly widespread type of suicide committed by older women. Acquiescent suicide is defined as "a form of suicide that emerges when women are absorbed by a physical and social context that simultaneously diminishes their worth and will not brook their release. . . . acquiescent suicide represents a form of suicide that occurs in relatively isolated settings with hierarchical patterns of interaction that intensify the powerlessness perceived and felt by residents'' (p. 366). Many older women, particularly those who are ill and institutionalized, acquiesce to serious illness (decline food and treatment, become uninterested in maintaining desired social relationships) and in doing so end their own lives quietly and slowly without the assistance of others. Acquiescent suicide is quiet, subtle, and an often-overlooked form of suicide. Osgood and Eisenhandler also discussed assisted suicide as a major form of suicide for older women. They pointed out that older women are the group most likely to be the ''victims'' of assisted suicide at the hands of their husbands or physicians. Compared to men, women are much more frequently the victims of assisted suicide (Canetto, 1995), deaths that are not usually recorded as suicides. When we consider suicide attempts, ILTBs, assisted suicides, and reported completed suicides, women actually exhibit a greater number of total suicidal behaviors than do men at all ages. Table 13.1 displays suicide rates by age and gender for young, middle-aged, and older individuals for the decade 1980–1990.

Explanations for Age and Gender Differences

Lewes (1857) attributed the cause for the lower suicide rate among women to women's ''greater timidity'' and ''their greater power of passive endurance'' of bodily and mental pain. Durkheim (1951) ascribed the lower suicide rate in women to their lack of intelligence and ingenuity. Lester (1972) attributed the lower rate of suicide in women to their smaller size and suggested that women are not strong enough to use violent and lethal methods of self-destruction. Others have attributed the lower rate of suicide in women to choice of method. Traditionally, women have chosen less lethal methods such as pills and poisons, while men have chosen more lethal methods such as guns. By 1988 only 31.9 percent of women completing suicide used firearms, compared to 65 percent of males who used firearms.

Bonnar and McGee (1977), Stengel (1964), and Lester (1969) suggested that women engage in suicide attempts to control, persuade, manipulate, or force others' behaviors or emotions or to express aggression against others. Canetto (1993) and Lewis and Shepeard (1992) attributed variations in rates of suicidal behaviors by gender to cultural variations in perceived acceptability of such behaviors. In Western cultures nonlethal suicidal behavior is seen as ''feminine'' and is common in women, while lethal suicides are seen as ''masculine.''

One explanation for age differences in completed suicide is that compared to younger individuals, older adults are more likely to live alone and are more socially isolated; therefore, clues to their suicide will not be as likely to be recognized by significant others or work associates, and there is less chance that they will be discovered or rescued before dying. Older adults also have fewer physical resources and poorer recuperative powers than do young people; thus they are more likely than younger people to die from suicidal behavior (Osgood

Health, Psychological, and Living Issues

Table 13.1
U.S. Suicide Rates by Age and Sex, 1980–1990

Males									
Year	15-24	25-34	35-44	45-54	55-64	65-74	75-84	85+	65+
1990	22.1	24.8	23.7	23.1	25.8	32.1	55.6	65.3	41.4
1989	21.5	24.7	22.8	22.6	25.1	34.2	51.5	68.2	41.7
1988	21.9	25.0	22.9	21.7	25.0	33.0	57.2	60.4	41.8
1987	21.3	24.8	22.9	23.8	26.6	34.8	57.1	66.9	43.4
1986	21.7	25.5	23.0	24.4	26.7	35.5	54.8	61.6	42.7
1985	21.4	24.5	22.3	23.5	26.8	33.3	53.1	55.4	40.4
1984	20.5	24.9	22.6	23.7	27.2	33.4	48.5	51.6	38.9
1983	19.4	24.9	22.0	23.8	25.8	31.2	49.2	53.7	37.8
1982	19.8	25.2	22.5	24.1	26.2	31.1	45.1	50.2	36.2
1981	19.7	25.5	23.2	22.5	25.0	28.4	41.4	50.2	33.4
1980	20.2	25.0	22.5	22.9	24.5	30.2	42.0	50.6	34.8

Females									
Year	15-24	25-34	35-44	45-54	55-64	65-74	75-84	85-	65+
1990	3.9	5.6	6.8	6.8	7.4	6.7	6.3	5.3	6.4
1989	4.2	5.7	6.7	7.4	7.4	6.0	5.9	5.9	5.9
1988	4.2	5.7	6.9	7.9	7.2	6.8	6.9	5.0	6.6
1987	4.3	5.9	7.2	8.5	7.7	7.2	7.0	4.6	6.8
1986	4.4	5.9	7.6	8.8	8.4	7.2	7.5	4.7	7.1
1985	4.4	5.9	7.1	8.3	7.7	6.9	6.8	4.6	6.6
1984	4.4	6.1	7.7	9.2	8.5	7.3	6.3	4.9	6.7
1983	4.3	6.5	7.6	9.0	8.4	7.3	6.4	5.1	6.8
1982	4.2	7.0	8.4	9.5	8.8	6.9	5.8	3.9	6.2
1981	4.6	7.4	8.9	10.1	8.8	6.8	5.2	3.8	6.0
1980	4.3	7.1	8.5	9.4	8.4	6.5	5.4	5.5	6.0

*Per 100,000 population.
Source: Table prepared by John L. McIntosh, Ph.D., Professor of Psychology, Indiana University,
South Bend, from data obtained directly from the National Center for Health Statistics (NCHS),
publications of NCHS (*Vital Statistics of the United States*, annual volumes; *NCHS Monthly Vital
Statistics Reports*, annual advance reports of final mortality statistics), and population figures
from U.S. Bureau of the Census (1993, *Current population Reports*, Series P-25, No. 1095). Only
part of the table is reported here.

& McIntosh, 1986). The final explanation for age differences in suicide and
attempted suicide is that older people are much more likely than younger people
to use the more lethal methods (Kaplan, Adamek, & Johnson, 1994). Over half
of those 65 or older use a gun to commit suicide, while young people much
more frequently use drugs or poisons.

FACTORS IN SUICIDE AND ATTEMPTED SUICIDE

Child Abuse

Abuse in early life may be a factor in subsequent depression and suicidal
behaviors for middle-aged and elderly women. Briere (1992) identified four

types of child abuse: sexual abuse, physical abuse, psychological abuse, and emotional neglect. Based on various prevalence studies, the rate of sexual victimization of girls is considered to be between 20 percent and 30 percent (Finkelhor, Hotaling, Lewis, & Smith, 1989; Russell, 1986). In clinical populations the rate is between 50 percent and 60 percent (Briere & Runtz, 1987; Chu & Dill, 1990). The incidence of physical abuse of children in the United States during the decade of the 1980s has been approximately 11–14 percent (National Center on Child Abuse and Neglect, 1988).

Finkelhor and Browne (1985) have proposed a framework in which to understand the serious negative effects of child sexual abuse on victims, which is also applicable to other forms of child abuse, particularly physical abuse. Four traumagenic dynamics—traumatic sexualization, betrayal, stigmatization, and powerlessness—are identified as the core of the psychological injury inflicted by abuse. These dynamics result in feelings of isolation, guilt, shame, low self-esteem, helplessness and hopelessness, a sense of being "different," grave disenchantment and disillusionment, difficulty in forming healthy, meaningful social relationships, distrust of and aversion to intimate relationships, and self-destructive behavior. Herman (1981) reported that many women who were sexually abused as children by their fathers suffer from feelings of loneliness and emptiness and see themselves as outsiders who are not normal.

Depression is the symptom most commonly reported among adults molested as children, and physical abuse is also more prevalent in the histories of depressed women than in those who do not suffer from depression. Stein, Golding, Siegel, Burnam, and Sorenson (1988) reported a lifetime risk of depression among women molested as children of 21.9 percent, compared to a lifetime risk of 5.5 percent for women not molested as children. In addition, Briere (1992) argued that in their desperation to deal with the acute abuse-related distress and emotional pain, adult victims of childhood abuse resort to alcohol and drugs to distract, calm, soothe, or anesthetize their pain. Furthermore, studies have linked childhood physical abuse with substance abuse later in life (Dembo et al., 1989; Gil, 1988).

Suicide represents the ultimate escape from psychic pain. Individuals who engage in self-destructive behavior are expressing a deep-seated rage. Women are more likely than men to turn their rage inward and attempt to punish or kill themselves. Stephens (1987, 1988), who examined the social relationships of 50 adult female suicide attempters ranging in age from 18 to 63, found that the female suicide attempters described their family life and teenage years as disruptive and unhappy and their childhood and adolescence as filled with feelings of failure and guilt. Thirty percent of them had been physically and/or sexually abused by their families. Many other studies have revealed that suicide attempts are much more prevalent in women who were sexually abused as children than among nonabused women (Briere & Runtz, 1987; Briere & Woo, 1992; Briere & Zaidi, 1989; Ensink, 1992).

Through reminiscence, a natural process of remembering the past, older women may uncover painful memories of early abuse. Feelings of helplessness, powerlessness, shame, guilt, humiliation, and degradation, denied or buried for many years, may surface for the first time in late life. Late life is also a period of multiple losses, shrinking finances, and physical decline, often accompanied by feelings of powerlessness, helplessness, and loss of control, which may bring back similar feelings from childhood.

Victimization in Adolescence and Adulthood

Rape and battering are two particularly damaging forms of assault against adolescent girls and adult females. Rape, the number one crime against women, is not a sexual act, but rather a hostile violent criminal act with sex as the weapon aimed at dominating, degrading, humiliating, and subjugating the victim (Medea & Thompson, 1974). According to the U.S. Department of Justice (1991), 102,555 rapes were reported in 1990, an overall incidence rate of 41.2 per 100,000 women, or 1 forcible rape every 5 minutes. The incidence rate for those 65 or older is 10 per 100,000.

Based on in-depth interviews with 92 adult women who were victims of forcible rape, Burgess and Holmstrom (1974) developed their concept of the "rape trauma syndrome." Interviewed women who had a past or current history of physical, psychiatric, or social difficulties developed additional symptoms such as depression, alcoholism, drug use, and suicidal behavior. Research on the impact of rape on victims has found that women who are raped have low self-esteem (Kilpatrick et al., 1985; Kilpatrick & Veronen, 1984) and increased risk of depression (Becker, Skinner, Abel, Axelrod, & Treacy, 1984; Burnam et al., 1988; Wirtz & Harrell, 1987) and suicide (Greenspan & Samuel, 1989; Myers, Templer, & Brown, 1984).

Wife abuse or wife battering is the other major form of victimization of women. Women seldom report physical abuse by a spouse or boyfriend, so it is impossible to estimate the prevalence of battering. Hilberman and Munson (1977–78), who studied 60 battered women, described a uniform psychological response that was identical for all the battered women in their sample. The women were in a constant state of terror, experienced agitation and anxiety regularly, and were very fearful and constantly vigilant, unable to relax or sleep, screaming and crying frequently. They had a deep sense of anger and rage, which they directed inward against themselves in the form of alcoholism, self-mutilation, and suicide.

In her study of 120 battered women Walker (1979) found that many suffered from low self-esteem and an overwhelming sense of helplessness and power-lessness. The battered woman's syndrome is the term used to describe the condition of these women. Researchers have found that battered women suffer from feelings of low self-esteem (Mills, Rieker, & Carmen, 1984) and depression (Rounsaville, 1978; Gayford, 1975) and are vulnerable to self-destructive behavior (Counts, 1987; Gayford, 1975; Hoff, 1990).

Interpersonal Difficulties

Interpersonal difficulties of suicidal individuals were noted by Lester (1972, cited in Lester, 1988), who reported isolation and disengagement of such individuals, even if they were married, and Maris (1989), who noted the negative quality of social relations among suicidal individuals. An analysis of suicide notes written by women (Leenaars, 1988) indicated unbearable psychological pain, interpersonal difficulties, rejection or aggression, and inability to adjust to personal difficulties. The childhoods of women who are suicidal often were characterized by nonnurturing, absent, alcoholic, abusive, or mentally ill parents (Stephens, 1988). Such pathological early interpersonal relationships are linked by researchers to later suicidal ideation (Cooley, 1992; Kaplan & Klein, 1989; Maris, 1989). Stephens concluded that the precipitating factors for suicidal behaviors by women "typically involve severe, often chronic interpersonal conflicts with significant others" (1988, p. 73).

The concept of social support has been widely investigated as a possible mediating or protective factor for depression and suicide. A 1993 study (Kendler et al.) concluded that social support, interpersonal difficulties, and parental warmth were interrelated predictors of depression, while other researchers (Aneshensel, 1986; Goodenow, Reisine, & Grady, 1990) concluded that the perceived quality of social support does affect women's psychological well-being. Females may be more adversely affected by the lack of such support. Kaplan and Klein (1989) acknowledged interpersonal stress as a factor in women's suicide attempts. Interpersonal conflict with family and friends has been investigated by Vega, Kolody, Valle, and Weir (1991), who noted that family support was more salient for emotional support than that of friends. Thompson and Heller concluded that "elderly women with low perceived family support had poorer psychological well-being regardless of perceived support from friends or network embeddedness" (1990, p. 535).

Suicidal behaviors for women have historically been interpreted as dyadic—involving difficulties with a spouse, partner, or significant other. Kiev (1976), in a cluster analysis of suicide attempters, determined through factor analysis that interpersonal conflict, social relations, and attitudes of significant others were significant prognostic factors. He noted that those who threaten or make less serious attempts may kill themselves in subsequent attempts.

More depressive symptoms were experienced by unhappily married women than either happily married or unmarried women or married men (Aneshensel, 1986). "Middle-aged women who kill themselves are often married" (Canetto, 1994, p. 89). Stephens (1988), who conducted life histories of 50 female suicide attempters, found that suicidal behaviors were facilitated by unhealthy relationships and unrealistic expectations of those love relationships. All of the suicidal women had "interpersonal histories of relentlessly negative relationships with the most important people in their lives" (Stephens, 1988, p. 84). Vanfossen

(1986) concluded that the quality of the marital relationship is crucial for emotional well-being.

Maris (1989) analyzed national data and determined that marriage in general does protect against suicide. The highest suicide rates are among the divorced, except for widowed 20–24-year-olds. Yang and Lester (1988) analyzed 1980 data from 48 states and concluded that for the females, the divorce rate, the degree of urbanization, and the amount of interstate migration were determined to be predictors of suicidal behavior. These factors can all be viewed as increasing social stress. While divorce is associated with suicide, the gap between the suicide rates of the divorced and the married has indeed narrowed as divorce has become increasingly more common (Stack, 1990). For divorced white females, from 1961 to 1979, the increasing divorce rates were not accompanied by increasing suicide rates, except for women aged 45–49 and 55–59. Stable suicide rates (or decreases) were noted for women aged 60 or above. With the exception of elderly males, divorced people have a suicide rate at least double that of married people. Divorce tends to worsen the economic position of women, thus leading to depression and role conflict (Weitzman, 1985, cited in Stack, 1990).

Widowhood is another factor contributing to suicide rates. Stack (1990) reported that for female widows aged 35–49 (middle aged) the suicide rate increased during the period 1959–79, while for those aged 70–75 the suicide rate fell. For other age groups the rates stayed stable or declined. The rates for the widowed overall are higher than for the married at almost all ages for both men and women. Widows were, on average, older, less satisfied with income, less healthy, and less happy than elderly married women (Greene & Feld, 1989). Blankfield (1989) reported that middle-aged and elderly widows admitted to alcohol dependence treatment programs were susceptible to abnormal grief reactions, such as depression, isolation, and substance abuse (all risk factors for suicidal behaviors). Although Roughan (1993) noted that elderly widows cope and adapt better than young widows, the impact of widowhood is significant. Osgood (1985) indicated that widows are sad, lonely, and anxious. The first year after bereavement is the time of greatest risk for suicide (MacMahon & Pugh, 1985, and Miller, 1979, cited in Osgood, 1985). The widowed person often loses friendship and associational roles, along with losing the role of spouse (Osgood, 1985). Finally, Canetto (1994) reiterated that females aged 65 or older are 3.5 times more likely to be widowed than elderly males, to have limited financial resources, and to live alone. These women often display high rates of indirectly suicidal behaviors. Canetto urged an awareness of such gender difference in order to counsel the suicidal elderly (Canetto, 1994).

Employment and Financial Difficulties

It was hypothesized by Neuringer and Lettieri (1982) that increasing numbers of employed women may lead to an increase in the numbers of women who complete a suicide act. However, Lester and Yang (1991) examined data from 1946 to 1984 and determined that female participation in the labor force was negatively associated with the suicide rates of women in the United States. Neuringer and Lettieri (1982) had speculated that gender equality and the assumption of previously male work roles may lead to women assuming male patterns of greater numbers of completed suicide, thus leading to "suicide [becoming] an equal opportunity death" (Neuringer & Lettieri, 1982, p. 23). This has not been true for all women. Current research supports the fact that suicide behaviors have increased for professional women (de Castro, Pimenta, & Martins, 1988; McGrath, Keita, Strickland, & Russo, 1990). Aneshensel (1986) determined that high levels of work strain combined with marital stress contributed to depression. Snapp (1992) investigated occupational stress and social support and depression among black and white professional managerial women through 200 life-history interviews. This study determined that levels of depression were related to marital and parental status. Trouble with boss or subordinates was directly related to depression. This study did not find that social support buffered the effects of occupational stress.

Characteristics of employment affect depression levels and psychological well-being. Braun and Hollander (1988) indicated that depression levels were related to high job demands coupled with low decision latitude, especially for women. Pugliesi (1988) determined that autonomy and complexity of work may affect social support, which in turn affects psychological well-being. There is evidence that there are lower rates of psychological distress and/or depression for employed married women than for unemployed married women, especially for women with supportive husbands (Kessler & McRae, 1982). These researchers found that the benefits of employment were greatest for older women.

If employment may be linked with mental health for some women, then unemployment may be a significant factor affecting rates of depression and suicide (Aneshensel, 1986; Hall & Johnson, 1988; Vanfossen, 1986). Women who are unemployed are three times more likely to be depressed than employed women, even those with high work strain (Aneshensel, 1986). Poor health and not currently working were independent predictors of depressed mood for elderly women (Siegel & Kuykendall, 1990). In another study (Pearlin & Johnson, 1977, cited in Aneshensel, 1986), the unemployed were determined more likely to experience economic strain, depression, and social isolation.

Social support and depression among unemployed workers were investigated by Rife (1990), who noted that depression and lengthy periods of unemployment are common for elderly workers. Finally, poverty is positively associated with mental health problems (Belle, 1990). The prevalence of poverty among women is on the rise in the United States, associated with divorce, widowhood, and unhappy marriages, thus providing a threat to mental health. Economic strain, helplessness, and failure in receiving assistance may lead to despair, depression, alcoholism, self-medication, and perhaps suicidal acts.

Alcoholism

Alcohol abuse has been related to depression and to suicidal behaviors. According to the National Council on Alcoholism (1987), of the approximately 10 million alcoholics in the United States, 30 to 50 percent are estimated to be women. The report of the White House Mini-Conference on Older Women (Older Women's League Educational Fund, 1981) noted that among women 44 to 55, 25 percent have drinking problems.

Depression occurs frequently in alcoholics. The incidence of depression in alcoholics ranges from 28 percent to 59 percent (Regier et al., 1984; Roy et al., 1991). The relationship between alcoholism and suicide is also well established. The National Institute on Alcohol Abuse and Alcoholism (NIAAA) estimates that more than one-third of all suicides in the United States are related to alcohol. In their comprehensive review of 46 studies from 14 countries, Murphy and Wetzel (1990) concluded that "the lifetime risk of suicide ranged from 2.2 percent for alcoholics with a history of outpatient treatment to 3.4 percent for alcoholics with a history of inpatient treatment," and the lifetime risk of persons with alcoholism is "twice that of the general population and 60 to 120 times higher than that of the nonpsychiatrically ill in the general population" (cited in Roy, 1992, p. 211). Clinical studies conducted in various countries have confirmed that alcohol use is associated with 25 percent to 50 percent of suicides (Dorpat & Ripley, 1960; Frances, Franklin, & Flavin, 1986). Data from recent international studies confirm the strong relationship between alcoholism and suicide among the elderly (Battle & Battle, 1991; Berguland, Bergman, & Lindberg, 1991; Clark & Clark, 1991).

Some empirical studies have specifically identified the important role alcoholism plays in the suicide of women. Dahlgren and Myrhed (1977), who compared the mortality of 100 female and 100 male alcoholics, found that excess mortality from suicides was significantly higher in female alcoholics than in male alcoholics. Lindberg and Agren (1988), who compared excess mortality among male and female hospitalized alcoholics in Stockholm from 1962 to 1983, also found excess mortality from suicide significantly more prevalent in female alcoholics than in male alcoholics. Roy, Lamparski, DeJong, Moore, and Linnoila (1990), who compared males and females with alcoholism ($N = 298$), found that significantly more of the females (30.6 percent) than of the males (14.6 percent) had attempted suicide.

Beck, Steer, and McElroy (1982) administered the Scale for Suicidal Ideation, the Beck Depression Inventory, and the Hopelessness Scale to 105 alcoholics (76 men, 29 women) who had attempted suicide and found that hopelessness was a much more significant predictor of suicidal ideation than was depression. They concluded that the hopelessness that accompanies alcoholism is a major factor in suicide.

Depression

One of the most consistent findings in research on depression is that more women than men are clinically diagnosed with depression. Data from clinical case studies and community surveys estimate that the female-to-male ratio for depression is at least two to one, with some reporting a ratio of five or six to one (Nolen-Hoeksema, 1987, 1990; Strickland, 1989). The American Psychological Association National Task Force on Women and Depression (McGrath et al., 1990) reported recently that there are currently at least 7 million women in the United States with a diagnosable depression. One in four women can be expected to experience at least one episode of major depression during her lifetime.

The most elaborate theory of depression is the learned helplessness theory (Seligman, 1975). Seligman reported that animals who received repeated inescapable shocks eventually became passive and gave up trying to escape the shocks. They learned to be helpless. Seligman ascribed three effects of repeated exposure to aversive situations: (a) a decreased motivation to take initiative; (b) a general expectation that one cannot avoid or stop aversive situations; and (c) feelings of depression. In 1978 Abramson, Seligman, and Teasdale introduced a revised theory, suggesting that it is not uncontrollable events per se, but cognitive attitudes that define events as uncontrollable that result in feelings of helplessness. A person feels depressed because she blames herself for negative events and thinks that these negative events will occur in the future. Abramson, Alloy, and Metalsky (1989) revised the 1978 theory of helplessness and depression and focused on the expectation of hopelessness as the major cause for what they called "hopelessness depression." Women who have been abused as children and/or raped or battered as adults are particularly vulnerable to feelings of low self-esteem, loss of control, powerlessness, helplessness, and hopelessness. Women who feel that they have failed as marriage partners and have lost a spouse and women who have lost a job and financial resources are also vulnerable to feelings of low self-esteem, loss of control, helplessness, hopelessness, and depression.

The psychological condition most frequently reported as a characteristic of individuals with alcoholism and people who are suicidal is depression. Studies of persons with alcoholism reveal that between 30 and 60 percent suffer from depression (Murphy, 1992). Lifetime risk for suicide in the general population is 1 percent, compared to 15 percent for depressives. Evidence from many earlier studies in various countries found that depression was a major factor in about half of the suicides (Beskow, 1979; Chynoweth, Tonge, & Armstrong, 1980; Dorpat & Ripley, 1960; Rich, Young, & Fowler, 1986). These studies found depression to be more predictive of suicide in those 60 and older than in younger age groups. Findings from studies in various countries provide additional support for the significant relationship between depression and suicide in late life (Cattel,

1991; Clark & Clark, 1991; Neng & Zhi-Xu, 1991; Nimeus, Alsen, Regnell, Traskman-Benda, & Ojehagen, 1991).

Neuringer and Lettieri (1982) compared four groups of suicidal women, defined in terms of lethality of suicidal intent. Compared to the other three groups, highly suicidal women were significantly more likely to describe life as empty, to have more feelings of inadequacy and guilt and less feelings of self-approval and self-confidence, and to be unhappy and depressed. Other studies have found a strong relationship between depression and suicidal behavior in women (Brown & Harris, 1978; Conwell, Rotenberg, & Caine, 1990; Sundqvist-Stensman, 1987).

These suicidogenic factors are evident in some well-known suicidal women, including Sylvia Plath, Virginia Wolff, Sara Teasdale, Dorothy Parker, and Anne Sexton. Figure 13.1 presents a heuristic model that demonstrates the various factors that contribute to suicide and attempted suicide in middle-aged and older women. While there is no demonstration of a causal relationship in figure 13.1, the key factors identified and the resultant emotional reactions have been consistently identified in the literature as precursors of both alcoholism and suicidal behaviors for women.

CONCLUSION

There is a paucity of research literature on suicide among middle-aged and older women, particularly older women. Adamek and Kaplan (1996) listed several reasons for the neglect of the older female population: "First, the suicide rate of older women is one-fifth the rate of older men; second, national mortality data is often not reported by gender and are subject to undercounts particularly for women; third, theories of elderly suicide seem to be either gender-neutral or male-oriented; and fourth, the prevailing view of women and suicide is that women use suicide attempts as a 'cry for help' and are much less determined to kill themselves" (p. 72). The rising trend in suicide rates among women 65 or over and the greater use of firearms by older women cast doubt on the long-accepted view that suicide is a masculine behavior. In future decades, as sociocultural beliefs about women and gender roles change and as women enter occupations traditionally reserved for men in our society, and as firearms become more readily available and acceptable to women of all ages, we can expect a significant rise in the rate of completed suicide among women 65 or over. It is possible that the suicide rate for women 65 or older might more closely approximate the currently high rate of suicide among women 45 to 54 years of age.

REFERENCES

Abramson, L. Y., Alloy, L. B., & Metalsky, G. L. (1989). Hopelessness depression: A theory-based subtype of depression. *Psychological Review, 96,* 358–372.

Figure 13.1
Model of Suicidal Behavior in Women

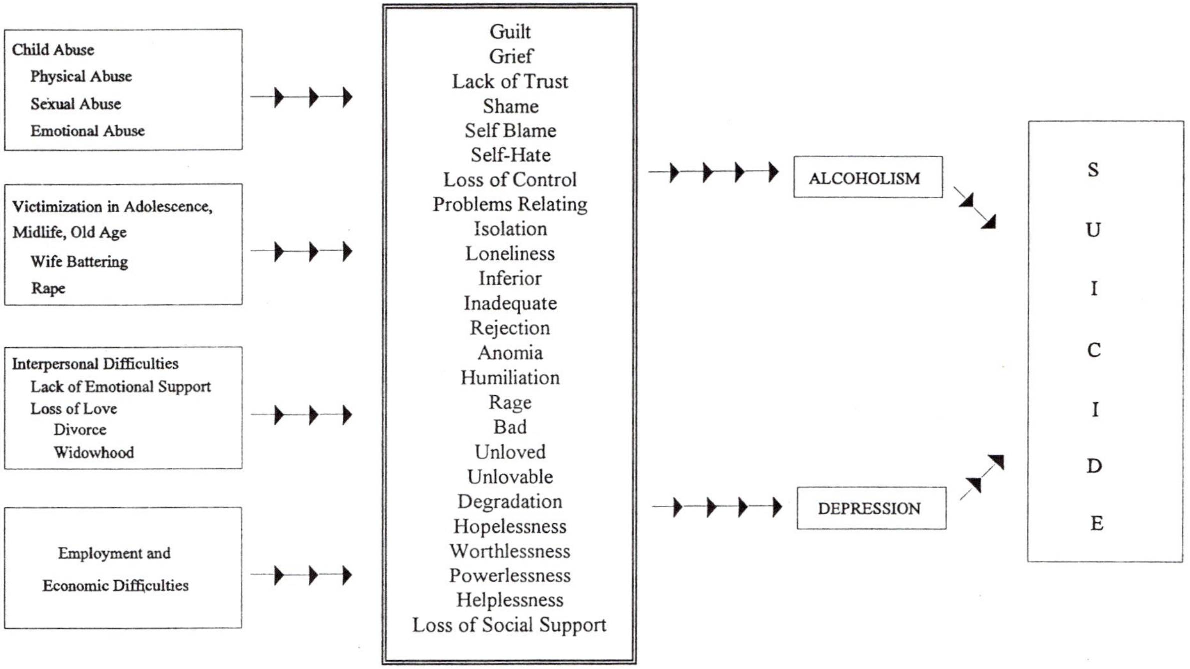

Abramson, L. Y., Seligman, M. E. P., & Teasdale, J. (1978). Learned helplessness in humans: Critique and reformulation. *Journal of Abnormal Psychology, 87*, 49–74.

Adamek, M. E., & Kaplan, M. S. (1996). The growing use of firearms by suicidal older women, 1979–1992: A research note. *Suicide and Life-threatening Behavior, 26*(1), 71–78.

Aneshensel, C. S. (1986). Marital and employment role strain, social support, and depression among adult women. In S. E. Hobfoll (Ed.), *Stress, social support, and women* (pp. 99–114). New York: Hemisphere Publishing.

Battle, A. O., & Battle, M. V. (1991). *Insights provided by survivors of elderly suicides.* Paper presented at the 16th Congress for the International Association of Suicide Prevention, Hamburg, Germany.

Beck, A. T., Steer, R. A., & McElroy, M. G. (1982). Relationships of hopelessness, depression, and previous suicide attempts to suicidal ideation in alcoholics. *Journal of Studies on Alcohol, 43*, 1042–1046.

Becker, J. V., Skinner, L. J., Abel, G. G., Axelrod, R., & Treacy, E. C. (1984). Depressive symptoms associated with sexual assault. *Journal of Sex and Marital Therapy, 10*(3), 185–192.

Belle, D. (1990). Poverty and women's mental health. *American Psychologist, 45*(3), 385–389.

Berguland, M., Bergman, H., & Lindberg, S. (1991). *Attempted suicide and other high-risk behaviors in alcoholics related to suicide and violent death.* Paper presented at the 16th Congress for the International Association of Suicide Prevention, Hamburg, Germany.

Beskow, J. (1979). Suicide and mental disorder in Swedish men. *Acta Psychiatrica Scandinavica* (Suppl. *277*), 1–138.

Blankfield, A. (1989). Grief, alcohol dependence, and women. *Drug and Alcohol Dependence, 24*, 45–49.

Bonnar, J. W., & McGee, R. K. (1977). Suicidal behavior as a form of communication in married couples. *Suicide and Life-threatening Behavior, 7*(1), 7–16.

Braun, S., & Hollander, R. B. (1988). Work and depression among women in the Federal Republic of Germany. *Women and Health, 14*(2), 3–26.

Briere, J. N. (1992). *Child abuse trauma: Theory and treatment of the lasting effects.* Newbury Park, CA: Sage.

Briere, J., & Runtz, M. (1987). Post-sexual abuse trauma: Data and implications for clinical practice. *Journal of Interpersonal Violence, 2*, 367–379.

Briere, J., & Woo, R. (1992). *Child abuse sequelae in adult psychiatric emergency room patients.* Paper presented at the Annual Meeting of the American Psychological Association, San Francisco.

Briere, J., & Zaidi, L. Y. (1989). Sexual abuse histories and sequelae in female psychiatric emergency room patients. *American Journal of Psychiatry, 146*, 1602–1606.

Brown, G. W., & Harris, T. O. (1978). *Social origins of depression: A study of psychiatric disorder in women.* New York: Free Press.

Burgess, A. W., & Holmstrom, L. L. (1974). Rape trauma syndrome. *American Journal of Psychiatry, 131*, 981–986.

Burnam, M. A., Stein, J. A., Golding, J. M., Siegel, J. M., Sorenson, S. B., Forsythe, A. B., & Telles, C. A. (1988). Sexual assault and mental disorders in a community population. *Journal of Consulting and Clinical Psychology, 56*(6), 843–850.

Canetto, S. S. (1994). Gender issues in counseling the suicidal elderly. In D. Lester & M. Tallmer (Eds.), *Now I lay me down: Suicide in the elderly* (pp. 88–105). Philadelphia: Charles Press Publishers.

———. (1995). Elderly women and suicidal behavior. In S. S. Canetto & D. Lester (Eds.), *Women and suicidal behavior* (pp. 215–233). New York: Springer.

Cattel, H. R. (1991). *Completed suicide in the elderly*. Paper presented at the 16th Congress for the International Association of Suicide Prevention, Hamburg, Germany.

Chu, J. A., & Dill, D. L. (1990). Dissociative symptoms in relation to childhood physical and sexual abuse. *American Journal of Psychiatry, 147*, 887–892.

Chynoweth, R., Tonge, J. I., & Armstrong, J. (1980). Suicide in Brisbane: A retrospective psychosocial study. *Australian and New Zealand Journal of Psychiatry, 14*, 37–45.

Clark, D. C., & Clark, S. H. (1991). *A psychological autopsy study of elderly suicide*. Paper presented at the 16th Congress for the International Association of Suicide Prevention, Hamburg, Germany.

Conwell, Y., Rotenberg, M., & Caine, E. D. (1990). Completed suicide at age 50 and over. *Journal of the American Geriatrics Society, 38*, 640–644.

Cooley, E. L. (1992). Family expressiveness and proneness to depression among college women. *Journal of Research in Personality, 26*, 281–287.

Counts, D. A. (1987). Female suicide and wife abuse: A cross-cultural perspective. *Suicide and Life-Threatening Behavior, 17*(3), 194–203.

Dahlgren, L., & Myrhed, M. (1977). Alcoholic females. II. Causes of death with reference to sex difference. *Acta Psychiatrica Scandinavica, 56*, 81–91.

De Castro, E. F., Pimenta, F., & Martins, I. (1988). Female independence in Portugal: Effect on suicide rates. *Acta Psychiatrica Scandinavica, 78*, 147–155.

Dembo, R., Williams, L., LaVoie, L., Barry, E., Getreu, A., Wish, E., Schmeidler, J., & Washburn, M. (1989). Physical abuse, sexual victimization, and illicit drug use: Replication of a structural analysis among a new sample of high-risk youths. *Violence and Victims, 4*, 121–138.

Dorpat, L., & Ripley, H. S. (1960). A study of suicide in the Seattle area. *Comprehensive Psychiatry, 1*, 121–138.

Durkheim, E. (1951). *Suicide* (J. Spaulding & G. Simpson, Trans.). Glencoe, IL: Free Press. (Original published in 1897).

Ensink, B. J. (1992). *Confusing realities: A study on child sexual abuse and psychiatric symptoms*. Amsterdam: VU University Press.

Finkelhor, D., & Browne, A. (1985). The traumatic impact of child sexual abuse: A conceptualization. *Journal of Orthopsychiatry, 55*, 530–541.

Finkelhor, D., Hotaling, G., Lewis, I. A., & Smith, C. (1989). Sexual abuse and its relationship to later sexual satisfaction, marital status, religion, and attitudes. *Journal of Interpersonal Violence, 4*(4), 379–399.

Frances, R., Franklin, J., & Flavin, D. (1986). Suicide and alcoholism. *Annals of the New York Academy of Sciences, 487*, 316–326.

Gayford, J. J. (1975). Wife battering: A preliminary survey of 100 cases. *British Medical Journal, 1*, 194–197.

Gil, E. (1988). *Treatment of adult survivors of childhood abuse*. Walnut Creek, CA: Launch.

Goodenow, C., Reisine, S. T., & Grady, K. E. (1990). Quality of social support and associated social and psychological functioning in women with rheumatoid arthritis. *Health Psychology, 9*(3), 266–284.

Greene, R. W., & Feld, S. (1989). Social support coverage and the well-being of elderly widows and married women. *Journal of Family Issues, 10*(1), 33–51.

Greenspan, G. S., & Samuel, S. E. (1989). Self-cutting after rape. *American Journal of Psychiatry, 146*, 789–790.

Hall, E. M., & Johnson, J. V. (1988). Depression in unemployed Swedish women. *Social Science and Medicine, 27*(12), 1349–1355.

Herman, J. L. (1981). *Father-daughter incest.* Cambridge, MA: Harvard University Press.

Hilberman, E., & Munson, K. (1977–78). Sixty battered women: A preliminary survey. *Victimology: An International Journal, 2*(3–4), 460–470.

Hoff, L. (1990). *Battered women as survivors.* New York: Routledge.

Kaplan, A. G., & Klein, R. B. (1989). Women and suicide. In D. Jacobs & H. N. Brown (Eds.), *Suicide: Understanding and responding* (pp. 257–282). Madison, CT: International Universities Press.

Kaplan, M. S., Adamek, M. E., & Johnson, S. (1994). Trends in firearm suicide among older American males. *Gerontologist, 34*(1), 59–65.

Kendler, K. S., Kessler, R. C., Neale, M. C., Heath, A. C., Phil, D., & Eaves, L. J. (1993). The prediction of major depression in women: Toward an integrated etiologic model. *American Journal of Psychiatry, 150*(8), 1139–1148.

Kessler, R. C., & McRae, J. A. (1982). The effect of wives' unemployment on the mental health of married men and women. *American Sociological Review, 47*, 216–227.

Kiev, A. (1976). Cluster analysis profiles of suicide attempters. *American Journal of Psychiatry, 133*(2), 150–153.

Kilpatrick, D., Best, C., Veronen, L., Amick, A., Villeponteaux, L., & Ruff, G. (1985). Mental health correlates of criminal victimization: A random community survey. *Journal of Consulting and Clinical Psychology, 53*, 866–873.

Kilpatrick, D. G., & Veronen, L. J. (1984). *Rape and post-traumatic stress disorder: A two-year longitudinal study.* Paper presented at the meeting of the American Psychosomatic Society, Hilton Head, SC.

Leenaars, A. A. (1988). The suicide notes of women. In D. Lester (Ed.), *Why women kill themselves* (pp. 53–71). Springfield, IL: Charles C. Thomas.

Lester, D. (1969). Suicidal behavior in men and women. *Mental Hygiene, 53*, 340–345.

———. (1972). *Why people kill themselves.* Springfield, IL: Charles C. Thomas.

———. (1988). Suicide in women: An overview. In D. Lester (Ed.), *Why women kill themselves* (pp. 3–15). Springfield, IL: Charles C. Thomas.

Lester, D., & Yang, B. (1991). The relationship between divorce, unemployment, and female participation in the labour force and suicide rates in Australia and America. *Australian and New Zealand Journal of Psychiatry, 25*, 519–523.

Lewes, G. H. (1857). Suicide in life and literature. *Westminster Review*, pp. 52–78.

Lewis, R. J., & Shepeard, G. (1992). Inferred characteristics of successful suicides as function of gender and context. *Suicide and Life-Threatening Behavior, 22*, 187–198.

Lindberg, S., & Agren, G. (1988). Mortality among male and female hospitalized alcoholics in Stockholm, 1962–1983. *British Journal of Addiction, 83*, 1193–1200.

McGrath, E., Keita, G., Strickland, B., & Russo, N. (Eds.). (1990). *Women and depression: Risk factors and treatment issues.* Washington, DC: American Psychiatric Association.

Maris, R. W. (1989). The social relations of suicide. In D. Jacobs & H. N. Brown (Eds.), *Suicide: Understanding and responding* (pp. 87–125). Madison, CT: International Universities Press.

Medea, A., & Thompson, K. (1974). *Against rape.* New York: Farrar, Straus, & Giroux.

Mills, T., Rieker, P., & Carmen, E. (1984). Hospitalization experiences of victims of abuse. *Victimology, 9,* 436–459.

Murphy, G. E. (1992). *Suicide in alcoholism.* New York: Oxford University Press.

Murphy, G., & Wetzel, R. (1990). The lifetime risk of suicide in alcoholism. *Archives of General Psychiatry, 47,* 383–392.

Myers, M. B., Templer, D. I., & Brown, R. (1984). Coping ability of women who become victims of rape. *Journal of Consulting and Clinical Psychology, 52,* 73–78.

National Center on Child Abuse and Neglect. (1988). *Study findings: Study of national incidence and prevalence of child abuse and neglect.* Washington, DC: author.

National Council on Alcoholism. (1987). *Facts on alcoholism and alcohol-related problems.* Washington, DC: author.

Neng, T., & Zhi-Xu, G. (1991). *Epidemiology of suicidal death of the elderly in Shanghai.* Paper presented at the 16th Congress for the International Association of Suicide Prevention, Hamburg, Germany.

Neuringer, C., & Lettieri, D. J. (1982). *Suicidal women: Their thinking and feeling patterns.* New York: Gardner Press.

Nimeus, A., Alsen, M., Regnell, G., Traskman-Benda, L., & Ojehagen, A. (1991). *Suicide attempters in Lund: Elderly versus young.* Paper presented at the 16th Congress for the International Association of Suicide Prevention, Hamburg, Germany.

Nolen-Hoeksema, S. (1987). Sex differences in unipolar depression: Evidence and theory. *Psychological Bulletin, 101,* 259–282.

———. (1990). *Sex differences in depression.* Stanford, CA: Stanford University Press.

Older Women's League Educational Fund. (1981). *White House Conference on Aging: Report of the Mini-Conference on Older Women, Des Moines, Iowa.* Oakland, CA: author.

Osgood, N. J. (1985). *Suicide in the elderly: A practitioner's guide to diagnosis and mental health intervention.* Rockville, MD: Aspen.

Osgood, N. J., Brant, B. A., & Lipman, A. (1991). *Suicide among the elderly in long-term care facilities.* Westport, CT: Greenwood Press.

Osgood, N. J., & Eisenhandler, S. A. (1994). Gender and assisted and acquiescent suicide: A suicidologist's perspective. *Issues in Law and Medicine, 9*(4), 361–374.

Osgood, N. J., & McIntosh, J. L. (1986). *Suicide and the elderly: An annotated bibliography and review.* Westport, CT: Greenwood Press.

Pugliesi, K. (1988). Employment characteristics, social support, and the well-being of women. *Women and Health, 14*(1), 35–58.

Regier, D. A., Myers, J. K., Kramer, M., Robins, L. N., Blazer, D. G., Hough, R. L., Eaton, W. W., & Locke, B. Z. (1984). The NIMH epidemiologic catchment area program: Historical context, major objectives, and study population characteristics. *Archives of General Psychiatry, 41*(10), 934–941.

Rich, C. L., Young, D., & Fowler, R. C. (1986). San Diego suicide study, I. Young vs. old subjects. *Archives of General Psychiatry, 43,* 577–582.

Rife, J. C. (1990). Clinical comments: Social support and depression among older unemployed workers. *Clinical Gerontologist, 10*(1), 42–45.

Roughan, P. A. (1993). Mental health and psychiatric disorders in older women. *Clinics in Geriatric Medicine, 9*(1), 173–190.

Rounsaville, B. J. (1978). Theories in marital violence: Evidence from a study of battered women. *Victimology: An International Journal, 3*(1–2), 11–31.

Roy, A. (1992). Suicide among alcoholics. *International Review of Psychiatry, 4*, 211–216.

Roy, A., DeJong, J., Lamparski, D., Adinoff, B., George, T., Moore, V., Garnett, D., Kerich, M., & Linnoila, M. (1991). Mental disorders among alcoholics: Relationship to age of onset and cerebrospinal fluid neuropeptides. *Archives of General Psychiatry, 48*, 423–427.

Roy, A., Lamparski, D., DeJong, J., Moore, V., & Linnoila, M. (1990). Characteristics of alcoholics who attempt suicide. *American Journal of Psychiatry, 147*, 761–765.

Russell, D. E. H. (1986). *The secret trauma: Incest in the lives of girls and women*. New York: Basic Books.

Seligman, M. E. P. (1975). *Helplessness*. San Francisco, CA: W. H. Freeman.

Siegel, J. M., & Kuykendall, D. H. (1990). Loss, widowhood, and psychological distress among the elderly. *Journal of Consulting and Clinical Psychology, 58*(5), 519–524.

Snapp, M. B. (1992). Occupational stress, social support, and depression among black and white professional-managerial women. *Women and Health, 18*(1), 41–79.

Stack, S. (1990). New micro-level data on the impact of divorce on suicide, 1959–1980: A test of two theories. *Journal of Marriage and the Family, 52*(11), 119–127.

Stein, J. A., Golding, J. M., Siegel, J. M., Burnam, M. A., & Sorenson, S. B. (1988). Long-term psychological sequelae of child sexual abuse: The Los Angeles epidemiological catchment area study. In G. E. Wyatt & G. J. Powell (Eds.), *Lasting effects of child sexual abuse* (pp. 135–154). Newbury Park, CA: Sage.

Stengel, E. (1964). *Suicide and attempted suicide*. London: Penguin.

Stephens, B. J. (1987). Cheap thrills and humble pie. *Suicide and Life-Threatening Behavior, 17*, 107–118.

———. (1988). The social relationships of suicidal women. In D. Lester (Ed.), *Why women kill themselves* (pp. 73–85). Springfield, IL: Charles C. Thomas.

Strickland, B. R. (1989). *Gender differences in depression*. Paper presented at the meeting of the Boulder Symposium on Clinical Depression, Boulder, CO.

Sundqvist-Stensman, U. B. (1987). Suicides among 523 persons in a Swedish county with and without contact with psychiatric care. *Acta Psychiatrica Scandinavica, 76*, 8–14.

Thompson, M. G., & Heller, K. (1990). Facets of support related to well-being: Quantitative social isolation and perceived family support in a sample of elderly women. *Psychology and Aging, 5*(4), 535–544.

Umberson, D., Wortman, C. B., & Kessler, R. C. (1992). Widowhood and depression: Explaining long-term gender differences in vulnerability. *Journal of Health and Social Behavior, 33*(1), 10–24.

U. S. Department of Justice. (1991). *Uniform crime reports, 1990* (282–0761/US 217). Washington, DC: U.S. Government Printing Office.

Van Casteren, V., Van der Veken, J., Tafforeau, J., & Van Oyen, H. (1993). Suicide and attempted suicide reported by general practitioners in Belgium, 1990–1991. *Acta Psychiatrica Scandinavica, 87*(6), 451–455.

Vanfossen, B. E. (1986). Sex differences in depression: The role of spouse support. In S. E. Hobfoll (Ed.), *Stress, social support, and women* (pp. 69–84). New York: Hemisphere Publishing.

Vega, W. A., Kolody, B., Valle, R., & Weir, J. (1991). Social networks, social support, and their relationship to depression among immigrant Mexican women. *Human Organization, 50*(2), 154–162.

Walker, L. E. (1979). *The battered woman*. New York: Harper & Row.

Wirtz, P. W., & Harrell, A. V. (1987). Effects of postassault exposure to attack-similar stimuli on long-term recovery of victims. *Journal of Consulting and Clinical Psychology, 55*(1), 10–16.

Yang, B., & Lester, D. (1988). Research note: The participation of females in the labor force and rates of personal violence (suicide and homicide). *Suicide and Life-threatening Behavior, 18*(3), 270–278.

Fourteen

Women Survivors: The Oldest Old

SALLY BOULD AND CHARLES F. LONGINO, JR.

This chapter considers the women at the apex of the population pyramid, America's oldest women. As a subpopulation, the arbitrary age boundary is drawn at age 85 (Bould, Sanborn, & Reif, 1989). One reason that the oldest women are now beginning to come into demographic consciousness is that the National Institute on Aging, in the mid-1980s (Suzman, 1984), generated a program announcement promoting research applications on a newly discovered subpopulation, the oldest old. Americans at these extreme ages were experiencing dramatic extensions of life. Gradually a small body of knowledge began to build around the oldest part of the American population and invariably to lead to the observation that this was largely a woman's territory. In 1990, 72% of Americans 85 or over were women.[1]

The oldest women are an interesting gerontological population because they form the boundary of longevity. They are the ultimate aging population, extending life to its chronological limit, and they hold the secret of what normal aging is at the extreme of old age. Does the aging process look different when viewed from the final part of the journey rather than from a stop along the way? In demographic terms, it is an unusually good perspective from which to consider aging and cohort effects. Extreme longevity, because it falls outside the statistical norm of expected limits, is an anomaly, something to be explained (Longino & Murphy, 1995). Why do the oldest Americans, especially women, live so long? What accounts for their survivability? Interest in this issue implies a grudging admiration of the long journey, a triumph of life over death. Physical reductionism in scientific medicine, however, draws research attention to genetic solutions and away from social and psychological factors embedded in the environment that would explain extreme longevity. Social gerontology takes a broader view and insists that capacity and environment are strongly implicated.

Furthermore, an understanding of women's survival is critical for social policy debates (Zones, Estes, & Birney, 1987).

Unfortunately, the broader gerontological view has often defined very old women as victims—victims of a system that leaves them with a high risk of disabilities and with neither a husband nor an adequate income (Hess, 1985; Minkler & Stone, 1985). Olson (1988) entitled her article "Aging Is a Woman's Problem" and stressed, in particular, women living alone as well as those in nursing homes. Very old women have a lower "quality of life" due to lower income, a higher risk of living alone, and a higher risk of disability than very old men (Haug & Folmar, 1986). Being old and female is referred to as "double jeopardy" (Payne & Whittington, 1976). This gloomy view needs to be contrasted with the counterpart that premature death is a "man's problem." The survival of women should be celebrated, given its potential.

Survivors are admired in American literature. They are the ones who remain to tell the story after the others have died. Herman Melville's protagonist, Ishmael, is an example of one who survived the cataclysmic self-defense of Moby Dick. The protagonist of Oliver Stone's film *Platoon* is another who endures to reflect on the meaning of life and death. But these are stories of heroic men, not ordinary men and women. To live through the normal struggles of life and to survive into advanced old age, however, is seldom considered heroic for women. When women survive, therefore, they are less often celebrated as victors than pitied as victims for having outlived their friends and family.

It is disturbing that the oldest old women, given their preponderance, have not been studied more extensively. One reason is that the biomedical interests have focused more on issues raised by death in men rather than survival in women. Both the Baltimore study and the Framingham study initially examined men exclusively. Disproportionate funding has gone into the diseases that are key causes of death among midlife and older men (e.g., heart disease), while research on breast cancer, a cause of death for midlife and older women, received substantial funding only after organized groups of women protested.

The perspective of older women as survivors needs to be given attention to counterbalance the discussion of older women as victims. This is especially true of very long-lived women. Their strength in surviving should be celebrated. These women are the true pioneers of the aging society, not its helpless victims. Nevertheless, being a pioneer involves hardship and requires that the society develop policies to ease the hardship of the current women pioneers in the territory of very old age. Furthermore, our understanding of these women's lives will enable better planning for the lives of women and men who come after them.

The eagerness of some researchers to claim victimhood for exceedingly old women must be tempered by caution against portraying persons in this age group as frail and dependent (Binstock, 1992; Estes, 1979). This is especially a risk for women who are subject to the cultural stereotypes of being more dependent than men at any age. Furthermore, women are often put in situations, such as labor-market circumstances and those concerning Social Security retirement benefits, that place them in positions subordinate to men and dependent upon them. It is important to reject the idea of the normal dependencies of old age and to stress the possibilities for productive lives even when one is in her late 80s and 90s. This chapter acknowledges the extreme difficulties of many women of great age, yet insists on the perspective of women as survivors. The preponderance of women at the top of the population pyramid is ipso facto proof of their biological and psychological strength in spite of a higher degree of disability. Furthermore, although objectively disadvantaged, women 75 or older report equal or higher levels of subjective well-being compared to men of the same age (Chappell & Havens, 1980). In spite of higher levels of widowhood, oldest old women are much less likely to commit suicide than men of the same age.

Physiological robustness is critical to all issues of personal autonomy and independence at any age. Robustness declines with the accumulation of chronic illnesses. Women suffer from higher disability levels than men and sustain these levels for a longer period in their lives. This occurs throughout the older ages, as demonstrated by cross-national studies (Rahman, Strauss, Gertler, Ashley, & Fox, 1994). In the 1990 U.S. census, 44% of women 85 or over but only 33% of men reported a self-care limitation, while 24% of the women but 36% of the men indicated no limitation of any kind. These data call attention to the need to study diseases that disable but do not kill. For example, women of all ages are twice as likely as men to report activity limitations due to arthritis (Centers for Disease Control, 1994). Oldest old women do have a higher risk of entering a nursing home because of their higher age-specific risk of disability, not simply because they live longer.

There is a widespread belief that women are relegated to nursing homes because they have no spouse (Hess, 1985, p. 322). Women widows are pitied because they have no one to care for them; yet their disproportionate risk of institutionalization can be simply attributed to the fact that they are disproportionately disabled. Furthermore, although men benefit more in terms of reduced nursing-home stay (of four months) if they have a spouse, men benefit not at all if they have an adult child. Women, on the other hand, benefit in terms of a reduced nursing-home stay (three months' reduction) if they have an adult child (Freedman, 1993). Men and women 75–84 living in the community were equally likely to be receiving help only from informal sources, but men were more likely to receive help from formal sources than women (Chipperfield, 1994). Clearly, widowed women are not being ''abandoned'' disproportionately in the community. It is time to cease pitying women who are widows and put research efforts into the diseases and disorders that result in institutionalization among the oldest old.

The effectiveness of women in marshaling interpersonal resources to obtain informal support and caregiving needs to be honored. Their effective strategies need to be studied in terms of learning how they cope with the thinning of their social support network because of death, disability, and geographical scattering

(Bould et al., 1989). Instead of approaching this issue with pity, we need to examine the lives of the oldest women for rich data for understanding strategies whereby the social and residential aspects of their environment can offset changes in physiological robustness in order to support personal autonomy (Lawton, 1985). In other words, the women at the apex of the population pyramid may provide for gerontology the richest data on effective survival strategies utilizing informal support.

Aging is a feminist issue, however (Hartman, 1990), and widows do suffer from the loss of their husbands in drastic financial ways. Retirement income is set up to reward the primary wage earner in the formal sector and his living spouse. Private pension plans, until 1984, could ignore any widows' benefits. Furthermore, the U.S. Social Security retirement program is set up in such a way as to protect a married couple from poverty with 150% benefit. That benefit drops by one-third for the husband's widow (Bould et al., 1989). These patterns of retirement funding have been especially harsh on the oldest old women because of their particular cohort experience as workers and family caregivers.

COHORT-SPECIFIC EXPERIENCE

Women in their late 80s and 90s are certainly a product of their life experiences. Those life experiences have been molded by the social history of their times. They are survivors of a specific birth cohort. Women who were 85 in 1990 were born in 1905. Nearly all of their older friends were born near the turn of the century. Thus their present circumstances reflect, to a large extent, the events of twentieth-century America. Preston (1992) put this point succinctly when he wrote, "Cohorts begin the march with their own unique endowment of social and biological attributes; ... they absorb the wars, epidemics, recessions, and booms of their time; and they witness the attrition of their members in ways that transform the composition of survivors" (p. 50).

In this context, Mary Grace Kovar and Robyn Stone (1992) have ably summarized the cohort experience of the oldest women in the 1990s. When they were born, infant mortality rates were much higher than they are now, and they were exposed to diseases in their childhood that are rarely encountered today. Death rates from infectious diseases such as tuberculosis and diphtheria were high. Indeed, at the turn of the century, life expectancy at birth was only 47 years, due primarily to a high prevalence of infant and child mortality. They were children or adolescents during the influenza epidemic following World War I that saw death rates double and double once again before returning to baseline in one year.

Furthermore, women of this cohort had fewer children than those in older and younger birth cohorts, and this fact may affect the availability of adult-child caregivers now, in their very old age. They were born into large families, but when they were in their own prime childbearing years, they lived through the Great Depression. Many couples felt that they could not afford to have and support large families. The depression was followed by World War II, which took many men away from their wives for several years. By the time the men returned home, it was late for this cohort of women to enlarge their families, and their childbearing years were cut short. Their children were born in the fertility low point just before the baby boom. Infant mortality rates also remained relatively high.

Work opportunities for women have also played out differently for different birth cohorts. Many of the oldest women in 1995 had work opportunities during World War II when the men were fighting overseas, but they tended to leave the work force when the men returned. Aside from the war years when child care was provided, the labor-force participation pattern was M shaped, with the highest labor-force participation rates before and after childbearing (Kovar & Stone, 1992). These patterns made it difficult to get vested for pensions or to gain high wages through a series of raises. African-American women, who had patterns of continuous labor-force participation, were not in formal-sector jobs covered by pensions or Social Security. As a result, retirement income for the oldest women relied far more heavily upon the work experience of their husbands than of themselves (O'Rand & Henretta, 1982). Their husbands, however, also suffered interrupted careers due to their military service, or if their husbands were African American, the husbands' jobs were often not covered by Social Security.

Historical and social context is important to understanding the personal resources of the oldest women. At the turn of the century, for example, America was a rural nation. It was not until the 1920 census that half of the population lived in urban places, that is, places with populations of over 2,500. Today more than half of the population lives in metropolitan statistical areas of over 1,000,000. In rural America an eighth-grade education was considered sufficient to handle the issues that one would face in work. School years were short, and school vacations coincided with the busy planting and harvest seasons. Many did not see a need for even eight years of formal schooling. In major urban areas immigrant boys and girls were also expected to work at an early age. America's oldest women have considerably fewer years of education, on the whole, than do their daughters or granddaughters who grew up in larger towns and cities or in second-generation immigrant families. The lack of education among the oldest women today impacted their work opportunities later in their lives as educational standards rose in many segments of the labor market. This is true even though more oldest old women (30%) than men (24%) graduated from high school.

In some rural regions of the nation education and race were very closely connected (Siegler, Longino, & Johnson, 1992). Formal education in the American South was legally segregated until 1954. The oldest African-American women today who grew up in the South were far too old in 1954 to benefit from changes in the educational system. In addition to differences in formal education opportunity, there has been a differential life history of coping patterns in terms of race in the American South. Furthermore, these oldest old African-American women were less likely to have left the South in the 1950s for Northern cities. The point here is that there are also regional differences in the cohort experience of older women that must be remembered and considered.

Although women had an edge in education, men had more income of all kinds, except for public assistance income. Social Security is the most widespread income source in this very old age group. Nearly three-quarters (73%) of women receive Social Security income, and four-fifths (79%) of men. Because men receive income from more sources and higher amounts from those sources, the personal income for the oldest women, on average, was only two-thirds of that of men their age. The greatest income gap was between men with no limitations ($10,992 in 1989) and women with no limitations ($7,400 in 1989). The smallest difference in median income was between men in institutions ($6,204 in 1989) and women in institutions ($5,760 in 1989). Women with low personal income are more likely to live alone, so that their one-person household income is more likely to be below poverty. Men, however, are much more likely to live with their wives, who will bring in income in terms of their spouse benefit under Social Security (the spouse benefit is 50% of the primary beneficiary amount). Nearly all of the oldest old women are widowed, but nearly half of the men are not. Unmarried women with very low incomes must often live with others; this is especially true if they are also disabled (Bishop, 1986). Elderly women living with others are more likely to report poor health than those living alone, especially after age 75 (Anson, 1988).

For all levels of disability among community dwellers, the poverty rates for women were 5% or more higher than for men. The largest difference in poverty rates, however, was for those with no limitation, where 20.3% of women were poor, but only 11.3% of men were poor. Here, of course, men have the advantage of living with a spouse and a spouse's Social Security check. Furthermore, although two cannot live as cheaply as one, it took $7,495 for an elderly couple to be above poverty but $5,947 for an elderly individual in 1989.

THE LIMITATIONS OF OLDEST WOMEN LIVING IN THE COMMUNITY IN 1990

The physical limitations of the oldest women can now be estimated using census data. For decades the census has examined work disability. For the first time in 1990, however, the census chose two general questions to measure functional stability. The mobility limitation asked, "Because of a health condition that has lasted for six or more months, does this person have any difficulty going outside the home alone (for example, to shop or visit a doctor's office)?" This item measures one dimension of instrumental activity limitation and indicates a possible need for help but not necessarily a need for care. The self-care limitation question asked if the person had any difficulty "taking care of his or her own personal needs (for example, bathing, dressing or getting around inside the home)?'' This measure is a global activities of daily living (ADL) measure and is an indicator of a possible need for long-term care, not just help. It is important to note very clearly that studies norming these census items against other measures in other national surveys have not yet appeared in the literature. The measure of disability also varies with the use of the words "difficulty" or "limitation" in contrast to the explicit wording of needing "the help of another person." For the oldest old, however, 90% of those with a health limitation need the help of another person in order to manage (Feller, 1986).

Those who are already institutionalized are classified separately. For this analysis, the disability items are arranged in a scale only for community-dwelling persons 85 or older. A person with a self-care limitation is considered to be the most disabled, followed by a person with a mobility limitation (but no problem with self-care), followed by a person with only a work limitation (and without the more severe restrictions). Those defined as "without limitations" have indicated having none of these limitations.

In 1990 there was a relatively high level of diversity in the population of women aged 85 or older where physical limitations were concerned. About a quarter of this population (26.8%) was institutionalized, nearly entirely in nursing homes. About the same proportion (25.4%) had no health conditions (lasting six months or longer) that limited their mobility or self-care. They could even imagine themselves working, if they chose to do so. Nearly half (47.6%) of the oldest women were living in the community with various levels of disability: about one-fifth (21.5%) had self-care limitations; nearly another fifth (18.1%) could not get out of the house on short trips without help, but they did not need help with personal care; 8%, who indicated neither type of these limitations, said that even though they were mobile and could care for themselves, they would be physically limited in work activity. Women at the apex of the population pyramid are relatively independent and robust. Even allowing for some underestimation of disability by these crude measures, this population is quite diverse in the members' levels of physical ability (Bould, Smith, & Longino, 1997).

How do very old women living in the community cope with self-care and mobility limitations? Part of the answer is found in the social support embedded in their living arrangements. As disability increases, some of the women adjust their resources, including their living arrangements, in order to get more help. Living alone has come to be an acceptable practice for the oldest women who are widowed, so long as they can cope by themselves. Mobility limitations do not interfere with independent residence, for example, so long as there is a taxi service, public transportation, or friends who will provide rides. In 1990 over half (58.6%) of women in the community who needed only help getting to the store or doctor's office lived alone. One would think, however, that self-care limitations would preclude a solo residence. Apparently this is not so. A surprisingly large population (44.4%) of women in the community who had self-care limitations also lived alone. The census item asks if one has difficulty performing personal care tasks, not whether one can perform them at all. If these tasks continue to become more difficult, a point is reached when care is needed. At this point an adjustment in living arrangements may bring the care that is needed. A higher proportion of the oldest women in the community with self-care limitations (31.4%) were living in the homes of children and other relatives than were those with only mobility limitations (22.4%). About a tenth of women with either type of limitation lived in their own home with a relative who lived with them.

For unmarried women, the least preferred arrangement is to live in the home of their children or other relatives. These living arrangements often make the person needing help feel like a burden (Bould, 1991). Household space may also be tight, leaving less privacy for everyone. These relatives, most often a daughter, have other demands on their time—husbands, children or grandchildren, work—and may feel stressed by the needs of the elderly parent. The daughter herself may have physical limitations.

Living in one's own home with relatives, on the other hand, is less likely to make the elder feel that she is a burden, and from the standpoint of the older woman, this arrangement is also less disruptive. Furthermore, the woman is providing shelter for relatives and thus is better able to think of the relationship as reciprocal. Because she is giving in return for care or help, she is less likely to feel like a burden to her relative (Bould et al., 1989). Overall issues of very old women living with relatives are intergenerational issues of mothers and daughters where the adult daughter is herself approaching old age (Sanborn & Bould, 1991). As noted earlier, the nursing-home stay is reduced by three months for mothers having an adult child (Freedman, 1993).

The two primary reasons that unmarried elderly live with relatives are poverty and disability. Living with relatives can ease the poverty of the one-person household by combining incomes as well as by providing help with the household. The poverty rate among women living alone is 31%, although there are many poor households where the elder lives with others.

SPECULATING ABOUT CHANGES IN THE OLDEST WOMEN OF THE FUTURE

If we become fixated on an age category and define it as a high-risk population for special care and help, as we tend to do with the oldest women, we run the risk of underestimating the effects of cohort changes in this population (Smith & Longino, 1995b). Whether the population will be less hardy as more survive into it, or more robust as the large baby-boom cohort enters it two generations from now because of its greater attention to healthy lifestyles, is an academic guessing game. It is most likely that there will be several offsetting factors at work in the process. The only confident guess is that the oldest women will be different in some ways that affect long-term care. Estimates based on population numbers alone, without considering carefully issues of population diversity within age categories, are doomed to be weaker predictors than any good planner would like to use, and the issue of cohort change compounds the problem.

Recent research using the 1982, 1984, and 1989 National Long-Term Care Surveys (Manton, Corder, & Stallard, 1993b) tells us, for example, that chronic disability prevalence among community-dwelling and institutionalized persons declined across the three panels, and that the declines in chronic disability prevalence were greatest among those over age 85. The authors speculated that these improvements may be due to higher levels of education and income in the later elderly cohorts as compared with earlier ones. Higher educational attainment and income levels contribute to greater understanding of dietary and lifestyle factors that impact health and well-being, a line of reasoning supported by the work of Maddox and Clark (1992), who found a strong negative association between both education and income and disability rates.

Higher educational and income levels of successive cohorts of the oldest women, along with biomedical advances in treating causes of disability, imply the possibility that chronic disability rates will continue to decline. Although such improvements would be welcomed by all concerned, modest declines in disability prevalence will not be enough to offset the increases in the growth of the elderly population. The absolute numbers of chronically disabled very old women will certainly continue to expand. This is especially true due to the disabling effect of osteoarthritis among very old women (CDC, 1994).

One of the progressive and relatively rapid changes for the oldest women is their trend toward independent residence and away from coresidence with children and other relatives. Rates of the oldest old women living alone increased between 1980 and 1990. Although those with mobility and self-care disabilities continue to live with others at a higher rate, because census measures of functional limitations are new, there is no way to tell if the shift over time to greater independent residence among the oldest women is found even among the disabled. If it is, this factor will force us to rethink informal caregiving and raise questions about the relative ability of caregivers in the community, particularly family members, as well as community resources.

Women in their retirement years, but not yet among the oldest women, are well endowed with family resources because they are the parents of the large baby-boom cohorts. Many analysts anticipate that the supply of family caregivers will decline in the future as the low-fertility baby-boom cohorts themselves age. Some have argued that even among baby-boom caregivers, because of increased labor-force participation, adult daughters, the traditional caregivers of the elderly, will be less available to their parents (Treas, 1977). Were this to happen, a substantial share of the costs of meeting dependency needs would be shifted either to the public sector or to the now-expanding fee-for-service home care industry in the private sector. Manton, Corder, and Stallard (1993a) also found evidence that the use of assistive devices and housing modifications to ease disability is up sharply, while personal assistance alone from family members and formal sources declined significantly between 1982 and 1989.

The trend toward greater residential independence, combined with the development and use of independence-supporting personal-assistance technologies, may be part of a long-term adaptive process (Manton et al., 1993a). Depending heavily on family members or others, unless the interdependence is the kind that preserves self-respect and self-determination, is a far less attractive alternative for those who can afford appropriate technology-supported self-care. As the number of the oldest women grows, as the demographic trends tell us that it will, a marketplace for assistive technology will grow proportionately. For the oldest old, these devices can reduce the need for a person to help, but they are not likely to eliminate that need; needing a device generally indicates the additional need of a person for those 85 or over (Feller, 1986).

It is easy to forget that the oldest women have been caring all of their long lives, and self-care is only a part of the whole. This is not to say that family members and others should not provide needed support. However, what we will call the "institutional" point of view is that problems can best be solved by individuals and their family members and friends in noninstitutional and informal ways. This appears to be especially true for older women. Older women appear to be better able to manage their interpersonal resources (Bould et al., 1989). We would argue that enriching the ability and honing the skills of informal caregivers, as well as those of the oldest women themselves, including effective devices, may reduce the strain as these women at the apex of the population pyramid continue to balance their changing physical limitations with their resources.

RESEARCH ISSUES IN STUDYING AMERICA'S OLDEST WOMEN

It is difficult to get representative samples of the oldest women in one's community. These women are the most available for research in institutional settings and most elusive in the community. Because of relatively low levels of education, they may not volunteer to participate in studies or may be reluctant to be put into situations where they could be made to seem foolish. Telephone surveys are least effective because many poor oldest old do not have telephones and many others are hearing impaired; 48% of the oldest old report some hearing impairment (National Center for Health Statistics, 1986). Children and others may be very protective of their very old parents and deny access to researchers when they cannot also be present. The oldest old living alone are often very reluctant to open their doors to an interviewer. Sampling a small segment of any population provides special challenges.

Census data are useful in making population estimates for this group, which is very difficult to interview. The census microdata files, the most flexible of all census products, are limited in terms of meaningful items with which to describe this population. The census can neither capture the relationships between older persons and others who do not live in the same household nor provide any depth to the relationships within the household.

Another great challenge in studying the very old is that of data quality. Memory problems become research problems in interviews with many very old persons (Siegler et al., 1992). When dealing with informants who may be having memory problems, how does one deal with cognitive decline? Colleen Johnson's experience in interviewing centenarians in San Francisco suggests that perceptions of the present and memories of the past may be two qualitatively different realms of data (Johnson & Barer, 1990).

A set of cognitive processes, commonly in action among the oldest women, is labeled as discourse strategies (Johnson & Barer, 1990). These strategies entail carrying on dialogues with themselves, and sometimes with others, to explain and interpret the events and experiences impinging upon their lives. If successful, they are able to maintain the mood and motivations of discourse in the face of a series of physical and social losses. An aura of survivorship appears to permeate these discourse strategies; having lived so long, one has outlived one's contemporaries. Such a status confers not only a sense of aloneness but also a sense of singularity. Detachment is also commonly discerned as individuals discuss their daily lives; such a stance permits them to withdraw voluntarily not only from the problems of others but also from social expectations. Life is freer and less problematic if less is expected of the very old. Living in a world with few normative constraints, one has outlived the worries that plague younger individuals.

It is best to keep a clear conceptual fix on the collective cohort experience of the oldest women being studied. Drawing a chart with demographic and historical facts for each five-year period of a cohort's collective life helps to provide a context for interview data. In addition, researchers who study the oldest part of the population must resist making comparisons with other persons of the same ages at earlier times unless such comparisons take into account the structural changes that could generate predictable differences between the two study populations. In this age group there is nearly complete turnover with every decade.

Overall research needs to develop a positive framework for understanding these women's lives. Matilda Riley (1985) suggested that ''longevity will give women a new capacity for selfhood—for independence, personal mastery, assurance.'' An emphasis on very old women's survival capacities should replace the current emphasis on pity and victimology. Simply the fact of survival for oldest old women should prompt the search for developing this new potential.

NOTE

1. The 1990 data presented here are drawn from the 5% sample of the 1990 census microdata files. See Bould, Smith, and Longino (1995) for further details.

REFERENCES

Anson, Ofra. (1988). Evidence that elderly women living alone may be in better health than their counterparts. *Sociology and Social Research, 72*(2), 114–115.

Binstock, R. H. (1992). The oldest old and "intergenerational equity." In R. M. Suzman, D. P. Willis, & K. G. Manton (Eds.), *The oldest old* (pp. 394–417). New York: Oxford University Press.

Bishop, C. (1986). Living arrangement choices of elderly singles: Effects of income and disability. *Health Care Financing Review, 7*(3), 65–73.

Bould, Sally. (1991). The oldest old: Caregiving or social support. In D. G. Unger & D. R. Powell (Eds.), *Families as nurturing systems: Support across the life span* (pp. 235–251). New York: Haworth Press.

Bould, S., Sanborn, B., & Reif, L. (1989). *Eighty-five plus: The oldest old.* Belmont, CA: Wadsworth Publishing.

Bould, Sally, Smith, Mark H., & Longino, Charles F., Jr. (1997). Ability, disability, and the oldest old. *Journal of Aging and Social Policy* (forthcoming).

Centers for Disease Control (CDC). (1994). Arthritis prevalence and activity limitations—United States. *Morbidity and Mortality Weekly Report, 43*(24), 433–438.

Chappell, Neena L., & Havens, Betty. (1980). Old and female: Testing the double jeopardy hypothesis. *Sociological Quarterly, 21*, 157–171.

Chipperfield, Judith G. (1994). The support source mix: A comparison of elderly men and women from two decades. *Canadian Journal on Aging, 13*(4), 434–453.

Estes, C. R. (1979). *The aging enterprise: A critical examination of social policies and services for the aged.* San Francisco: Jossey-Bass.

Feller, B. A. (1986). Americans needing home care, United States. In National Center for Health Statistics, *Vital and Health Statistics*, Series 10, No. 153. DHHS Pub. No. (PHS) 86–1581. Public Health Service. Washington, DC: U.S. Government Printing Office.

Freedman, Vicki. (1993). Kin and nursing home lengths of stay: A backward recurrence time approach. *Journal of Health and Social Behavior, 34*, 138–152.

Hartman, Ann. (1990). Aging as a feminist issue. *Social Work, 35*(5), 387–388.

Haug, Marie R., & Folmar, Steven J. (1986). Longevity, gender, and life quality. *Journal of Health and Social Behavior, 27*, 332–345.

Hess, Beth B. (1985). Aging policies and old women: The hidden agenda. In Alice S. Rossi (Ed.), *Gender and the life course* (pp. 319–332). New York: Aldine.

Johnson, C. L., & Barer, B. M. (1990). Families and networks among older inner-city blacks. *Gerontologist, 30*, 726–733.

Kovar, M. G., & Stone, R. (1992). The social environment of the very old. In R. M. Suzman, D. P. Willis, & K. G. Manton (Eds.), *The oldest old* (pp. 303–320). New York: Oxford University Press.

Lawton, M. P. (1985). Housing and living environments of older people. In R. H. Binstock, & E. Shanas (Eds.), *Handbook of aging and the social sciences* (pp. 450–478). New York: Van Nostrand Reinhold.

Longino, C. F., Jr. (1988a). A population profile of very old men and women in the United States. *Sociological Quarterly, 29*, 559–564.

———. (1988b). Who are the oldest Americans? *Gerontologist, 28*, 515–523.

Longino, C. F., Jr., & Murphy, J. W. (1995). *The old age challenge to the biomedical model.* Amityville, NY: Baywood Press.

Maddox, G. L., & Clark, D. O. (1992). Trajectories of functional impairment in later life. *Journal of Health and Social Behavior, 33*, 114–125.

Manton, K. G., Corder, L. & Stallard, E. (1993a). Changes in the use of personal assistance and special equipment from 1982 to 1989: Results from the 1982 and 1989 National Long Term Care Surveys. *Gerontologist, 33*, 168–176.

———. (1993b). Estimates of change in chronic disability and institutional incidence and prevalence rates in the U.S. elderly population from 1982, 1984, and 1989 National Long Term Care Surveys. *Journal of Gerontology: Social Sciences, 48*, S153–S166.

Minkler, M., & Stone, R. (1985). The feminization of poverty and older women. *Gerontologist, 25*(4), 351–357.

National Center for Health Statistics. (1986, September 19). Aging in the eighties, impaired senses for sound and light in persons age 65 years and over. *Advance Data from Vital and Health Statistics, 125*. Hyattsville, MD: U.S. Department of Health and Human Services.

Olson, Laura Katz. (1988). Aging is a woman's problem. *Journal of Aging Studies, 2*(2), 97–108.

O'Rand, A. M., & Henretta, J. C. (1982). Midlife work history and retirement income of older single and married women. In M. Szinovacz (Ed.), *Women's retirement*. Beverly Hills, CA: Sage Publications.

Payne, B., & Whittington, F. (1976). Older women: An examination of popular stereotypes and research evidence. *Social Problems, 23*, 488–504.

Preston, S. H. (1992). Cohort succession and the future of the oldest old. In R. M. Suzman, D. P. Willis, & K. G. Manton (Eds.), *The oldest old* (pp. 50–57). New York: Oxford University Press.

Rahman, Omar, Strauss, John, Gertler, Paul, Ashley, Deanna & Fox, Kristin. (1994). Gender differences in adult health: An international comparison. *Gerontologist, 34*(4), 463–469.

Riley, Matilda W. (1985). Women, men, and the lengthening life course. In Alice S. Rossi (Ed.), *Gender and the life course* (pp. 333–348). New York: Aldine.

Sanborn, Beverly, & Bould, Sally. (1991). Intergenerational caregivers of the oldest old. *Marriage and Family Review, 16*(1–2), 125–142.

Siegler, I. C., Longino, C. F., Jr., & Johnson, C. (1992). The Georgia centenarian study: Comments from friends. *International Journal of Aging and Human Development* (Special Issue: The Georgia Centenarian Study), 77–82.

Smith, M. H., & Longino, C. F., Jr. (1995a). The demography of caregiving. *Educational Gerontology, 20*, 633–643.

———. (1995b). Matching people with services in long-term care. In Z. Harel & R. Dunkle (Eds.), *Long-term care, people, and services* (chap. 2). New York: Springer.

Suzman, R. M. (1984). *Background memorandum on the oldest old*. Bethesda, MD: National Institute on Aging.

Suzman, R. M., & Riley, M. W. (1985). Introducing the "oldest old." *Milbank Memorial Fund Quarterly, 63*, 177–186.

Treas, J. (1977). Family support systems for the aged: Some social and demographic considerations. *Gerontologist, 17*, 486–491.

Zones, Jane S., Estes, Carroll L., & Birney, Elizabeth A. (1987). Gender, public policy, and the oldest old. *Aging and Society, 7*, 275–302.

Fifteen

Religion and Faith Development of Older Women

BARBARA PAYNE-STANCIL

A human being would certainly not want to grow to be seventy or eighty years old if this longevity had no meaning. . . . The afternoon of human life must have a significance of its own and cannot be merely a pitiful appendage to life's morning. (Jung, 1933)

Women's search for the meaning of their lives begins long before they become "older women." Even as teenagers they begin to raise questions about the meaning of life and the impact of their own lives (Gallup, 1993). The search continues and expands until as older women they are seeking to find the meaning of their long lives and long life in general. They are seeking, as Carl Jung observed, to find that the afternoon of life has a significance of its own and is not just some pitiful appendage to life's morning (Jung, 1933), or, as Anne Morrow Lindbergh (1975) found in her quest, that "the active years before forty or fifty are outlived. But there is still the afternoon opening up, which one can spend not in the feverish pace of the morning, but in having time at last for those intellectual, cultural and spiritual activities that were pushed aside" (p. 80). The search for meaning, then, is a lifelong religious quest. With apologies to Robert Browning, it may be in growing older that we discover that he was right, the last of life was that for which the first was made. It may be that in the afternoon of life the meaning becomes clearer and complete.

Women's search for the meaning of their lives is reflected in their involvement in religious activities and practices. Women are more religious than men—at every age. Women attend and support their churches more than men. Even when religious activities decline with age, they decline less for women, and religion becomes more important to them.

Compared to men, women participate in more devotional, private religious practices, and as older women they are twice as likely to consider themselves to be "very religious" (Gallup, 1994). What men and women have in common is that religion becomes more important with age, and private practices increase.

Early studies of religion and aging consistently supported these observations (Orbach, 1961; Moberg, 1965; Payne & Whittington, 1976; Wingrove & Alston, 1971; Argyle & Beit-Hallahmi, 1975; Blazer & Palmore, 1976; Alston & Alston, 1980; Young & Dowling, 1987). The more recent Gallup surveys (1991) and faith-development studies (Stokes, 1990; Faracasin, 1992; Thompson, 1991) are finding the same gender differences in levels of religiosity. Although these studies do report higher religiosity among women, they do not mean that men do not experience increases in religiosity and faith changes as they grow older (Payne, 1994). Men seem to experience faith in different ways than women.

This chapter is not about gender differences in religiosity and faith development. It is about the religiosity and faith development of older women and the forces affecting their religious life, including gender, the aging process, and social forces; it includes some short vignettes of how religious experience and practices change as women age; it identifies the religious and spiritual experiences of baby boomers that will affect the religiosity and faith development of older women; and, finally, it presents implications for practice and future research.

RELIGIOSITY AND FAITH DEVELOPMENT

The methodological differences between religiosity and faith-development studies yield different types of information. The religiosity studies based on survey research of "outer" aspects of religion tell us about beliefs, practices, and selected faith responses (Payne, 1982). Religiosity is measured by frequency of church attendance, adherence to traditional beliefs, and practices. These studies do track the continuation of these practices and commitments. However, information about shifts in the spiritual quest and faith development is limited (Payne, 1990a).

Faith-development researchers, on the other hand, may include religiosity measures, but only as they contribute to the investigation of the dynamics by which women find and make meaning of life's significant issues, events, and transitions. Faith-development studies, then, provide more about the dynamics of faith experiences and help us understand more about the "inner aspect" of women's spiritual journey.

FAITH DEVELOPMENT

Faith-development studies are based on the concept of earlier developmental theory that human beings move through life according to regular and known principles of stability and change (Havighurst, 1948). To the developmental concept investigators added Fowler's (1982) processual concept that faith is something that one does, not has; faith is a process of becoming; it is active. Faith is used as a verb to capture the dynamic and changing quality of one's religiousness, or "faithing."

Faith stages are hierarchical and build on one another, but are not age-specific, and there is no right or wrong faith or assumptions that some people have "more" or "less" faith than others. As Stokes (1990a) explained, "Each (developmental) stage is a point in our faith and aging journey and experience. It represents the dimensions of faith appropriate for our needs."

Fowler's stages are briefly summarized in table 15.1 and fully developed in *Stages of Faith* (1982). The stages demonstrate the principle that faith development moves from ritualistic faith to expressions of connectedness. Interestingly, they are compatible with the gerontological concept of aging differently (Maddox, 1987). We age differently and we "faith" differently. We do not all enter our older years at the same faith stage or at the same level of religious maturity.

The major sources about the variations in older women's faith development are (1) the Faith and Development in the Life Cycle study supported by the Religious Education Association of the United States and Canada (Stokes, 1990a) and (2) Benson and Elkin's (1990) national study of 11,122 churchgoers in six Protestant denominations. Other significant sources are the dissertations of Faracasin (1992) and Shulik (1979) that examine how gender and age jointly impact the faith development of men and women. Shulik's study was the first to focus on the faith stages of older men and women and to make an effort to identify the stage of each older person in the study.

Benson and Elkin contributed further to the understanding of faith development by devising two dimensions of faith maturity, the horizontal and vertical maturities. Horizontal maturity is described as prochurch involvement that results in acts of love, mercy, and justice. Vertical faith is defined as devotionalism (prayer, meditation) and a deep personal relationship with God: having a faith that shapes thinking, determines moral action, and provides meaning and purpose to life (Benson & Elkin, 1990).

Faracasin's (1992) secondary analysis of a selected sample of churchgoers over 60 years of age from the Benson and Elkin study of gender differences in faith development provided additional insight into the religiosity and faith development of older women. Most of those included in the study were over 60, women (78%), white, and with some college or more education (52%). He found that "women have the highest level of maturity at every age. The level of maturity not only persists, but increases. The highest level was among those over 70" (Faracasin, 1992, p. 119). Women's higher involvement in vertical religious practices was found to be related to their faith maturity. Faracasin interpreted this as evidence that older women are not "reflecting on how well they have lived with regard to people and things, but how well they have lived in relation to God" (Faracasin, 1992, p. 121).

Table 15.1
Fowler's Stages of Faith Development

Stage 1: Intuitive-Projective Faith
Almost totally limited to children (to age 6), individuals in Stage 1 reflect the faith attributes of parents and family as perceived by that person. Typically, at this time of life, the preschool child accepts parental faith attitudes without question.

Stage 2: Mythic-Literal Faith
In later childhood, the person becomes aware of and begins to internalize the faith attitudes and views of persons, primarily adults, other than family members. There is an increasing awareness of different faith attitudes in society, but the individual still tends to hold to those of family and religious traditions. Some adults remain in this stage through much of their lives.

Stage 3: Synthetic-Conventional Faith
The attitudes and values of peers (or the "gang") are major determinants of one's values at this stage, including those related to faith. Adherence to the "norm" is paramount as life's increasing complexities are perceived as necessitating the set of values held in common by the others close to the individual. This affiliation with a community continues for many into adulthood, where a large percentage of people find a faith, or security, in their relationship with a church, synagogue or religious body.

Stage 4: Individuative-Reflective Faith
As adolescents move into adulthood and assume adult responsibilities—marriage and family, vocation, financial interdependency—they often again question some of the fundamental faith assumptions of their parents or religious tradition. For many, the need to doubt, question, and even reject elements of one's faith traditions is necessary for further faith development. This phenomenon is not restricted to young adulthood; an increasing number of persons in the middle and later years are faced with the need to rethink their faith.

Stage 5: Conjunctive Faith
Usually no earlier than the middle years, some adults are able to bring into meaningful reconciliation the variety of faith dynamics that have played important roles in previous stages of their faith development; their faith roots of family and church, the beliefs of others, and the answers they have found in their own questions are all tempered with the maturity that comes only with the experiencing of life. Individuals are able to identify beyond boundaries of race, class, or ideology to understand and integrate the views of others into their own expression of faith, arrived at individually as a mature expression of a faith that is wholly their own.

Stage 6: Universalizing Faith
Persons in Stage 6 are rare. They are, however, those whose lives are so attuned to the ultimate meaning of life that their faith expression is beyond self-interest, taking on a universalizing quality. Fowler theorizes that this stage "represents the culmination of growth in faith, brought about by human fidelity and Divine grace and revelation."

Source: From Bruning (1982, pp. 35–37).

In the prochurch horizontal dimension women showed a consistent and continuous involvement. The increased involvement compared to their younger years suggests that performing acts of love, justice, and mercy increased in importance in their later years. They remained actively involved in church-related functions despite increases in physical limitations. There were no indications of disengagement from the church. On the contrary, there was continuity and stability. This may indicate that the church and related activities remain especially useful to women in their religious growth and take on additional importance as they encounter the various events related to living longer.

Most older women can expect to live from 10 to 18 years as widows. How they cope with being single in their older years and how they use alone time are challenges to their vertical and horizontal faith life. They have the opportunity to turn their time alone into creative solitude (Payne & McFadden, 1994).

FACTORS INFLUENCING FAITH DEVELOPMENT IN OLDER WOMEN

Historical and Social Forces

Despite women's greater religious devotion, commitment, and participation in church and synagogue, historically, the major religious traditions have granted the higher spiritual privileges and leadership positions, clerical and lay, to men. Women have been viewed or treated as second-class participants.

Two historical events began to change women's religious status—World War II and the women's movement. During World War II women assumed new nontraditional roles, and many wanted to continue in the new occupational roles. The women's movement introduced major changes in the image of appropriate roles for women—and men—that have led to a new status for women. These events are period effects that made second-class participation or exclusion in any area no longer acceptable.

In 1949 Doris Lockerman, an *Atlanta Constitution* feature writer, related the new status of women to the churches. She reported that "many leaders are uneasy about the status of women who are almost universally barred from participation in the business of the church, and in clerical conclaves over the land the issue rears its insistent head with more and more frequency" (Lockerman, 1949). Lockerman further cited the rector of a major Atlanta Episcopal church as saying, "If we expect women to finance us, they should have the privilege and responsibility of representation." This was the same year I was admitted on special status as the first woman to attend Candler School of Theology, Emory University. Eight years later (1957) the first woman was ordained in the North Georgia Conference of the United Methodist Church. Reverend Ruth Rogers was an older woman. Beginning at age 54, she served local churches and became the North Georgia Conference Evangelist until her retirement at age 65.

There have been significant changes since Rogers's ordination and Lockerman's article. Women's professional roles in the church began to change rapidly and significantly. Significant numbers of women have been ordained in Protestant and Jewish bodies. Women entered seminaries of all the Protestant denominations and Hebrew seminaries, and by the 1990s they accounted for over 50% of seminaries' enrollment. All the major Protestant faiths and the Jewish rabbinate are accepting women into full clergy relationships. Only the Catholic church continues to deny the admission of women. In 1994 the pope made it clear that there will be no female Catholic priests. Women's roles are restricted to religious orders.

Changes also occurred among the lay leadership. The role of laywomen in the church began to change. Men were no longer the only ones appointed to the major boards and committees making the important congregational decisions. Women were no longer relegated to the kitchen to make coffee or to bake cookies and covered dishes for social events, or to teach the children.

The impact of the women's movement was also evident in theological schools. Women faculty members were added in all theological disciplines, including systematic theology. These women theologians and clergy provided the stimulus for the development of feminist theology. They led with renewed vigor the work of Elizabeth Cady Stanton in the 1890s to draw attention to the sexist treatment and injustices against women by established patriarchal religions. They built on Stanton's work to produce the *Woman's Bible* and to remove sexist language from many rituals, hymns, and religious writings. These changes are opening up new opportunities for women's faith experiences that extend into later life. Given their longer life, women have the opportunity to interpret the differences these changes make to the meaning and development of faith in late life.

Gender

We have seen from a review of the research that gender makes a difference in the way women experience and act out their faith. These gender differences in religiosity and faith development of older women are better explained by sociocultural, economic, and educational status than by biologically determined physical distinctions. Frequent assumptions about behavioral differences are that "boys are independent, girls are dependent; boys are aggressive, girls are more passive; boys have stronger visual abilities, girls have stronger verbal abilities" (Renzetti & Curran, 1992). Although research on biological differences in male-female behavior has been inconsistent (Maccoby & Jacklin, 1974), there is no biological evidence for the religiosity differences of men and women.

Although the social roles assigned to women in the church limited their professional and lay leadership, their participation and commitment did not decline. Psychological and sociological research used to explain the effects of limited social roles on the religiosity of women has relied on some aspect of the deprivation compensation concept. Some (Gari & Scheinfeld, 1968) argued that pre–World War II women were socialized to submissiveness and expressiveness, which made the emotional and authoritarian aspects of religion more likely to appeal to them. Others, like Glock, Ringer, and Babbie (1967), attributed women's religiosity to the secondary position they held in society. As powerless women denied access to the economic, political, religious, and socially prestigious roles, they turned to religion as compensation for depreciation. The churches, these researchers argued, offer alternative rewards to those deprived of status gratification in the social world.

Since the period of "deprivation" is over and women are in the work force and accepted in all social roles, were these only period effects? Or are there other forces and period effects that will contribute to the continuation of women's high level of religiosity and faith maturity? What will be the period effects on the religiosity and faith practices of working single and married women and shared parenting? Will their patterns of response become more like those of men?

Women not only live longer than men, they are most likely to spend an average of 10 to 18 years single due to widowhood and divorce, and be a part of disproportionately female generations. Will this be another period of deprivation, one of age and marital status? Will the church offer alternative rewards for this new gender deprivation? These trends pose questions for future investigators.

Retirement

Transition periods and crisis events play an important role in faith development at any age. Retirement is one of those transition and crisis events that is more age-specific and usually occurs after age 60. The altered lifestyle patterns and social networks require restructuring accompanied by a crisis of meaning and identity of self as a retiree. Retirees face the questions Who am I now? and Of what value is an adult who is no longer a productive worker?

Until recently, the impact of retirement on women has been altered lifestyles because husbands were home every day. The jokes about the stress this caused are numerous. The most frequently quoted is "My wife told me she married me for breakfast and dinner, but never for lunch." The husband's retirement interfered with the household and social patterns of the homemaker woman. This is another one of those period effects that is changing and will continue to change as the numbers of retired women increase dramatically into the next century.

Another form of the crisis comes when the husband (usually a few years older) retires before his wife. The woman may face an early-retirement decision. Regardless of whether it is the husband's retirement, the woman's, or both, it is a period of transition accompanied by a loss of work identity and power, a loss of the social network of coworkers. It is an emptying out of one's work life. It is a form of death. Adjustments to the new lifestyle require a search for new meanings, values, and social structure (Stokes, 1990b; Szinovacz, 1982).

The retirement experience of professional women varies. Biographical and autobiographical accounts of their experiences are important sources of the impact on their faith practices and contribution to their faith development. The retirement experiences of two professional women illustrate these differences. The first is Maggie Kuhn, whom you may recognize as the "Gray Panther." Maggie's experience is an example of how a single religious professional reacted to her retirement and the faith-development consequences. Maggie was a staff person for the Council of Churches and the Presbyterian Office for Church and Society. Her mandatory retirement from the National Council of Churches made her very angry. She reacted by using her new freedom, skills, and knowledge of involvement in social issues to organize the Gray Panthers, an intergenerational organization to eradicate ageism and promote peace and justice (Bianchi, 1994). She refused to retire from life and continued to speak out for important causes, try new roles, and take new risks. Her work after retirement had more social impact and received more recognition than any of her earlier work. She is credited with making advocacy for the rights of older persons an integral part of aging organizations affecting public policy. Most of all, she has made it clear that older people, and women in particular, are major resources for active change in congregations and society. She sounded the call for more intergenerational collaboration in responding to social injustices (Hessel, 1977). It seems safe to say that Maggie's experience moved her into Fowler's fifth stage as she identified beyond the boundaries of race, class, age, or ideology to understand and integrate the views of others into her own expression of faith and the role of congregations.

The second retiree is Sarah Payton (Patty) Boyle. Her case is not as politically spectacular as it is insightful into the spiritual crisis accompanying retirement—the pain, trauma, and despair felt by many older women. The spiritual needs of older women are often overshadowed by the perceived social, physical, and economic needs. Patty recorded her retirement spiritual experience in *The Desert Blooms* (Boyle, 1983). When Patty retired as a respected college professor, honored for her prominent role in the civil rights movement, a wife of 33 years, mother of adult children, and a committed church person, she knew what she wanted to do—to bring into full function the person she was created to be. She felt that she was moving toward such fulfillment. She described her feelings at the time as "a strong outward thrust of accumulated wisdom and practical know-how. I expected to reap a good harvest by using them. The future was out there waiting. It didn't occur to me that I might not be able to deal with it" (Boyle, 1983, p. 20). But her life did not work out as she envisioned. Her expected closer relationship with her husband was dashed when he suddenly left her. Her children were married and in other parts of the country. She was a single older woman. She determined not to focus on what she had lost, but on what she would gain—a new freedom and independence. Still filled with optimism and a strong sense of her ability to adapt, she decided to move to another city.

She thrust herself into a totally different physical and social environment to begin this new phase of her life. She moved from being a homeowner in a college town to being an apartment renter in the suburbs of Washington, D.C., and from a mountain view to that of a rooftop and an asphalt parking lot. Typical of Patty, she ignored the negatives and focused on a few token trees and the stimulus of a new environment. What she found was that the roles and responsibilities that seemed limiting were not as limiting as having no responsibility to significant others. The newfound freedom impeded her creativity more than overwork and a tight schedule. Her efforts to structure a new role were not so simple. All the relationships were new and had to be renegotiated with people who did not see the real "Patty," but a single, old woman.

Her choice of a church mirrored her decision for new directions and change. She chose an ecumenical, well-known Washington church rather than one of her own denomination. She soon felt like she had alien status in a strange land. Seeking stability in the midst of change, she moved to a church of her own denomination to meet her need for shared meanings, rituals, and a church family. She found some of this friendliness, self-recognition, group identity, and a feeling of being needed. However, her identity began to change. She was being treated differently within the church and in all social interactions in a phony, condescending, and overly solicitous manner. In fact, some acted toward her as though she were economically, physically, and psychologically deficient. She felt denigrated. Slowly she realized that her identity was spoiled as she learned that she was one of those "oldpeople" (spelled as one word) and not the creative, exciting, competent, outgoing Patty.

This realization resulted in a period of deep depression, disengagement, and despair that lasted for four years. It was out of this deep despair, lost faith in the clergy, and alienation from the church, a feeling that her faith was dead, that she had a new experience in her relationship with God and others that created a new "Patty." She related that so unbearable did the situation become that one day she cried out in her pain, "God help me," but she heard nothing but awful silence. She turned on the television, and a representative of Alcoholics Anonymous was explaining the use of St. Francis's serenity prayer as a key to recovery. This prayer is a well-known faith symbol, "God grant me the serenity to accept the things I cannot change, the courage to change the things I can, and the wisdom to know the difference." This became the turning point. She accepted her feelings of being old, tired, lost, and with no home, as well as the views of others about older people as a nuisance, an impediment and not a resource in the church, and her own desire to die.

She took positive action steps to change what she could. She enrolled in continuing-education classes and changed the stereotypes about older learners by making the highest grade; she served on jury duty and became a general volunteer in her church and a volunteer visitor in retirement homes and nursing homes. Slowly, positive feelings about herself and others emerged as she acted on now, not yesterdays or tomorrows. She learned to help her peers (other older people) by confirming the person, not directing her or him; she learned the art of listening (Payne, 1990b). The next section includes a description of one more major experience on her faith journey that was related to health, dying, and grief.

Health

Among the early explanations for the anticipated decline of older persons' attendance and participation in church activities was that of physical limitations due to health and the aging process. Obviously, those who were institutionalized or confined to their homes due to health problems were going to be limited in these church-related activities. However, it was soon observed that interest and participation in private practices of their faith did not accompany physical limitations. On the contrary, these became the stimulus to further faith development (Blazer & Palmore, 1976; Stark, 1968).

The case of Ruth Gray helps us understand how change in health affects women. Ruth was a single, older woman, the widow of a minister, retired from her work in the Christian education of children for her denomination. At age 85 her health required that she enter a retirement home. This was not a happy decision. However, she responded to it by keeping a diary of her social and spiritual struggle to maintain her individuality and personhood. For this struggle for the survival of the spirit, she drew on her resources of a lifetime of involvement in the church and as a professional in religious education. Her diary became a book that continues to help others understand what the journey involves and that it can be victorious.

But it is not always the change in a woman's health that creates a social and spiritual struggle with her faith. It may be the change in the health of her husband, parents, or other relatives, even an older son or daughter. It is the traditional assumption that as a woman, she will shoulder the majority of the caregiving responsibilities (Kaye & Applegate, 1994). Age does not exempt her from this expectation. While experiencing her own aging, the older woman becomes *the* caregiver. The role of caregiver is isolating and involves a twenty-four-hour day for an indefinite period of time, from months to years. Her normal routine is interrupted, and she disengages from her social network of friends and church activities. The resulting social isolation makes the physical and emotional stress greater and frequently leads to the likelihood that she will develop physical and psychological problems.

Caregiver depression is not unusual and is a serious factor in the care of the patient and the physical health of the caregiver. Cohen and Eisdorfer (1993) observed that "caregivers frequently view themselves as the sole provider for almost all the older person's needs, stretch themselves out and become more and more isolated and vulnerable to problems of their own." The depression that may result is not always recognized. Cohen and Eisdorfer believed that "physicians' recognition of mental health problems is notoriously poor . . . and recognition of depression is suboptimal." This situation makes it even more critical that the older woman caregiver maintain her church ties and that her pastor recognize her spiritual needs as well as the needs for caregiver support services.

We pick up the final account of the faith development of Patty thirteen years after her retirement. Those years had been the richest of her life, filled with a sense of belonging, contributing, loving, and being loved. Never had she felt a greater sense of progress, autonomy, and security; her coping skills were steadier, her goals clearer, and the meaning of her life better understood. Then a series of events began to occur that were unlike anything she had ever experienced. She became the caregiver of her single, favorite, 82-year-old cousin Frank (known in theological circles in the 1950s and 1960s as Stringfellow Barr). He had Alzheimer's disease and could no longer care for himself. Patty learned all about this disease and how to relate to a loved one with it. She used many creative ways of communicating with him and trying to help him, only to be helped herself as she learned that it is not so much our ability to reason as how we respond to our world that makes us human. Frank taught her what being truly human meant. Through her care for him she learned more about losses, disease, dying, death, and grief. She became a part of a small sharing group of dying persons to discuss the meaning of dying and death, the fears, and the needs of the dying person in relation to her or his faith. Her spiritual breakthrough was to know that the substance that sustains us in earthly life is love, and we need not fear the source of all love. Patty had learned to face and accept her own mortality, death, and the final meaning of her life: to give and receive love.

There is not space here to repeat more of Patty's spiritual journey, but I recommend it for more complete and in-depth reading. It is also a methodological example of the significance of the spiritual autobiography in understanding the inner-space dynamics of the faith development of older women.

Involvement in Organized Religion

Lifelong membership and involvement in a church along with strong family involvement play a major role in the faith development of older women (Stokes, 1990a), in their continued engagement in church life, and in social issues. Elizabeth Welch is one of those lifelong active church persons who refuse to retire, but choose to reinvest their lives in making a dynamic career out of aging. She is sounding the call for other older adults to join her in responding to the opportunity to exercise great political power and religious leadership. She is redirecting her energies to defining a new role for all older people and especially older women. This effort has included writing her autobiography, *Learning to Be 85*, in which she identified a particular event in each age that indicates a learning that has proved to be not only beneficial, but crucial to her becoming 85. She summarized that learning:

They arose from where I was and what my identity had to do with my name; my understanding of how important a sense of humor is; my realization of the real meaning of giving; my learning how to grow into responsibility; I must also acknowledge the power of prayer and a personal spiritual faith. Certainly, I also benefited from the un-learning of prejudice, from giving others the respect they are due; from realizing what personal relationships mean to me, and from seeing how teaching translates into being taught. (Welch, 1991, p. 13)

For the lifelong members, the desire to participate in the life of the church remains constant (Ainlay & Smith, 1984). Lifestyle changes in retirement years make it possible to exercise that participation in new and creative ways. The barriers to participation may be restrictions due to health problems, or they may be due to ageism that blinds congregational leaders to the untapped resources and skills of older women for creative service.

One Methodist minister discovered that his presuppositions about older church members as barriers to the progress of the church were wrong. Blaine Taylor was assigned to an urban church where over half of the members were "old people" over 65. He described his experience:

I had been conditioned to see them only in terms of the old stereotypes generated by society's prejudices. AGEISM was not in my vocabulary. . . . My congregation helped me to understand that those over sixty-five were just people, special only in the extent of their experience, wisdom, and self-understanding. They had all the strengths and weak-nesses, all the hopes and fears, and all the cares and concerns of people everywhere. . . . I began to see them as individuals. (Taylor, 1984, p. 13)

Taylor discovered that these older members were a remarkable resource and had strengths that most of us do not recognize. He recorded his experiences in de-veloping a ministry with, by, and for older persons that is a testimony not only of the desire of older persons to participate in their church, but how they did. Taylor's experience reinforces the observation of Ainlay and Smith (1984) that we do not know enough about the qualitative age differences of religious par-ticipation of older persons, much less the gender differences in their experiences.

FAITH DEVELOPMENT OF THE NEW OLDER WOMAN

No discussion of religiosity and faith development in older women can be confined to existing studies and data because a new older woman is coming. In just fourteen years the first baby-boomer woman will be eligible to receive her Social Security check and retire on a pension. She will be joined over the next two decades by about 40 million more women. The baby boomers born between 1946 and 1964 are no longer babies, but "preretirees." How will this group whose members have already shaped our national life shape the religious life and faith development of future older women? Gallup (1994) said that the baby boomers have already created their own religious shock wave, and sociologist Wade Roof (1993) contended that they are transforming and will transform America's religious landscape.

What constitutes this religious shock wave? Those who are studying the religious behavior of baby boomers (Gallup, 1994; Roof, 1993; C. K. Miller, 1992) agree that they have a unique worldview—a baby-boomer spirituality. Gallup found that in many ways they are no different from their parents (the older women of the 1990s). Their parents took them to Sunday School and church, and they dropped out as teenagers and young adults (like all the generations before them), although their form of dropping out was more visible and dramatic. They protested everything from civil rights to the Vietnam War to California lettuce and grapes, and they explored alternative lifestyles and alternative religions—Hare Krishna, Moonies, Jesus freaks, and so on. Gallup studies in the 1980s found that religious beliefs among the boomers were true to traditional levels of American participation, beliefs, and practices. In 1994 Gallup reported that they are "statistically unremarkable, mirroring the religious characteristics of the general population—church membership, attendance, religious preference, and other measures." Then what is different? It is primarily the movement from religiosity to spirituality.

The baby-boomer woman is a working woman (72%), and gender equality permeates her culture. She is viewed as an autonomous, competent person defined in her own right and not by a husband's role or her family roles. Roof (1993) pointed out that women structure their lives, including how they spend Sundays, more and more as do working men. Conditions of work, not gender, have the greater influence on religious life. They are more likely to drop out altogether or attend services irregularly, pray less, or report fewer memorable religious experiences. Roof reported that "they find the existing programs in most congregations, including many of the older gender-based men's and women's groups, inadequate for their needs. Rather, they look for more specific type of programs organized around career concerns, women's issues and lifestyles" (p. 222). There is a definite generational break between the baby-boomer woman and the older woman.

Along with these religious interests and patterns of involvement, the baby-boomer women are seeking a transforming, unifying vision of life as a spiritual journey. They separate the spiritual from the religious. They define religious as the traditional congregational organization, worship, and ritual. The spiritual is the direct experience with God. They are looking for relationships and experiences of sharing, caring, accepting, and belonging. The baby-boomer woman's spiritual journey is to find a connection between life and meaning and about finding a way to express it. She finds her religious quests supported in small, intentional groups formed within a congregation or in the community, and they may be found in new forms of community. Roof (1993) predicted that boomers will create new forms of community already seen in new village forms, co-housing movements, and cooperative housing.

Among the baby boomers in his study, Roof found that 80% believe in God or a higher power, but they want to make a direct contact with the sacred without commitment to institutions, rituals, or orthodox beliefs. They have "an open, exploring approach to religion. They are seeking meaning in relationships and have a strong desire for commitment to others and the community" (p. 5). They portend an emerging elder culture much like the subculture of the aging predicted by Arnold Rose in 1962 (Rose, 1965) that cherishes the bonds people form with one another. Given the numbers of older persons and especially older women, such values and actions form the social and spiritual supports in old age.

CONCLUSION AND IMPLICATIONS FOR RESEARCH AND PRACTICE

Although the religiosity research shows that older women's interest, their participation in church activities, and the value they place on religion continue to increase into their 70s and beyond (Faracasin, 1992), information about the dynamics of their faith development in late life is limited. There are few studies on the relation of religion to their aging experience, especially among those over 85.

The continued organizational participation of older women raises Ainlay and Smith's (1984) question concerning the qualitative age difference in the structure of that participation. It also raises the question of the inclusiveness of older women in the total life of the organization.

The need for more research is obvious, especially studies that focus on the dynamics of faith development and change. Psychologist James Birren (1990) and survey researcher George Gallup (1992) referred to this as research on the inner space as contrasted to the outer space (religiosity) of older persons. If we focus on inner space, do we get a complete picture if we neglect the outer space?

What we may need is research that combines the outer and inner faith-life data and a theoretical framework for interpretation. Gallup's survey research provides a still picture of the outer space, and the spiritual autobiography provides a moving picture. We may have expected these to be mutually exclusive when they are inclusive. The whole story may require bringing the outer and inner faith life together with a faith-development theory such as Fowler's for interpretation. This is the design adopted by Faracasin (1992).

In any event, the shift in research interest to spirituality that studies the human spirit, religious or God consciousness, and the search for meaning and purpose in life (Ellison, 1983) coincides with the baby boomers' spiritual quest. If the search for meaning is a lifelong journey, the journey is not over until the last miles are recorded. The question is, "What have older women found to be the meaning and purpose of life?"

The vignettes and several excerpts from spiritual autobiographies of older women were included in our discussion to suggest the insights that spiritual autobiographies provide and to propose the development of the spiritual autobiography as a research methodology begun by Birren (1990), Clements (1994), and Bianchi (1982). Such studies are needed in response to the interests of baby boomers in spirituality, small special-interest groups, and community building reported by Roof (1993). The inclusion of two or more generations of women would make it possible to project future trends in religiosity and faith development of older women.

Research on the response of congregations to older persons, and older women in particular, would provide an understanding of organizational constraints and opportunities for older women. We know more about the older women's religiosity and faith development than we do about the religious organizational responses to the older woman. Implications for practice are directed to older women themselves and to local congregational program planners. Older women need to be taught and encouraged to write their own spiritual autobiographies. Congregational program planners need to create ways these experiences can be shared, especially in intergenerational groups. Recording and sharing spiritual autobiographies tell us where we have been in our journey and where we are now and motivate us to go where we want to go.

SPIRITUAL AUTOBIOGRAPHICAL POSTSCRIPT

Several valued colleagues, in discussing this chapter with me, encouraged me to add this part of my own spiritual autobiography as a postscript. I do not know whether I am "more religious" at 74 than I was at 34. I do know that the practice is different, that I do not need certain religious expressions to maintain the strength of my faith. I do know that I still need my church and want to be a part of it.

I greet each day with rejoicing for the present and God's presence in and within my life, my new home and public life. Somehow I am discovering spiritually that this is the last for which the first experiences were made. Is this perhaps maturity of faith?

I went through the period of learning about Jesus and the Bible stories; I went to seminary and received my formal theological and biblical training; I went through the period of trying to "walk in Jesus' steps" and found that I neither had the spiritual strength nor was I supposed to—I could not be God or Jesus (what a relief!). I went through the period of structured, designated, daily times for prayer and meditation; I even kept Baillie's (1949) *Diary of Private Prayer* for three years. I served in professional and lay leadership positions within my denomination. I made a religious pilgrimage to the Holy Land and learned the role geography plays in faith development; I became a caregiver and learned about the spiritual nature of dying; I became a care-receiver and learned about interdependence and hope; I had an out-of-body experience and learned that my physical body did not define me, but who I am does. Now, in the present, all of the past steps are leading me to need less ritual, but increased creative solitude time, to new relationships and active concern about the social and physical world. I have found that loving and being loved by family and friends bring joy, peace, and security. I find opportunities to continue to make some contribution to the understanding of long life and the last meaning and purpose in my life—and I'm not through. I don't expect, as Martin Kahler (1967) observed, to become fully serene or mature in my faith; I expect the inner struggle to go on to my last day no matter how old I become. Am I more religious? I don't think so. I am just religiously different.

REFERENCES

Ainlay, S. C., & Smith, D. R. (1984). Aging and religious participation. *Journal of Gerontology, 39*(3), 357–363.

Alston, J. P., & Alston, L. T. (1980). Religion and the older woman. In M. M. Fuller & C. A. Martin (Eds.), *The older woman: Lavender rose or Gray Panther* (pp. 262–278). Springfield, IL: Charles C. Thomas.

Alston, J. P., & Wingrove, C. R. (1974). Cohort analysis of church attendance. *Social Forces, 53*(2), 324.

Argyle, M., & Beit-Hallahmi, B. (1975). *The social psychology of religion.* Boston: Routledge & Kegan Paul.

Baillie, J. (1949). *A diary of private prayer.* New York: Charles Scribner's Sons.

Benson, P. L., & Elkin, C. H. (1990). A national study of Protestant congregations: A summary report on faith, life, loyalty, and congregational life. Minneapolis: Search Institute.

Bianchi, E. C. (1982). *Aging as a spiritual journey.* New York: Crossroad.

———. (1994). *Elder wisdom: Crafting your own elderhood.* New York: Crossroad.

Birren, J. E. (1990). Spiritual maturity in psychological development. In J. J. Seeber (Ed.), *Spiritual maturity in the later years.* New York: Haworth Press.

Blazer, D. G., & Palmore, E. (1976). Religion and aging in a longitudinal panel. *Gerontologist, 16*(1), 82–85.

Boyle, S. P. (1983). *The desert blooms.* Nashville: Abingdon Press.

Bruning, C., & Stokes, K. (1982). The hypotheses paper. In K. Stokes (Ed.), *Faith development in the adult life cycle* (pp. 35–37). New York: W. H. Sadlier.

Clements, W. M. (1994). *Making the last the best: Meaning for life's fourth quarter of life.* Keynote address. South Eastern jurisdiction older adult conference of the United Methodist Church, August 14, 1994. Lake Junaluska, North Carolina.

Cohen, D., & Eisdorfer, C. (1993). *Seven steps to effective parent care.* New York: Tarcher Putnam.

Cornwall, M. (1989). Faith development of men and women over the life span. In S. Bahr & E. Peterson (Eds.), *Aging and the family* (pp. 115–139). Lexington, MA: Lexington Books.

Ellison, G. W. (1983). Spiritual well-being: Conceptualization and measurement. *Journal of Psychology and Theology, 11*(4), 330–340.

Faracasin, T. W. (1992). The relationship of gender differences to adult religious development (Doctoral dissertation, University of Minnesota, Minneapolis). *Dissertation Abstracts International*, DAI-536–02B-0377, (University Microfilms No. AAI 9220254).

Fowler, J. (1982). Stages of faith in the adult life cycles. In K. Stokes (Ed.), *Faith development in the adult life cycle* (pp. 179–298). New York: W. H. Sadlier.

———. (1987). *Faith development in the adult life cycle: The report of a research project*. New Haven, CT: Religious Research Association.

Fuller, M. M., & Martin, C. A. (Eds). (1980). *The older woman: Lavender rose or Gray Panther*. Springfield, IL: Charles C. Thomas.

Gallup, G. (1985). *Faith development and your ministry*. Princeton, NJ: Princeton Religion Research Center.

———. (1987). Age, a key factor in comparing religiousness of men and women. *Emerging Trends, 9*(9). Princeton, NJ: Princeton Religion Research Center.

———. (1991). What every pastor should know about the average American. *Emerging Trends, 13*(3). Princeton, NJ: Princeton Religion Research Center.

———. (1992). Surveys reveal religious "inner life." *Emerging Trends, 14*(10). Princeton, NJ: Princeton Religion Research Center.

———. (1993). Teens want answers to hard questions of life. *Emerging Trends, 15*(7). Princeton, NJ: Princeton Religion Research Center.

———. (1994). Baby boomers have created their own religious shock wave. *Emerging Trends, 16*(2). Princeton, NJ: Princeton Religion Research Center.

Gari, J. E., & Scheinfeld, A. (1968). Sex differences in mental and behavioral traits. *Genetic Psychology Monographs, 77*,(2) 169–299.

Gilligan, C. (1982). *In a different voice: Psychological theory and women's development*. Cambridge, MA: Harvard University Press.

———. (1986). In a different voice: Visions of maturity. In J. W. Conn (Ed.), *Women's spirituality: Resource for Christian development* (pp. 63–87) New York: Paulist Press.

Glock, C. Y., Ringer, B. B., & Babbie, E. R. (1967). *To comfort and to challenge*. Berkeley: University of California Press.

Goodwen, W. (1982). Responses from an adult development perspective. In K. Stokes (Ed.), *Faith development in the adult life cycle* (pp. 85–120). New York: W. H. Sadlier.

Havighurst, R. (1948). *Developmental tasks and education*. Chicago: University of Chicago Press.

Hessel, D. (1977). *Maggie Kuhn on aging: A dialogue*. Philadelphia: Westminster Press.

Jung, C. (1933). *Modern man in search of a soul*. New York: Harcourt, Brace, & World.

Kahler, M. (1967). Justification by faith. Lecture in P. Tillich (Ed.), *Perspectives on 19th and 20th century Protestant theology*. New York: Harper & Row.

Kaye, L. W., & Applegate, J. S. (1994). Older men and family caregiving orientation. In E. H. Thompson, Jr. (Ed.), *Older men's lives* (pp. 218–236). Thousand Oaks, CA: Sage Publications.

Koenig, H., Smiley, M., & Gonzales, J. A. P. (1988). *Religion, health, and aging: A review and theoretical integration*. Westport, CT: Greenwood Press.

Lindbergh, A. M. (1975). *Gift from the sea*. New York: Pantheon Books.

Lockerman, D. (1949, October 17). Church's headache, women's freedom. *Atlanta Constitution*.

Maccoby, E., & Jacklin, C. (1974). *The psychology of sex differences.* Stanford, CA: Stanford University Press.

Maddox, G. L. (1987). Aging differently. *Gerontologist, 27*(5), 557–564.

Miller, B. (1987). Gender and control among spouses of the cognitively impaired: A research note. *Gerontologist, 27,* 447–453.

————. (1990). Gender differences in spouse management of caregiver role. In E. K. Abel & M. K. Nelson (Eds.), *Circles of care: Work and identity in women's lives* (pp. 92–104). Albany: State University of New York Press.

Miller, C. K. (1992). *Baby boomer spirituality.* Nashville: Disciples Resources.

Moberg, D. O. (1965). Religiosity in old age. *Gerontologist, 5,* 78–87.

Orbach, H. L. (1961). Aging and religion: Church attendance in the Detroit metropolitan area. *Geriatrics, 16,* 530–540.

Payne, B. P. (1982). Religiosity. In D. J. Mangen & W. A. Peterson (Eds.), *Social roles and social participation* (pp. 342–388). Minneapolis: University of Minnesota Press.

————. (1990a, Fall). Research and theoretical approaches to spirituality and aging. *Generations,* 11–16.

————. (1990b). Spiritual maturity and meaning-filled relationships: A sociological perspective. In J. J. Seeber (Ed.), *Spiritual maturity in the later years* (pp. 25–40). New York: Haworth Press.

————. (1993). *Faith development among older men: Case studies.* Unpublished papers.

————. (1994). Faith development in older men. In E. H. Thompson, Jr. (Ed.), *Older men's lives* (pp. 85–103). Thousand Oaks, CA: Sage Publications.

Payne, B. P., & McFadden, S. H. (1994). From loneliness to solitude: Religious and spiritual journeys in late life. In L. E. Thomas & S. A. Eisenhandler (Eds.), *Aging and the religious dimension* (pp. 13–28). Westport, CT: Auburn House.

Payne, B. P., & Whittington, F. J. (1976). Older women: An examination of popular stereotypes and research evidence. *Social Problems, 23,* 488–504.

Renzetti, C. M., & Curran, D. J. (1992). *Women, men, and society* (2nd ed.). Boston: Allyn & Bacon.

Roof, W. C. (1993). *A generation of seekers.* San Francisco: Harper.

Rose, A. M. (1965). The subculture of the aging: A framework for research in social gerontology. In A. M. Rose & W. A. Peterson (Eds.), *Older people and their social world* (pp. 3–16). Philadelphia: F. A. Davis Company.

Shulik, R. N. (1979). Faith development, moral development, and old age: An assessment of Fowler's faith development paradigm (Doctoral dissertation, University of Chicago). *Dissertation Abstracts International,* ABI 0531731 (University Microfilms No. DA 140–06–2907–0613–2907).

Stark, R. (1968). Age and faith: A changing outlook at an old process. *Sociological Analysis, 29,* 1–10.

Stokes, K. (Ed.). (1982). *Faith development in the adult life cycle.* New York: W. H. Sadlier.

————. (1990a). Faith development in the adult life cycle. *Journal of Religious Gerontology, 7,* 167–184.

————. (1990b). *Faith is a verb.* Mystic, CT: Twenty-third Publications.

Szinovacz, M. (Ed.). (1982). *Women's retirement.* Beverly Hills, CA: Sage.

Taylor, B. (1984). *The church's ministry with older adults.* Nashville: Abingdon Press.

Thompson, E. H., Jr. (1991). Beneath the status characteristic: Gender variations in religiousness. *Journal of the Scientific Study of Religion, 30*, 381–394.

Welch, E. (1991). *Learning to be 85*. Nashville: Upper Room Resources.

Wingrove, C. R., & Alston, J. P. (1971). Age, aging, and church attendance. *Gerontologist, 11*, 356–358.

Young, G., & Dowling, W. (1987). Dimensions of religiosity in old age: Accounting for variation in types of participation. *Journal of Gerontology, 42*(4), 376–380.

Sixteen

Voluntarism among Older Women

WINIFRED DOWLING

Voluntarism has been an essential part of American life since Europeans began migrating to America. From the first permanent settlement in Virginia in 1607, mutual self-help has been essential to American survival.

The early immigrants of the seventeenth and eighteenth centuries had left their homeland almost never to return. They left behind both the social support structure of extended families and the technical support structure that provided the necessities of everyday life. Thus they were far more dependent on the voluntary help of other people in the colony than they would have been in their native land. There were simply not as many grandparents, aunts, uncles, and cousins to help till the fields, bring in the harvest, educate the children, or assist in times of sickness. Although society and voluntary organizations were male dominated, women volunteers played a significant part (Dowling, 1992; Nemschoff, 1981).

Older women, in this preindustrial age, were involved in the activities of everyday life, but were circumscribed by both law and custom. Women were dependent on men for their legal identity and economic support throughout their lifespan. Furthermore, aging women were expected to be passive, and it was widely assumed that an active old age for women was inappropriate (Premo, 1990). Although there were older women who managed to exercise independence and to serve both family and others, they remained highly unusual. One impressive example is part of a 1798 compilation of writings by Judith Sargent Murray in which she described the achievements of an elderly Massachusetts woman as a "marvel of self-education, industry, and strength." Her knowledge of farming was so complete that farmers throughout the vicinity sought her advice; her neighbors consulted her on "every perplexing emergency"; and she served others as a "valuable nurse" (Premo, 1990).

Women's role remained largely domestic until the latter part of the nineteenth century. The rapid industrialization of the United States and the flood of immigrants brought vast changes in social roles. The great surge of immigration that took place from 1880 to 1914 totaled 18 million immigrants. These immigrants tended to settle in the cities rather than on farmland. Most were poor and lived in crowded slums with terrible public health problems. Charitable organizations, staffed by volunteers, cared for the "worthy poor." Many of the organizations were religious; others were begun by wealthy individuals or groups; still others sprang from ethnic roots—self-help for the many nationalities and races among immigrants.

A great many of the national voluntary agencies that are significant in American life were begun between 1880 and 1920, including Girl Scouts, Junior League, the National Council of Jewish Women, the American Red Cross, the American Cancer Society, and Community Chests, the forerunner of United Way (Dowling, 1992). Most of these organizations were begun and run by women. As service by women volunteers became more significant, there developed a stereotypical image of the volunteer as an upper- or middle-class white homemaker (Chambre, 1987; Nathanson & Eggleton, 1993; Nemschoff, 1981). That portrait of a volunteer was probably never accurate; research in the last decade shows how widespread volunteering is. Describing the typical volunteer as "the older matron living in the suburbs" tells only part of the story (Taylor, 1990). Data from a number of large studies show that older women are only slightly more likely to volunteer than older men and that, in general, older people are less likely to volunteer than younger age groups (Chambre, 1987; Fischer & Schaffer, 1993; Hayghe, 1991; Herzog, Kahn, Morgan, Jackson, & Antonucci, 1989; Independent Sector, 1990, 1992).

Although there is a growing body of research on voluntarism, the difficulty of definition remains. Most studies have defined voluntarism to mean formal volunteering for an organization. However, the Gallup surveys for the Independent Sector (a private nonprofit group encouraging giving, volunteering, and other not-for-profit initiatives) include informal volunteering (Hayghe, 1991). "Informal" volunteering means the nonorganizational help that people offer to friends and neighbors, from taking soup to a sick neighbor to baby-sitting for a friend.

It is sometimes difficult to distinguish between formal and informal volunteering: If a volunteer regularly visits a homebound neighbor, why does this not "count" as volunteering as much as, for example, a Retired Senior Volunteer Program (RSVP) volunteer who is part of a home-visitation program? Further, informal volunteering is more often done by certain groups. For instance, women and minorities are more likely to be in these informal helping networks that do not show up on volunteer studies (Fischer & Schaffer, 1993).

Because of the difficulty of definition of voluntarism, the percentage of older people shown to be volunteers varies from 11% to 52% (Fischer & Schaffer, 1993). Even comparing just two surveys—the Current Population Survey (CPS) of May 1989 and the 1990 Gallup Organization Survey for the Independent Sector—showed a difference from 10.9% (the CPS supplement on volunteers) to 41% in the Gallup poll for people over 65 years of age (Hayghe, 1991). Overall, the trend seems to be that the rate of volunteering for both young and old is increasing. Interestingly, among older people, it appears that the rate of voluntarism is increasing for men, but not for women (Chambre, 1984; Hamilton, Frederick, & Schneider's Company, 1988; Herzog et al., 1989; Fischer & Schaffer, 1993).

In the last thirty years there has been a significant shift in attitudes about volunteering by older people. There used to be a sense that retirement meant not being involved; volunteer organizations did not reach out to older people; and there was often a lack of interest in voluntarism among older people, perhaps because of the lack of opportunity. Now, on the contrary, older people are seen as a valuable resource to be cultivated for their own benefit and that of society (Chambre, 1987; Costello, 1990; Keller, 1981).

Although it appears from most studies that older men and women volunteer in about equal proportions, numerically there are more older women volunteers simply by the fact that there are more women over the age of 65 (Chambre, 1987). That single fact may reinforce the perception that a higher percentage of older women are volunteering, since they are more numerous.

Major studies point to level of education and economic status as being the major predictors of volunteer service for older women. Since higher education tends to relate to higher income, it is not clear which is the more predictive variable (Hayghe, 1991; Independent Sector, 1992). One practical factor is that volunteering often includes some out-of-pocket expenses that lower-income people may not be able to afford. In addition, older people with higher educational skills tend to be more attractive to volunteer organizations (Chambre, 1984).

Age also predicts the level of volunteering for both men and women. The Independent Sector survey of 1992 showed that 42% of people aged 65–74 said that they had volunteered in the previous year. The figure for people 75 or over was 26.6%. Other studies show comparable rates of decline (Chambre, 1987; Herzog & Morgan, 1992; Ishii-Kuntz, 1990). It seems that increasing age influences volunteering independently of health status. But the decline in volunteering seems to be occurring at much later ages, after 75 or 80 (Chambre, 1987; Fischer & Schaffer, 1993; Herzog et al., 1989). One study found that the rate of voluntarism after age 80 declined much more sharply for men than it did for women: 14% of women were still participating in volunteering, compared to only 7% of men (Chambre, 1987). It has been pointed out that it may not be age itself that influences the rate of volunteering. The intervening factors may be income and education. The older a woman is, the more likely she is to have fewer years of schooling and lower income (Chambre, 1987).

One could logically assume that declining health would be strongly associated with a decline in volunteering, yet survey results are contradictory (Chambre, 1987). When people over 65 were asked why they did not volunteer, health reasons were cited by 31.4% of nonvolunteers, but another reason, "personal schedule too full," was mentioned more often (32.2%) (Independent Sector, 1992). Health reasons may also be considered an acceptable explanation for not volunteering and may not reflect actual health status.

One health-related question is not usually asked on volunteer surveys: whether the health of a spouse affects the ability to begin or continue volunteer work. In a nationwide panel study it was found that the physical health of family members was implicated about 28% of the time when health reasons were cited for dropping out (Booz-Allen & Hamilton, 1985). Thus older women may be obliged to leave volunteer work more often for caregiving reasons than older men do.

Work has a definite effect on volunteering by older women, but not in the expected direction. Although retired women and lifelong homemakers have the most disposable time, they are not the most likely to volunteer. Employed older people, especially those who work part-time, have the highest volunteer rates. One major study showed that older homemakers are least likely to volunteer (Chambre, 1987; Fischer, Mueller, & Cooper, 1991; Fischer & Schaffer, 1993; Independent Sector, 1992).

Susan Chambre, in *Good Deeds in Old Age*, noted that the effect of retirement differs markedly between retired professional men and women. When professional women retired, they were twice as likely to volunteer as were professional men (49% as compared to 25%). Among women who retired from clerical, blue-collar, service, and farm jobs, the rate of volunteering was about 1 in 5, about the same level as men retiring from similar jobs (Chambre, 1987).

Marital status can have an effect on volunteering. Studies tend to show that older married people are more likely than unmarried to volunteer. Since married people usually have higher income levels, this may explain the difference (Fischer et al., 1991; Fischer & Schaffer, 1993; Independent Sector, 1992). The effect of widowhood on volunteering is mixed. Some studies demonstrate that widows have a higher rate of voluntarism (Booz-Allen & Hamilton, 1985; Hayghe, 1991; Ishii-Kuntz, 1990). If age is controlled, it seems that widowhood for women is not a significant factor in volunteer participation, but that for men it appears to be associated with lower levels of volunteering (Chambre, 1987).

Volunteer service has often been discussed as a substitute for role loss, and early studies sometimes assumed that voluntarism was, above all, compensatory. The hypothesis was that older women who had lost a spouse, work, or family roles would have a higher rate of voluntarism. This compensatory view of older women and voluntarism has not been borne out. On the contrary, it seems that better-off older women—those with higher education and income, stronger family ties, higher activity levels, and better mental health and life-satisfaction ratios—are most likely to volunteer (Booz-Allen & Hamilton, 1985; Chambre, 1984, 1987; Fischer & Schaffer, 1993; Independent Sector, 1992).

There remains the question whether volunteering enhances life satisfaction and activity levels or whether the opposite is true—that volunteering attracts people who are active and satisfied with their lives (Chambre, 1987; Fischer & Schaffer, 1993). A Retired Senior Volunteer Program study (women comprised 80% of the sample) compared RSVP volunteers and nonvolunteers over time on each of five measures: social resources, mental outlook, physical health, economic resources, and overall functioning. While RSVP attracted a healthier group of seniors, it was also found that RSVP participation was associated with improved or stable levels of functioning, while noticeable declines in functioning were evident among nonvolunteers (Booz-Allen & Hamilton, 1985). The study concluded that it was virtually impossible to discover whether the volunteer program keeps seniors at a higher functioning level or whether the higher functioning enabled volunteers to stay in the program. It may be that the self-selection process attracts and keeps volunteers. On the other hand, it may be that volunteer service is the cause of improved or at least stabilized functioning (Booz-Allen & Hamilton, 1985).

There are distinct gender differences between older women and men volunteers. Women tend to be involved in the more expressive volunteer jobs, while men are more instrumental. Older women as volunteers are more often caregivers, social organizers, social service providers, and tutors, while men are more often board members, fundraisers, and recreational and technical volunteers. In an American Red Cross study (1988) on its volunteers (where the majority are over the age of 55), there were significant differences in the gender of volunteers, particularly at the leadership level. Women are underrepresented among governance-level volunteers (the chairpersons of Red Cross chapters, for example). These differences reflect both societal expectation and the experience of older women and men throughout their lifetimes when gender roles were more distinct than they are now (Chambre, 1987; Fischer et al., 1991; Fischer & Schaffer, 1993). In the past twenty-five years women's participation in the work force has changed markedly, and older women are increasingly retirees rather than homemakers. It appears that gender differences are becoming smaller, especially when men and women in similar occupations and job levels are compared (Chambre, 1987).

Older women are active across the whole spectrum of volunteer service. Government programs that include older volunteers run the gamut from the Corporation for National and Community Service to SCORE (Service Corps of Retired Executives) to the Peace Corps. The expansion of volunteering has been a goal of public policy at least since the 1960s. President John F. Kennedy inaugurated the Peace Corps in 1961. President Lyndon Johnson started VISTA (Volunteers in Service to America) and the Foster Grandparent Program. Richard Nixon started ACTION, the federal volunteer agency. President George Bush began the Points of Light Foundation. President William Clinton established the Corporation for National and Community Service to encourage voluntarism at all levels and all ages (Dowling, 1992).

There are a number of federal volunteer programs designed specifically for older people. They include the Retired Senior Volunteer Program, the Foster

Grandparent Program, and the Senior Companion Program. These three programs comprise the National Senior Service Corps, part of the Corporation for National and Community Service. Interestingly, the proportion of women in the National Senior Service Corps is much higher than that of men, which does not reflect the statistics of other major studies (Independent Sector, 1990, 1992). RSVP's 430,000 volunteers are made up of 75% women; Foster Grandparents, 90% female; Senior Companions, 85% female. Although the roles of both Foster Grandparents and Senior Companions might be considered an extension of women's roles of child care and caregiving, that is not true of the Retired Senior Volunteer Program.

The Service Corps of Retired Executives, with nearly 3,000 volunteers, has, not unexpectedly, only 12% women. In the private sector older women are involved in large numbers in the national health organizations like the American Red Cross, the American Heart Association, the American Cancer Society, and United Way (American Red Cross, 1988). The American Association of Retired Persons (AARP) conducted an informal count of four field volunteer groups in 1992 and found that 42% of the AARP volunteers were women.

Corporate retiree programs are another growing area for older women's involvement. The National Retiree Volunteer Center helps corporations develop volunteer programs for retirees; it estimates that one-third of the volunteer retirees' leadership are women. In the corporate retiree programs men outnumber women at the outset, but more and more women are taking leadership positions. There is some evidence that women in the program are developing leadership skills in retirement that were not available during their work life.

Corporations ranging from Levi Strauss to Honeywell have women retiree volunteers. The AT&T and Bell Telephone companies across the country have had the Telephone Pioneer of America volunteer program in place since 1911. With 850,000 members, it is the largest industry-related volunteer organization in the world. An estimated 25% of all Telephone Pioneers are older women.

The biennial surveys by the Independent Sector show that more volunteers serve religious organizations than in any other area. A close second is informal volunteering, with education third (Independent Sector, 1990, 1992). The major difference between older and younger women is that there are fewer older women involved in schools and other educational institutions. In the Current Population Survey of 1989, the percentage of people 65 years of age or older who volunteered in schools was only 4.3%, compared to 20.3% of volunteers between ages 35 and 44 (Hayghe, 1991).

Adults of all ages report volunteering for religious organizations as the most common volunteer activity. Surveys report that among older people, about two out of five volunteer for a religious organization (Fischer et al., 1991; Hayghe, 1991; Independent Sector, 1992).

Churches, synagogues, and mosques are inextricably connected with volunteer work. They would not be viable organizations without volunteers, and they spawn other volunteer activity, like visits to the homebound and support for the homeless. National movements have been fostered by church volunteers: the civil rights movement and the peace movement during the Vietnam War, for example (Fischer et al., 1991). Most of all, religious values are congruent with the primary motivations that respondents report as their reasons for volunteering (Fischer et al., 1991; Independent Sector, 1990, 1992). According to the Gallup polls for the Independent Sector (1990, 1992), the greatest personal motivation for giving and volunteering was feeling that those who had more should help those who had less (53%, 55%). The second- and third-highest reasons were gaining a sense of personal satisfaction (50%, 43%) and meeting religious beliefs and commitment (43%, 41%).

Some studies suggest that there may be differing motivations when comparing older and younger women, with younger women more likely to cite gaining knowledge or advocacy as a motive. Older women may be more motivated by the traditional desire to give back to the community (Nathanson & Eggleton, 1993). One study of volunteers pointed up the difference in motivation between older women and men. The women gave dual reasons for volunteering, both altruism and socializing. The men described only altruism as a motive (Morrow-Howell & Mui, 1989).

Lucy Rose Fischer and Kay Banister Schaffer outlined the research and theories on volunteer motivation and identified eight categories: altruism, ideology, egoism, material/reward, status/reward, social relationship, leisure time, and personal growth (Fischer & Schaffer, 1993). As noted earlier, respondents to volunteer surveys most often give an altruistic reason for volunteering: "to help those who have less," "to give back to the community." Older people may be more likely to believe that they should contribute to the community (Herzog & House, 1991). Many volunteers have ideologic concerns: they want to work on the environment, or for the Democratic party, or for the Alzheimer's Association, or the prolife movement. Older volunteers more often give "religious concern" as a motive (Independent Sector, 1990).

Egotistic motivation refers to the self-oriented aspect of volunteering, not only wanting to help others, but to respond to personal psychological needs. People may volunteer because they want to feel better about themselves, gain approval, avoid feelings of guilt, and so on (Fischer & Schaffer, 1993). Material reward means that the volunteer receives some benefit, including privileges (such as a museum volunteer might have), tax deductions, possible gifts, or certain material advantages (like volunteering in one's neighborhood association or school Parent Teacher Association). Older volunteers are much less apt to mention material rewards as a motive for volunteering than younger people (Independent Sector, 1990). Status remarks were described by Fischer and Schaffer (1993) as "enlightened self-interest," as in the cases of the businessman who may donate time to a charity that may indirectly benefit his business or a volunteer who wants to gain job skills. Not surprisingly, older volunteers are least likely to say that getting experience is a motivation (Independent Sector, 1990).

Social relationship motivations fit into the fabric of volunteer service, which is nearly always involved with other people. Survey results of volunteers often mention "to meet people" or "to make friends" as a motive. The social motive is important in recruiting volunteers and may be even more so in retaining them (Daniels, 1985; Fischer & Schaffer, 1993; Morrow-Howell & Mui, 1989). Leisure-time motivations mean the amount of disposable time given up for voluntarism. Independent Sector (1990) reported that older volunteers, unsurprisingly, are more likely to cite free time as a motivation for volunteering. Personal growth motivations, according to Fischer and Schaffer (1993), are some of the intangible benefits of volunteering, like having learning opportunities, the chance to grow personally, strengthening a sense of meaning and purpose, and even a "helper's high."

Whatever mix of motives older women volunteers may have, they are insufficient if there are inadequate volunteer opportunities. What is the likely future for older women volunteers? Volunteering is such an integral part of the American psyche that we know that it will not disappear. Most older women have past volunteer experience, even if they are not current volunteers. Their widely varying backgrounds range from the traditional to those that reflect the great changes in women's roles in the past twenty-five years (Kieffer, 1986).

We can expect that older women's volunteer roles will change significantly in the next decade or two. For example, only 12% of SCORE (the Service Corps of Retired Executives) members are women, accurately reflecting the past, where few women could become executives. The number of women in SCORE is bound to rise, as it will in other programs that have in the past heavily recruited volunteers to fill men's traditional roles. As the population continues to age, the proportion of women is expected to increase among both the young-old and the old-old. We can assume a greater number of potential volunteers among the young-old, but possibly among the old-old as well. Although there is a distinct downturn in the rate of volunteering as people reach their late 70s (Chambre, 1987), this may be caused by lack of opportunity as well as the limitations that usually accompany the later stages of life. One large volunteer program, the Retired Senior Volunteer Program (RSVP), makes a special effort to recruit the disabled. Thousands of RSVP volunteers are visually and hearing impaired, in wheelchairs, homebound, and even bedridden (Dowling, 1988).

To look at the future of America is to know that we will have an increasing number of minority elderly. In the past, minority elderly have been less likely to volunteer because of low income, language and cultural differences, and lower education levels. The lower rate of voluntarism may stem more from low income and less education than from the fact of being a minority person. For instance, several studies have shown that when social class is controlled for, blacks are more likely to volunteer than whites (Fischer & Schaffer, 1993). Older volunteers—women and men, minorities and the white majority—all have to contend with the dual attitudes of ageism and undervaluing volunteer work. Our country has devalued the skills, capacities, and experience of older people for fifty years or more (Kieffer, 1986; Myers, Manton, and Bacellar, 1986). As Susan Chambre

(1994) put it, "We live in a society where voluntarism is applauded and seen as distinctly American, and yet volunteers themselves are often treated with less respect than they might be." Being "just a volunteer" is often the way older women report their activities and similarly is how volunteer work is viewed: less important than paid work, a time-filler, another aspect of leisure. A woman of 65 has an average life expectancy of 16 years, yet the increasing number of years that older people will spend being "old" has not been translated into enough opportunities and understanding of the possibilities of old age (Fischer & Schaffer, 1993). Our social and psychological adjustment to longer lives lags behind the medical and physical realities.

It appears that most of the free time that becomes available for retired people is taken up with passive, solitary activities, mostly watching television and listening to the radio (Chambre, 1987), despite the research suggesting that older people are not as active and productive as they would like (Fischer & Schaffer, 1993). So our challenge is to understand better our own aging and the changes that older women have undergone in the last three decades and to search out the opportunities of voluntarism that bring meaning to older women's lives. As Maggie Kuhn and Tish Sommers wrote during the 1981 White House Conference on Aging, "Volunteers can create their own jobs, take vacations at will, choose priorities, work on causes of deep concern, and select tasks for self-actualization. Such volunteerism provides joyous occupations . . . the pearl of leisure-time activities."

REFERENCES

ACTION, the Federal Domestic Volunteer Agency. (1988). *An evaluation of family caregiver services.* Washington, DC: Author.

American Red Cross. (1988). *Volunteer 2000 study: Volume 1. Findings and recommendations.* Washington, DC: Author.

Booz-Allen & Hamilton. (1985). *National Retired Senior Volunteer Program participant impact evaluation.* Washington, DC: ACTION, the Federal Domestic Volunteer Agency.

Bull, C. Neil, & Levine, Nancy D. (1993). *The older volunteer: An annotated bibliography.* Westport, CT: Greenwood Press.

Bull, C. Neil, & Payne, Barbara (1988). *Brief bibliography: A selective annotated bibliography for gerontology instruction: The older volunteer.* Washington, DC: Association for Gerontology in Higher Education.

Chambre, Susan M. (1984). Is volunteering a substitute for role loss in old age? An empirical test of activity theory. *Gerontologist, 24,* 292–298.

———. (1987). *Good deeds in old age: Volunteering by the new leisure class.* Lexington, MA: Lexington Books.

———. (1994). Review of older volunteers: A guide to research and practice. *Contemporary Gerontology: A Journal of Reviews and Critical Disclosure, 1,* 14–15.

Costello, Cynthia B. (1990). Resourceful aging: Mobilizing older citizens for volunteer service. In *Resourceful aging: Today and tomorrow.* Conference proceedings, volume 1, executive summary. Washington, DC: American Association of Retired Persons.

Daniels, Arlene K. (1985). Good times and good works: The place of sociability in the work of women volunteers. *Social Problems, 32,* 363–374.

Dowling, Winifred. (1988). *Testimony before the Federal Council on Aging.* Chicago: Gerontology Center at the University of Illinois.

———. (1992). *Volunteerism in the U.S.A.* Paper presented at the First Japan Volunteer Festival, International Symposium, Kobe, Japan.

Fischer, Lucy R., Mueller, Daniel P., & Cooper, Philip W. (1991). Older volunteers: A discussion of the Minnesota Senior Study. *Gerontologist, 31,* 183–194.

Fischer, Lucy R., & Schaffer, Kay B. (1993). *Older volunteers: A guide to research and practice.* Newbury Park, CA: Sage Publications.

Hamilton, Frederick, & Schneider's Company. (1988). *Attitudes of Americans over 45 years of age on volunteerism.* Washington, DC: American Association of Retired Persons.

Hayghe, Howard V. (1991). Volunteers in the U.S.: Who donates the time? *Monthly Labor Review, 114,*(2) 17–23.

Herzog, A. Regula, & House, James S. (1991). Productive activities and aging well. *Generations, 15,* 49–54.

Herzog, A. Regula, Kahn, Robert L., Morgan, James N., Jackson, James S., & Antonucci, Toni C. (1989). Age differences in productive activities. *Journal of Gerontology: Social Sciences, 44,* S129–S138.

Herzog, A. Regula, & Morgan, James N. (1992). Age and gender differences in the value of productive activities: Four different approaches. *Research on Aging, 14,* 169–198.

Independent Sector. (1990). *Giving and volunteering in the United States.* Findings from a national survey conducted by the Gallup Organization, Washington, DC.

———. (1992). *Giving and volunteering in the United States.* Findings from a national survey conducted by the Gallup Organization, Washington, DC.

Ishii-Kuntz, Masako. (1990). Formal activities for elderly women: Determinants of participation in voluntary and senior center activities. *Journal of Women and Aging, 2,* 79–97.

Keller, John. (1981). Elders and volunteerism. *Generations, 4,* 4–5.

Kieffer, Jarold A. (1986). The older volunteer resource. In Committee on an Aging Society (Ed.), *Productive roles in an older society* (pp. 51–72). Washington, DC: National Academy Press.

Morrow-Howell, Nancy, & Mui, Ada. (1989). Elderly volunteers: Reasons for initiating and terminating service. *Journal of Gerontological Social Work, 13,* 21–33.

Myers, George C., Manton, Kenneth G., & Bacellar, Helena. (1986). Sociodemographic aspects of future unpaid productive roles. In Committee on an Aging Society (Ed.), *Productive roles in an older society* (pp. 110–149). Washington, DC: National Academy Press.

Nathanson, Ilene L., & Eggleton, Elizabeth. (1993). Motivation versus program effect on length of service: A study of four cohorts of ombudservice volunteers. *Journal of Gerontological Social Work, 19,* 95–114.

National Eldercare Institute on Employment and Volunteerism. (1992a). *An annotated bibliography on volunteerism and aging.* College Park, MD.

———. (1992b). *Directory of resources: Volunteerism and aging.* College Park, MD.

Nemschoff, Helene L. (1981). Women as volunteers: Long history, new roles. *Generations, 5*, 35, 48.

Ozawa, Martha N., & Morrow-Howell, Nancy. Services provided by elderly volunteers: An empirical study. *Journal of Gerontological Social Work, 13*, 65–80.

Premo, Terri L. (1990). *Winter friends: Women growing old in the new republic, 1785–1835.* Urbana: University of Illinois Press.

Taylor, S. (1990, April/May). Talents, tools, and time. *Modern Maturity*, 79–84.

Seventeen

Living Arrangements for Midlife and Older Women

FRANCES M. CARP

The living environment is important at all ages (Blank, 1988). Qualities of housing and neighborhood gain saliency as age-related decrements in sensory-motor processes, strength and endurance, and health, financial, and transportation resources interact with thinning social networks to constrict the environment accessible for meeting life-maintenance and psychosocial needs. Satisfaction with one's living arrangements is important in its own right and because it is consistently found to be strongly related to well-being, mental health, and life satisfaction (Carp & Christensen, 1986; McAuley & Offerle, 1983; Scheidt & Windley, 1983).

REVIEW OF RESEARCH

Thirty years ago, to stimulate research in this area, a national conference on "Patterns of Living and Housing of Middle-Aged and Older People" was convened by three federal entities: the Housing and Home Finance Agency, the Administration on Aging, and the National Institute of Child Health and Human Development Institute's Program on Aging (Carp, 1966). The titles of the 1965 conference and this chapter are strikingly similar except for the final words, "people" in the former and "women" in the latter. In fact, the majority of persons in studies reported at the conference were women, as a reflection of gender differences in the population accentuated by the segments of that population that were studied.

Early research was on persons in special projects (public housing and retirement centers) or institutions, due largely to federal policies and funding resources and ease of collecting data (Carp, 1976). Later attention turned to living arrangements of the majority of older persons (Carp, 1987). This made clear the wide diversity among older persons and the need for a variety of living housing for them. Individual differences widen with age; the older the group, the greater the span among its members in any characteristic. Heterogeneity is further increased among "the elderly" by their much greater age span compared to other groups (e.g., preschoolers, adolescents).

Definitions of middle and old age vary widely. Much research follows Bismarck when he established social security in Germany and uses age 65 as the demarcation. In Bismarck's day few persons lived long beyond 65. In 1900, 1 in 25 Americans reached age 65, but in 1990, 1 of every 8 Americans was at least that old (*Aging America*, 1991; U.S. Bureau of the Census, 1993). In this century nearly 25 years of average life expectancy has been gained, which is nearly equal to the gain during the previous 5,000 years (R. N. Butler, 1994).

Today, persons 65 and older encompass more than a generation in age, with attendant differences in competence in dealing with living arrangements, life experience with homes and neighborhoods, and expectations and preferences regarding them. In 1900 a person aged 65 could expect to live nearly 12 more years, but today a person who reaches 65 can expect to live more than 17 additional years. By the year 2030 the number of Americans 65 or older will nearly double and will comprise 20% of the population. The fastest-growing segment of the older population is the "oldest old." By the turn of the century 26% of Americans will be 80 or older. The number of Americans aged 85+ increased by 50% between 1960 and 1970, then by 60% from 1970 to 1980, and is expected to triple between 1980 and 2030 (*Aging America*, 1991; U.S. Bureau of the Census, 1993).

Women and men age differently (Barer, 1994). In terms of longevity, in 1989 women aged 65 averaged about 19 years of life expectancy, and men, about 14 (National Center for Health Statistics, 1992). Most persons in the fastest-growing segment, those 85 or older, are women. In 1982 persons 100 or older numbered about 32,000, and every day about 30 people turned 100. By 2030 about 280 will do so. By 2090 centenarians will number about 1.9 million. This disproportionately female population explosion will further widen diversities and emphasize the need for heterogeneous living-arrangement options suitable to the needs and desires of that expanding population that is becoming increasingly female with added years of life.

WHERE DO OLDER WOMEN LIVE AT PRESENT?

In Their Own Homes in the Community

Stereotypes have the "young-old" (vigorous, active) in retirement communities and the "old-old" (frail, unwell) in nursing homes. In reality, the vast majority of older people live in ordinary housing, most of them in the same units they occupied earlier (Blank, 1988; Carp, 1987). There are significant sex differences in living arrangements.

Living Alone. In recent years the percentage of older women living alone has grown precipitously (Wolf, 1990). In 1983, for the 65–74 age bracket, 36% of women but only 12% of men lived alone; and for the 75+ age bracket, 42% of women but only 19% of men lived alone (U.S. Senate, 1985–86). In 1988, 38% of older women lived alone (Schwenk, 1991). Among women 75+, percentages living alone were 30% in 1965 and 50% in 1984, and the projection for 1995 was 60% (National Research Council, 1988). This trend reflects to some extent the prevailing desire to live independently, enabled by improvements in financial status and health. However, living alone entails diminished social networks and especially the lack of a special support person and is associated with depression in women (but not men) (Palinkas, Wingard, & Barrett-Connor, 1990).

Loss of spouse is a major cause of living alone. Due to sex differences in life expectancy and the tendency of brides to be younger than their bridegrooms, women are far more likely to be widowed. In 1984, for the 65–74 group, less than half the women but 80% of the men were living with spouses; and for those 75+, only 23% of the women but two-thirds of the men lived with spouses (U.S. Senate, 1985–86). Living with one's spouse is a positive factor in longevity and well-being, and loss of the spouse is probably the most traumatic life event (Holahan & Holahan, 1987).

Many older women live alone not by choice but for lack of alternatives. They tend to be economically deprived, to have chronic and multiple health problems and inadequate health care, to be socially isolated, and to suffer lives of very poor quality (Mason, 1994; U.S. Congress, 1989). If life is to be more than mere existence and have acceptable quality, the environment must provide resources for meeting not only life-maintenance needs but also psychosocial needs (Carp, 1987). Living alone increases the difficulty of meeting needs that enable existence in the community (food, clothing, medical care, banking) and needs for personal interaction, social support, and self-realization whose satisfaction determines the quality of life.

Suburban/Central City/Rural. Suburbs are "graying" steadily, mostly as the result of "aging in place." After World War II there were general population shifts from rural to urban areas and from central cities to suburbs. Once in the suburbs, people tended to remain there as they grew older. For persons 65 or older, from 1960 to 1980 there was steady growth in the suburban population and steady decline in the city centers. This trend is expected to continue well into the next century (National Research Council, 1988).

The flight to the suburbs is attributed to "push" factors associated with inner cities (lack of low-cost housing, less attractive housing stock, undesired changes in neighborhoods, and scarcity of nearby family members) and "pull" factors associated with suburbs (newer and available housing, less traffic congestion, and the perception of lower crime rates). However, in two major metropolitan areas in Texas and California, proximity to the city center was positively related to active, autonomous, and satisfying use of time, space, and the social network by the elderly (Carp, 1979). In the eyes of elderly residents of the most deteriorated parts of New York City, access to services, facilities and amenities, and the "many possibilities for satisfying personal tastes, desires, and needs" outweighed the negative considerations of personal danger, environmental deterioration, dirt, the fast tempo of life, living among persons different from oneself, and the high cost of living (Cantor, 1979). Single-room occupants (SROs) (43% of them women) strongly prefer to remain in centrally located areas where apartments are beyond their means. They do not want shared housing. By remaining in centrally located areas, SROs meet personal needs they cannot by available alternatives (Crystal & Beck, 1992).

In the suburbs facilities for shopping and other tasks of daily living tend to be distant from homes, and public transit is sparse or nonexistent. When today's graying suburbanites bought their homes, they were young automobile drivers who did not think twice about going wherever and whenever they desired. As aging suburbanites become ex-drivers, their ability to meet even their subsistence needs becomes restricted. Community resources for meeting basic needs for food, clothing, and medical care and supplies lie at some distance from home. Walking to medical/dental buildings and shopping facilities is rarely possible for young and vigorous suburbanites. Public transportation is designed for the work commuter and does not provide service to places and at times suitable for older suburban residents (Carp, 1988).

Loss of the driver's license is highly correlated with age and is usually attributable to sensory-motor decrements, most often visual (National Research Council, 1988). This loss is traumatic both as official documentation of obsolescence and because it removes accustomed means of meeting subsistence needs and higher-order needs of sociability, service, recreation, and religious and esthetic experience (Carp, 1988). Among current suburban elderly the situation is especially poignant for women, who are likely never to have been automobile drivers and are likely to be widows used to being driven by their husbands to places they wanted to go.

Advocates for the elderly as well as scholars have viewed the farm household nostalgically but incorrectly as the ideal for elderly women (Gratton & Haber, 1993). In actuality, rural women are the most disadvantaged. They lack the autonomy of urban women due to their lesser financial security and are unable to retain their own households and maintain the desired "intimacy at a distance" with their children. They become dependent members of children's households or live in the poor-quality housing available to them. Their poverty is linked to poorer economic opportunity for women in nonmetropolitan areas and to the greater costs to women for nontraditional life-cycle patterns (e.g., divorce, separation) in rural areas (McLaughlin & Holden, 1993).

For older residents of rural areas, housing is poor, and resources for meeting subsistence needs (the grocery store, the physician's and dentist's offices, drug stores, and banks) and psychosocial needs that are equally important if life is to have acceptable quality (other people, place of worship, library, senior center, friends' homes) are difficult or impossible to reach (Carp, 1988). Public transit does not exist. Elderly farm women are unlikely to have cars, and rural roads are narrow and poorly maintained and lighted. The outflow of younger residents to urban areas reduces availability of rides with others, as well as visits from younger relatives and acquaintances.

Distribution across the Nation. Older persons are less likely to move than are younger people. From 1975 to 1980 only 21% of persons aged 65 and older moved, compared to 48% of those under 65 (American Association of Retired Persons, 1982). In 1983, 5% of Americans over 65 moved, compared to the national average of 16.6% (U.S. Senate, 1985–86). Elderly movers usually do not go far. The small percentage who move to another state generally go from the Northeast and Midwest to "Sun Belt" states. Half go to six states: Florida (which receives more than the other five states combined), California, Nevada, Arizona, Texas, and New Jersey (National Research Council, 1988).

Migration patterns of the young affect the living arrangements of older generations. The moving of younger persons to metropolitan areas created high concentrations (15%+) of elders left behind in 500 rural counties. America's heartland felt the results of this differential mobility most strongly; six of the ten states with the highest percentages of elderly residents are agricultural midwestern states. The ten are Florida, Arkansas, Rhode Island, Iowa, Missouri, South Dakota, Nebraska, Kansas, Pennsylvania, and Massachusetts (National Research Council, 1988).

The Quality of Their Housing

Housing quality is generally inferior for older people and more so for women alone than for couples or men alone. Housing quality also differs, objectively and subjectively, between owners and renters (Christensen, Carp, Cranz, & Wiley, 1992).

Homeowners. Most older persons want to remain in their own homes as long as possible. Nearly three-quarters own their homes, and they represent a quarter of the nation's homeowners (Carp, 1987; Christensen et al., 1992).

Many live in old houses that need repairs. Households headed by persons 62 or older are almost twice as likely as households headed by persons under 62 to live in homes rated by the Annual Housing Survey (AHS) conducted by the U.S. Census Bureau as inadequate in at least one major characteristic (kitchen equipment, water, heat, electricity, structure) (Christensen et al., 1992).

Older households occupy 40% of the nation's homeowner living units with an AHS-defined inadequacy. Moreover, they are much more likely to occupy units with multiple deficiencies, which entail greater threat to the safety and health of occupants than does deficiency in one characteristic. Older householders occupy 44% of the homeowner units in the United States that have multiple deficiencies according to AHS standards.

A disproportionately large number of older women live in substandard units. More than half the AHS-defined inadequate housing is owned by women living alone. The housing of older women living by themselves is more dilapidated, and occupants are less likely to make needed repairs (Mayer & Olson, 1980).

Renters. Older renters are in housing of even poorer quality (Carp, 1987; Christensen et al., 1992). Old women living alone in rented facilities are generally in housing of the poorest quality, with the most structural deficiencies and poorest maintenance.

Reasons for Inadequate Housing for Independent Living

The deficiencies in housing for the elderly stem largely from their inadequate economic resources and the lack of suitable housing stock.

Economic Resources. Prior to 1960 many older persons suffered severe economic deprivation due to lack of Social Security or other retirement-benefit programs and to the Great Depression, which had made it impossible for them to build up savings. Between 1960 and 1974 there were large reductions in the percentage of older persons living in poverty because of the general rise in the standard of living, improved Social Security benefits, and the spread of private retirement plans. The legislated cost-of-living increases for Social Security between 1968 and 1971 were especially helpful. After 1974 the poverty rate for the elderly remained stable, and it is not expected to diminish (U.S. Senate, 1985–86) without major policy changes.

Though incomes decline at retirement, the majority of young-old married couples have financial resources sufficient to live comfortably. The old-old are poorer. The median income for households with heads 75 or older is three-fourths that for households with heads 65–74 (National Research Council, 1988). This difference is due to smaller retirement benefits. Salaries and wages were lower when they retired. The longer since a person retired, the lower the current income. Retired people over age 75 are much more likely to be poor than are retirees 55 to 75. About 17% of Americans over 75 and about 22% of those 85+ live below the poverty line (U.S. Senate, 1985–86).

At all ages, poverty rates are higher for women, and that differential is increasing (McLanahan, Sorensen, & Watson, 1989). The most impoverished of the old are women living alone (Carp, 1987). The situation is exacerbated in today's cohort by reduction of income from spouses' retirement benefits at widowhood, and lack of benefits of their own for the many who were never employed (U.S. Congress, May 1990, July 1990, 1992). Retirement incomes of women who worked are low because they had low-paid jobs and because their working-life expectancy has declined while their life expectancy has increased. Stone (1987) wrote of "the feminization of poverty" especially among older women, and Hardy and Hazelrigg (1993) of the "gender of poverty in an aging population."

Elderly persons pay higher proportions of their incomes for housing than do younger generations (Carp & Christensen, 1986). Many of those incomes are small, particularly among women, and especially among the old-old and women alone, which leaves little money for other budgetary categories. As age advances, health problems increase, with consequently greater need for physicians' and dentists' services and pharmaceuticals. Women in general have been short-changed on medical research and treatment (U.S. Congress, July 1991). Women at midlife receive second-rate health care (U.S. Congress, May 1991). In an aging America women receive inequitably poor health care (Lamphere-Thorpe & Blandon, 1991). The failure of the rapidly growing percentage of older women who are alone to seek medical care is due to financial rather than health status (Keith, 1987). "Discretionary funds" for sociability, recreation, religious participation, and other meaningful activities are scant or absent. The quality of life is very poor (Carp & Christensen, 1986).

Suitable Housing Stock. An innovative study to estimate the housing needs of the elderly in quantitative terms took as criteria (1) the national goal of independent living for elders who want it, (2) elimination of substandard housing occupied by the elderly, and (3) replacement of units occupied by older persons that are removed from the housing inventory (Handler, 1981). The conclusions were as follows: (1) In 1980 there was need for independent housing for 2.3 million elderly; and by 2000 nearly 2.8 million additional units will be needed. An average of 139,000 dwelling units would have to be added to the stock of housing suitable for the elderly every year beginning in 1980 if the goal were to be met by 2000. (2) In 1980, 1.3 million units occupied by the elderly were substandard, and by the year 2000 the number will increase to 1.9 million units. If a twenty-year program had begun in 1980 to eliminate or improve substandard units, an annual average of 32,000 units would have to be replaced and another 64,000 rehabilitated by 2000. (3) A minimum of 104,000 units destroyed annually by fires, floods, and other disasters or torn down by a public agency or the owner would have to be replaced. Overall, then, 275,000 units would have to be added to the housing stock for the elderly, and another 64,000 units would have to be replaced every year over a twenty-year period beginning in 1980. It is fifteen years since those projections were made, and no program has been put in place.

"Standard" housing may not be appropriate in assessing living arrangements for older people (Carp, 1994a). A conference of experts convened by the American Association of Retired Persons (1993) focused on how to design new housing and retrofit old housing to promote independence over the years of longer living. They concluded that "special" features old people need (e.g., grab bars) are also beneficial for others, and that original design should include provision for easy modifications.

There are tools to help older people assess and improve their own arrangements. Pynoos and Cohen (1992a) prepared a checklist guide for a tour of one's home, specifying hazards for particular areas (entry, kitchen, bathroom, bedroom, living areas) as well as general concerns (fire safety, fall prevention, security, cleaning, dressing). The resident marks each item "Yes" or "No," then sets priorities among "Yeses." The publication suggests solutions by environmental and behavioral alterations, includes a resource guide that gives names and addresses of organizations and publications, and suggests types of local stores helpful with various problems.

Another Pynoos and Cohen device (1992b) takes the person on an imaginary tour of six houses and apartments with a volunteer at an agency that helps older persons make their homes more livable. Readers help the character identify problems and solutions that might apply to their own homes. This attractive publication presents problems and solutions in cartoons; tasks are presented as games and puzzles. There is a quiz on myths and realities about the home; a list of sources of products, information, and funding; and tips on how to locate reliable repair services.

In the Homes of Relatives

Some aging persons become incapable of sustaining independent living in the housing available to them. The "fit" between personal competence and environmental demand, and that between personal needs and environmental resources, is too poor. America has a long tradition stressing the importance of the family taking care of its own, and kin are the caregivers for most "frail elderly" (80%). An older man is more likely to be taken into a relative's home than is an older woman (Schwenk, 1991). However, due to the uneven gender distribution in the population segment, more frail elderly women live with kin.

Another societal assumption—that all families can and will provide adequate care—may be a myth. It might seem that provision of care and assistance by younger adults to aging parents would be rewarding to both generations. However, research suggests that such benefits accrue to neither generation. Children of the elderly tend to be in two-job couples or single-parent situations. An increasing proportion are themselves retired. Caring for an elderly parent is a difficult and unremitting task that falls ordinarily on a daughter or daughter-in-law. Conflict between the roles of worker and caregiver to an elderly parent has negative effects: increased absenteeism from work, psychological stress, and strains on relationships with husbands and children (Barling, MacEwen, Kelloway, & Higginbottom, 1994). Absenteeism negatively affects current income and job advancement and security and future retirement benefits. These negative effects do not occur among working women who assist aging parents who do not live with them. It may not be lack of concern for elderly parents but stress on their own lives and families that impedes children from taking them into their homes or impels moving them out to nursing homes.

In addition, being a relative does not guarantee willingness or ability to provide suitable care, or even a loving attitude. Domestic elder abuse—physical injury, emotional stress, neglect, misappropriation of funds, rape—occurs in "situations in which the assumption of loving, competent family care is not appropriate" (Sengstock, 1991). In population studies estimates of abuse by "loved ones" range from 0.5% to 32% (Haviland & O'Brien, 1989). Reports of practitioners support the high end of the range of estimates based on self- and caregiver-report studies. Among community physicians, nurses, and social workers, 32% reported observing physical, psychological, or financial abuse among patients 56 or older (Sadler & Kurrie, 1993).

Most domestic elder abuse occurs when the older person lives with family members (Lachs & Pillemer, 1995). Elders are reluctant to complain about kin caretakers, and caretakers are unlikely to report misbehavior on their own part or that of their spouses or other family members. The costs of domestic elder abuse to society are high in terms of "intergenerational transmission of violence." "Elder abuse holds a pivotal position in the family life cycle of violence. Adults, perhaps themselves abused as children, become the abusers of their aged and infirm parents, while their own children watch, learn, and wait their turn" (Costa, 1993, p. 377). Societal costs are high in caring for victims. Nearly 50% of the cases of domestic elder abuse lead to physically apparent trauma that often requires hospitalization and sometimes results in death (Costa, 1993). In one hospital over a six-month period, 63% of the admissions for elder abuse (brutal beatings, rapes, burns, fractures) were repeat visits (Fulmer, McMahon, Baer-Hines, & Forget, 1992). Domestic abuse is ongoing and chronic.

In Institutions

The vast majority of admittants to nursing homes do not come on their own or from homes of their own but are brought by family members with whom they were living (Lachs & Pillemer, 1995). About 4% to 5% of persons aged 65 or older are in nursing homes at any time. The rate of nursing-home residence has remained the same in many analyses of various sets of data over the past thirty years. Likelihood of institutionalization increases with age, from about 2% for those under 75 to as much as 16% for those 85 or older. Most nursing-home residents (70%) are women, three-quarters of whom do not have husbands, compared to only 40% of their age peers outside institutions (U.S. Senate, 1985–86). There is a sharply increasing population of single, older women who are economically and socially deprived. They suffer chronic health problems and are more likely than are old men to have multiple health problems (Ory, Cox, Gift, & Abeles, 1994), and many of those over 85 need some type of help in daily functioning (Mason, 1994). Yet they face government cost-containment measures that deny them medical care and home services. Thus many are forced into nursing homes (Olson, 1988). Demographic changes and increasing divorce and nonmarriage rates foretell that more women will live alone in the future, and the means and success with which they will cope are problematic (Uzawa, 1993).

The prospect of placement in a long-term-care facility is met with aversion and resistance by older people, and the move often results in their more rapid physical and cognitive deterioration (Teresi, Holmes, & Monaco, 1993). Aides, the staff who have the most contact with residents, are inadequately screened and trained and poorly paid. The work is physically demanding and intrinsically unrewarding. Turnover is very high. In addition to negative aspects of institutional living such as depersonalization, regimentation, quality of food, and isolation, abuse—physical, sexual, and emotional—by staff occurs. Its incidence is difficult to determine and is probably vastly underestimated (Haviland & O'Brien, 1989). Residents are hesitant to complain or even respond to questions about abuse, fearing retaliation, and any complaints they voice are easily attributed to their "senility." Aside from humane considerations, nursing-home care is far more expensive than community-based services at home (Green, Lovey, & Ondrich, 1993).

Those without Homes

Estimates of the number of elderly among the homeless vary widely (Keigher & Greenblatt, 1992). Studies of shelter data report 14.5%–28% of the homeless to be 50 or older, and as many as 27% to be 60 or older. Street surveys and outreach programs report as high as 50%. Of a random sample of elderly homeless persons, 45% were in that status due to problems with their previous living environments (fire, "deplorable conditions," utility shutoff, eviction). Sandra Butler (1993) found middle-aged homeless women to be very similar to other middle-aged women in such variables as relationships, resiliency, normalcy, and political awareness. Poverty and shortage of low-cost housing left them homeless.

Summary

Currently, young-old women who live with their husbands, in reasonably good health and with adequate financial resources, have opportunities to meet both their basic, subsistence needs and the psychological needs that give quality to life. Older-old women, likely to be widowed and to live alone, with lesser economic resources and more health problems, are likely to be in living arrangements that make it difficult to meet the basic needs that must be met if they are to sustain existence, let alone the higher-order needs for sociability, service to others, recreation, and religious and esthetic experience whose satisfaction makes life more than mere existence. The most deprived community residents are older women who live alone.

For those not able to afford or find arrangements compatible with their abilities to conduct the necessary activities of daily living, options are not attractive. Some move into the homes of relatives, usually children. At best this imposes a severe burden on the caretaker and her family and causes feelings of dependency and shame in the older woman. Usually the primary caretaker is a woman, and, if she works, the demands may jeopardize her job security and advancement and reduce her own later retirement benefits. This is likely to cause deterioration in her well-being and in relationships with her spouse and children. These effects on the caregiver must take their toll on the older woman. At worst, a relative's home can be a traumatic setting for an elderly woman, create guilt in family members, and teach the youngest generation to continue the pattern of domestic violence. In any given case, nursing-home placement or even living on the streets may be better or worse.

WHAT AWAITS FUTURE COHORTS OF OLD WOMEN?

Consequences of the Population Age Structure

Several future cohorts of older Americans are alive. The comparisons that were drawn between today's elderly and today's younger age groups and projections of changes in these comparisons suggest what the future holds.

Aging of the Population. The elder segment of the population will continue expanding dramatically, in absolute numbers and relative to the total. Soon "baby boomers" will be retirees, producing seismic shifts. The most obvious implication for housing is that a large number and proportion of units should be prepared that are suitable to the needs and abilities of the older American population as it evolves. The present housing stock is insufficient and inadequate for today's elderly, and future demand will be drastically greater. Guidelines for construction and renovation of suitable housing exist. The lack is not so much in information as in policy and funding to implement that knowledge.

The size of the older population may increase its influence on societal decisions. The political clout of the elderly is being felt already. The augmenting size of the older population may increase attention to its needs. On the other hand, effects on the dependency ratio (the proportion of nonworking to working-age persons) must be considered. The elderly dependency ratio is at an all-time high and is expected to nearly double within a few decades. Then the elderly dependency ratio will exceed that of the youthful dependency ratio, while presently it is less than half as large (U.S. Bureau of the Census, 1993). When most of the "dependent" are old people, issues of intergenerational equity may become inflammatory. For example,

Since the late 1970s, in the context of growing federal deficits and spiralling health care costs, an artificially homogenized group—"the elderly"—has become a scapegoat for a variety of American problems that have been rhetorically unified as issues of intergenerational conflict and equity. As expenditures on benefits to the aging have climbed . . . older people have become increasingly stereotyped as prosperous, hedonistic, selfish, and politically controlling "greedy geezers." They have been blamed for problems of children, the declining strength of the U.S. economy, and the nation's general disability to free up resources for use in a variety of worthy causes. (Binstock, Jahnigen, & Post, 1994, p. 360)

Differential Patterns of Aging for Women and Men. The increase in life expectancy is not constant between sex groups or among age groups within "the elderly.'' The preponderance of women over men is apparent at all older age levels and accelerates with advancing age. Population aging does not necessarily lead to increasing disability rates (Ory et al., 1994). Projections of life expectancy now include the number of years before death and the number of active, healthy years. A healthy man at age 65 may expect at least 15 more years of life, with good health for 13 of those years. A healthy woman at 65 can expect to live as many as 20 more years, but she may have good health and be able to live independently only during 16 of those years (Suzman, Willis, & Manton, 1992). Thus increasing numbers of aging women will need arrangements for independent living for more years than will men, and more women will need some form of assisted living for more years than will their male counterparts.

A large increase in the number of elderly women living alone lies ahead. By 2020 probably only about 9% of elderly men will live alone, while the proportion of elderly women living alone will have increased to 41%. The age of widowhood is expected to increase only slightly, much less than women's life expectancy. There will be more widows than widowers, and widows will have more years after loss of their husbands, leaving a much greater proportion of the expanding aging population in widowhood for much longer periods, during most of which they will be competent to live in their own homes, if such homes are available and affordable. Women are no longer as dependent as in previous times upon marriage for financial security, and future cohorts may have higher percentages of women who never marry. The divorce rate shows no sign of diminishing, and differential longevity will result in a preponderance of women among the divorced. Currently, poverty is related to living alone, especially for women. It is not clear how long this will persist.

Other Cohort Changes

Health and Health Care. As life expectancy has risen, so have improvements in health and health care as new cohorts enter old age (Binstock et al., 1994). Older people are in increasingly good physical and mental health due to advances in medical sciences and technologies and changes in lifestyles. Attention has been forced to the inequitable treatment of women in medical research and service (U.S. Congress, July 1991). One significant result was creation of the Office of Research on Women's Issues within the National Institutes of Health (Thomas, 1990). It was necessary for the Congress to hold up the annual appropriation for the U.S. Public Health Department before that office was made operational, and its effectiveness in improving women's health research and practice remains to be seen.

Many doctors attribute symptoms of older people to "age," and their inability to "cure" old age renders older persons unsatisfying as patients. Typically, physicians were not trained to deal with a multiplicity of disorders such as occur with advancing age nor to understand the complex interactions of drug therapies for multiple disorders (Binstock et al., 1994). Older persons' primary-care physicians should be "generalists." Currently, specialists are in relative oversupply due to differential fees, and they tend to be highly "specialized" as a result of medical-school curricula. Medical schools are now attempting to attract students to general practice and to include in their requirements some introduction to geriatric medicine, multiple disorders, and drug interactions. More women are entering the field of medicine. It is too soon to assess the effects of these trends, but they should be beneficial to the physical and mental competence of women in regard to their living arrangements.

However, Callahan (1987) labeled health care expenditures for the elderly "a great fiscal black hole" (p. 17) that will shortly absorb an unlimited amount of national resources. He and others, including politicians, argue that the federal government should set limits on benefits for older persons. One suggestion is that life-saving care be denied to persons at some arbitrary age cutoff. Aside from the ethical and moral considerations, rationing health care to older Americans does not seem to economists to have a significant impact on aggregate health costs. Analyses suggest that the most extreme scenario would save about 5% of national health care expenditure (Jahnigen & Binstock, 1991). "It is doubtful that the American public, if reasonably informed about the negligible fiscal impact that could be achieved, will support policy proposals for drastically rationing acute health care for older people" (Binstock et al., 1994, pp. 360–361). These authors believed that the most likely change will be redistribution of financial burdens among persons eligible for Medicare in accordance with their ability to pay—which would simply extend a trend begun with the Social Security Reform Act of 1983 and built upon in subsequent legislation. Refusal or rationing of health care to those over any given age would jeopardize more older women for longer periods of time as compared to men.

Currently, people enjoy improved mental and physical health during most of the expanding years of life. Various programs are in place to improve health care and research, especially in regard to women. In planning housing for future elderly, it is essential to keep in mind that the vast increase among the "oldest old," most of whom will be women, does not suggest construction of institutions for the frail and demented. This author knows well one centenarian who lives on the second floor of an apartment building without elevators in Boston, keeps up with the world and national news and her very large family, and can beat anyone at gin rummy. Today, she is not unique, and in future cohorts women like her will be legion.

Education, Jobs, and Retirement Income. Young women continue to pursue educational goals and to enter the labor force in greater numbers, increasingly in fields once reserved to men (Carp, 1992). As yet, they have not caught up with men in career advancement and pay, but these differences show some signs of narrowing. An increasing number of women will have retirement benefits of their own, which will be higher than at present because of their better jobs, giving them better financial resources for housing.

Homeownership and Attachment to Place. Today's young—tomorrow's old—

have much higher rates of residential mobility and less attachment to particular places. Today's elderly own their homes at a far higher rate than do younger persons and are more likely to have remained at one address for many years. Young people are finding it difficult to buy homes, so homeownership may decline among future cohorts. Renters are less attached to their homes and more likely to move. The life experience of future elderly will have been largely with apartments or condominiums.

Attachment to place will be further weakened by the tendency of young adults to move greater distances and many times for career purposes. Thus the reluctance of current older persons to leave their homes may become a thing of the past. Future old people, particularly widows, will not be trapped by habit in overlarge homes they are unable (financially and/or physically) to maintain.

CONCLUSION

These considerations point to a future in which a larger age span and greater numbers of more competent older women will be personally able to maintain that highly desired state, independent living in the community. However, availability of appropriate living arrangements is crucial. Such arrangements include not only housing but also access to services and facilities necessary for continued existence and to resources for meeting the psychosocial needs whose satisfaction determines life quality. Community services to meet the needs of aging women are a potentially powerful mechanism for extending the years of independent living. Even for the frail elderly, community services with home delivery are cost-effective for society (Green, Lovey, & Ondrich, 1993) as well. Provision of appropriate housing and access to services and facilities for older persons were major societal concerns in the 1960s and 1970s. However, as a woman who devoted a long life to research and service in this area pointed out, the political climate "changed radically" about 1982, so that provision of appropriate living arrangements for the aging was "no longer a priority" (Donahue, 1992). Currently, the political arena seems even less receptive, despite clear evidence of the fiscal soundness of these humane programs.

These considerations point also to a future in which expanding numbers of increasingly competent older women will increasingly meet their needs for sociable interaction, nurturance (helping and being helped by others), and satisfying use of leisure time in groups of nonrelated persons, building or having already built their own nonkin social support systems. The rise in the numbers of older women living alone and the disadvantages of that arrangement have been discussed. There is no reason to expect a change in the lesser likelihood of an old woman alone than of an old man alone to be taken into the home of a relative, and some question whether this is a good solution, anyway. Birthrates were higher when today's old-old were born, so their children and grandchildren have fewer siblings and extended-family members for a support system based on kinship. Mobile lifestyles have dispersed what family members there are.

These changes in kinship norms and societal organization, in addition to the changing cohort patterns in housing tenure and mobility, point to easier acceptance of some form of congregate housing (Streib, 1990) that provides social contact and access to services and facilities that enable residents to meet their subsistence and psychosocial needs and to continue living independently in the community with a high quality of life. On-site facilities for the few final years in which protected living is requisite may be desirable (Carp, 1994b).

Aging has been dubbed "a women's problem," the sources of which lie in the socially systemic problems of younger women (Olson, 1988). Lifelong patterns of women's roles (at home as unpaid caregivers and in the work force receiving inequitable pay) are causal to the deprived status of older women today. Solutions lie in redressing the structural inequities that limit options for today's older women, so that upcoming cohorts of women will have the financial and experiential resources to secure living arrangements that enable them to have good, long lives (Arendell & Estes, 1991; Rix, 1993).

REFERENCES

Aging America: Trends and projections. (1991). Prepared by the U.S. Senate Special Committee on Aging, the American Association of Retired Persons, the Federal Council on the Aging, and the U.S. Administration on Aging. Washington, DC: U.S. Department of Health & Human Services.

American Association of Retired Persons. (1982). *A profile of older Americans.* Washington, DC: Author.

————. (1993). *Life-span design of residential environments for an aging population.* Washington, DC: Author.

Arendell, Terry, & Estes, Carol. (1991). Older women in the post-Reagan era. *International Journal of Health Services, 21*(1), 59–73.

Barer, Barbara. (1994). Men and women aging differently. *International Journal of Aging and Human Development, 38*(1), 29–40.

Barling, Julian, MacEwen, Karyl E., Kelloway, E. Kevin, & Higginbottom, Susan F. (1994). Predictors and outcomes of elder-care-based interrole conflict. *Psychology and Aging, 9*(3), 391–397.

Binstock, Robert H., Jahnigen, Dennis W., & Post, Stephen G. (1994). Exploring the future of health care for older people. In Ronald P. Abeles, Helen C. Gift, & Marcia G. Ory (Eds.), *Aging and Quality of Life* (pp. 350–366). New York: Springer.

Blank, Thomas O. (1988). *Older persons and their housing—today and tomorrow.* Springfield, IL: Charles C. Thomas.

Butler, Robert N. (1994). Historical perspectives on aging and quality of life. In Ronald P. Abeles, Helen C. Gift, & Marcia G. Ory (Eds.), *Aging and quality of life.* New York: Springer.

Butler, Sandra S. (1993). Listening to middle-aged homeless women talk about their lives. *Affilia, 8*(4), 388–409.

Callahan, Daniel. (1987). *Setting limits: Medical goals in an aging society.* New York: Simon & Schuster.

Cantor, Marjorie H. (1979). Life space and social support. In Thomas O. Byerts, Sandra C. Howell, & Leon A. Pastalan (Eds.), *Environmental Context of Aging*. New York: Garland.

Carp, Frances M. (1966). *Patterns of living and housing of middle-aged and older people*. Washington, DC: U.S. Government Printing Office.

———. (1976). Housing and living environments of older people. In Robert Binstock & Ethel Shanas (Eds.), *Handbook of aging and the social sciences* (pp. 244–263). New York: Van Nostrand Reinhold.

———. (1979). Life-style and location within the city. In Thomas O. Byerts, Sandra C. Howell, & Leon A. Pastalan (Eds.), *Environmental context of aging* (pp. 16–32). New York: Garland.

———. (1987). Environment and aging. In Daniel Stokols & Irwin Altman (Eds.), *Handbook of environmental psychology* (Vol. 1, pp. 329–360). New York: Wiley.

———. (1988). Significance of mobility for the well-being of the elderly. In National Research Council, *Transportation in an aging society* (Vol. 2, pp. 1–21). Washington, DC: Transportation Research Board.

———. (Ed.) (1992). *Lives of career women: Approaches to work, marriage, children*. New York: Plenum.

———. (1994a). Assessing the environment. In M. Powell Lawton & Jeanne A. Teresi (Eds.), *Annual review of gerontology and geriatrics: Focus on assessment techniques* (pp. 302–323). New York: Springer.

———. (1994b). *Victoria Plaza revisited: Lessons for the evaluation of housing for the elderly*. Milwaukee: University of Wisconsin–Milwaukee, Center for Architecture & Urban Planning Research.

Carp, Frances M., & Christensen, David L. (1986). Older women living alone. *Research on Aging, 8*, 407–425.

Christensen, David L., Carp, Frances M., Cranz, Galen L., & Wiley, James A. (1992). Objective housing indicators as predictors of subjective evaluations of elderly residents. *Journal of Environmental Psychology, 12*, 225–236.

Costa, A. J. (1993). Elder abuse. *Primary Care, 20*, 375–389.

Crystal, Stephen, & Beck, Pearl. (1992). A room of one's own: The SRO and the single elderly. *Gerontologist, 32*(5), 684–692.

Donahue, Wilma T. (1992). A survivor's story. In Frances M. Carp (Ed.), *Lives of career women: Approaches to work, marriage, children* (pp. 23–41). New York: Plenum.

Fulmer, T., McMahon, D. J., Baer-Hines, M., & Forget, B. (1992). Abuse, neglect, abandonment, violence, and exploitation: An analysis of all elderly patients seen in one emergency department during a six-month period. *Journal of Emergency Nursing, 18*, 505–510.

Gratton, Brian, & Haber, Carole. (1993). In search of intimacy at a distance: Family history from the perspective of elderly women. *Journal of Aging Studies, 7*(2), 183–194.

Green, Vernon L., Lovey, Mary E., & Ondrich, Jan I. (1993). The cost-effectiveness of community services in a frail elderly population. *Gerontologist, 33*, 177–189.

Handler, Benjamin. (1981). *Housing needs of the elderly*. Ann Arbor: National Policy Center on Housing & Living Arrangements for Older Americans.

Hardy, Melissa A., & Hazelrigg, Lawrence. (1993). The gender of poverty in an aging population. *Research on Aging, 15*(3), 243–278.

Haviland, Sue, & O'Brien, James. (1989). Physical abuse and neglect of the elderly: Assessment and intervention. *Orthopaedic Nursing, 8*(4), 11–18.

Hayward, Mark A., Grady, William R., & McLaughlin, Steven A. (1988). Recent changes in mortality and labor force behavior among older Americans: Consequences for nonworking life expectancy. *Journals of Gerontology, 43*(6), S194–S199.

Holahan, Carole K., & Holahan, Charles J. (1987). Self-efficacy, social support, and depression in aging. *Journal of Gerontology, 42*, 49–74.

Jahnigen, Dennis W., & Binstock, Robert H. (1991). Economic and clinical realities: Health care for older people. In Robert H. Binstock & Stephen G. Post (Eds.), *Too old for health care? Controversies in medicine, law, economics, and ethics* (pp. 13–43). Baltimore: Johns Hopkins University Press.

Keigher, Sharon M., & Greenblatt, Sadelle T. (1992). Housing emergencies and the etiology of homelessness among the urban elderly. *Gerontologist, 32*(4), 457–465.

Keith, Pat M. (1987). Postponement of health care by unmarried older women. *Women and Aging, 12*(1), 47–60.

Lachs, Mark S., & Pillemer, Karl A. (1995). Abuse and neglect of elderly persons. *New England Journal of Medicine, 332*, 437–443.

Lampere-Thorpe, Jo-Ann, & Blandon, Robert J. (1991). *Years gained and opportunities lost: Women and health care in an aging America.* Southport, CT: Institute for Policy Analysis.

McAuley, William J., & Offerle, Joan M. (1983). Perceived suitability of residence and life satisfaction among the elderly and handicapped. *Journal of Housing for the Elderly, 1*, 63–75.

McLanahan, Sara S., Sorensen, Annette, & Watson, Dorothy. (1989). *Sex Differences in Poverty, 1950–1980.* Ann Arbor: University of Michigan Press.

McLaughlin, Diane K., & Holden, Karen. (1993). Nonmetropolitan elderly women: A portrait of economic vulnerability. *Journal of Applied Gerontology, 12*(3), 320–334.

Mason, James O. (1994). Foreword. In Ronald P. Abeles, Helen C. Gift, & Marcia G. Ory (Eds.), *Aging and quality of life* (pp. ix–xi). New York: Springer.

Mayer, Neil, & Olson, Lee. (1980). *The effectiveness of federal home repair and improvement programs in meeting elderly homeowner needs.* Washington, DC: Urban Institute.

National Center for Health Statistics. (1992). *Health data on older Americans, United States.* Washington, DC: U.S. Government Printing Office.

National Research Council. (1988). *Transportation in an aging society.* Washington, DC: National Transportation Research Board.

Olson, Laura K. (1988). Aging is a woman's problem: Issues faced by the female elderly population. *Journal of Aging Studies, 2*(2), 97–108.

Ory, Marcia G., Cox, Donna M., Gift, Helen C., & Abeles, Ronald P. (1994). Introduction. In Ronald P. Abeles, Helen C. Gift, & Marcia G. Ory (Eds.). *Aging and quality of life* (pp. 1–18). New York: Springer.

Palinkas, Lawrence A., Wingard, Deborah L., & Barrett-Connor, Elizabeth. (1990). The biocultural context of social networks and depression among the elderly. *Social Science and Medicine, 30*(4), 441–447.

Pynoos, Jon, & Cohen, Eli. (1992a). *Home safety guide for older people.* Washington, DC: Serif Press.

————. (1992b). *The perfect fit: Creative ideas for a safe and livable home.* Washington, DC: American Association of Retired Persons.

Rix, Sara B. (1993). Women and well-being in retirement: What role for public policy? *Journal of Women and Aging, 4*(4), 37–56.

Sadler, P. M., & Kurrie, S. E. (1993). Australian service providers' responses to elder abuse. *Journal of Elder Abuse and Neglect,* 1993, *5*(1), 57–75.

Scheidt, Rick J., & Windley, Paul G. (1983). The mental health of small-town rural elderly residents. *Journal of Gerontology, 38,* 472–479.

Schwenk, Frankie N. (1991). Women 65 years or older: A comparison of economic well-being by living arrangements. *Family Economics Review, 4*(3), 2–8.

Sengstock, Mary C. (1991). Sex and gender implications in cases of elder abuse. *Journal of Women and Aging, 3*(4), 25–43.

Stone, Robyn. (1987). *The feminization of poverty and older women: An update.* Rockville, MD: U.S. Department of Health and Human Services.

Streib, Gordon F. (1990). Congregate housing: People, places, and policies. In David Tilson (Ed.), *Aging in place: Supporting the frail elderly in residential environments.* Glenview, IL: Scott, Foresman.

Suzman, Richard M., Willis, David P., & Manton, Kenneth G. (1992). *The oldest old.* New York: Oxford University Press.

Teresi, Jeanne A., Holmes, Douglas, & Monaco, Charlene. (1993). An evaluation of the effects of commingling cognitively and noncognitively impaired individuals in long-term care facilities. *Gerontologist, 33*(3), 350–358.

Thomas, Amelia. (1990, September 10) For release. *HHH News.* Washington, DC: U.S. Department of Health and Human Services.

U.S. Bureau of the Census, (1993). *Sixty-five plus in America.* Current Population Reports. Special Issue. P25–1092. Washington, DC: U.S. Government Printing Office.

U.S. Congress, House Select Committee on Aging. (1989). *Quality of life for older women: Older women living alone.* Washington, DC: U.S. Government Printing Office.

————. (1990, May). *Women in retirement: Are they losing out?* Washington, DC: U.S. Government Printing Office.

————. (1990, July). *Retirement income for women.* Washington, DC: U.S. Government Printing Office.

————. (1991, May). *Women at midlife: Consumers of second-rate health care?* Washington, DC: U.S. Government Printing Office.

————. (1991, July). *Women health care consumers: Short-changed on medical research and treatment.* Washington, DC: U.S. Government Printing Office.

————. (1992). *Income and employment.* Washington, DC: U.S. Government Printing Office.

U.S. Senate, Special Committee on Aging. (1985–86). *Aging America.* Washington, DC: U.S. Government Printing Office.

Uzawa, Martha N. (1993). Solitude in old age: Effects of female hardship on elderly women's lives. *Affilia, 8*(2), 136–156.

Wolf, Douglas A. (1990). *Household patterns of older women.* Washington, DC: Urban Institute.

Part IV

Racial, Ethnic, and
Demographic Issues

Eighteen

Midlife and Older Black Women

PENNY A. RALSTON

Nearly thirty years ago Jacqueline Johnson Jackson (1967), in the first known literature review on black aged, presented the case that the field of gerontology had systematically excluded older blacks. She argued that there was a need to know more about this population, and further, there was a need to study subgroups of black aged because of the possible differential effects of socioenvironmental and psychological conditions. Over the years there has been considerable attention given to providing empirical knowledge regarding older blacks (see, e.g., Harel, McKinney, & Williams, 1990; J. J. Jackson, 1980; J. S. Jackson, 1988; J. S. Jackson, Chatters, & Taylor, 1993; Manuel, 1982). Concurrently, our knowledge of subgroups of older blacks has also increased.

One subgroup of older blacks that has received increased attention in the gerontological literature is midlife and older black women, paralleling the burgeoning literature base on black women in general (see, e.g., Bell-Scott, 1984; Bracey, 1986–87; Busby, 1992; Giddings, 1984, hooks, 1981; Jones, 1995; Ladner, 1971; Lerner, 1972; Noble, 1978; Vaz, 1995). Although our knowledge has been advanced regarding midlife and older women, we are, to a large extent, still unclear about the lives of this group and the resulting individual and societal consequences. We know, for example, that historically, these women faced social, economic, and political challenges that resulted in a socioenvironment characterized by frequent poverty and discrimination. But we also know that many black women have somehow "beaten the odds" and have reached old age after productive lives of working, raising families, and supporting communities

A portion of this chapter was taken from J. P. Dancy and P. A. Ralston, "Health promotion: The needs of black elders," paper presented at the Gerontological Society of America Annual Meeting, San Francisco, November 1991. Research for that paper was supported in part by the Center on Rural Elderly, University of Missouri at Kansas City.

(Jones, 1995). While other scholars have noted this contradictory phenomenon in older blacks in general (J. S. Jackson et al., 1993; Stanford, 1990), few have seen older black women as a distinctive case (Jones, 1995; Edmonds, 1990).

Given this discussion, it would be easy to portray black women across the life course as victims of the socioenvironmental conditions of their lives. In fact, earlier works by gerontologists did discuss older black women within the context of their "plight" and "coping capacities" (see, e.g. Lindsay, 1975). This discussion could also portray black women as martyrs or superhuman individuals who have overcome obstacles through hard work and a good heart (Ladner, 1971; Jones, 1995) and who receive large amounts of social and economic support from a broad array of kin (Kivett, 1993).

However, between these two obviously stereotypical views is another perspective: black women over the life course assume roles that may compensate for the limitations of their socioenvironment. As workers, child rearers, wives/companions, and community volunteers, black women make substantial contributions to society. Assuming these roles has been dictated not only by their own desires but also by societal imposition. For example, historically, whether or not to work outside the home was, for most black women, not a choice because of black male unemployment and underemployment (Jones, 1995). Child rearing in black families sometimes was expanded to include fictive kin, thus increasing child-care responsibilities (Billingsley, 1968; Shimkin, Shimkin, & Frate, 1978). Marital relations were often complicated by economic limitations, lack of suitable partners, and role strain (Staples, 1981). Organizations in the black community, such as black churches, have relied on black women for sustainability (Hine, 1993).

The roles assumed by black women, whether self-initiated or imposed by society, may have resulted in two outcomes. On the one hand, roles assumed by black women may have led to the development of human capacities that compensate for limitations in the socioenvironment. On the other hand, these roles, coupled with socioenvironmental limitations, may have detrimental effects on black women's health and personal well-being. In midlife and old age these detrimental effects may be somewhat cumulative and thus more pervasive.

The purpose of this chapter is to present and review the extant literature to explore this conceptual perspective of midlife and older black women. Specifically, this chapter begins with a discussion of the sociohistorical context for black women. Then roles and supports are examined, including family, community, and work and retirement roles. Health, both physical and mental, is discussed in relation to health behaviors. The chapter concludes with an analysis of the literature in relation to the conceptual perspective presented and areas of additional research that are needed.

SOCIOHISTORICAL CONTEXT

Black women who are now 70 years of age or older were born during the 1920s. The majority of these women were born in the southeastern region of the United States and lived in racial segregation (Edmonds, 1990; Richardson, 1990). Between 1900 and 1930 the great migration of blacks from the South to the North occurred, and in total two million blacks were relocated (Jones, 1995). Black women participated in this migration to a large extent, sometimes following their trailblazing husbands who moved to urban settings to find better opportunities for employment. Single black women also moved north, often to find domestic servant positions that paid higher wages than in the South (Jones, 1995).

The primary employment black women were able to obtain was in domestic service, although a small number worked in black-owned businesses or as black professionals (teachers, nurses). For example, in 1910 there were approximately 2 million black female workers, and over 1.8 million or 91 percent worked in agriculture, as servants, or in laundries. Only 1 percent of the working population were teachers (22,000), and only a few were physicians and lawyers (333 and 2, respectively) (Edmonds, 1990). Although black women desired to move into other types of employment such as clerical and salesclerk positions, this was not possible due to overt racism in society at the time that led to white immigrants being selected for these positions (Jones, 1995). Jones (1995) pointed out that an extraordinarily high proportion of black women worked and served as primary or supplementary breadwinners in their households and often took home wages more nearly equal to those of their male counterparts. Thus the progress of black families as a group was linked to the job status of the black female, who, unlike her white counterparts, could rarely indulge in romantic fantasies about marriage that would end her days as a worker. Even black women with formal educations were relegated to menial jobs because of racial discrimination (Edmonds, 1990; Jones, 1995).

Historically, black women, like blacks in general, have had fewer opportunities for educational attainment and thus lower educational levels. Zopf (1986) pointed out that education of today's elderly black people still bears the mark of "separate-but-equal" schools, general discrimination, and social expectations for blacks in the early 1900s. Regarding the latter, education had less relevance for blacks, many of whom were born and reared in the South and whose future was enmeshed in agriculture. Education reflected a time investment that black families could ill afford when survival was the greater need. Yet black Americans have historically valued education as a means to improve their lives and to overcome the oppression and social control of dominant society (Anderson, 1988). Thus black educational attainment has steadily increased throughout the years. For example, median years of school completed for blacks 65–69 years of age increased from 3.8 years in 1940 to 8.4 years in 1982 (compared to 8.2 to 12.2 years for whites) (Zopf, 1986). For black women, educational attainment has been greater than for black men, with black women being less represented in the group of functional illiterates, more likely to have gone to college and to have finished four years of college, and more likely to have obtained college and postgraduate degrees (Zopf, 1986).

Although educational attainment may have increased over the years for blacks in general and black women in particular, the resulting lack of employment and other economic opportunities has led to incomes for blacks that are lower than those of whites. Moreover, black women's income is lowest in comparison to white males and females and black males. Using U.S. Bureau of the Census data, Zopf (1986) reported that the median income for black females aged 65 or over was $3,558, compared to $4,219 for Black males, $5,186 for white females, and $6,161 for white males. How, then, have black women, particularly older black women, coped with such limited economic resources? Zopf (1986) indicated that because per capita incomes for blacks have remained low throughout their lifetimes, the drop-off in old age is less of an adjustment than for whites. In addition, Parks's (1988) study of older rural blacks in three Southern states showed that assistance from family may buffer poverty, with 67% of the older black females having assistance provided by relatives (in comparison to 33% for black males).

Regardless of their social and economic disadvantages, black women historically have had broad participation in society that is documented in black historical and anthropological literature (Aschenbrenner, 1975; Gutman, 1976; Hine, 1993; Jones, 1995; Shimkin et al., 1978; Stack, 1975). These works demonstrate that black women's involvement and activism in communities, to a large extent, sustained the entire institutional infrastructure of black life and culture in this society. Hine (1993), in the introduction to *Black Women in America, An Historical Encyclopedia*, where she described her initial foray into black women's history, said it best:

Black women . . . ha[ve] founded schools and settlement houses, provided welfare for orphaned children, homes for the aged, clinics for the sick, and money for scholarships. They were tireless political workers, and librarians on the one hand and domestic servants, laundresses, and beauticians on the other. Black churches were utterly dependent on their fundraising labors. They organized celebrations, festivals, balls, symposia, lectures, and recitals. (p. xx)

In sum, the sociohistorical context for older black women is indeed a distinctive one. They are products of postslavery America, including overt as well as covert attempts by dominant society to limit their social involvement and economic opportunities. Tied to older black women's sociohistory is that of older black men, many of whom were unable to secure economic resources during their younger lives to solely support their families. Thus black women became partners with black men to provide economic resources for their families, even though their employment was often in low-paying domestic service jobs and often required migration to geographical areas where more opportunities were available. Black women's sociohistory also shows a collective industriousness and a desire for individual, family, and community development, as demonstrated by their progress in educational attainment and their work to enhance community well-being. Black women, then, have had a unique history in the twentieth century that has impacted their lives as they have aged. With this as a backdrop, the next two sections of this chapter present a review of the literature related to key aspects of older black women's lives, including their roles, supports, and health and health behaviors. This review will help to identify the extent to which members of this group have been impacted by the socioenvironmental conditions of their lives.

ROLES AND SUPPORTS

Family

Black women engage in a variety of roles across the lifespan, including roles involving family, community, and work. There is considerable evidence that broad kin as well as nonkin networks provide a rich source of support for black families (Billingsley, 1968; Shimkin et al., 1978; Stack, 1975). Black families appear to be more involved in exchanges of help across generations, and older blacks, in comparison to older whites, give more help to children and grandchildren (Cantor, 1979; Mutran, 1985; R. J. Taylor, 1988). Older black women have more contact with adult children than black men, with factors such as number of sons and daughters, proximity to nearest child, and parental education all influencing frequency of contact (Chatters & Taylor, 1993).

Although there is documentation of the role of family member for black women in their earlier lives (Aschenbrenner, 1975; Jones, 1995; Shimkin et al., 1978; Stack, 1975; Vaz, 1995), the nature of this role in later life is less well known. The focus of research on family life for older black women has been help seeking and receipt of support (R. J. Taylor, 1988). Mutran (1985), however, found that help from older to younger generations does occur in black families and is often related to the number of children within the household. Because of extended-family households, older blacks are more likely to be involved in child care and other family support activities. Supporting cultural distinctions, Mutran (1985) also found that black elderly persons who feel that the older generation deserves more respect are also those more involved in helping other members of their family.

Kivett (1993) documented the important grandmother-grandchild relationship, including black and white comparisons, in a rural sample of elderly. She found that there were racial similarities in household density and amount of association with grandchildren when socioeconomic status was controlled. Proximity of grandchildren was also similar for both groups and was related to association with and help received from grandchildren. However, she also found cultural distinctions in grandmother-grandchild exchanges. Black grandmothers both gave and received more help from grandchildren than white grandmothers, supporting the cultural versus socioeconomic basis for intergenerational exchanges. These data also support the strong female ties within the black extended family (Dilworth-Anderson, 1992; Martin & Martin, 1978). As Kivett (1993) pointed out, "Young females may be singled out more frequently by grandmothers in a socialization-to-role process" (p. 170).

Other relationships, such as male-female relationships, have received little attention in the literature on older black families. This may be partially due to older blacks being less likely to have a spouse—they are twice as likely as whites to be divorced or separated and proportionately more likely to be widowed (Engram & Lockery, 1993). For older black women, remarriage is less likely because older black men marry younger women and because there are fewer black men who reach old age (Engram & Lockery, 1993). Interestingly, black male-female relationships as a topic have engaged much debate because, across the life cycle, black males and females are often viewed as unable to perform societally prescribed roles because of economic and social conditions for blacks. Black women as "matriarchs" and black men as exploitative are the resulting stereotypes (Ladner, 1971).

Despite these views, older black males and females do share intimacy, in marital relations as well as in other relationships. For example, Engram and Lockery (1993) found in their national sample of older blacks that 26.6 percent of the older black women were married and 9 percent of those not married had romantic involvement, compared to 59.8 percent and 40.2 percent, respectively, for older black men. Moreover, 71.1 percent of the married older black women felt that a good love life was very important, compared to 80.2 percent of the older black men (43.5 and 63.5 percent, respectively, for older black women and men romantically involved). While these data reflect perceptions rather than observed behaviors of this population, they do give an indication of the values older black males and females have regarding intimacy.

Community

Older black women are involved in selected community organizations, and the extent of this involvement is related to several factors. Gibson (1993) found, in a national sample of retired black Americans aged 55–101, that 7.1 percent and 2.8 percent, respectively, were involved in church-related activities and clubs/organizations (male involvement was 9.6 and 2.9 percent, respectively). Ralston and Mercier (1984) found that "going to church" was one of the frequent activities in a national sample of black women aged 66 to 71. Parks (1988), in a multistate sample of rural older blacks in the Southeast region, found that 62.4 percent of the women were involved in church work, 65.2 percent gave money to the church, and 60.7 percent were involved in community work (male involvement was 37.6, 34.8, and 39.3 percent, respectively). Factors related to community involvement include educational level (Gibson, 1993) and health (Ralston & Mercier, 1984), in that those with more education and those who perceived their health as better than others appeared to have higher levels of involvement. Gibson (1993) found that income and gender were not related to church and other community involvement, although Parks's (1988) data revealed clear gender differences.

There is a paucity of data regarding participation of midlife and older black women in age-segregated community organizations. In general, some of the literature shows that participation rates for older blacks in senior centers are high in comparison to those of whites and other ethnic groups (Harris & Associates, 1981). However, other data suggest that race is not a significant factor in senior-center participation (Krout, Cutler, & Coward, 1990), although methodological issues have been raised about these findings (Ralston, 1991). Black women's involvement in senior centers has not been examined, although more females than males participate in senior centers because demographically more women are available to participate.

Work and Retirement

Work and retirement roles for midlife and older black women are characterized by a lack of clear definition between when work ends and retirement begins. Gibson (1987, 1988, 1993), who has written extensively on the need to reconceptualize retirement for black Americans, argued that new social trends may be creating a new type of black retirees, the "unretired-retired." This group is composed of individuals 55 years of age or older who are not working but who do not call themselves retired. The creation of this group reflects trends of declining labor-force participation of middle-aged and older blacks, increases in physical disability, and increases in availability of disability pay (Gibson, 1987).

Gibson's research showed that nearly 40 percent of blacks aged 55 or over do not view themselves as retired (Gibson, 1988). For older blacks, subjective retirement is predicted by age, subjective disability, and work history. Those who are older, who view themselves as disabled, or who worked full-time over the life course considered themselves retired. Gender, as well as urbanicity and social class, were not predictors of subjective retirement (Gibson, 1988). Although research on white populations notes significant gender differences in the predictors of subjective retirement (Murray, 1979; Irelan & Bell, 1972), black men and women have been lifetime workers with similarly discontinuous work patterns, and thus gender for aged blacks is not an important factor (Gibson, 1987, 1988).

For older blacks who continue to work in old age, work status is predicted by health, age, family income, marital status, and region of country (Coleman, 1993). Specifically, those who have fewer health problems, are younger, have higher incomes, are widowed, and live in the western region of the country are more likely to be in the labor force before or after retirement age. Gender was not a significant predictor of work status, although black males did work more hours, indicating that they may be participating in more flexible, part-time work (Coleman, 1993). Coleman (1993) suggested that most black women 55 or older may have been restricted to domestic work in their earlier years. In midlife and old age these women may not have the physical strength to continue working in this occupation.

HEALTH AND HEALTH BEHAVIORS

In asking the question how black women fare when they age with regard to economics, loneliness, mortality, and isolationism, J. J. Jackson (1976) concluded: "Generally, the aggregated conditions of older Black women which were prevalent when they were younger continue into old age, merely becoming more exacerbated" (p. 54). What would be her response to the topic of health and midlife and older black women?

Perhaps due to their life circumstances, black women have developed certain attitudes toward how they perceive their health. Edmonds (1990) pointed out that for many midlife and older black women today, health is self-perceived as "good" even when it is not. Their norms for what is "good health" reflect sociocultural and historical influences and the mindset that not feeling well is "the cross one must bear" (Edmonds, 1990). Although a plausible explanation for overestimation of health status may be that older black women have limited awareness of signs and symptoms of disease, there is evidence that they do have a great deal of experiential health information (Edmonds, 1992) and that playing down their health problems may be a coping mechanism. Another explanation for overestimation of health status may be that, considering the multiple roles they have in families, "there is no time to be sick." Knowing the "truth" about their health could impact the well-being of a whole family, and even talking about one's health becomes taboo. Thus black women often live in a "conspiracy of silence."

One can speculate that these attitudes of denial and silence, complicated by a sometimes inaccessible and sometimes racist health care system, may have resulted in a cohort of older black women who are at risk in terms of health. Thus J. J. Jackson's conclusion is possibly true for health status as well: The aggregated health conditions of older black women when they were younger have continued and become more exacerbated in old age.

Richardson's (1990) extensive review of aging and health among black American elders pointed out in a startling way the health condition of older black women in comparison to their black male and white counterparts. The summary of her review, along with additional sources, shows the following:

- Coronary heart disease and stroke account for 41 percent of the excess mortality observed in black women (Richardson, 1992). Coronary heart disease prevalence and mortality are higher in black women than in white women even after age 65 (Richardson, 1992). Until age 75, black females appear to have a higher incidence of stroke than black males (Gillum, 1988).

- Older black females who routinely receive treatment for chronic illness fail to have routine Pap smears, and they are dying from cancer in disproportionate numbers. An examination of excess cancer deaths indicates that a greater percentage of black women die between the ages of 45 and 69 years than any other age group (Richardson, 1992).

- Breast cancer is the leading cause of cancer among black women in the United States (Burack & Liang, 1989). Black females appear to have a poorer breast cancer survival rate than either white or Hispanic women, even when controlling for age, socioeconomic status, stage, and delay in seeking treatment (Vernon, Tilley, Neale, & Steinfeldt, 1985).

- Although older black women's rate of suicide is the lowest in comparison to black males and white males and females, the rate of suicide for older black women per 100,000 increased from 1.4 in 1980 to 2.4 in 1986 (Meehan, Saltzman, & Sattin, 1991).

- There is a 50 percent higher rate of diabetes among black females and a 16 percent higher rate of diabetes in black males than in their white counterparts (Lieberman, 1988; Report of the Secretary's Task Force on Black & Minority Health, 1985; Roseman, 1985). Black females appear to have the highest rate of both diagnosed and undiagnosed diabetes (Roseman, 1985), and it is the fourth leading cause of death for this group (Glaser, Molnar, & Bleich, 1995).

- Black women have significantly lower caloric intake than white women between the ages of 46 to 65 and over 65 years (Gartside, Khoury, & Glueck, 1984). Compared to whites, the diets of black females are the most nutritionally inadequate, followed by the diets of their male counterparts (Jerome, 1988).

- For the category of senile and presenile dementia, nonwhite females had higher average annual mortality rates than white females in the age groups of 45–49, 65–69, and 70–74 (Harper & Alexander, 1990).

- The only good news for black women: Black females at every age have approximately one-half as many hip fractures as white females (White, Farmer, & Brody, 1984).

The health problems of older black women are exacerbated by a health care system that cares little about them. Lewis (1992) pointed out that access to all areas of health care is difficult for minority women, especially those who are poor. Once health care services are used, women sometimes feel neglected and disrespected, with their chronic diseases ignored or undertreated (Lewis, 1992). Moreover, women in general and minority women in particular suffer from poor treatment from underpaid and undertrained health workers who many times have not had the opportunity to resolve their own personal feeling about working with sick elderly (Lewis, 1992). Racist behaviors of health care workers affect use of health services. S. Taylor (1992) pointed out that community mental health care facilities are often underutilized by older black women because of the racist attitudes the clients feel in therapy sessions. Thus the long-standing racial tensions in a community can spill over into the health care system.

Older black women, who are many times already at risk economically, find themselves in a difficult situation when costs for health care rise beyond capacity to pay. When faced with a major illness, older black women who have any accumulated income must spend a significant portion of their overall resources in order to receive Medicaid benefits (Lewis, 1992). When faced with such choices, it is understandable that older black women decide to delay formal health care or to seek only intermittent treatment.

For older black women, social supports are both a comfort and a source of strain. Watson (1990) pointed out that living arrangement is a crucial exogenous factor bearing on the incidence of poverty among women and especially black women. Black single female heads of households who have dependent children, other relatives, and/or nonrelatives living with them are more likely to have more economic problems than those who live alone. Taylor (1982) found that 94 percent of the older black women interviewed for her study described the family as the most dependable source of aid. However, there was also evidence in a small portion of cases that conflict in intergenerational households was identified as a source of stress. Learner and Kivett (1981) indicated that household composition and family structure could be factors predisposing elderly blacks to greater dietary problems due to limited economic resources needing to be shared in those households with other family members. Older black women, particularly those who are heads of households, must cope with the responsibilities and demands that come with being the primary household manager. With regard to health and health care, there clearly may be ''no time to be sick'' or ''no money to get well.''

CONCLUSIONS

In the beginning of this chapter, a conceptual perspective relating roles of older black women to their socioenvironment was presented. Specifically, the argument was made that black women over the life course assume roles (family, community, work) and, in so doing, develop human capacities that may compensate for the limitations in their socioenvironment, including social, economic, and political factors affecting their personal development and well-being. The literature revealed in this chapter indeed shows that historically as well as presently, older black women have limitations in their socioenvironment. Yet the roles that midlife and older black women have performed in family, community, and work suggest that they are productive citizens who have acquired the human capacities to compensate for limitations in their socioenvironment. Older black women are involved in exchanges across generations (i.e., grandmother to grandchild), are involved in intimate relations (marriage or ''romantic'' involvements), and feel that a good love life is important (although less so than black men). Community participation of older black women includes churches, clubs, and senior centers and varies by educational level and health. Work and retirement patterns of older black women are similar to those of black men, with a large percentage (40 percent) of those 55 or older considered ''unretired-retired.''

This review also shows, however, that performing family, community, and work roles within the context of the socioenvironment may be related to the health status of midlife and older black women. The data clearly indicate that this group is at risk for health problems. In comparison to black males and whites of both sexes, they are more likely to suffer from strokes, cancer, diabetes, and poor nutrition, among other problems. Their attitudes toward health, shaped from a long history of limited access to education and employment opportunities, are characterized by an overestimation of health, a denial of the sick role, and often an unwillingness to discuss health problems (i.e., a "conspiracy of silence"). They find the health care system at times inaccessible and have little confidence in the treatment they may receive there. Their socioeconomic status, sometimes exacerbated by being heads of households, often prevents use of health care as frequently as needed. Family as well as other supports can be a source of comfort, but also may cause stress, particularly if the older black woman is heading a household comprised of other dependents.

Given the profile of older black women presented in this chapter, it is clear that there is a collective resilience in this group to perform the necessary roles in their families and communities, regardless of socioenvironmental factors that could inhibit their performance. Midlife and older black women are key givers and receivers of help in their families, and they participate to a greater extent than black males in churches, clubs, and other organizations. In addition, black women have historically been involved in paid work activity. Do these multiple roles come at a price in terms of their health?

With the current debate regarding health care, there are attempts at the societal level to bring about changes in the health care system. However, whether these changes will be of help to the bulk of older black women is in question. Given older black women's reluctance to use the established health care system, the movement toward managed care and the restrictions that this type of structure may impose on consumer choice may only serve to decrease use of health care by older black women. Concurrently, the need for midlife and older black women to take preventive steps in health maintenance needs to be stressed. Concerns about diet and nutrition and getting regular checkups (e.g., Pap smears, breast examinations) would, to a great extent, reduce major health problems for black women as they age. Perhaps most important, black women need to be empowered to care for themselves first.

This concluding section also addresses research needs as they relate to midlife and older black women. As demonstrated by this chapter, the literature on midlife and older black women has grown a great deal since the late 1960s when Jacqueline Johnson Jackson wrote her first review on black aged. However, there are some noticeable gaps that will be outlined here.

First, because of the diversity of occupations black women now hold, additional research is needed to tease out how current and future cohorts of black women with different occupations view retirement. Gibson (1993) pointed out that in past cohorts of older blacks, occupation may not have been a relevant factor in retirement research because racial discrimination placed a ceiling on their occupational mobility. Moreover, black women's occupations have become more diverse over the years. Whereas 49 percent of black female employees worked in domestic service in 1949, only 27 percent had this occupation in 1990. In 1990, 39 percent were in technical or administrative positions, 19 percent were in managerial and professional positions, 12 percent were in semi-skilled labor, 2 percent were in skilled labor, and 0.3 percent were in agriculture (O'Hare, Pollard, Mann, & Kent, 1991). These patterns vary in comparison to black males, whose occupations reflect more semiskilled labor and fewer technical/administrative and managerial/professional positions than those of black females (33, 17, and 13 percent, respectively) (O'Hare et al., 1991). Thus subjective retirement and work status for women may be less similar to men in future cohorts of black Americans. Investigating black women with diverse occupations (see, e.g., Carlton-LaNey, 1992; Fontaine & Greenlee, 1993; Perkins, 1993) will add to our understanding of their work and retirement roles as they age.

Second, as indicated in this chapter, the bulk of the literature on family life for older black women has concerned help seeking and receipt of support. Even in the literature on community participation, where the emphasis has been on black women's involvement, the data are sketchy regarding the nature and type of this involvement. In essence, the focus in the gerontological literature has been on older black women as a group in need of help and support. Yet historically as well as presently, it is clear that black women as they age have considerable capacity to provide help and assistance to others. Chronicling this assistance is necessary to give a more accurate picture of black women as they age as a resource to themselves, their families, and their communities. This approach to ethnogerontological research is particularly important considering that future cohorts of midlife and older black women will have higher educational levels and may be more involved in assistance giving. Various research methodologies, including ethnographic and other qualitative methodologies along with longitudinal quantitative studies, will help to enrich the data base on midlife and older black women and to expand our conceptual knowledge about their everyday lives.

In summary, this chapter has presented and reviewed extant literature on midlife and older black women, examining their lives in relation to their socioenvironment, which, historically, has been disadvantaged economically, socially, and politically. The data reported here show that for the most part, black women as a group still have many disadvantages. Yet black women as they age overcome many of these limitations and not only become productive workers, family members, and community participants, but also frequently are the vital link for others in these roles. There are, however, consequences for midlife and older black women assuming these various roles, perhaps exacerbated by the socioenvironmental conditions of their lives. Poor health is clearly one of these consequences.

Does the future bode well for midlife and older black women? This question may be difficult to answer. The current cohort of young and midlife black women includes a diverse group, especially in terms of socioeconomic level.

O'Hare et al. (1991) pointed out that African Americans experienced growing polarization during the 1980s, widening the split between rich and poor. In 1989 nearly one in seven black families had an income of $50,000 or more (in constant dollars), compared with one out of every seventeen in 1967. The number of affluent black families increased from 266,000 in 1967 to just over one million in 1989, nearly a fourfold increase (O'Hare et al., 1991). In contrast, in 1989 the median annual income for black families was $20,000, slightly below the comparable figure for 1969. Black family income was 61 percent that of whites in 1969, but only 56 percent as high in 1989. One reason for black families losing ground economically is the growth in female-headed families, which pulled a larger proportion of black families into the lowest income group. In 1989 black female-headed families had only a third the annual income of black married-couple families, $11,600 compared with $30,700 (O'Hare et al., 1991).

In addition to socioeconomic level, black women also are impacted by recent phenomena such as the role of drugs and gang violence in the structure and functioning of black families; the changing policies in welfare, Medicaid, food assistance, and other government programs; and the high rates of teenage pregnancy, which often serves as the precursor to female-headed families. In sum, with the socioeconomic diversity in black families, coupled with the economic and social uncertainty of some of these families, the future for midlife and older black women may reflect differential jeopardy (Dancy & Ralston, 1991), with some subgroups of this population faring worse than others. However, increased research efforts are needed that will help the gerontological community, including scholars, policy makers, and practitioners, grow in their understanding and appreciation of midlife and older black women and work toward enhancing their well-being.

REFERENCES

Anderson, J. D. (1988). *The education of blacks in the South, 1860–1935*. Chapel Hill: University of North Carolina Press.

Aschenbrenner, J. (1975). *Lifelines: Black families in Chicago*. New York: Holt, Rinehart & Winston.

Bell-Scott, P. (1984). Black women's education [Special issue]. *Sage: A Scholarly Journal on Black Women, 3*(1).

Billingsley, A. (1968). *Black families in white America*. Englewood Cliffs, NJ: Prentice-Hall.

Bracey, J. (1986–87). Afro-American women: A brief guide to writings from historical and feminist perspectives. *Contributions in Black Studies, 8*, 106–110.

Burack, R. C., & Liang, J. (1989). The acceptance and completion of mammography by older black women. *American Journal of Public Health, 79*(6), 721–726.

Busby, M. (Ed.). (1992). *Daughters of Africa*. New York: Ballantine Books.

Cantor, M. H. (1979). Neighbors and friends: An overlooked resource in the informal support system. *Research on Aging, 1*, 434–463.

Carlton-LaNey, I. (1992). Elderly black farm women: A population at risk. *Social Work,* *37*(6), 517–523.

Chatters, L. M. and Taylor, R. J. (1993). Intergenerational support: The provision of assistance to parents by adult children. In J. S. Jackson, L. M. Chatters, & R. J. Taylor (Eds.), *Aging in black America*. Newbury Park, CA: Sage.

Coleman, L. M. (1993). The black Americans who keep working. In J. S. Jackson, L. M. Chatters, & R. J. Taylor (Eds.), *Aging in black America*. Newbury Park, CA: Sage.

Dancy, J., & Ralston, P. (1991, November). *Health promotion: The needs of black elders*. Paper presented at the Gerontological Society of America Annual Meeting, San Francisco.

Dilworth-Anderson, P. (1992). Extended kin networks in black families. *Generations,* *16*(3), 29–32.

Edmonds, M. M. (1990). The health of the black aged female. In Z. Harel, E. A. Mc-Kinney, & M. Williams (Eds.), *Black aged: Understanding diversity and service needs*. Newbury Park, CA: Sage.

———. (1992, November). *The influence of social history on the health and illness behaviors of the aged black female*. Paper presented at the Gerontological Society of America Annual Meeting, Washington, DC.

Engram, E., & Lockery, S. A. (1993). Intimate partnerships. In J. S. Jackson, L. M. Chatters, & R. J. Taylor (Eds.), *Aging in black America*. Newbury Park, CA: Sage.

Fontaine, D., & Greenlee, S. (1993). Black women: Double solos in the workplace. *Western Journal of Black Studies, 17*(3), 121–125.

Gartside, P. S., Khoury, P., & Glueck, C. J. (1984). Determinants of high density lipo-protein cholesterol in blacks and whites: The Second National Health and Nutri-tion Examination Survey. *American Heart Journal, 108*(3, pt. 2), 641–652.

Gibson, R. C. (1987). Reconceptualizing retirement for black Americans. *Gerontologist,* *27*(6), 691–698.

———. (1988). The work, retirement, and disability of older black Americans. In J. S. Jackson (Ed.), *The black American elderly: Research on physical and psycho-social health*. New York: Springer.

———. (1993). The black American retirement experience. In J. S. Jackson, L. M. Chatters, & R. J. Taylor (Eds.), *Aging in black America*. Newbury Park, CA: Sage.

Giddings, P. (1984). *When and where I enter: The impact of black women on race and sex in America*. New York: Morrow.

Gillum, R. F. (1988). Stroke in blacks. *Stroke, 19*, 1–9.

Glaser, J. F., Molnar, I. G., & Bleich, D. (1995). Older white and black women with diabetes: Some nutritional comparisons. *Journal of Family and Consumer Sci-ences, 87*(3), 19–24.

Gutman, H. G. (1976). *The black family in slavery and freedom, 1750–1925*. New York: Pantheon Books.

Harel, Z., McKinney, E. A., & Williams, M. (Eds.). (1990). *Black aged: Understanding diversity and service needs*. Newbury Park, CA: Sage.

Harper, M. S., & Alexander, C. D. (1990). *Minority aging: Essential curricula content for selected health and allied health professions* (DHHS Publication No. HRS-P-DV 90–4). Washington, DC: U.S. Department of Health and Human Services.

Harris, L., & Associates, Inc. (1981). *Aging in the eighties: America in transition.* Washington, DC: National Council on the Aging.

Hine, D. C. (Ed.). (1993). *Black women in America, An historical encyclopedia.* Brooklyn, NY: Carlson.

hooks, b. (1981). *Ain't I a woman? Black women and feminism.* Boston: South End Press.

Irelan, L. M., & Bell, D. B. (1972). Understanding subjectively defined retirement: A pilot analysis. *Gerontologist, 12,* 354–356.

Jackson, J. J. (1967). Social gerontology and the Negro: A review. *Gerontologist, 7,* 168–178.

———. (1971). The Blacklands of gerontology. *Aging and Human Development, 2,* 156–171.

———. (1976). The plight of older black women in the United States. *Black Scholar, 7,* 47–55.

———. (1980). *Minorities and aging.* Belmont, CA: Wadsworth.

———. (1982). The black elderly: Reassessing the plight of older black women. *Black Scholar, 13*(1), 2–4.

Jackson, J. S. (Ed.). (1988). *The black American elderly: Research on physical and psychosocial health.* New York: Springer.

Jackson, J. S., Chatters, L. M., & Taylor, R. J. (Eds.). (1993). *Aging in black America.* Newbury Park, CA: Sage.

Jerome, N. (1988). Dietary intake and nutritional status of older U.S. blacks: An overview. In J. S. Jackson (Ed.), *The black American elderly: Research on physical and psychosocial health.* New York: Springer.

Jones, J. (1995). *Labor of love, labor of sorrow: Black women, work, and the family from slavery to the present.* New York: Vintage.

Kivett, V. (1993). Racial comparisons of the grandmother role: Implications for strengthening the family support system of older black women. *Family Relations, 42,* 165–172.

Krout, J., Cutler, S. J., & Coward, R. T. (1990). Correlates of senior center participation: A national analysis. *Gerontologist, 30,* 72–79.

Ladner, J. (1971). *Tomorrow's tomorrow: The black woman.* Garden City, NY: Doubleday.

Learner, R. M., & Kivett, V. R. (1981). Discriminators of perceived dietary adequacy among the rural elderly. *Journal of the American Dietetic Association, 78*(4), 330–337.

Lerner, G. (1972). *Black women in white America: A documentary history.* New York: Pantheon.

Lewis, I. (1992, November). *Health issues of older black women* (Discussant). Symposium presented at the Gerontological Society of America Annual Meeting, Washington, DC.

Lieberman, L. S. (1988). Diabetes and obesity in elderly Black Americans. In J. S. Jackson (Ed.), *The black American elderly: Research on physical and psychosocial health.* New York: Springer.

Lindsay, I. (1975). Coping capacities of the black aged. In *No longer young: The older woman in America.* Proceedings of the 26th Annual Conference on Aging, Institute of Gerontology, The University of Michigan–Wayne State University.

Manuel, R. (Ed.). (1982). *Minority aging: Sociological and social psychological attitudes*. Westport, CT: Greenwood Press.

Martin, E., & Martin, J. (1978). *The black extended family*. Chicago: University of Chicago Press.

Meehan, P., Saltzman, L., & Sattin, R. (1991). Suicides among older United States residents: Epidemiologic characteristics and trends. *American Journal of Public Health, 81*(9), 1198–1200.

Murray, J. (1979). Subjective retirement. *Social Security Bulletin, 42*(11), 20–25, 43.

Mutran, E. (1985). Intergenerational family support among blacks and whites: Response to culture or to socioeconomic differences. *Journal of Gerontology, 40*(3), 382–389.

Noble, J. (1978). *Beautiful, also, are the souls of my black sisters: A history of the black woman in America*. Englewood Cliffs, NJ: Prentice-Hall.

O'Hare, W. P., Pollard, K. M., Mann, T. L., & Kent, M. M. (1991). *African Americans in the 1990s. Population Bulletin, 46*(1).

Parks, A. G. (1988). *Black elderly in rural America: A comprehensive study*. Bristol, IN: Wyndham Hall.

Perkins, K. (1993). Working-class women and retirement. *Journal of Gerontological Social Work, 20*(3/4), 129–146.

Ralston, P. (1991). Senior centers and minority elders: A critical review. *Gerontologist, 31*(3), 325–331.

Ralston, P., & Mercier, J. (1984, November). *Older black women: Relationship of activity to retirement attitudes and life satisfaction*. Paper presented at the Gerontological Society of America Annual Meeting, San Antonio.

Report of the Secretary's Task Force on Black and Minority Health. (1985). *Cardiovascular and Cerebrovascular Disease* (Vol. 4, Part 2). Washington, DC: DHHS; U.S. Government Printing Office.

Richardson, J. (1990). *Aging and health: Black American elders*. Stanford, CA: Stanford Geriatric Education Center.

———. (1992, November). *Physical health perspective of older black women*. Paper presented at the Gerontological Society of America Annual Meeting, Washington, DC.

Roseman, J. M. (1985). Diabetes in Black Americans. In National Diabetes Data Group (Eds.), *Diabetes in America* (NIH Publication No. 85–1468, pp. 1–24). Washington, DC: U.S. Government Printing Office.

Shimkin, D. B., Shimkin, E. M., & Frate, D. A. (1978). *The extended family in black societies*. Chicago: Aldine.

Stack, C. (1975). *All our kin: Strategies for surviving in a black community*. New York: Harper.

Stanford, P. (1990). Diverse black aged. In Z. Harel, E. A. McKinney, & M. Williams (Eds.), *Black aged: Understanding diversity and service needs*. Newbury Park, CA: Sage.

Staples, R. (1981). *The world of black singles: Changing patterns of male/female relations*. Westport, CT: Greenwood Press.

Taylor, R. J. (1988). Aging and supportive relationships among black Americans. In J. S. Jackson (Ed.), *The black American elderly: Research on physical and psychosocial health*. New York: Springer.

Taylor, S. (1982). Mental health and successful coping among aged black women. In R.

Manuel (Ed.), *Minority aging: Sociological and social psychological issues.* Westport, CT: Greenwood Press.

————. (1992, November). *African American women and the mental health system.* Paper presented at the Gerontological Society of America Annual Meeting, Washington, DC.

Vaz, K. M. (Ed.). (1995). *Black women in America.* Thousand Oaks, CA: Sage.

Vernon, S. W., Tilley, B. C., Neale, A. V., & Steinfeldt, L. (1985). Ethnicity, survival, and delay in seeking treatment for symptoms of breast cancer. *Cancer, 55,* 1563–1571.

Watson, W. H. (1990). Family care, economics, and health. In Z. Harel, E. A. McKinney, & M. Williams (Eds.), *Black aged: Understanding diversity and service needs.* Newbury Park, CA: Sage.

White, L., Farmer, M., & Brody, J. (1984). Who is at risk? Hip fracture epidemiology report. *Journal of Gerontological Nursing, 10*(10), 26–29.

Zopf, P. E. (1986). *America's older population.* Houston: Cap & Gown.

Nineteen

Hidden Lives: Aging and Contemporary American Indian Women

ROBERT JOHN, PATRICE H. BLANCHARD, AND CATHERINE HAGAN HENNESSY

Since few works have specifically addressed the lives of American Indian women elders, the initial impression is that information on older Indian women does not exist. Our final conclusion, however, is that a fair amount of information does exist, but in anecdotal and hidden form. Because so little has been written about aging and American Indian women and most of the existing information is concealed or in obscure places, the lives of older American Indian women are also hidden.

Information on aging American Indian women can be classified into five types: basic demographic data, scholarly articles, review essays and bibliographies, autobiographies and biographies, and literature (fiction/poetry). Each of these sources of information has its strengths and weaknesses, but all of them together do not present a comprehensive portrait of the lives of American Indian women elders.

Demographic data provide a good starting point in understanding the basic features of any population. The strength of demographic information is that it permits an objective description of population characteristics and an assessment of the prevalence of certain conditions, such as widowhood or poverty. Although demographic information is essential to our understanding, it misses the individual experience and the richness and complexity of life in a cultural context.

Scholarly articles normally constitute the basis of knowledge on any given topic. However, scholarly articles about American Indian women elders tend to focus on narrow issues and generally use small samples that certainly are not representative of the diversity of Indian cultures. The number of demographic studies and scholarly articles on older Indian women is especially limited, leading to the conclusion that most American Indian aging researchers consider gender differences unimportant.

In recent years review essays and bibliographies have appeared that contribute to our understanding by devoting exclusive attention to American Indian women's issues. These works have been important in raising relevant contemporary issues and have done more to shape thinking and discussion about Indian women than any of the other genres. However, these articles are primarily social commentary, contain little empirical evidence about contemporary American Indian women, and treat aging issues superficially or not at all. For example, in one comprehensive bibliography of 672 entries (Green, 1983), there were only 7 works with aging themes.

Autobiographies and biographies are also a significant source of information about American Indian women. Autobiographies and, to a lesser extent, biographies are rich in anecdotal data. Radin (1920, p. 2) maintained that "personal reminiscences and impressions, inadequate as they are, are likely to throw more light on the workings of the mind and emotions of primitive man [sic] than any amount of speculation from a sophisticated ethnologist." Undoubtedly, this genre is useful in developing understanding and insight. However, many autobiographies are tainted by the cultural biases of Western editors or ghost writers. Citing a work by Gusdorf (1980), Eakin (1985, p. 199) noted "that autobiography is not a universal phenomenon, and that the 'conscious awareness of the singularity of each individual life' which autobiography assumes 'is the late product of a specific civilization.'" Sands (1992, p. 270) reinforced this point by saying that "autobiography is not an indigenous form of literature for American Indian peoples," whom Culley (1992, p. 25) described as "communal and oral, expressive of a culture that did not and does not place particular value on the individual." Although it is reasonable to question whose voice is heard through these words, Brumble (1981, p. 6) maintained that "an autobiography is at least *claiming* to be told from the point of view of an Indian."

However, as Green (1980, p. 252) lamented, even in this, "the sturdiest branch of the scholarly tree," the life stories of older Indian women are missing. For example, fewer than one-fourth of 577 autobiographies summarized by Brumble (1981) were about Indian women. Moreover, as with review articles and bibliographies, although biographical material on American Indian women exists, very little of it addresses the aging process or discusses issues that affect elderly Indian women. Works with promising titles (Bataille & Sands, 1984; Brumble, 1988; Green, 1992) did not contain any aging key words in their subject indexes. Even historical overviews (Niethammer, 1977) had limited discussion of widowhood and old age, and only a few pages, if any, were devoted to the later stages of life in various life histories (Qoyawayma, 1964; Landes, 1971; Stewart, 1980; Welch, 1985). In addition, this genre, while it provides examples of older Indian women's roles and status, tends to concentrate attention on women who are noteworthy for their achievements as artists, political leaders, or educators—again hiding the lives of ordinary aging American Indian women.

In contrast to the other genres, a large body of recent literary works by Native American women exists. Fiction and poetry add an unmistakable indigenous female voice to the literature on women's experience and can lend color and depth to the few academic descriptions of the lives of older Indian women. *Love Medicine* (Erdrich, 1984) vividly described the lives of two of the major characters in their old age, from their decisions to move to a senior citizens' home to the emotional upheavals of widowhood and to their influence in managing a reservation factory. Although many important issues are addressed obliquely in fiction and poetry, others such as the roles played by Indian grandmothers are clearly depicted. For instance, Wilson (1980) portrayed a special relationship between grandmother and granddaughter, while Silko (1980a) gave a heartrending illustration of the child-rearing role of some older Indian women.

At best, however, fictional characters and situations are what Max Weber (1949, p. 49) called "ideal types" or the "one-sided accentuation of one or more points of view and by the synthesis of a great many diffuse, discrete, more or less present and occasionally absent concrete individual phenomena" useful "for heuristic as well as expository purposes." Although literary works can enhance our perception and ability to give elegant expression to an issue, ultimately, literature blurs the demarcation between fact and fantasy and cannot substitute for social scientific understanding. Unlike fiction and poetry, the purpose of which is to entertain and leave much to the interpretation of the reader, the purpose of social scientific writing is to communicate a single interpretation clearly and unambiguously and offer convincing evidence for that view.

THEMES AND INTERPRETIVE FRAMEWORKS

There are a number of general difficulties encountered in doing research on American Indians: if and how ethnic categories are affected by urban or rural residence, the continuum of "progressive" versus "traditional" value sets, tribal affiliation, degree of Indian blood (Weibel-Orlando, 1988; cf. Wagner, 1976), if and how research tools or researchers are culturally biased (Barón, Manson, Ackerson, & Brenneman, 1990), and the limited amount of census information for the Indian population, especially breakdowns by sex and age for a statistically invisible population.

In addition, in researching Indian aging, several cultural value differences become important: the individual view of self, the focus of life importance, and Indian attitudes toward aging. One possible explanation of why so little has been written about the later years of Indian life, even in autobiographies, is that the individual "self" is considered a small part of the tribe in most Indian cultures. The tribe continues even after the self has died, so the emphasis of individual Indian life stories has not been on the end of life, but on the individual as a cultural conduit of the ongoing tribe. For example, Annie Ned (Cruikshank, 1990), telling her life story in her mid-90s, refused to include "unimportant" and "trivial" personal experiences such as her thirty-year marriage to a white man and the loss of her home in a fire. She focused instead on tribal teachings learned as a child and those teachings she could pass on as an elder. Generally, this lack of self-reflection and revelation leaves a Western audience dissatisfied. Recognizing the difficulty posed by the lack of emphasis on individual experience considered important in Western culture, Cruikshank (1990, p. x) noted that "autobiography is a culturally specific narrative genre rather than a universal form for explaining experience."

Even the organizing principle of autobiographies is a concept foreign from an American Indian worldview. Chronological time as the frame for life history is a Western idea; the Indian concept of time is cyclic. Descriptions of Indian lives place more emphasis on the quality of action than on linear progression, a form of expression more akin to the long-standing American Indian tradition of storytelling. This may also be a possible reason for the lack of information on the aging process and aging issues. Many American Indian cultures see aging as a natural process, not worthy of examination as a distinct stage of life.

Gender Relations in American Indian Cultures

Much of the literature exclusively about American Indian women has addressed the issue of gender relations based on historical accounts and anthropological evidence. Although there were a few exceptions noted within American Indian cultures, this literature suggests that gender relations prior to contact with Euro-Christian cultures tended to be egalitarian in nature (Green, 1980; Allen, 1986; Tsosie, 1988; Bonvillain, 1989; LaFromboise, Heyle, & Ozer, 1990; Gutiérrez, 1991). These writers share the view that Native American women in general, and older Native American women in particular, had much higher status prior to contact with Euro-Christian culture. This body of literature persuasively argues that contact with patriarchal Anglo-European Christian culture undermined the status of women, especially in the public sphere.[1] Their analysis suggests that Anglo-European men viewed Indian men as having the same status difference and gender roles as they had with Anglo-European women. It is unclear whether or how Indian men might have resisted this assignation, but this process disenfranchised Indian women and changed gender roles within Indian societies as many Indian men accepted a patriarchal worldview introduced from outside.

These authors conclude that culture contact greatly deformed gender relations in American Indian cultures and created stereotypical views of Indian women that continue today. This tendency of Anglo-European thought has led to the dichotomous view of Indian women as either a "princess" or a "squaw" (Green, 1980; Albers, 1983; Tsosie, 1988; Bataille & Sands, 1991) or other "distorted images" (Medicine, 1988), the aged equivalents of which are the wise and respected elder or the useless old woman.

Many suggest that after a 500-year decline, the status of Indian women is on the rise (Green, 1980, 1992; Bataille & Sands, 1984; Allen, 1986, 1991; Tsosie, 1988; LaFromboise et al., 1990; Jaimes & Halsey, 1992). Each of these authors observed that gender roles within Indian societies are in the process of changing back to more traditional egalitarian forms that some (Tsosie, 1988; LaFromboise et al., 1990) labeled "retraditionalization." However, as Medicine (1988, p. 89) noted, "Native women must deal with the chauvinism and gender bias of the Native American leadership: men."

Heterogeneity among American Indians

Another important consideration in establishing a valid interpretive framework is the cultural heterogeneity among American Indians. In addition to contemporary gender differences, which have been neglected to a large degree, tribal diversity and the rural/urban bifurcation of the American Indian population are important factors to recognize. As Rapp (1979, p. 511) pointed out, the multitude of differences and similarities must be understood, "not by reducing them to one simple pattern," but simultaneously as a complex totality.

Despite the growth of Pan-Indianism (Hertzberg, 1971), especially in urban environments, tribal identity remains the most important anchor of self-identity among American Indians. There are approximately 300 federally recognized reservations; 500 tribes, bands, or Alaska Native villages; and an estimated 100 nonrecognized tribes in the United States. To a large degree, each of these rural and reservation groups continues to practice a unique cultural heritage.

Another factor to be considered in developing our understanding of American Indian aging is the rural/urban bifurcation of the American Indian population. The urbanization of the American Indian population during and after World War II has created two worlds of aging among American Indians (John, 1991) and constitutes a substantial impediment to our knowledge of American Indian aging, including issues relevant to the lives of Indian women elders. Approximately half of all American Indian elders live in urban environments, and very little is known about their status, characteristics, or experiences. Unlike their rural and reservation counterparts, American Indian elders who live in urban environments are dispersed among the general urban population. They have no tribal community or tribal government concerned with their welfare, nor do they have special governmental institutions such as the Indian Health Service (IHS) or Bureau of Indian Affairs (BIA) that are responsible for aspects of their well-being.

All of these themes and interpretive issues are linked together as powerful crosscurrents that affect the values, norms, behaviors, and experiences of American Indian women as they age. A number of authors have raised these issues in the context of a discussion of acculturation or assimilation (Wagner, 1976; Hanson, 1980) or, more appropriately, biculturation. For example, Wagner (1976) constructed a three-category typology based on the degree of acculturation among seventeen urban American Indian women. However, issues and implications of cultural values have not been fully investigated. Separately and together these issues are extremely important in any attempt to understand the aging of contemporary American Indian women.

DEMOGRAPHIC DATA

No work has yet addressed the gender differences among American Indian elders that can be documented by use of the 1900 U.S. census. Unfortunately, the Census Bureau has made it more difficult to ascertain gender differences among American Indian elders because of a decision to eliminate publication of the *Detailed Population Characteristics* volume that contained a great deal of information by age, sex, and race from previous census surveys (John, 1995). As a result, very little information is easily accessible by age, sex, and race from the 1990 data. However, a number of the basic features of the American Indian population can be ascertained.

In 1990 American Indian elders aged 60 or over comprised approximately 8.5% of the total American Indian population. Of the total American Indian population, approximately 3.7% were male elders and 4.8% were female elders (U.S. Department of Commerce, 1992). Based on this difference in survivorship, the median age of the female American Indian population was 27.2 years, compared to 25.3 years for American Indian males (U.S. Department of Commerce, 1992).

Sex Ratio

In 1990 the sex-ratio imbalance among American Indian elders was not as great as in the white elderly population. Approximately 56% of the American Indian population aged 60 or over was female, compared to 59% of the white elderly population (U.S. Department of Commerce, 1992). However, there are important sex-ratio differences between urban and rural American Indian elderly populations. In fact, the sex-ratio imbalance is particularly pronounced among urban American Indian elders aged 60 or over. Females comprised 58% of the urban American Indian elderly population but only 54% of the rural Indian elderly population. This represents a small convergence in the sex-ratio imbalance between 1980 and 1990 (John, 1995). The most obvious consequence of the sex-ratio difference is that urban American Indian female elders have substantially fewer American Indian male elders available as potential companions compared to their rural counterparts.

Marital Status

Higher male mortality greatly reduces the likelihood that American Indian female elders will have a spouse in later life. Among female Indian elders aged 60 or over, only 38% are currently married, 45% are widowed, 10% are divorced, 3% are separated, and 4% never married (U.S. Department of Commerce, 1992, table 34). In contrast, among American Indian male elders aged 60 or over, 66% are currently married, 15% are widowed, 10% are divorced, 3% are separated, and 7% never married. Overall, female American Indian elders aged 60 or over were far less likely than male Indian elders to be married (38% versus 66%) and three times more likely to be widowed (45% versus 15%). The most telling gender difference among American Indian elders aged 60 or over is that 66% of males have a spouse, while 62% of female elders do not.

By age 65–74 female elders are as likely to be widowed (42%) as currently married (41%). By age 75–84 female Indian elders are nearly three times as likely to be widowed (65%) as currently married (23%), and among elders over 85 years of age 83% of American Indian female elders are widowed. Female Indian elders, therefore, are at significant risk of social isolation and economic hardship as they age, a pattern evident in the general population as well.

Living Alone

American Indian female elders aged 60 or over are 1.7 times as likely as their male age peers to live alone (U.S. Department of Commerce, 1992, table 30). Differences in the proportion of male and female elders who live alone are relatively small between 60 and 64 years of age. However, after age 65 a disproportionate number of female American Indian elders live alone. After age 75, 43% of all female American Indian elders live alone. Indeed, after age 75, 75% of all elders who live alone are female. While living alone is an established risk factor to well-being in old age, support from family members does help to maintain some elders in the community. Beckett and Dungee-Anderson (1992) offered a positive resolution in the case study of 70-year-old Anita Thundercloud, who lived alone, became too ill to take care of herself, and was admitted to a rest home by a social worker without objection by her family. After regular visits, it was decided that Anita should return home with support of ten households close to her home. "Service providers ranged from 13 year-old grandchildren to 58 year-old children" (Beckett & Dungee-Anderson, 1992, p. 315).

Economic Status

According to the 1990 census (U.S. Department of Commerce, 1993, table 49), 29% of all American Indian elders aged 65 or over live in poverty. However, it is well known that marital status (McLaughlin & Holden, 1993) and living arrangements greatly influence the likelihood of experiencing economic deprivation. Among families headed by an American Indian householder aged 65 or over, 25% live in poverty. However, closer examination reveals the economic disadvantage of female elders and elders who live alone, the great majority of whom are female. Although the figure is high in comparison to the general elderly population, only 20% of married-couple families headed by an American Indian elder aged 65 or over live in poverty. In comparison, 37% of households headed by an American Indian female elder aged 65 or over with no husband present live in poverty, as do 43% of unrelated individuals.[2] Red Horse (1990) illustrated the extreme consequence of the impoverished situation of an 80-year-old Indian woman whose vision was impaired by glaucoma. She had led an active life and worked hard until shortly before her death, but according to Red Horse (1990, p. 2), she "died of conditions aggravated by poverty" when she tripped on the uneven floors of her "ramshackle" house and hit her head.

Educational Attainment

An important determinant of individual life chances, educational attainment is low and inversely related to age among American Indian elders. This trend favors succeeding generations of American Indian elders since educational attainment is highly correlated with socioeconomic status and other measures of well-being in later life. As among other groups, educational attainment and income are positively related among American Indian elders (John, 1995, p. 37). However, male Indian elders derive greater economic benefit from a given level of education than female elders, and the discrepancy between the genders increases as educational attainment increases.

PHYSICAL AND MENTAL HEALTH

American Indians are living longer because of improvements in health care during the last half century. According to the IHS (1991), life expectancy at birth increased by 20 years for American Indians (from 51 years to 71.1 years) during the 40-year period between 1940 and 1980. In comparison, life expectancy at birth for the white population increased by only 10 years (to 74.4 years) during the same period. For both populations, this increase in life expectancy was greater for females than for males. By 1980 life expectancy at birth for American Indian females had increased by 23 years (to 75.1 years), while American Indian male life expectancy had increased by approximately 16 years (to 67.1 years). The gap between American Indian and white life expectancy at birth has narrowed so that life expectancy at birth is only 3.6 years less for American Indian males and 3 years less for American Indian females.

Physical Health

Representative data on the health status of a portion of American Indians— including older women—has only recently become available from the 1987 Survey of American Indians and Alaska Natives (SAIAN). This survey, which parallels the 1987 National Medical Expenditure Survey for the U.S. adult population, included a sample of approximately 6,500 individuals who were eligible for care from the Indian Health Service and living on or near federally recognized reservations, the historic areas of Oklahoma, or in Alaska.

To date, the few published reports from the SAIAN data that allow us to characterize the health status of older American Indian women show that, relative to older American Indian men and to their female peers in the general U.S. population, this group experiences a number of advantages as well as disadvantages in terms of the prevalence of chronic diseases (Johnson & Taylor, 1991). American Indian females aged 45 to 64 had significantly lower rates of cardiovascular disease than their male counterparts (10% compared to 21%). These differences persist into old age, with 24% of American Indian women aged 65 or older suffering from cardiovascular conditions, compared to 35% of American Indian men in this age group. The rate of heart disease for older American Indian women also compares favorably to that of women aged 65 or older in the U.S. population as a whole (33%).

According to the SAIAN data, older American Indian women also enjoy a comparative advantage over older U.S. women in the occurrence of arthritis, the most prevalent chronic condition and source of activity limitation among the elderly (Institute of Medicine, 1991). Among middle-aged and aging women (ages 45–64), rates of arthritis were 34% for American Indians and 40% for women in the U.S. population. Likewise, arthritis was reported by 52% of American Indian women aged 65 or older and 61% of their U.S. female counterparts.

The lower incidence of arthritis should not be interpreted as lessening the impact of this disease on older Native American women. They, even more than the general population, depend on the use of their hands for the various art forms and craftwork deemed important in Indian life, as well as to perform a number of activities of daily living in rural areas such as chopping wood or hauling water, not commonly performed by elders in the general population. In fact, powerful descriptions of arthritis and its effects were found in stories by Native American women:

She was tired of being alone with the old woman whose body had been stiffening for as long as the girl could remember. Her knees and knuckles were swollen grotesquely and the pain had squeezed the brown skin of her face tight against the bones; it left her eyes hard like river stone. The girl asked once, what it was that did this to her body, and the old woman had raised up from sewing a sealskin boot, and stared at her. "The joints," the old woman said in a low voice, whispering like wind across the roof, "the joints are swollen with anger." (Silko, 1980b, p. 71)

U.S. women in the oldest age group also had a substantially higher prevalence of hypertension (53%)—the next most common chronic condition among the elderly—than did women in the SAIAN (38%). In terms of health disadvantages, the SAIAN study confirms a well-established epidemiologic fact that American Indian women (as well as men) suffer disproportionately from diabetes at all ages, with the highest rates occurring among women aged 65 or over (32%). Finally, American Indian women at all ages, and especially in old age, surpass American Indian men and the general population in rates of gallbladder disease.

Findings from the SAIAN on personal health practices (Lefkowitz & Underwood, 1991) also indicate that older Native American women less frequently avail themselves of several recommended health-screening services than do women in the general U.S. population. These services, including clinical breast examination and mammography to detect breast cancer and Pap testing for cervical cancer, are among those targeted by federal health objectives for the reduction of morbidity and mortality among older women in *Healthy People 2000* (U.S. Department of Health and Human Services, 1991). Of particular interest is the fact that the difference in utilization of periodic screening between women in the SAIAN and in the U.S. population increases with age. Although women in both groups are less likely to be screened at older ages, the decrease in rates of screening for breast and cervical cancer with age is even more pronounced for older American Indian women.

While the rate of breast examination among women in the U.S. population drops from 93% for those aged 50 to 59 to 86% for those 60 or older, the rate for American Indian women declines from 70% to 66% for the respective age groups. A similar pattern can be observed for the use of mammography. Screening rates for U.S. women decrease from 48% (ages 50 to 59) to 38% (ages 60 or older), compared to from 19% to 17% across the two age groups for women in the SAIAN. The nearly ubiquitous prevalence of Pap screening among U.S. women in their 50s (92%) is far less common among American Indian women at these ages (76%). Similarly, the comparative rates for women 60 years of age or older are 83% for the U.S. population and 64% for American Indians. These findings are significant in light of the heightened risk of cervical cancer among Indian women over the age of 60 compared to Caucasians, as demonstrated in previous epidemiologic research (Jordan & Key, 1981).

The issue of health screening is extremely important since American Indians had the worst five-year survival rate for lung, stomach, and breast cancer of the eight ethnic groups on which comparative information is available (Boss, 1990). Although it is unknown whether differences in later-life health practices between American Indian and non-Indian women result from issues of health care access or culture, or both, it is clear that older American Indian women experience a number of excess health risks through lack of periodic screening in comparison to their counterparts in the general population.

Accidental injuries among American Indian elders also reveal a significant gender difference. According to an IHS study of injuries between 1981 and 1985, female American Indian elders over 65 years old were less likely to die from an accident that involved a motor vehicle than were male Indian elders. According to this study (IHS, 1990, p. 46-A), 29% of injury deaths among American Indian males over 65 years old were the result of motor-vehicle accidents, compared to 25% of injury deaths among American Indian female elders. In contrast, falls accounted for approximately 15% of injury deaths among Indian male elders and 24% of injury deaths among Indian female elders.

Other health-status indicators document broader health differences between male and female American Indian elders. For the first time, the 1990 census included questions about the existence of two types of disability: a mobility or

Figure 19.1
American Indian Elders Aged 65 Years or Over with a Mobility or Self-Care Limitation by Sex, 1990

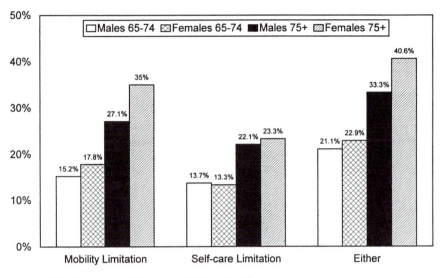

Source: U.S. Department of Commerce (1993), table 40.

self-care limitation. Either of these conditions was defined as the result of the existence of a physical or mental health condition that lasted for six months or more. A mobility limitation is a global measure of the ability to perform instrumental activities of daily living outside the home, such as shopping or going to the doctor's office. A self-care limitation is a global measure of the ability to perform personal activities of daily living inside the home, such as dressing or bathing. As seen in figure 19.1, data suggest that health-related limitations on mobility or self-care are more common among females than males. This gender difference is particularly pronounced for a mobility limitation. Overall, the differences in the percentages of elders with self-care limitations were quite small.

Other information on the physical health status of American Indian elders does not add greatly to our understanding of older Indian women. One common problem with much of the scholarly literature about the health of aging American Indian women is a small sample size and/or a very narrow focus that precludes valid generalization. For example, a study of bone density in postmenopausal American Indian females (Evers, Orchard, & Haddad, 1985) found that the Indian women in the study had less bone mass than Caucasian women of similar age. In addition, the predictors and primary determinants of bone density were not the same for Caucasian and Indian women. However, the sample included only 34 Indian women from three tribes (Oneida, Chippewa, and Muncey). Although pioneering and suggestive, this study and others like it are hardly enough to extrapolate the findings to American Indian women in general.

Mental Health

Very little is known about the mental health status of older American Indian women. Barón et al.'s (1990) study of depressive symptomatology in 314 adults aged 45 or older with chronic disease among four Pacific Northwest tribes constitutes the only source of sex-specific information on the prevalence of a mental disorder among older Indian women. Analysis of scores obtained for the sample using the Center for Epidemiologic Studies Depression Scale (CES-D) demonstrated that females were significantly more likely than males to exceed the threshold score for depression (38% versus 16%). This finding of the higher prevalence of depression among Indian women is consistent with findings for the general U.S. population. However, although the prevalence estimates for depression in this sample of American Indians exceeds those found for older whites with chronic illness (Berkman et al., 1986), because these estimates are not broken down by both age and sex, we do not know how women in this sample compare in their experience of depression to various age groups of non-Indian women.

Other indicators of the mental health status of older American Indian women can be discerned from attitudinal studies. Despite a generally positive portrayal of the roles and status reserved for old age among American Indians, two studies of aging among American Indian women revealed negative views of the aging process. Hunter, Linn, and Pratt's (1979) study of married white, black, Cuban, Indian, and Chicano women aged 35 through 45 found that the 57 Indian women had the most negative attitude toward death, the least favorable views of old age, and the most negative view of the family of the groups studied. These findings, however, must be approached with caution because the authors provided little information on the details of their methodology and little interpretation of their findings.

Richek, Chuculate, and Klinert (1971), using a retrospective technique, found that "healthy" Indian women become significantly less optimistic as they age and that the disengagement process is different for Indian and Caucasian women. They found that Indian women disengage from peers and work first, while Caucasian women disengage from children and authority figures. Their most valid findings, based solely on an analysis of current attitudes, were that aged Indian women had significantly more positive attitudes toward children and authority figures and less positive attitudes toward work than their Caucasian age peers. In addition, this study of 35 Indian women and 15 Caucasian women, mean ages 71.7 and 73.9, respectively, found that the Indian women chose their mean happiest age to be 32, a full 10 years younger than the age chosen by the Caucasian women.

However, Harris, Page, and Begay (1988) in their study of a convenience sample of 257 American Indian, Hispanic, and Anglo subjects (median age 60), which included 82 Indian women, found no ethnic differences in mean happiest ages. Although there were significant ethnic differences in number of children, household size, educational attainment, and subjects' ages, few ethnic differences in attitudes toward aging were found. The only significant between-group difference was that American Indians were more likely to enjoy spending time with old people than were Anglos.

Life satisfaction is the only other mental health issue that has been researched among American Indian elders. Johnson et al. (1986) examined the life satisfaction of 58 elderly American Indians (76% of whom were female) between the ages of 51 and 85 who resided on two midwestern reservations. These authors tested the relationship between seventeen independent variables and life-satisfaction scores. Their analysis revealed that the frequency of conversations with others, loneliness, the extent to which illness impaired the ability to perform activities of daily living, condition of eyesight and hearing, and subjective assessment of physical health were the best predictors of life satisfaction.

Using the same data for American Indians, Johnson et al. (1988) compared life satisfaction and mental health among white, black, Hispanic, Jewish, and American Indian elders. Although the limitations of this study make any conclusions tentative, American Indian elders had the second-worst life satisfaction of the five groups. Only Hispanic elders reported lower life satisfaction than Indian elders. However, Indian elders differed from Hispanics on only one of the four measures of life satisfaction. Compared to Hispanics, Indian elders reported higher levels of zest, which was defined as enthusiasm and interest in life.

Johnson et al. (1986) suggested that variables associated with health may be useful as indicators of life satisfaction in elderly reservation American Indians. Moreover, they also suggested that subjective measures of life satisfaction may be more predictive of mental health status than objective measures. Although sufficient research findings are lacking, mental health, happiness, and life satisfaction for many older American Indian women may be tied, even more so than among females in the general population, to physical health status. Davidson's (1982, pp. 137–138) description of the enigma of growing old is a good synopsis of this relationship:

You see how it is to be old, real hard. If my hands were all right [arthritis], I could do so much weaving. If my ears were all right I could be so happy. *Q'edaəng e?du ijing*— "old and good for nothing." I'm just like an old tree. Nothing's good for it. Sunshine makes it crack, and then the rain soaks in the cracks. But as long as you stay healthy you don't feel old. I know I'm old but I still enjoy myself. What I see still makes me happy.

STATUS AND ROLES

According to Green (1980, p. 263), most "Native American women look forward to being old—an elder—when their words, actions, and leadership come to be respected." Block (1979, p. 188), however, felt that traditional respect for older people "is fast eroding" in contemporary Indian societies because of federal program emphasis on the young. John (1988) also argued that the historical existence of increased status with age may be changing due to the increasing acculturation of young American Indians; that is, they may adopt the negative view of age of the dominant culture. Barber, Cook, and Ackerman (1985), however, in a study of 83 Navajo youth found no correlation between acculturation and attitude toward filial responsibility, connoting a continued endorsement of traditional values and respect for elders.

Unfortunately, very few studies have investigated status issues or how status has been changing. Shepardson's (1982) interviews of 27 Navajo women, a few Navajo men, and a few "others" exemplifies the state of research as well as the mixed opinions on the contemporary status of Indian women. The three basic views on the current status of Navajo women include the following: (1) conditions are better and status is higher now; (2) economic improvements have occurred, but women's overall status is the same; and (3) the "old days" were better for women.

Status

Many Native American legends and creation stories support powerful and influential status for women (Fisher, 1980; Tsosie, 1988; Allen, 1991). The Navajo's Changing Woman is responsible for all new life as well as successful crop growth; she taught customs to the People, just as older women of the tribe do today. In the Cheyenne legend "Old Woman of the Spring," it is the old woman who has the knowledge and power to restore the buffalo to the people. Grandmother Spider, despite the infirmities of old age, succeeded in bringing firelight to the world when younger males had failed and taught the Cherokee the art of pottery making. The power of women depicted in these and other stories helps create strong self-images for Indian women and continues to enhance the position of older women in Indian society today.

Historically, the status of women in general, and older women in particular, was higher in matrilocal/matrilineal societies than in patrilocal/patrilineal ones. Regardless of inheritance and residence patterns, however, most scholars agree that age did, and still does, enhance a woman's status in Indian culture. Two things occur with age to enhance the status of older Indian women: increased life experiences that empower elders to provide guidance for the young and the removal of certain ritual and social taboos associated with the reproductive cycle. For example, Hammerschlag (1988, p. 105) explained that the "Indian worldview is pragmatic—you can't know anything until you've done it. . . . knowledge from experience is why you have to be gray to be able to heal." Advancing age also weakens social constraints or provides new social opportunities. For instance, Cypress (1993) described the restrictions traditionally placed on Indian women during menstruation, and although she said that many young women disregard the taboos today, she noted that there is certain medicine work that only elderly women may do. Crowley (1994) pointed out that in contrast to the Western view that menopause is a bleak event, for Native Americans it can be viewed favorably because it entitles women to participate in previously restricted activities.

Economic change has also altered the status of American Indian females. In general, the shift that occurred during the twentieth century from subsistence economic activities to wage work initially undermined Indian females' traditional roles and status, even within the family. However, the negative consequences of economic change on the status of Indian females were short term because of their adaptation to the wage economy and the broader economic shift from manufacturing to service occupations in which females are able to find employment. Now, with employment opportunities in the service sector as well as status derived from traditional roles and activities, the overall status of American Indian women is probably better than before wage work altered economic patterns in Indian Country. The loss of traditional sources of income for older Indian women has also been offset by the institution of federal aid programs. In 1949 Indians became eligible for several types of federal aid: to dependent children, to the blind, and to the aged. Since Indian women outlive Indian men and are far more likely to raise children or grandchildren as a single head of household, they especially benefit from these income supports. The receipt of regular income—whether from wage work, federal programs, or traditional economic activities—is definitely advantageous for older American Indian women and helps secure their status.

Roles

Along with the status of aging women, role is a much-discussed theme in almost every genre of the literature. An important issue that has not been fully researched, however, is role change. The few scholars who have studied this issue differ on whether men's or women's roles have changed the most. Some observers of the Navajo (Witherspoon, 1975; Christopherson, 1981) suggest that men's gender roles have changed more than women's because women continue to exercise economic power in subsistence residential units that have been the basis of the traditional Navajo tribal economy for over a century. Blanchard (1975), however, maintained the opposite for the Navajo. He claimed that Protestant sects have afforded Indian women new gender roles and statuses to compensate for the loss of roles and prestige that has accompanied economic change. Blanchard found that Navajo women who had joined either of the Protestant churches on the Ramah Reservation had twice the formal education, were twice as likely to work outside the home, were more likely to have lived and worked off the reservation, were more likely to live in a neolocal situation and in smaller households, were more likely to have fewer children, and were less likely to honor traditional social obligations than their more traditional counterparts. Although opinions of older Indian women's status varied, there was general consensus about their main roles: grandmother/caregiver, educator/wisdom keeper, leader, artist, and dependent old woman.

Grandmother/Caregiver. Among the important features of American Indian families in which extended-family relationships are present are the special nature of the grandparent-grandchild relationship (Tefft, 1968; Ball, 1970; Lewis, 1981; Ryan, 1981) and the singular importance of the grandmother in the family network (John, 1988). Indeed, the grandmother is the center of American Indian family life, and she holds the family together. Many authors (Fisher, 1980; Shomaker, 1989; Crow Dog & Erdoes, 1990; Bradford & Thom, 1992; Green, 1992) described the grandmother's role as primary caregiver for grandchildren, especially on reservations. Given the tendency among American Indians to begin childbearing at a very early age, it is common for a woman to be a grandmother by the time she is 40 and often by the time she is in her mid-30s.

Although motherhood is an important transition in the life course, marking the status of becoming a woman, grandmotherhood may be an even more important transition because of the additional family and other responsibilities a woman assumes (both real and symbolic). A young Cherokee medicine woman, Dhyani Ywahoo (Perrone, Stockel, & Krueger, 1989, p. 68), said, "I learned constantly from the elders. Even now, because by our tradition, you're not really manifest as an adult until you're fifty-one. . . . [Women] are usually beyond individual family bearing at age fifty-one and able to be mother for all things."

Grandmothers also provide tangible support. Women who have children while they are teenagers frequently have little inclination or preparation for motherhood, and some irresponsibility is anticipated and tolerated (Metcalf, 1979), as long as it does not endanger the well-being of the child. Generally, the young woman looks to her mother for assistance and training and frequently passes a great deal of responsibility for the care of the child to her mother. In fact, on occasion the grandmother takes over rearing one or more grandchildren because she or other family members feel that the child is not being raised properly or the parent(s) decide that it will benefit the child (Guillemin, 1975; Miller, 1979; Shomaker, 1989). A child may also go to live with a family member who needs help that the child can provide or if a family member would like to have a child around (Underhill, 1965), a process that Shomaker (1989) has documented among contemporary Navajo grandmothers. It is also not unusual for a child to ask to live with grandparents, a request that is honored if it is not a manifest impossibility. Shomaker (1989) also acknowledged that a child's desires are an important consideration among the Navajo in the unlikely event that a grandchild no longer wishes to live with her or his grandmother.

Despite the centrality of grandmotherhood in the family life of American Indians, very few scholarly studies have investigated the topic. Shomaker (1989, 1990) produced two closely related works about Navajo grandmothers that provide some insight into this role. Her first effort characterized the circumstances surrounding the placement of one or more grandchildren ($N = 98$) with their grandmother. The types of situations that most commonly precipitated the placement of grandchildren in the care of their grandmother included "a deficit in parenting skills" that created an "unhealthy living environment for the grandchildren" (36% of the cases); a change in the parent's lifestyle, including death of a parent, an off-reservation job, or remarriage (32% of the placements); a family work load that was too heavy for the mother, who was often unwed and unable to provide adequate care to the children (18% of the cases); and the "grandmother's needs" (14% of the cases). In this last instance, grandchildren were sometimes given to the grandmother as a sign of respect. Grandmothers were also given children because they said that they were lonely and wanted to have a child around for companionship or that they would like to raise another child.

Shomaker's second article (1990) introduced some confusion into the characterization of the role of Navajo grandmothers and the transfer of grandchildren to their care. Her thesis was that grandchildren are transferred to the care of grandmothers on the conscious expectation that this will secure care in old age when the grandmother becomes frail. She admitted (1989, 1990), however, that frequently this arrangement does not result in care by the grandchildren in later life. The difficulty with her thesis and the representation of the situation is the explicit nature of the exchange she posited. As her previous work has shown, only a small percentage of cases of fosterage (14%) occur because the child will serve to meet a need of the grandmother. In the great preponderance of cases, the child is provided care because of family problems that the grandmother is not willing to let adversely affect her grandchild. Our experience suggests that interventions by the grandmother to provide care to her grandchildren are based, at best, on a sentiment of generalized reciprocity, rather than a rational calculation of some expected future benefit.

Although it is frequently described in autobiographies and literature, far less has been documented about the personal relationship between grandmothers and grandchildren. Citing work by Leighton and Kluckhohn (1948), Shomaker (1989, pp. 6–7) characterized the relationship between grandmother and grandchild as "very warm, loving, solicitous, and indulgent." The degree to which this is typical of the grandmother-grandchild relationship and whether and how this may differ from the stereotypical grandmother role in American culture is yet to be fully investigated.

Based on a study of only 28 grandparents living in 17 households composed of elders who had returned to tribal homelands from urban areas, Weibel-Orlando (1990) identified five common and sometimes overlapping grandparenting styles. These were the "cultural conservator" grandparent (35% of the households) who eagerly seeks to care for grandchildren for extended periods of time in order to socialize them into American Indian lifeways; the "custodial grandparent" (18% of the households) who is thrust into this caretaking situation because of some type of family disruption; the "ceremonial grandparent" (12% of households) who has face-to-face interaction with grandchildren (and children) at regular intervals and otherwise maintains contact throughout the year during holidays, birthdays, and other special occasions; the "distanced grand-parent" (18% of households) whose visits are infrequent, not tied to family events or holidays, and reflect the growing divergence between the values and lifestyles of some portions of urban and rural-reservation populations; and the "fictive grandparent" (18% of households) who forms relationships with nonkin because of the lack or absence of biological grandchildren.

The only challenge to this general consensus about the preeminent position of the Indian grandmother has been offered by Bea Medicine. According to Medicine (1981, p. 19), the literature may popularize the role of grandmother at the expense of the socialization provided by a broader kin group: "More data are needed on the frequency of child care exchange and the utilization of kinship networks for child care in most Indian groups. There is always mention of 'Grandmother' as a primary socializer in current native rhetoric, but little about the utilization of kin groups in the socialization process of children."

Educator/Wisdom Keeper. It is hard to separate the role of "grandmother" from that of educator and storyteller who passes on tribal traditions and knowl-edge. Shomaker (1990) mentioned the grandmother's role in dispensing wisdom about developing and maintaining a household and in child rearing. However, Bradford and Thom (1992, p. 24) summed up the most frequent contemporary viewpoint: "At the end of a woman's life she was still useful to her family and tribe. She was respected for her knowledge, wisdom and power. Today, mothers and grandmothers continue to teach generations worth of traditions to their chil-dren and grandchildren." Fisher (1980) agreed, calling the grandmother the "supreme storyteller" in many Plains and Pueblo cultures and "integral to the oral tradition."

Life sketches also provide examples of older Indian women's contemporary role as educator and wise elder. According to Morez (1977, p. 126), "In Navajo society, the woman is the dominant figure who becomes the wise one in her old age." In another example, Painter and Valois (1985) described a Sioux Indian woman elder who now lives in the San Francisco Bay area serving urban Indians as healer, spiritual leader, and teacher.

Political Leader. Historically, Indian women have exercised political leader-ship within Indian cultures, whether such leadership was manifested formally in the public sphere or in less obvious, but no less important, ways within family and clan structures. One sign of the rise of Indian women to public leadership positions within American Indian tribes is their election to tribal chairperson. A number of well-known examples of this exist. However, a more important and prevalent contemporary sign is the number of mature Indian women who direct tribal health, social service, and other governmental agencies. Women leaders in midlevel administrative and managerial positions are quite common through-out Indian Country. Irene Stewart's (1980, p. 84) participation in tribal programs for elderly Navajos—she was described as "a senior citizen herself, playing her part as always in the planning and execution of programs to benefit her peo-ple"—illustrates the formal and informal leadership role elders frequently play within tribal political and service systems. Hanson (1980) depicted a similar process of increasing educational attainment, labor-force participation, and political leadership by urban American Indian women.

Women's political leadership is also a common theme in other types of literature. Crow Dog and Erdoes (1990, p. 113) pointed out an example of the leadership role older American Indian women played in the Wounded Knee struggle: "Wounded Knee was not the brainchild of wild, foaming-at-the-mouth militants, but of patient and totally unpolitical, traditional Sioux, mostly old Sioux ladies." Jaimes and Halsey (1992, p. 328) agreed, saying, "The staunchest and most active traditionalist support came from elder Oglala women." Jaimes and Halsey (1992) gave a number of other examples of older Indian women providing contemporary political leadership during the struggles over northern California land claims, western Washington fishing rights, and the Navajo-Hopi land dispute.

Artist. Another salient historical and contemporary contribution of American Indian women is the creation of decorative and ceremonial objects (Schneider, 1983). As Woodhead (1994, p. 129) noted, despite "declining physical ability, many Indian artisans reach an artistic peak late in their lives." There are many examples of the craftsmanship of older contemporary Indian women. For example, Albers and Medicine (1983) documented the uses, meaning, and significance of the star quilt in understanding the continued importance of female art in Sioux ceremonial life. In other cases artistic accomplishments by older women artists have broken gender barriers rather than reinforcing traditional gender activities. For instance, Sands (1992), in her review of a Haida woman's autobiography, noted that it was only in her later years that Davidson broke the sexual barrier and asserted herself as an artist in the male form of decorative painting.

In addition to breaking gender barriers, art has often been critical to the economic support of older Indian women. During World War II many Zuni women took up the craft of jewelry making to support their families while Zuni men were overseas fighting (Adair, 1944). In a study of elderly Shonto weavers, Russell and McDonald (1982) noted that weaving contributed almost half of the women's incomes. Craft production of secular or sacred objects (whether beadwork, basketry, rug weaving, pottery, or leatherwork) continues to provide prestige and financial rewards for Indian women.

Dependent Old Woman. The roles previously discussed all involve active contributions on the part of the older woman to the life of the extended family and the tribe. In fact, as Trimble (1993, p. 115) pointed out, "As long as the community recognizes elders and gives them opportunities to fulfill their roles in tribal and ceremonial life, elders remain vital and purposeful." The issue of the inevitable dependencies of old age and their consequences for the contemporary American Indian woman are highlighted in the distinction between "elders" and "elderlies" (Weibel-Orlando, 1989; Trimble, 1993). While the former category indicates persons to whom esteem is accorded due to their experience and wisdom, the latter, somewhat pejorative, category denotes older persons who, because of their dependencies, are the recipients of various government services.

This distinction between elders and elderlies is simplistic and overdrawn. If the term "elder" only applies to an exceptionally limited number of persons in each tribe who are the preeminent bearers and exemplars of the culture and the alternate assignation applies to dependent older persons, then many older Indians fit neither category. Frequently, "elderlies" is simply used as a plural noun by people who work in aging services and who clearly intend to make no invidious distinction or show the least disrespect. Moreover, "elders" can be highly dependent on a variety of aging services and age-based entitlement programs. Indeed, the desire to preserve Indian cultures is a frequently mentioned motivation behind the development of comprehensive aging services for American Indians.

We suggest that the Indian values related to these issues of culture and aging are more complex. In American Indian societies total dependence is no more valued than total independence. However, evidence suggests that where traditional American Indian values are operating, dependence and need in old age are perhaps less harshly judged than in Anglo culture (Clark & Anderson, 1967). For example, in a qualitative study of family caregiving among Pueblo Indians, Hennessy and John (1995) highlighted the culturally patterned attitudes toward dependency and the expectation, ready acceptance, and assumption of the role of primary or main caregiver to a frail elderly relative among Pueblo women. For the caregivers in the study, providing care to functionally dependent elders was a significant expression of their identity as American Indians and reflected the importance of interdependence, or connectedness and reciprocity, within the extended family and the tribe that continues into dependent old age.

CONCLUSION

It is only in the last twenty-five years that gender studies have begun to focus proper attention on the contributions of women to society. This effort, especially among Anglo women, has led to important philosophical debates, theoretical developments, and increased research on women's issues. Without doubt, more basic and applied research needs to be done. With the changes in consciousness and a growing research momentum, future advances in knowledge of women's issues are to be expected.

Unfortunately, Indian women in general, and aging Indian women in particular, have not fully profited from increased research attention. This chapter reflects the deficits in our knowledge. Single, exploratory studies of particular topics are the norm, and many studies rely on convenience samples, employ small sample sizes, use questionable analytic techniques, and make unwarranted generalizations. Moreover, many of the researchers who have attempted to contribute to our knowledge have not shown the sustained intellectual commitment necessary to produce enduring results on any topic. In addition, the research has not adequately addressed the implications of the cultural diversity within the Indian population. As a consequence, very little research has produced solid, much less definitive, results. Assembling a picture of aging and American Indian women currently requires an iterative process of culling information and triangulating data from a variety of sources (both empirical and literary). Advancing our research knowledge of aging American Indian women requires the use of a variety of methods, research designs, and analytic techniques, in addition to greatly increased and sustained scholarly efforts.

What can be documented of the gender differences between aging American Indian women and men suggests that more attention needs to be given to the status, characteristics, and experiences of aging American Indian women. Although American Indian women obviously share common experiences and problems with American Indian men, such as the experience of a cultural minority in an aggressive, dominant culture, our research also documents significant gender differences that merit further study. As is true of the general population, American Indian women have higher life expectancy than American Indian males, a consequence of lower mortality over the life course. However, they also report a higher incidence of impairment that limits their ability to perform activities of daily living, experience greater poverty, are three times more likely to be widowed, and are more likely to live alone than American Indian male elders.

However, broad areas of interest and concern are yet to be fully investigated. Certainly, this statement is true of Indian women's physical and mental health status. A variety of family issues also need to be investigated. Among these, the changing status of Indian women and the means by which status is achieved, gender relations, and many important aspects of recognized roles (e.g., caregiver or grandmother) need concerted attention. Without a greatly expanded and refined research agenda, the lives of aging American Indian women will remain hidden, and the stereotypes that dominate conceptualizations of Indian women will go unchallenged and uncorrected.

NOTES

1. Albers (1983) and Albers and Medicine (1983, p. 137) pointed out that in Indian societies ''there has never been a clear-cut separation between public and domestic spheres. In the Sioux scheme of things, family and community are one and the same thing.''

2. According to the U.S. Bureau of the Census definition, an unrelated individual is someone who lives alone or with nonrelatives, is not related to the householder, or is a person living in group quarters who is not living in an institution.

REFERENCES

Adair, J. J. (1944). *The Navaho and Pueblo silversmith*. Norman: University of Oklahoma Press.

Albers, P. (1983). Introduction: New perspectives on Plains Indian women. In P. Albers & B. Medicine (Eds.), *The hidden half: Studies of Plains Indian women* (pp. 1–26). Washington, DC: University Press of America.

Albers, P., & Medicine, B. (1983). The role of Sioux women in the production of ceremonial objects: The case of the star quilt. In P. Albers & B. Medicine (Eds.), *The hidden half: Studies of Plains Indian women* (pp. 123–140). Washington, DC: University Press of America.

Allen, P. G. (1986). *The sacred hoop: Recovering the feminine in American Indian traditions.* Boston: Beacon Press.

———. (1991). *Grandmothers of the light: A medicine woman's sourcebook.* Boston: Beacon Press.

Ball, E. (1970). *In the days of Victorio: Recollections of a Warm Springs Apache.* Tucson: University of Arizona Press.

Barber, C. E., Cook, A. S., & Ackerman, A. (1985). The influence of acculturation on attitudes of filial responsibility among Navajo youth. *American Indian Quarterly, 9*(4), 421–432.

Barón, A. E., Manson, S. M., Ackerson, L. M., & Brenneman, D. L. (1990). Depressive symptomatology in older American Indians with chronic disease: Some psychometric considerations. In C. C. Attkisson & J. M. Zich (Eds.), *Depression in primary care: Screening and detection* (pp. 217–231). New York: Routledge Chapman & Hall.

Bataille, G. M., & Sands, K. M. (1984). *American Indian women: Telling their lives.* Lincoln: University of Nebraska Press.

———. (1991). *American Indian women: A guide to research.* New York: Garland.

Beckett, J. O., & Dungee-Anderson, D. (1992). Older minorities: Asian, Black, Hispanic, and Native Americans. In R. L. Schneider & N. P. Kropf (Eds.), *Gerontological social work: Knowledge, service settings, and special populations* (pp. 277–322). Chicago: Nelson-Hall.

Berkman, L. F., Berkman, C. S., Kasl, S., Freeman, D. H., Leo, L., Ostfeld, A. M., Cornoni-Huntley, J., & Brody, J. A. (1986). Depressive symptoms in relation to physical health and functioning in the elderly. *American Journal of Epidemiology, 124,* 372–388.

Blanchard, K. (1975). Changing sex roles and Protestantism among the Navajo women in Ramah. *Journal for the Scientific Study of Religion, 14,* 43–50.

Block, M. R. (1979). Exiled Americans: The plight of Indian aged in the U.S. In D. E. Gelfand & A. J. Kutzik (Eds.), *Ethnicity and aging: Theory, research, and policy* (pp. 184–192). New York: Springer.

Blowsnake, S. (1963). *The autobiography of a Winnebago Indian,* P. Radin, Trans. New York: Dover.

Bonvillain, N. (1989). Gender relations in Native North America. *American Indian Culture and Research Journal, 13*(2), 1–28.

Boss, L. (1990). Cancer. In *Indian health conditions* (pp. 23–69). Washington, DC: Indian Health Service.

Bradford, C. J., & Thom, L. (1992). *Dancing colors: Paths of Native American women.* San Francisco: Chronicle Books.

Brumble, H. D. (1981). *An annotated bibliography of American Indian and Eskimo autobiographies.* Lincoln: University of Nebraska Press.

———. (1988). *American Indian autobiography.* Berkeley: University of California Press.

Christopherson, V. A. (1981). The rural Navajo family. In R. T. Coward & W. M. Smith, Jr. (Eds.), *The family in rural society* (pp. 105–111). Boulder, CO: Westview Press.

Clark, M., & Anderson, B. G. (1967). *Culture and aging: An anthropological study of older Americans.* Springfield, IL: C. C. Thomas

Crow Dog, M., & Erdoes, R. (1990). *Lakota woman.* New York: Harper Collins.

Crowley, S. L. (1994, May). The menopausal puzzle: Much ado about menopause. *AARP and NRTA Bulletin,* p. 2.

Cruikshank, J. (1990). *Life lived like a story: Life stories of three Yukon Native elders.* Lincoln: University of Nebraska Press.

Culley, M. (Ed.). (1992). *American women's autobiography: Fea(s)ts of memory.* Madison: University of Wisconsin Press.

Cypress, A. (1993). Men were taught more than women. In S. Wall, *Wisdom's daughters: Conversations with women elders of Native America* (pp. 85–90). New York: Harper Collins.

Davidson, F. E., as told to M. Blackman. (1982). *During my time.* Seattle: University of Washington Press.

Eakin, P. J. (1985). *Fictions in autobiography: Studies in the art of self-invention.* Princeton, NJ: Princeton University Press.

Erdrich, L. (1984). *Love medicine.* New York: Harper Collins.

Evers, S. E., Orchard, J. W., & Haddad, R. G. (1985). Bone density in postmenopausal North American Indian and Caucasian females. *Human Biology, 57*(4), 719–726.

Fisher, D. (Ed.). (1980). *The third woman: Minority women writers of the United States.* Boston: Houghton Mifflin.

Green, R. (1980). Native American women. *Signs: Journal of Women and Culture in Society, 6*(2), 248–267.

————. (1983). *Native American women: A contextual bibliography.* Bloomington: Indiana University Press.

————. (1992). *Women in American Indian society.* New York: Chelsea House.

Guillemin, J. (1975). *Urban renegades: The cultural strategy of American Indians.* New York: Columbia University Press.

Gusdorf, G. (1980). Conditions and limits of autobiography. In J. Olney (Ed.), *Autobiography: Essays theoretical and critical* (pp. 28–48). Princeton, NJ: Princeton University Press.

Gutiérrez, R. A. (1991). *When Jesus came, the Corn Mothers went away: Marriage, sexuality, and power in New Mexico, 1500–1846.* Stanford, CA: Stanford University Press.

Hammerschlag, C. A. (1988). *The dancing healers: A doctor's journey of healing with Native Americans.* San Francisco: Harper & Row.

Hanson, W. (1980). The urban Indian woman and her family. *Social Casework, 61*(8), 476–483.

Harris, M. B., Page, P., & Begay, C. (1988). Attitudes toward aging in a Southwestern sample: Effects of ethnicity, age, and sex. *Psychological Reports, 62,* 735–746.

Hennessy, C. H., & John, R. (1995). The interpretation of burden among Pueblo Indian caregivers. *Journal of Aging Studies, 9*(3), 215–229.

Hertzberg, H. W. (1971). *The search for an American Indian identity.* Syracuse: Syracuse University Press.

Hunter, K., Linn, M. W., & Pratt, T. C. (1979). Minority women's attitudes about aging. *Journal of Experimental Aging Research, 5*(2), 95–108.

Indian Health Service. (1990). *Injuries among American Indians and Alaska Natives.* Rockville, MD: Author.

———. (1991). *Trends in Indian health.* Rockville, MD: Author.

Institute of Medicine. (1991). *Disability in America: Toward a national agenda for prevention.* A. M. Pope & A. R. Tarlov (Eds.). Washington, DC: National Academy Press.

Jaimes, M. A., with Halsey, T. (1992). American Indian women at the center of indigenous resistance in contemporary North America. In M. A. Jaimes (Ed.), *The state of Native America: Genocide, colonization, and resistance* (pp. 311–344). Boston: South End Press.

John, R. (1988). The Native American family. In C. H. Mindel, R. W. Habenstein, & R. Wright, Jr. (Eds.), *Ethnic families in America: Patterns and variations* (3rd ed., pp. 325–363). New York: Elsevier.

———. (1991). The state of research on American Indian elders' health, income security, and social support networks. In *Minority elders: Longevity, economics, and health* (pp. 38–50). Washington, DC: Gerontological Society of America.

———. (1995). *American Indian and Alaska Native elders: An assessment of their current status and provision of services.* Rockville, MD: Indian Health Service.

Johnson, A., & Taylor, A. (1991). *Prevalence of chronic diseases: A summary of data from the survey of American Indians and Alaska Natives* (AHCPR Pub. No. 91-0031). Rockville, MD: Public Health Service, Agency for Health Care Policy and Research.

Johnson, F. L., Cook, E., Foxall, M. J., Kelleher, E., Kentopp, E., & Mannlein, E. A. (1986). Life satisfaction of the elderly American Indian. *International Journal of Nursing Studies, 23,* 265–273.

Johnson, F. L., Foxall, M. J., Kelleher, E., Kentopp, E., & Mannlein, E. A., Cook, E. (1988). Comparison of mental health and life satisfaction of five elderly ethnic groups. *Western Journal of Nursing Research, 10*(5), 613–628.

Jordan, S. W., & Key, C. R. (1981). Carcinoma of the cervix in southwestern American Indians: Results of a cytologic detection program. *Cancer, 47,* 2523–2532.

LaFromboise, T. D., Heyle, A. M., & Ozer, E. J. (1990). Changing and diverse roles of women in American Indian cultures. *Sex Roles, 22*(7/8), 455–476.

Landes, R. (1971). *The Ojibwa woman.* New York: W. W. Norton.

Lefkowitz, D. C., & Underwood, C. (1991). *Personal health practices: Findings from the Survey of American Indians and Alaska Natives* (AHCPR Pub. No. 91–0034). Rockville, MD: Public Health Service, Agency for Health Care Policy and Research.

Leighton, D., & Kluckhohn, C. (1948). *Children of the people.* Cambridge, MA: Harvard University Press.

Lewis, R. (1981). Patterns of strength of American Indian families. In J. Red Horse, A. Shattuck, & F. Hoffman (Eds.), *The American Indian family: Strengths and stresses* (pp. 101–106). Isleta, NM: American Indian Social Research and Development Associates.

McLaughlin, D. K., & Holden, K. C. (1993). Nonmetropolitan elderly women: A portrait of economic vulnerability. *Journal of Applied Gerontology, 12*(3), 320–334.

Medicine, B. (1981). American Indian family: Cultural change and adaptive strategies. *Journal of Ethnic Studies, 8*(4), 13–23.

———. (1988). Native American (Indian) women: A call for research. *Anthropology & Education Quarterly, 19*(2), 86–92.

Metcalf, A. (1979). Family reunion: Networks and treatment in a Native American community. *Group Psychotherapy, Psychodrama, and Sociometry, 32*, 179–189.

Miller, D. (1979). The Native American family: The urban way. In E. Corfman (Ed.), *Families today: A research sampler on families and children* (pp. 441–484). Washington, DC: U.S. Government Printing Office.

Morez, M. (1977). The woman is the dominant figure. In J. B. Katz (Ed.), *I am the fire of time: The voices of Native American women* (pp. 126–127). New York: E. P. Dutton.

Niethammer, C. (1977). *Daughters of the earth: The lives and legends of American Indian women.* New York: Collier Books.

Painter, C., & Valois, P. (1985). *Gifts of age.* San Francisco: Chronicle Books.

Perrone, B., Stockel, H. H., & Krueger, V. (1989). *Medicine women, curanderas, and women doctors.* Norman: University of Oklahoma Press.

Qoyawayma, P., as told to V. Carlson. (1964). *No turning back.* Albuquerque: University of New Mexico Press.

Rapp, R. (1979). Anthropology. *Signs: Journal of Women in Culture and Society, 4*(3), 497–513.

Red Horse, J. G. (1990). *American Indian aging: Issues in income, housing, and transportation.* Research paper presented at Minority Affairs Initiative Empowerment Conferences. Washington, DC: AARP.

Richek, H. G., Chuculate, O., & Klinert, D. (1971). Aging and ethnicity in healthy elderly women. *Geriatrics, 26*, 146–152.

Russell, S. C., & McDonald, M. B. (1982). The economic contributions of women in a rural western Navajo community. *American Indian Quarterly, 6*(3&4), 262–282.

Ryan, R. A. (1981). Strengths of the American Indian family: State of the art. In J. Red Horse, A. Shattuck, & F. Hoffman (Eds.), *The American Indian family: Strengths and stresses* (pp. 25–43). Isleta, NM: American Indian Social Research and Development Associates.

Sands, K. M. (1992). Indian women's personal narrative: Voices past and present. In M. Culley (Ed.), *American women's autobiography: Fea(s)ts of memory* (pp. 268–294). Madison: University of Wisconsin Press.

Schneider, M. J. (1983). Women's work: An examination of women's roles in Plains Indian arts and crafts. In P. Albers & B. Medicine (Eds.), *The hidden half: Studies of Plains Indian women* (pp. 101–121). Washington, DC: University Press of America.

Shepardson, M. (1982). The status of Navajo women. *American Indian Quarterly, 6*(1&2), 149–169.

Shomaker, D. M. (1989). Transfer of children and the importance of grandmothers among the Navajo Indians. *Journal of Cross-Cultural Gerontology, 4*, 1–18.

———. (1990). Health care, cultural expectations, and frail elderly Navajo grandmothers. *Journal of Cross-Cultural Gerontology, 5*, 21–34.

Silko, L. M. (1980a). Gallup, New Mexico—Indian capital of the world. In D. Fisher (Ed.), *The third woman: Minority women writers of the U.S.* (pp. 49–53). Boston: Houghton Mifflin.

————. (1980b). Storyteller. In D. Fisher (Ed.), *The third woman: Minority women writers of the United States* (pp. 70–83). Boston: Houghton Mifflin.

Stewart, I. (1980). *A voice in her tribe: A Navaho woman's own story.* Socorro, NM: Ballena Press Anthropological Paper No. 17.

Tefft, S. K. (1968). Intergenerational value differentials and family structure among the Wind River Shoshone. *American Anthropologist, 70,* 330–333.

Trimble, S. (1993). *The People: Indians of the American southwest.* Santa Fe: SAR Press.

Tsosie, R. (1988). Changing women: The cross-currents of American Indian feminine identity. *American Indian Culture and Research Journal, 12*(1), 1–37.

Underhill, R. M. (1965). The Papago family. In M. F. Nimkoff (Ed.), *Comparative family systems* (pp. 147–162). Boston: Houghton Mifflin.

U.S. Department of Commerce. (1992). *General population characteristics: United States.* Washington, DC: U.S. Government Printing Office.

————. (1993). *Social and economic characteristics: United States.* Washington, DC: U.S. Government Printing Office.

U.S. Department of Health and Human Services. (1991). *Healthy people 2000: National health promotion and disease prevention objectives.* Washington, DC: U.S. Government Printing Office.

Wagner, J. K. (1976). The role of intermarriage in the acculturation of selected urban American Indian women. *Anthropologica, 18*(2), 5–29.

Weber, M. (1949). *The methodology of the social sciences* (E. A. Shils & H. A. Finch, Trans. and Eds.). New York: Free Press.

Weibel-Orlando, J. (1988). Indians, ethnicity as a resource, and aging: You can go home again. *Journal of Cross-Cultural Gerontology, 3,* 323–348.

————. (1989). Elders and elderlies: Well-being in Indian old age. *American Indian Culture and Research Journal, 13*(3&4), 149–170.

————. (1990). Grandparenting styles: Native American perspectives. In J. Sokolovsky (Ed.), *The cultural context of aging: Worldwide perspectives* (pp. 109–125). New York: Bergin & Garvey.

Welch, D. (1985). *Zitkala-Sa: An American Indian leader, 1876–1938.* Unpublished doctoral dissertation, Department of History, University of Wyoming, Laramie.

Wilson, R. C. (1980). Keeping hair. In D. Fisher (Ed.), *The third woman: Minority women writers of the United States* (p. 103). Boston: Houghton Mifflin.

Witherspoon, G. (1975). *Navajo kinship and marriage.* Chicago: University of Chicago Press.

Woodhead, H. (Ed.). (1994). *The American Indians: Cycles of life.* Alexandria, VA: Time-Life Books.

Twenty

Issues and Trends Affecting Asian Americans, Women, and Aging

DARLENE YEE

BACKGROUND

This chapter examines the aging of Asian-American women in our society. While the primary purpose of this chapter is to discuss what is known about Asian-American women and aging, it is important to emphasize that the studies needed to produce understanding of ethnic variations are yet to be completed. This chapter presents the literature available and identifies key categories in which Asian Americans have been, or could be, studied.

Asian Americans are classified by the U.S. Bureau of the Census as those native Americans or immigrants whose family origins are Asian or Pacific Island ethnicities, including Chinese, East Indian, Filipino, Indochinese (e.g., Cambodian, Hmong, Laotian, Mien, Vietnamese), Japanese, Korean, and Pacific Islanders (e.g., Fijians, Guamanians, Hawaiians, Samoans). There is no consistent or specific differentiation of past ethnic migration within these Asian and Pacific Island countries. Chinese from China and those residing in another country prior to emigration to the United States are not specifically differentiated (e.g., a Chinese woman from China versus Hong Kong versus Taiwan). Throughout the chapter the term "Asian Americans" is used interchangeably with the term "Asian-American women"; but unless it is clear by context or otherwise specified, it may refer to Asian-American women (and men) of all age intervals.

Asian Americans were not included in the decennial census as a separate category until 1980 (Hendricks & Hendricks, 1986). As a result, there is inadequate information about Asian Americans to detail past characteristics or to form a baseline upon which to estimate future changes as health and socioeconomic norms vary. Furthermore, we have insufficient knowledge of Asian Americans and their aging to determine how they have coped with living and working in a minority status. Even less is known about Asian-American women; and knowledge of Asian-American women and aging is limited at best. In view of the paucity of data, we can only coordinate what information exists on this specific population and make inferences from related literature and research studies.

As we discuss Asian-American women and aging in our society, it is important to recognize the diversity included in the demographic description of Asian Americans. Asian Americans are not a homogeneous group and are composed of people from diverse cultural and ethnic backgrounds. Data available on Asian Americans do not typically address the component ethnic groups, only the broad categorization of Asian-American descent. This categorization creates multiple problems in trying to understand the aging of Asian-American women: (1) there are limited data on Asian Americans and their aging, (2) ethnicity has been pooled into one large category, (3) gender differentiation has been limited, and (4) age grading and generational information is limited. This situation produces a dilemma; we can either avoid the topic because of lack of specific information or present the available data and point out deficits as a guide for future studies. The latter option is presented in this chapter.

In selecting this option, it is important to remember that women age through the same basic biological process regardless of ethnicity. What we can draw from the limited data available are some of the different effects that social and cultural variations have on the biological process, as inferred from the general categorization of Asian Americans and/or data on Asian-American men. Given the intertwining of female and male lives, the use of these data is not always a major obstacle, but they do severely limit how some gender-specific issues can be addressed (e.g., breast and cervical cancers, postmenopausal conditions such as osteoporosis, and social isolation in late life).

Equally important in the interpretation of aging and cultural and ethnic variations are the length of time (and generational cohort) in this country (Kiefer, 1974), regional differences, and socioeconomic status in the United States. Economic, health, psychological, and social well-being is a function of acculturation and generational cohort. The generational cohort should be supplemented by information about the time of emigration for émigrés and first-generation women and about the region of the country and its acceptance of Asian and Pacific Island émigrés. Ultimately, individuals and groups and the needs and problems in their lives are what we seek to understand.

The discussion in this chapter presents available information on some of the major characteristics used to describe the general population of which Asian-American women are a part. In the presentation of each characteristic, the influences on the aging of Asian-American women are presented and some of the specific limitations in the source data are highlighted. A summary discussion at the end of the chapter underscores the key issues and trends that are known and not known about the aging of Asian-American women.

DEMOGRAPHIC CHARACTERISTICS

Because related literature and research studies on Asian Americans have applied different age intervals to denote elderly, no consistent criterion for "aged" has been used in this chapter. In many cases, however, age 55 has been the lower age limit in denoting elderly. The chronological age at which individuals become "elderly" has been changing and is related to life expectancy.

With increased life expectancy, the terms "middle age" and "old age" have simultaneously changed their limits, and a range of added descriptors (e.g., young-old, middle-old, old-old) has proliferated. These differentiations have been cited in the literature on aging (Neugarten & Moore, 1968), but should not be applied retroactively to studies prior to their definition, or to more general demographic studies in which these differentiations have not been applied.

This terminology issue causes additional problems in consideration of the aging of Asian-American women. The cultural, social, and economic conditions of the countries from which they or their parents originated may vary greatly. These variations alter life expectancy, health, and well-being (particularly in new immigrants, and to a lesser extent in first-generation Asian Americans). We must attempt to address both age differentiation and ethnic variation.

In any review of the demography of the elderly population, ethnicity is emerging, along with gender, as an important variable in understanding the needs and problems of an aging population. The graying of America has been compared to the feminization of America; older women tend to outnumber older men in the United States by a ratio of three to two. However, older Asian Americans have higher proportions of men than the general population does because early immigration laws that allowed men to enter as laborers did not permit like entry of women and children. Among those aged 60–64, there are 84 men for every 100 women. The sex ratio actually increases in the 70–74-year-old age group, then declines at age 85 and over (AARP, 1987).

Asian Americans are the third-largest, and the fastest-growing, minority group in the United States. Data from the 1980 census indicated 135,022 Asian Americans aged 55 to 59; 183,479 aged 60–69; 102,009 aged 70–79; and 38,395 aged 80 or over. These numbers contributed to an overall increase of 120% since 1970, compared to a 6.4% increase for whites, a 17.4% increase for blacks, and a 60.8% increase for Hispanics. This growth reflects the consolidation of families through immigration, and higher birthrates in many of the groups (Sakauye, 1990). From 1980 to 1985 this population increased 48.5% (about 5.1 million), compared to a 3.3% increase in the general population. Table 20.1 depicts the projected numbers and percentages of Asian Americans in the United States by group in the year 2000 (Kitano, 1990). Table 20.2 illustrates the Asian-American population by sex, 1990 and 2010, and percentage change, 1990–2010. Among older Asian Americans, 10% live in rural areas; over 55% live in California, Hawaii, and Washington (AARP, 1987). Life expectancy is rising and birthrates

Table 20.1
Projected Numbers and Percentages of Asian Americans in the United States by
Group in the Year 2000

Group	Number	Percentage of Total Asian Population
Filipino	2,070,571	21.0
Chinese	1,683,537	17.1
Vietnamese	1,574,385	16.0
Korean	1,320,759	13.4
Asian Indian	1,006,305	10.2
Japanese	856,619	8.7
Other Asian	1,338,188	13.6
Total	9,850,364	

Source: Gardner, R. W., Robey, B. & Smith, P. C. (1985, October). Asian Americans: Growth, change, and diversity. *Population Bulletin, 40* (4), p. 37, table 16, Asian American Population: 1980, Projected for 1990 and 2000.

are falling throughout Asia, resulting in a growing percentage of people over 60. Life expectancy for women in selected countries is portrayed in table 20.3.

ECONOMIC CHARACTERISTICS

As with most immigrants from non-English-speaking countries, the first generation of Asian Americans has lived with difficulties associated with limited or no English. Older immigrants have not yet overcome their so-called accents and communication problems, which limited their education, employment, and income opportunities. In later generations Asian Americans have often been able to assimilate better than most other ethnic minorities. As a group, they appear to do rather well economically compared to other ethnic groups. In general, Asian Americans are more likely to have a college education and/or graduate degree; they have lower unemployment rates and a higher median income; and poverty rates among Asian Americans are slightly above those among Caucasian Americans. Some consider Asian Americans a "model minority" on the basis of these economic characteristics; however, this designation perpetuates inattention to their actual needs and problems—particularly for first-generation Asian Americans who are at risk of multiple jeopardy—old, minority, and poor (Hendricks & Hendricks, 1986).

By combining the data from tables 20.1 and 20.2, an inference can be drawn about the life expectancies of Asian-American women, and with it, a related

Table 20.2
Asians: The Next Two Decades

(Numbers in Thousands)

	1990		2010		Percentage Change	
	Men	Women	Men	Women	Men	Women
All Ages	3,403	3,871	8,069	9,043	137%	134%
Under age 5	340	331	731	704	115%	113%
5 to 14	579	597	1,478	1,437	155%	141%
15 to 24	547	588	1,369	1,372	150%	133%
25 to 34	736	749	1,320	1,382	79%	85%
35 to 44	573	671	1,182	1,344	106%	100%
45 to 54	283	424	961	1,155	240%	172%
55 to 64	181	267	626	836	246%	213%
65 to 74	118	171	277	501	135%	193%
75 and older	46	73	125	312	172%	327%

Source: The Urban Institute, and Survey Sampling, Inc. (1993).

inference about their health and well-being. The translation of life expectancy from a country of origin is tenuous, because the modernity and standard of living of the nation of origin and of the United States can differ greatly and also typically vary with time (e.g., the change in life expectancy from 1950 to 1994). Third-world nations are modernizing more quickly than before, but we must differentiate when (and at what age) an émigré left that country and became exposed to culture, health care, lifestyle, and standard of living in the United States. It is also important to identify the American standard of living for the émigré and subsequent generational cohorts, as there is a significant difference in our own society by socioeconomic circumstances.

The differences for new émigrés are less; for example, life expectancy changed in China from 42 years in 1950 to 71 years in 1994. A woman emigrating in 1950 would have grown up in different circumstances than a like-aged woman emigrating in 1994. Second, there is a general shrinkage of difference by country of origin from 1950 to 1994, with life expectancy in many countries approaching that of the United States. Some notable exceptions are India, Indonesia, Pakistan, and the Philippines. Although data are limited, the cultures and lifestyles of these nations have changed as the global community has shrunk, making comparisons of like-aged women emigrating in 1950 versus 1994 more difficult.

Table 20.3
The Graying of Asia by Life Expectancy (LE)

Country	1950 LE	1994 LE	Percentage over 60
Brunei	62.10	72.69	4.3
China	42.30	70.90	8.6
Hong Kong	64.90	80.05	11.5
India	38.00	62.00	6.5
Indonesia	38.10	62.00	6.4
Japan	59.61	81.81	17.5
S. Korea	49.00	74.96	6.8
Malaysia	50.00	71.60	5.8
Myanmar	43.80	61.80	6.4
Pakistan	37.60	56.50	6.9
Philippines	47.72	66.10	5.3
Singapore	62.10	76.40	9.1
Sri Lanka	55.50	72.50	6.6
Thailand	49.10	68.85	7.3

Source: Los Angeles Times and San Jose Mercury News (1994, August 28).

AARP (1987) stated that more older Asian Americans lack formal education than Caucasians (13% versus 1.6%); fewer older Asian Americans hold high-school diplomas than Caucasians (26% versus 41%); more older Asian Americans continue working after age 65 than Caucasians; many older Asian Americans (25%) are self-employed as farmers or in small business; more older Asian Americans are unemployed as opposed to Caucasians (8% versus 5%); median income for older Asian-American men (65 years or over) is less than that of Caucasian men in the same age group ($5,551 versus $7,408); and median income for older Asian-American women is less than that of Caucasian women ($3,476 versus $3,894). Given that these differentiations, except for median income, are for the general population without gender identification, we can infer yet poorer rates for Asian-American women who combine the negative rates for both women and Asian-American descent.

Cabezas (1980) described frequent myths regarding the economic success of Asian Americans. To dispel the myth that Asian Americans do well because they go to college and their income exceeds that of Caucasian Americans, he presented data showing that Asian Americans receive inadequate returns of income for their educational levels, and that higher family incomes among Asian Americans are, in part, the result of more family members working many jobs with long hours. To dispel the myth that Asian Americans are not discriminated against in employment and are found in all business sectors, Cabezas presented information from studies by the United States Equal Employment Opportunity Commission showing significant discrimination against Asian Americans in the labor market. To dispel the myth that Asian Americans are in commerce for themselves and are very successful, he presented statistics showing that many Asian-American firms are in retail and service industries with modest gross receipts.

According to Kim (1986), it is not uncommon that both husband and wife are employed in the labor market. Consequently, Korean-American families enjoy a higher income than average American families. Two-thirds (66%) of Korean Americans in the Los Angeles area had an annual income that exceeded the national median income, and more than four in five (85%) had income that exceeded the median income of other ethnic minorities. However, many married Korean women pay the heaviest toll in the family by performing two or three jobs every day. Although married individuals demonstrate a higher level of life satisfaction, 91% of married women experience negative emotional experiences with their husbands, including alcoholism and gambling; moreover, if they live with their parents-in-law, their level of life satisfaction is low. In the New York area 80% of the clients of a Korean-American family service agency were women (Yum, 1986). Among the fastest-growing groups of older Americans are Korean elderly. They numbered 798,847 in 1990, a 125.3% increase since 1980. A Puget Sound area survey found that 75.5% did not speak English; and next to health, their greatest concern was the language barrier (National Resource Center: Diversity and Long-Term Care, 1994).

Chow (1987) examined the relationship of sex-role identity to occupational attainment, self-esteem, and work satisfaction for 161 employed Asian-American women. Androgynous Asian-American women and those with high occupational attainment had higher self-esteem and greater work satisfaction than those with other types of sex-role identity. The Women's Bureau (1989) reported that women-owned, nonfarm sole proprietorships increased 62.5% between 1980 and 1986. Women's share of total nonfarm sole proprietorships increased from 26.1% in 1980 to 29.9% in 1986. In 1982 black women owned 2.7% of all women-owned nonfarm sole proprietorships, Hispanic women owned 2.1%, and Asian-American women owned 1.6%. Opportunities for women business owners of all ethnic minority groups should be enhanced by the Women's Business Ownership Act of 1988. The National Institute of Education (1980) formulated a research agenda to shape policy on Asian-American women's educational and occupational needs.

Social inequality has a great influence on aging through its effect on jobs and lifetime earnings and through their consequent impact on health and retirement income in later life. The picture for older Asian Americans is mixed, although all groups show some negative effects of racism. Older Japanese Americans have had jobs that closely parallel those of Caucasian Americans and as a result have retirement incomes closer to those of Caucasian Americans than any other racial category. There is great diversity among older Chinese Americans in terms of jobs and retirement income. Older Filipino Americans are more likely to have had low-paying jobs and, thus, low retirement incomes. Despite their lower incomes, older Asian Americans tend to be in better health than older Caucasian Americans.

HEALTH CHARACTERISTICS

Socioeconomic factors differentiate health potential and life expectancy. Each minority group in the United States has its own set of health characteristics, problems, and needs. Based on the *Report of the Secretary's Task Force on Black and Minority Health* (U.S. DHHS, 1985), a series of fact sheets on each of the six priority areas in minority health has been prepared (Office of Minority Health Resource Center, 1990). Five of these priority areas (AIDS/HIV, cancer, chemical dependency, diabetes, and heart disease/stroke) in minority health are summarized here as they pertain to Asian Americans. Little research has been conducted on the health status of this population, but cancer (Japanese, Chinese, Native Hawaiians), diabetes (Japanese, Filipinos, Chinese, Koreans, Native Hawaiians), heart disease (Japanese, Native Hawaiians), and hypertension (Filipinos, Japanese, Native Hawaiians, Chinese) are significant problems (AARP, 1990). The prevalence of osteoporosis (Chinese) as evidenced by osteoporotic fractures is high (Woo et al., 1994).

AIDS/HIV Infection

Asian Americans make up about 2% of the population but only about 1% of all AIDS cases in the United States. AIDS rates are still low among Asian Americans compared to those for black and Hispanic Americans, but there has been a fast increase in the number of new cases. From 1985 to 1988 reported new cases escalated by more than 150%, the highest rate of increase among all American racial and ethnic groups. The incidence of AIDS among Asian Americans is less than half that of other racial and ethnic groups, but the apparent upward trend has raised concern that HIV infection may be occurring at rates undetected by estimates related to AIDS cases (Office of Minority Health Resource Center, 1990). The risk of AIDS/HIV infection for Asian-American women would be projected to be lower than for all women, but to follow the increasing trend seen for all women.

Cancer

Cancer rates are rising for Chinese Americans and Japanese-American men in the United States. But Asian Americans, who come from many different countries and cultures, have dissimilar cancer rates. These dissimilarities reflect genetic and cultural influences that often appear in diet. Typically, changes occur in activity and diet across the first generations that obscure direct comparison between émigré groups and long-term residents. Chinese Americans living in the United States have a high incidence of cervical cancer, esophageal cancer, multiple myeloma, and pancreatic cancer. Filipino Americans living in the United States have low survival rates for colon cancer. Hawaiians have a high incidence of breast cancer and lung cancer. Japanese Americans have a high incidence of stomach cancer, and Japanese-American men have a higher incidence of esophageal cancer than Caucasian Americans. Diet may be a factor in both cases, as evidenced in studies showing that as Japanese Americans adopt a Western diet, their incidence of stomach cancer declines (Office of Minority Health Resource Center, 1988a).

Chemical Dependency

Chinese and Japanese Americans living in the United States face a greater risk than Caucasian Americans of developing two cancers linked to smoking: cancer of the esophagus and cancer of the pancreas. The incidence of esophageal cancer is 2.5 times higher for Japanese-American men, 1.8 times higher for Chinese-American men, and 1.6 times higher for Chinese-American women than for their Caucasian-American counterparts. Cancer of the pancreas is 20% higher among Chinese-American women than among Caucasian-American women, and this cancer is increasing in both Chinese-American men and women. Native Hawaiians have an excess incidence and mortality for lung cancer.

Data are scarce on alcohol and other drug abuse among Asian Americans. A few studies indicate lower rates of alcohol and drug use than in the general population, but others indicate that problems do exist among some Asian-American groups. For example, Native Hawaiians are reported to drink more heavily than other groups in Hawaii and appear to be at greater risk of automobile accidents, injuries, and fatalities that result from driving under the influence of alcohol (Office of Minority Health Resource Center, 1988b).

What the data do not communicate are gender differences, socioeconomic information, and social stress levels. In addition, Asian-American women tend to have lower chemical dependencies than Asian-American men; hence some of the reported rates for Asian Americans as a group may overstate the risk for women. The data also provide little or no intergenerational information on chemical dependencies.

Diabetes

Diabetes is a significant problem among at least four groups of Asian Americans in the United States. Although data are scarce, one study has shown that Chinese, Filipino, Japanese, and Korean Americans living in Hawaii have double to triple the diabetes rates of Caucasian Americans. Most other studies concerned Japanese Americans; among Japanese-American men in the United States aged 40 or older, researchers found the diabetes rate to be as high as 10% to 14%. Another study suggests that Japanese Americans living in the United States have, as a group, more than twice as much diabetes as Japanese living in Japan. Still another reveals that Chinese, Filipino, and Japanese Americans who were born in the United States have higher death rates from diabetes than their native-born counterparts. Japanese-American diets in the United States are generally much higher in fat—both animal fat and total fat—than in Japan. Also, Japanese Americans in the United States tend to have a higher proportion of fatty tissue, even though they are not overweight. This suggests that a high-fat Western diet could be the culprit (Office of Minority Health Resource Center, 1988c).

We can infer that the risk of diabetes for an Asian-American woman varies by ethnic affiliation, generational cohort, diet, and lifestyle. Individual risk can be more accurately assessed through a medical history and clinical testing. If diet, weight, and lifestyle are the epidemiological risk factors, then risk varies with length of time (generational cohort) in the United States and the woman's change to a normative American lifestyle.

Heart Disease/Stroke

Japanese-American men in the United States stand out from most other groups in having very high death rates from stroke. The reasons are not clear, although studies suggest that Japanese-American men in Hawaii smoke more than Japanese men in Japan. Other Asian Americans have stroke rates similar to those of Caucasian Americans. Another gap involves Filipino Americans, in whom high blood pressure is a significant public health problem.

Filipino-American women, especially, are much more likely than Caucasian Americans to have uncontrolled high blood pressure. Some medical problems are seen in increased frequency due to higher-sodium diets, which increase the rates of hypertension and arteriosclerotic disease as a cause for dementia (Liu, 1985). Other risk factors, such as smoking and cholesterol levels, appear to be low among Asian Americans, especially among Asian-American women. Asian Americans have slightly lower death rates from heart disease than the general population in the United States (Office of Minority Health Resource Center, 1988d).

Lubben, Weiler, and Chi (1988) analyzed the health practices of a sample of elderly Medi-Cal recipients, including 123 (12%) of sampled Asian Americans. Asian Americans significantly differed from Caucasian Americans in ten of the thirteen health practices. Asian Americans did not smoke or drink alcohol, exercised regularly, avoided snacks, ate sufficient breads, cereals, and whole grains, and limited their intake of caffeine. However, contrary to the previous study, they tended to have more limited social networks and had more difficulty in sleeping than Caucasian Americans. The lack of social networks was attributed to foreign birth, immigrating to the United States at a young age, and remaining single. Generalizations from both of these studies may be limited because the samples were drawn from those seeking public assistance.

Two-thirds (66%) of the elderly living in San Francisco's Chinatown are in poor health and consequently have limitations in physical activities; many regularly visit physicians, including herbalists. More than two-thirds (70%) of Filipino-American elderly sustain fair to poor health condition, suffering most frequently (19%) from high blood pressure. Indochinese refugees from Southeast Asia brought their belief in supernatural powers, including the ancestral spirits and the spirits of nature, trees, and forests; their practice of such ethnic beliefs can be observed in dealing with their health problems (Murase, 1987). Most Korean Americans (80%) have chronic diseases such as diabetes, eye problems, high blood pressure, neuralgia, and stomach problems for which they receive treatment by Korean-American physicians (84%) and Korean-American herbal doctors (14.4%) (Korean-American Senior Citizens Society of the Greater New York, 1987).

The data suggest a generally higher risk of hypertension for Asian-American women immigrants, but data do not support extrapolating this risk to subsequent generations. The extrapolation would be yet weaker with changes in life circumstances and assimilation to mainstream life. The exceptions would be a more similar pattern to the general population of women with genetic differences superimposed. One concern is that any women maintaining belief in herbalists and/or folk medicine may experience later detection of cancer and, thus, lower survival rates than women using more traditional Western medical practices.

PSYCHOLOGICAL CHARACTERISTICS

At the present time, there are no accurate breakdowns of prevalence rates of psychopathology in Asian Americans (Sue & Monishima, 1982). Culturally unique syndromes of mental illness associated with Asian Americans include *amok* (Southeast Asian males showing sudden assaultive behavior), *hwa-byung* (a Korean response to prolonged suppressed anger causing epigastric distress and fears of death), and *latah* (an exaggerated startle response to minimal stimuli in Japanese and Southeast Asian women) (Lin & Finder, 1983; Westermeyer, 1985). Culturally unique syndromes and language barriers are not maintained in later generations who have assimilated, leading one to speculate that the initial clash of divergent cultures contributes to *amok, hwa-byung*, and *latah*.

Although dose levels administered for psychotropic medications often have been reported to be lower for Asian Americans (Yamamoto, James, & Pally, 1968), empirical research to establish differing dose requirements for Asian-American elderly and any sex differentials have not been reported. Dietary differences (e.g., high sodium and tyramine intake through soy sauce) may influence the effects of psychotropic medications (e.g., lithium and MAO inhibitors). Training programs in mental health should first sensitize caregivers to

differences in working with Asian Americans and to the need to become experienced in the needs and problems of a specific group (Sakauye, 1990).
Homma-True (1990) addressed the problems of Asian-American women and the
difficulties they may encounter in psychotherapy.

Although the Chinese-American elderly experience the lowest level of depression as compared to their Asian-American counterparts (Kuo, 1984), they
have more mental health problems than their Japanese-American counterparts;
emotional and mental health problems in Chinatown are apparent (Lum, Cheung,
Cho, Tang, & Yau, 1980). Korean immigrants have the highest incidence of
depression among their Asian-American counterparts (Kuo, 1984). Korean-
American elderly appear to be independent and internalize their problems with
concern about *che-myun* (face-saving). Korean Americans are highly competi-
tive even among their family members; the Korean-American support system is
much weaker than that of other Asian-American groups. Asian Americans often
pride themselves on their independence and self-sufficiency. Consequently, some
are particularly reluctant to seek health services, especially for counseling and
mental illness. The family is very important to many Asian Americans, and
family reliance can strengthen an individual's social support resources, but it
may also pose a barrier to care when it is truly needed (Office of Minority
Health Resource Center, 1990).

Suicide rates for Asian Americans in the United States are lower than rates
for other groups until middle age. But at about age 45 the rate for Chinese-
American women begins to rise with each successive age group after 45 and
reaches its peak in the oldest age groups. Japanese-American women have a
suicide rate higher than that of Caucasian-American women after age 75. Chi-
nese-, Japanese-, and Filipino-American male suicide rates are low, except in
the very oldest groups. The reasons for the gap between Caucasian and Chinese-
American women are unknown; one factor could be the strong stigma attached
to mental health problems in Chinese communities. This can prevent Chinese-
American women who are suffering from anxiety, depression, and displaced
homemaker syndrome from seeking much-needed care (Office of Minority
Health Resource Center, 1990).

Suicide rates vary greatly by race and sex, but the suicide methods of choice
employed by these groups have not been studied closely and across time. Annual
official national statistics for specific methods of suicide by race and sex were
examined from 1923 to 1978. During this time period, shifts occurred in the
proportions of suicides by method, most notably for women and Asian-American
groups. Although women continued to kill themselves with solid and liquid
poisons more often than men, firearms became a more frequent method in later
years. Among Chinese and Japanese Americans, the most common methods of
suicide were hanging, strangulation, and suffocation. However, the proportions
declined over time, while those for methods such as firearms increased. Firearms
continued to be the method most often used in completed suicides by black,
Caucasian, and Native American males. Results suggest that acculturation,

changing societal roles, and problems with the compilation of official statistics may be possible factors affecting changes in the suicide method of choice (McIntosh & Santos, 1981).

Acculturation and the development of positive self-concept among Asian-American women are both complicated by factors associated with their ethnicity and gender. Cultural barriers, physical differences, and racial and sex discrimination have made difficult the complete assimilation of Asian females into American society. Furthermore, failure to recognize sociocultural diversity within Asian-American groups has perpetuated the myth of Asian-American women's success and has led to the exclusion of Asian women as a whole from programs to aid minorities and women. In developing self-concept, Asian-American women confront the problem of integrating often-conflicting American and Asian cultural elements. Sex identity further complicates the process of self-concept development, because sex roles may also conflict in American and Asian cultures. In addition, Asian-American women's self-concept is shaped by others' negative perceptions and stereotypes of them. Needed are both further research to understand the determinants of Asian-American women's self-concept and policies that address the problems of developing a new image for this group (Chow, 1981).

Yamauchi (1981) examined the communication behavior of Asian-American women who held male-dominated, nontraditional jobs. Two hundred and eighty-seven Asian-American women of Chinese, Japanese, Korean, and Filipino descent in both traditional and nontraditional occupations were interviewed in San Francisco and Washington, D.C. In the interviews various instruments were utilized to determine the participants' ethnic identity, sexual identity, interracial identity, and verbal and nonverbal communication patterns. Analysis of the data led to a number of findings.

Yamauchi's results indicated that holders of nontraditional occupations displayed a combination of American and Asian value orientations; more masculine tendencies or the perceived ability associated with masculine-related orientations such as being more decisive and ambitious; a rejection of stereotypes attributed to them by white members of society; more situation- and person-specific assertive verbal behavior; and a trend toward more nonverbal assertive behavior. The pattern of multicultural adjustment of the Asian-American women in nontraditional occupations consisted of their being more highly educated and older than their counterparts in traditional occupations, and in their displaying an additional set of communication behavioral skills to deal with a variety of individuals of different sexes and cultures.

SOCIAL CHARACTERISTICS

There is a common tendency to discuss all Asian Americans as a monocultural group. Asian Americans constitute an extremely diverse population of different ethnic groups of native and foreign-born Americans. They differ substantially in customs, language, participation in American life, and social class structure. The percentage of elderly in each group varies. It is lowest in the Indochinese (2%), where the predominantly refugee status has limited elderly immigration, and highest in long-standing American groups (10.3% in Filipinos) (Liu, 1985). Older Asian Americans have unique cultural, dietary, and language barriers that make public programs and services for the elderly more difficult for them to use.

Heightened adaptational problems and culture shock exist for older Asian-American immigrants. Lower stamina or reduced sense of need to acculturate may increase adaptational problems and isolation compared to their younger counterparts. Cultural values often lead to minimizing psychiatric problems or to attributing them to external causes or to personality. Caregiving is often handled by the family system without assistance from mental health professionals. Community education and outreach are often crucial to access this heterogeneous population of older Asian Americans.

The majority of Asian-American men aged 65 or over are married, while the majority of Asian-American women 65 or over are widowed. Asian-American women are much more likely to be married than their Caucasian counterparts, with a smaller proportion remaining single in their later years. Only 19% of older Asian Americans live alone, whereas 30% of older Caucasian Americans live alone. Only 2% of older Asian Americans live in nursing homes, whereas 5% of older Caucasian Americans live in nursing homes. This difference is even more pronounced among the oldest old (85+), with 10% of Asian Americans in nursing homes as compared to 23% of Caucasians.

Empirical studies covering most older Asian Americans are lacking, although there are studies on older Chinese and Japanese Americans. Lubben and Becerra (1987) conducted a study of California seniors that included a sample of older Chinese Americans. The older Chinese and Mexican Americans were more likely to reside with other persons than the sample of older black and Caucasian Americans. The older Chinese and Mexican Americans were more likely to share housing and receive help from an adult child. The ties were the result of two major factors: cultural values and economic need. Close ties to the traditional culture meant a higher degree of parent-child supportive behavior.

Ujimoto (1987) studied several generations of Japanese Canadians in order to ascertain the general satisfaction and well-being of the aged respondents. The *issei*, or original immigrant generation of Japanese, felt that perseverance was the key to successful aging, while the *nissei*, or second generation of Japanese, stressed discipline and filial aspects. There were no significant differences between the three generations on such variables as group loyalty, moral obligations, pride, sense of duty, and thriftiness in the Japanese culture. The elderly Japanese belonged mainly to organizations composed of Japanese Canadians. However, there was little active participation in these organizations; membership was based primarily on moral or social gratitude and obligations. There was agreement that one cultural factor, that of *enryo* (reserve), was a hindrance toward successful aging. Japanese Canadians seek help only when they are in a desperate situation; their frequency of utilizing social services is apparently very low. As they grow older, more older Japanese-Canadian men than women visit Caucasian friends and *nisseis* (Ujimoto, 1987).

Asian-American communities with such names as Chinatown, Little Tokyo, Korea Town, and Little Saigon have fostered and maintained ethnic identity, insularity, and solidarity among themselves and consequently have established the reputation that they are nonacculturative (Markides & Mindel, 1987). Additional information and resources pertaining to Asian Americans, women, and aging may be acquired from various organizations identified in the Appendix to this chapter.

SUMMARY

It is important to acknowledge the differences and similarities between and within various ethnic minority groups. Questions are still being posed and answers sought. However, perhaps we have indicated categories in which information should be collected. Obviously, more research is needed, not only on ethnicity but also on gender (i.e., Asian-American women). The inclusion of women and minorities in research is important, both to ensure that they receive an appropriate share of the benefits of research and that they do not bear a disproportionate burden. To the extent that participation in research offers direct benefits to the participants, underrepresentation of women or minorities denies them the opportunity to benefit. Moreover, for purposes of generalizing research results, investigators must include the widest possible range of population groups (Office for Protection from Research Risks, 1994).

However, the examination of Asian Americans, women, and aging is complicated by a number of factors. A review of related literature suggests that ethnic origin, gender differentials, generational differences, acculturation, socioeconomic status, and regional differences in this country impact upon this investigation. The difficulty of examination also is compounded by other social trends such as affirmative action and the women's movement. As the health care delivery system changes, health potential and longevity will be affected by differences in preventive health and medical treatment. In studying Asian Americans, women, and aging, it is important to realize that they are part of a changing society like any other group.

The development of new studies needs to include information differentiated by age, ethnicity, gender, generational differences, and socioeconomic status; these studies must also reflect the changing trends brought about by both new levels of immigration and general social change. Without these data, the problem of ascribing appropriate characteristics to specific groups of Asian-American women will continue to be difficult; consequently, the identification and resolution of their needs and problems will be equally challenging. One solution would be a general epidemiological study designed to survey the aforementioned variables and identify lifestyle, standard of living, and health risks and behaviors. A second solution would be to identify differences by subgroupings from population norms and then to project subgroup characteristics. The former is desirable, but less feasible given current resources and the scope of this type of study (even in a cross-sectional versus a longitudinal design).

There also is a lack of focused collaboration and leadership to initiate such studies, and typically they fall into one of the subclasses of studies under culture and health in gerontology. The ethnic diversity of the groupings of Asian-American women produces less of a focus (e.g., there are no general studies on aging of European-American women who have a similar ethnic diversity). What is needed is a coherent policy statement to guide research. In the interim, the problems can be addressed on an individual basis in clinical situations, but not adequately even for the general population of Asian-American women, much less for the more correct and effective differentiation by ethnic group and generational cohort.

APPENDIX: ORGANIZATIONS PERTAINING TO ASIAN AMERICANS, WOMEN, AND AGING

Asian and Pacific Islander's American Health Forum
116 New Montgomery Street, Suite 531
San Francisco, CA 94105
Phone: 415–512–2710

The Association of Asian Pacific Community Health Organizations
1440 Broadway, Suite 510
Oakland, CA 94612
Phone: 510–272–9536

National Pacific/Asian Resource Center on Aging
Melbourne Tower
1511 3rd Avenue, Suite 914
Seattle, WA 98101
Phone: 206–624–1221

National Resource Center on Minority Aging Populations
University Center on Aging
College of Health and Human Services
San Diego State University
San Diego, CA 92182–0273
Phone: 619–594–2813

Office of Minority Health Resource Center
P.O. Box 37337
Washington, DC 20013–7337
Phone: 800–444–6472

REFERENCES

American Association of Retired Persons (AARP). (1987). *A portrait of older minorities.* Washington, DC: Author.

————. (1990). *Healthy aging: Making health promotion work for minority elders.* Washington, DC: Author.

Atchley, R. C. (1988). *Social forces and aging: An introduction to social gerontology.* 5th edition. Belmont, CA: Wadsworth Publishing Company.

Bass, S. A., Kutza, E. A., & Torres-Gil, F. M. (1990). *Diversity in aging: Challenges facing planners and policymakers in the 1990s.* Glenview, IL: Scott, Foresman & Company.

Bourliere, F. (1978). Ecology of human senescence. In J. C. Brocklehurst (Ed.), *Textbook of geriatric medicine and gerontology* 2nd edition, (pp. 71–85). Edinburgh: Churchill Livingstone.

Cabezas, A. (1980). Presentation on employment issues, U.S. Commission on Civil Rights. In *Civil Rights Issues of Asian and Pacific Americans: Myths and Realities* (pp. 389–393). Washington, DC: U.S. Government Printing Office.

Chow, E. (1981). Acculturation and self concept of the Asian American women. In P. Reid & G. Puryear (Eds.), *Minority women: Social and psychological perspectives* (pp. 1–35). New York: Holt, Rinehart & Winston.

————. (1987). The influence of sex-role identity and occupational: attainment on the psychological well-being of Asian American women. *Psychology of Women Quarterly, 11*(1), 69–81.

Hendricks, J., & Hendricks, C. D. (1986). *Aging in mass society: Myths and realities.* Boston: Little, Brown.

Homma-True, R. (1990). Psychotherapeutic issues with Asian American women. *Sex Roles: A Journal of Research, 22*(7–8), 477–486.

Huang, I. J. (1981). The Chinese American family. In C. H. Mindel & R. W. Habenstein (Eds.), *Ethnic families in America.* New York: Elsevier.

Kiefer, C. W. (1974). Lessons from the issei. In J. F. Gubrium (Ed.), *Late life: Communities and environmental policy* (pp. 167–200). Springfield: Charles C. Thomas.

Kim, J. S. (1986). *Social support among Korean immigrants in the Greater Atlanta area.* Doctoral dissertation. Atlanta University School of Social Work, Georgia.

Kim, P. K. H. (1990). Asian-American Families and the Elderly. In M. S. Harper (Ed.), *Minority aging: Essential curricula content for selected health and allied health professions* (pp. 349–363). Washington, DC: U.S. Government Printing Office.

Kitano, H. (1969). Japanese Americans and Mental Illness. In S. C. Plog & R. B. Edgerton (Eds.), *Changing perspectives in mental illness* (pp. 68–73). Englewood Cliffs, NJ: Prentice-Hall.

————. (1990). Values, beliefs, and practices of the Asian-American elderly: Implications for geriatric education. In M. S. Harper (Ed.), *Minority aging: Essential curricula content for selected health and allied health professions* (pp. 341–348). Washington, DC: U.S. Government Printing Office.

Kitano, H., & Daniels, R. (1988). *Asian Americans.* Englewood Cliffs, NJ: Prentice-Hall.

Korean-American Senior Citizens Society of the Greater New York. (1987). *Korean-American elderly in New York: Problems and prospects.* New York: KASCS.

Kuo, W. H. (1984). The prevalence of depression among Asian Americans. *Journal of Nervous and Mental Disease, 172*, 449–457.

Lee, J. J. (1986). Asian American elderly: A neglected minority group. *Journal of Gerontological Social Work, 9*(4), 103–117.

Lin, K. M., & Finder, E. (1983). Neuroleptic dosage for Asians. *American Journal of Psychiatry, 140*(4), 490–491.

Liu, W. T. (1985). Asian/Pacific American elderly: Mortality differentials, health status, and use of health services. *Journal of Applied Gerontology, 4*(1), 35–64.

Lubben, J. E., & Becerra, R. M. (1987). Social support among black, Mexican, and Chinese elderly. In D. E. Gelfand & C. M. Barresi (Eds.), *Ethnic dimensions of aging* (pp. 130–144). New York: Springer.

Lubben, J. E., Weiler, P. G. & Chi, I. (1988). Gender and ethnic differences in the health practices of the elderly poor. *Journal of Clinical Epidemiology, 42*(8), 725–733.

Lum, D., Cheung, L. Y., Cho, E. R., Tang, T. & Yau, H. B. (1980). The psychosocial needs of the Chinese elderly. *Social Casework, 61*, 100–105.

McIntosh, J. L., & Santos, J. F. (1981). *Changing patterns in methods of suicide by race and sex.* Paper presented at the annual meeting of the American Association of Suicidology, Albuquerque, NM.

Markides, K. S., & Mindel, C. H. (1987). *Aging and ethnicity.* Beverly Hills, CA: Sage Publications.

Markson, E. W. (Ed.). (1983). *Older women: Issues and prospects.* Lexington, MA: Lexington Books.

Marmot, M. G., et al. (1979). Japanese culture and coronary heart disease. In H. Orimo, K. Shimada, M. Iriki, & D. Maeda (Eds.), *Recent advances in gerontology* (pp. 476–479). Amsterdam: Excerpta Medica.

Morioka-Douglas, N., & Yeo, G. (1990). *Aging and health: Asian/Pacific Island American elders.* Stanford, CA: Stanford Geriatric Education Center.

Murase, K. (1987). *Indigenous healers in Southeast Asian refugee communities.* Paper presented at the Annual Meeting of the National Association of Social Workers, New Orleans, LA.

National Institute of Education. (1980). Proceedings of a Conference on the Educational and Occupational Needs of Asian-Pacific-American Women. San Francisco, CA.

National Resource Center: Diversity and Long-Term Care. (1994). *Diversity and long-term care news.* San Diego, CA: Author.

Neugarten, B. L., & Moore, J. W. (1968). The changing age status system. In B. L. Neugarten (Ed.), *Middle age and aging.* Chicago: University of Chicago Press.

Office for Protection from Research Risks. (1994). *NIH guidelines on the inclusion of women and minorities as subjects in clinical research.* Washington, DC: Author.

Office of Minority Health Resource Center. (1988a). *Closing the gap: Cancer and minorities.* Washington, DC: Department of Health and Human Services.

———. (1988b). *Closing the gap: Chemical dependency and minorities.* Washington, DC: Department of Health and Human Services.

———. (1988c). *Closing the gap: Diabetes and minorities.* Washington, DC: Department of Health and Human Services.

———. (1988d). *Closing the gap: Heart disease, stroke, and minorities.* Washington, DC: Department of Health and Human Services.

———. (1990). *Closing the gap: AIDS/HIV infection and minorities.* Washington, DC: Department of Health and Human Services.

Sakauye, K. (1990). Differential diagnosis, medication, treatment, and outcomes: Asian American elderly. In M. S. Harper (Ed.), *Minority aging: Essential curricula content for selected health and allied health professions* (pp. 331–339). Washington, DC: U.S. Government Printing Office.

Sue, S. & Monishima, J. K. (1982). *The mental health of Asian Americans.* San Francisco: Jossey-Bass Publishers.

Turner, B. F. & Troll, L. E. (Eds.). (1993). *Women growing older: Psychological perspectives.* Thousand Oaks, CA: Sage Publications.

Ujimoto, K. V. (1987). Organizational activities, cultural factors, and well-being of aged Japanese Canadians. In D. E. Gelfand & C. M. Barresi (Eds.), *Ethnic dimensions of aging* (pp. 145–160). New York: Springer.

U.S. Department of Health and Human Services. (1985). *Report of the secretary's task force on black and minority health,* Volume 1, Executive Summary. Office of the Secretary, Washington, DC.

Westermeyer, J. (1985). Psychiatric diagnosis across cultural boundaries. *American Journal of Psychiatry, 142*(7), 798–805.

Women's Bureau. (1989). *Women business owners.* Washington, DC: Author.

Woo, J., Lau, E., Swaminathan, R., MacDonald, D., Chan, E., & Leung, P. C. (1994). Association between calcium regulatory hormones and other factors and bone mineral density in elderly Chinese men and women. *Journal of Gerontology,* 49(4), M189–M194.

Yamamoto, J., James, Q. C., & Palley, N. (1968). Cultural problems in psychiatric treatment. *Archives of General Psychiatry, 19,* 45–59.

Yamauchi, J. S. (1981). *The cultural integration of Asian American professional women: Issues of identity and communication behavior.* Washington, DC: National Institute of Education.

Yum, J. (1986). Exploration of the Korean immigrant family. In Korean Association of New York (Ed.), *The Korean community in America.* New York: Korean Association of New York.

Twenty-One

Chicanas and Aging: Toward Definitions of Womanhood

ELISA FACIO

The growth of the aging enterprise took place with limited attention to ethnicity and minority-group status. It was not until the 1960s that notable studies of older African Americans appeared. Attention to Latinos/Latinas came even later, during the 1970s. Most of this attention was given to Chicanos/Chicanas, who constitute the largest proportion of Latinos/Latinas. Social scientists gave little attention to older Latinos/Latinas in part because of misconceptions and stereotypes about their place in society and the family, misperceptions that continue today. Much of the social science literature has painted a rather romanticized picture of the extended Latino family, which has been thought to support and protect the aged from a "hostile" world. As a result, the problems of older Latinos/Latinas, unlike their counterparts in some other racial/ethnic groups, were thought to be minimized by the "supportive qualities" of the Latino family. Recently this position has attracted critical attention.[1]

However, the great bulk of research gave little or no attention to critical gender analyses or gender differences. With respect to gender distinctions, differences among Latinos are similar to those among other groups of elderly. For example, women live longer and outnumber men, more often remaining widowed and living alone than men do. Older Latino men marry or remarry more often than men in other racial/ethnic minority groups; 83% of older Latino men are married, but only 33% of older Latinos live with a spouse (Lacayo, 1982). Critical gender analyses did not surface until the mid-1980s. Sanchez-Ayendez (1986) studied "the interplay between values and behavior in family and community of a group of older Puerto Rican women living on low incomes in Boston" (1986, p. 239). Sanchez-Ayendez described how women create and utilize familial and community networks in a supportive productive nature. Bastida (1984) explored age- and gender-linked norms among Mexican, Puerto Rican, and Cuban women. Her findings suggested that core cultural elements of the collective identity system exist among these three populations. In other words, women's lives are shaped by sex-appropriate behavior and the pursuit of realism: being realistic about age and aging (1984, p. 9). The most recent work on older Latinas, edited by Marta Sotomayor (1995), is entitled *In Triple Jeopardy: Aged Hispanic Women: Insights and Experience*. This rich volume of work increases mainstream society's understanding of research and its implications for policy development for older Hispanic women. Particular advice is made available for program administrators, psychologists and counselors, doctors, nurses, and service providers.

Espin's work (1992) focused on contemporary sexuality and the Hispanic woman. Espin's work suggested that "the honor of Latin families is strongly tied to the sexual purity of women. And the concept of honor and dignity is one of the essential distinctive marks of Hispanic culture" (1992, p. 149). The Hispanic woman's sexuality, as defined by culture, is linked to the roles she assumes in both the family and community throughout her life. In many instances she occupies roles that render her both powerful and powerless. For example, middle-aged and elderly Hispanic women retain important roles in their families, even after their sons and daughters are married. "Grandmothers are ever present and highly vocal in family affairs. Thus older women have much more status and power than their white American counterparts, who at this age may be suffering from depression due to what is commonly known as *empty-nest syndrome*" (1992, p. 150). It is unclear to which Hispanic group(s) Espin was referring, thus making it difficult to generalize her findings to a particular Latino group or groups. Nonetheless, Espin is one of the few writers who have critically looked at the relationship between sexuality, gender, and women's roles in old age. Facio's work (1996) focused particularly on older women of Mexican descent living in the United States. Her work showed how older Chicanas cope with economic and cultural marginality and how they gain the personal and financial resources they require to define womanhood in old age.[2]

In general, research on older "Hispanic" women remains scarce. Additionally, critical gender analyses continue to be limited. Given the diversity of the Hispanic population (which technically includes all Spanish-speaking people in the United States, representing some twenty countries throughout the Americas), one cannot easily generalize one set of research findings to the entire population categorized as "Hispanic." It is possible, however, to conduct comparative research among the major "Hispanic" groups, which include Cuban Americans, Puerto Ricans, and Chicanos/Mexican Americans. Thus this chapter will focus on older women of Mexican descent, or Chicanas, living in the United States. The following discussion is based on research conducted in northern California by Facio (1996).

OLDER CHICANAS

Ironically, Chicano aging has been viewed as a uniform process. Minority and Chicano aging research has failed to critically address the lives of older Chicanas. In minority aging women's issues have been addressed using a needs-assessment approach. In Chicano aging research the plight of older women has been masked with notions of familism. Familism, as defined in Chicano aging literature, embraces cultural values of family unity and expected mutual aid, respect for the aged, and a positive gender hierarchy considered specific to Chicano families.[3] The concept of familism has been used to explain the status of the elderly, how they cope with aging, and how gender dynamics among the elderly are constructed.

Over the last two decades studies guided by the concept of familism have described characteristics of strength and vitality among older Chicanas, who, nonetheless, defer to their husbands and male relatives (Boone, 1980; Coles, 1989; Sanchez-Ayendez, 1986; Sotomayor, 1973). Generally, older Chicanas have been viewed from a traditional perspective where gender differences are neither challenged nor questioned (Alvirez, Bean, & Williams, 1981; Mirande & Enriquez, 1979). Within this perspective, the older Chicana has been described as the expressive individual in the family. More specifically, the role of the Chicana grandmother has been portrayed as the nurturing elderly child-care provider and facilitator of religious and cultural values (Boswell & Curtis, 1984; Fitzpatrick, 1971; Perez, 1986).

Older Chicanas have been overwhelmingly portrayed as focal individuals in the extended family. Households have formed largely around women, mainly because of their role in child care. Alignments between women, both within the family and outside of it, often constitute the core of family networks. Scholars claim that older women perform a variety of tasks for their families (Markides, Boldt, & Ray, 1986; Schmidt & Padilla, 1983).

The Chicano family has been portrayed as a strong, resourceful unit with the Chicana as its center. For example, according to Zepeda (1979), "The role of 'la abuela' (grandmother) in the family is something most Mexicanos/Chicanos treasure" (p. 11). Notably, Chicana grandmothers have been considered "the backbone of family endurance and the symbol of cultural survival" (p. 12). The stories of two women embody these values:

Louisa . . . is the matriarch of her family. A woman with strong ideas and a wealth of practical knowledge, she is regarded as the family advice giver and chief storyteller.

At 56, Esperanza Salcido has always planned her life around her family. Her children are grown now, but her work of caring for others has changed very little. Today she looks after her young grandchildren. "Recently my dad got sick," she said, "so I'm taking care of him, too. . . . Yes, it's hard sometimes, but that's what families are all about." (Elsasser, MacKenzie & Tixier y Vigil, 1980, pp. 18, 62)

Social scientists have interpreted the role of older Chicanas as active and dominant. Chicanas appear to play an increasingly dominant role in the extended family as they grow older. Some scholars note that this contradicts the myth that the Chicano family is a patriarchal structure. This paradox has been explained by Maldonado (1975) as the consequence of high early death rates among Chicanos. Others attempt to explain it by simply noting that women weather the transition into old age better than men do. Male roles are seen as more tenuous and less well defined, providing fewer opportunities for older men to make themselves useful in their families in nontraditional, noneconomic ways (Cuellar, 1978; Velez, 1978).

This perspective implies that the older Chicana's subordinate status is vital for the physical and cultural survival of the family. Hence, for advocates of this approach, the cultural continuity of the Chicano family appears to be embedded in the Chicana's domestic and caregiving role. The continuity of the life course for older Chicanas is interpreted as remaining family centered. Whether familism is conceptualized as a structural, cultural, or combined phenomenon, studies consistently project the family as the most, and many times the only, important force in the lives of older Chicanas.

Rather than considering familism largely as an empirical or structural phenomenon, this concept must also be conceptualized as an ideological force. Casting familism as an ideology would help redefine the study of older Chicanas in broader sociological terms. In other words, it is important to look to ideology to understand where familism is rooted with respect to class, race/ethnicity, gender, and culture. To do this, we must identify the ideological components associated with familism and older Chicanas.

In previous research conducted by Facio (1996), her findings refuted the empirical evidence in Chicano aging literature surrounding this preceding debate. First, let us refer to the notion of the multigenerational household or extended family. According to Facio's study, familism as an empirical phenomenon, a manifestation of expected mutual aid and support, appears to have changed, although certain elements of familism, namely, family unity, have remained. In other words, the multigenerational household and extended family do not operate as the literature would lead us to believe. The study further suggested that older Chicanas have established modified networks with other older Chicanas and not necessarily with their own family. They still value family unity, but this unity may stem not from familism or culture, but from gender and age dynamics. Thus the data call for broadening our conceptualization of social networks among older Chicanas according to age and gender.

Second, the application of familism in explaining the gender hierarchy associated with the aged is the most ambiguous and limiting discussion in Chicano aging literature. In order to get a clearer sense of this hierarchy, we need to explore those aspects of familism that are rooted in gender. Studies by de la Torre and Pesquera (1993) and Segura (1986) have illustrated that motherhood and male authority are considered ideological components of familism, along with family unity. Male authority or patriarchy bonds women to motherhood and family caregiving roles (Segura, 1986, p. 199). The ideology of familism values these roles as beneficial to the maintenance of the family.

The value placed on motherhood continues with the transition to grandmotherhood. In other words, the values associated with motherhood legitimate the status of grandmotherhood. What we then have is the continued reproduction of gender. How older Chicanas respond to grandmotherhood is interesting. Facio's findings (1996) suggested that older Chicanas found grandmotherhood "confining" and "limiting" and that they sought ways to avoid meeting the expectations associated with grandmotherhood. Many women expressed joy and pride in being grandmothers, but they were not willing to take on the expectations associated with grandmotherhood, namely, child care. Thus a clearer identification of the values and expectations associated with the ideological component of familism and older Chicana lives is in order.

Male authority becomes a complex issue, as many of these women are widows and no longer have to deal with male authority at home as they did earlier. Undoubtedly, however, interactions with male relatives and male individuals in various settings take on a particular character shaped by patriarchy. In addition, the value that patriarchy places on motherhood and grandmotherhood appears to manifest itself during the Chicana's later years.

This discussion leads us to look further at gender. Such an analysis will illuminate the ideological premises and underlying implications of familism, namely, the value of male authority over females. However, this is not specific to Chicano families. Nonetheless, gender is a major component or dynamic of Chicano familism that continues to manifest itself throughout the Chicana's life course. Familism as proposed in Chicano aging literature has only served to explain and understand women as wives, mothers, and grandmothers.

This chapter focuses on women whose lives are no longer solely centered in the family. It focuses on older Chicanas who are no longer married, who no longer mother in their family of procreation, or who are not strictly involved in traditional family networks. Theoretically, it is important to stop "lumping" married and unmarried women together as if all women were alike. This analytical separation allows for a better understanding of older Chicana lives, as many no longer directly identify themselves in relationship to a traditional family structure. In other words, the lives of older Chicanas encompass much more than simply family relationships.

As a means of transcending the limited focus of familism, rather than rejecting the concept completely, sociological approaches such as political economy and feminist theory should be considered. The political economy approach generally takes the structural forces of social organization as its level of analysis. Rather than looking to individuals or technology as primary causal forces in society, political economy is ultimately concerned with the social relations of production (Alford & Friedland, 1985). The aged, in a political economy analysis, are a group of people who are used in helping to stabilize the capitalist mode of production by regulating the work force and maximizing productivity (Minkler & Estes, 1991).

Chicanos have also been analyzed as fulfilling the needs of capitalism by occupying low-wage jobs in a segmented labor force (Almaguer, 1975; Barrera, 1979). The political economy approach helps to illustrate how older Chicanos/ Chicanas are influenced by the political and economic position that Chicanos have historically held in the production process. Also, political economy analysis focuses on social power and inequality. This changes the focus of study from how individuals can adapt to aging to what political and economic changes can optimize the aging process. Furthermore, a political economy analysis of older Chicanos/Chicanas provides an understanding of how the Chicano family is shaped by its position in the system of production. This perspective highlights how the role of the elder in the family results from the economic exploitation of Chicanos, showing how the family mediates capitalism and aging.

Feminist theories vary as to whether the central social force that creates social differentiation based on gender is patriarchy, capitalism, or both. Theorists who use an analysis of patriarchy describe and explain how male dominance has been practiced historically under different social and economic systems. Early Marxist feminism described how women as a group had a definite relationship to the means of production and how their place in the home was economically necessary for the operation of a capitalist system. Later Marxist feminism has brought the consideration of patriarchy back into the analysis, looking at the dynamic relation between women's work in the home and productive forces outside of the home. Both capitalists as a class and men as a class are seen to benefit from the social relations of patriarchy and capitalism.

Feminist theory could draw studies of older Chicanos/Chicanas away from a concern with how the structure and functions of the family benignly benefit older people and toward an identification of how gender and class dominance transcends the family and continues into old age. Under feminist theory, Chicana grandmothers would be more than matriarchs; they would also take their place as players in the historical and societal process of gender oppression.

In general, the present generation of older Chicanas has been socialized to assume traditional tasks of child care and household maintenance. For many women of this generation, school was a luxury and privilege. In previous re-search, many women stressed how much they wanted to attend school. However, their parents, in particular their fathers, did not see the long-term benefits but only the immediate necessity of their labor. The "real" skills they were expected to need when they were no longer girls were those they learned at home.

Women's work consisted of growing and preparing food, making children's school clothes, and teaching children the hymns and prayers of the church. (The Catholic church held and continues to hold a special importance in the lives of many older Chicanas.) They learned to deliver babies and treat illnesses with herbs and patience. In almost every town one or two women, in addition to working in their homes, served other families in the community as *curanderas* (healers) or *parteras* (midwives).

During the childhood of today's older Chicanas, grandparents were a vital part of the family. Many women lived with their grandparents, where they were culturally educated with respect to food, traditional customs and beliefs, and the struggles that relatives experienced during and after the Mexican Revolution. By an early age, most older Chicanas had married, going straight from their fathers' to their husbands' homes. They moved from being daughters to being wives and mothers, with little, if any, time in between. Some of these women tell of early married life where they played games (e.g., skipping rope with their girlfriends) while cooking a pot of beans.

Older Chicanas, in general, find themselves struggling with past traditions in the midst of contemporary realities, creating contradictions and challenges in their old age. They were socialized with certain ideas about old age: that it would bring harmony, status, respect, and solace. However, the reality of their present lives' poverty, family structural changes, differential life expectancies, and longevity calls for the aged to reassess their expectations and thus redefine their old age. Older Chicanas, in particular, must also deal with traditions that reinforce a gender hierarchy. This is one aspect of older Chicanas' lives that has not been critically examined.

In the preceding discussion this author has attempted to introduce readers to older Chicanas, both past and present. This brief introduction touches on their early socialization regarding old age and subsequently their particular expectations about growing old. Given the realities of their present lives and their expectations of old age, what are the challenges that confront older Chicanas in socially constructing their old age? In other words, what is their social, economic, and cultural context?

This chapter argues that old age for Chicanas is largely determined by structural and cultural constraints. Structurally, older Chicanas are placed in poverty. Culturally, they are prescribed to remain without companionship and as caretakers. In other words, they are consigned to grandmotherhood. Older Chicanas, however, have taken measures to deal with conflicting cultural traditions and structural constraints through community organizations, such as senior-citizen centers and the church, and their own families. Within these contexts older Chicanas have actively defined or constructed varied meanings of their old age, their womanhood.

This chapter focuses on the cultural expectations or constraints older Chicanas face in constructing their old age, or womanhood, within the institution of the family and the larger Chicano/Chicana community. Facio's research suggested that Chicano culture requires that older women, whether they are biological or surrogate grandmothers, conform to the role of caregivers. Generally, cultural norms discourage older Chicanas from seeking male companionship but steer them toward an old age spent as caregivers, more commonly known as *las abuelas*. However, older Chicanas desire to be more than simply grandmothers, as currently proposed by the Chicano community. Older Chicanas also want to establish their identities as cultural teachers and older women. The cultural context of aging, primarily familism or *respeto*, and cultural values of women as caregivers or nurturers, is analyzed. In this chapter we clearly see how familism, ageism, and gender influence the Chicana's social definition of old age.

The older Chicana's attempt to redefine her womanhood conflicts with cultural expectations of older women's lives. For older Chicanas who are grandmothers or *abuelas*, Chicano culture imposes the traditional role of caregiving. This chapter is concerned with cultural expectations placed on older women who are grandmothers, not the familial or community roles for which many older Chicanas are recognized. For example, Espin (1992) said that "middle-aged and elderly Hispanic women retain important roles in their families even after their sons and daughters are married" (p. 142). Generally, opinions and advice of older Latinas or grandmothers are sought in major family decisions, thus rendering these women integral members in family affairs. Some may also act as providers of mental health services in an unofficial way as *curanderas* "for those people who believe in these alternative approaches to health care" (Espin, 1992, p. 142). Also, some Latina grandmothers have knowledge of herbal remedies for physical ailments. Some of these women can play a powerful role in their communities, given their reputation for being able to heal mind and body. Espin (1992) further argued that older Latina women may have more status and power than their Anglo counterparts. However, unlike the role of caregiver, these roles are not culturally prescribed.

As older Chicanas attempt to define and resolve their womanhood, they question and challenge cultural expectations, at the risk of being disrespected. Capitalizing on this respect is critical, as this facilitates the process of defining their womanhood. The family simultaneously presents a means of support, love, and respect, while stressing conformity and ultimately control. The older Chicana's self-aspiration as a cultural teacher threatens to alter tradition, as cultural expectations imposed on older Chicanas are antithetical to her desired existence.

To begin the examination of this dialectic, our discussion focuses on grandmotherhood. Based on Facio's research (1996), grandmotherhood can be defined as a stage in the life course when women, based on their age and sex, are expected to conform primarily to a caregiving and nurturing role. Thus grandmotherhood essentially involves "grandmothering," where older Chicanas provide care and nurture for grandchildren and/or great-grandchildren. In general, older Chicanas welcome grandmotherhood; at the same time they hope to redefine and broaden their relationship to the family. Chicana grandmothers are willing to assist with child care when necessary, but they object to the idea of grandmothers as convenient "baby-sitters." An important issue these women clarified was the distinction between "raising" (*crear*) grandchildren and providing "child care" (*cuidar*). For example, Concepcion said, "I didn't raise my grandchildren, but took care of them when I had to" (Facio, 1996, p. 92).

Experiences of grandmotherhood no doubt varied. Generally, women in Facio's study stated that they were satisfied with their relationships to their children and grandchildren. However, it was clear that they did not see themselves solely as caregivers. For example, Maria said, "I love it, but I'm not the kind of grandma where I'm going to sit down and only knit little things for my grandkids or nothing" (Facio, 1996, p. 92). Not all grandmothers have positive familial relationships, as the literature would lead one to believe. A few women have little or no contact with their grandchildren because of geographical distance or poor familial relationships.

Chicana grandmothers do not feel obligated to provide child care, although in times of need they provide care for their grandchildren and great-grandchildren. Many women said that they wanted to use the independence that old age has brought them in ways other than caregiving. For many, this is the first time they have had the opportunity to define or construct their own lives without the responsibility of caring for a parent, spouse, or children. Antonia described her expectations and obligations as a Chicana grandmother:

I thought that if I'm gonna be a grandma I could help mi'ja when she needed my help, but I was not obligated to stay home and take care of children so she could have a good time . . . because the grandparents have the right to be free and enjoy themselves when they're old or young or whatever. You have to have some consideration for your parents, not load them with children because they're grandparents or they're old. (Facio, 1996, p. 92)

Beyond the desire to establish themselves as cultural teachers, these women are no doubt influenced by their age. Many of these women are great-grandmothers and no longer have the energy to care for grandchildren or great-grandchildren. With their first grandchild they were elated. In many cases, these women admitted to wanting to have the grandchild daily. But they have very strong feelings about the obligations of grandmothers, particularly that of baby-sitting.

According to the older women in Facio's study (1996), grandmotherhood should not mean an obligation to perform tasks associated with mothering, caregiving, and nurturing. If the caregiver role is culturally valued, caregiving and nurturing should be regarded as the *abuela*'s contribution to mutual forms of assistance within familial networks. However, given the existence of patriarchy, caregiving and nurturing are not valued in society, thus contributing to women's oppression. Because of traditional socialization with respect to female/male roles, older Chicanas are accepting of the caregiver role when it is respected and not taken for granted, thus continuing to define grandmotherhood within a traditional context. Facio's research did not suggest that grandmotherhood be defined in relationship to a traditional role of caregiving. On the contrary, her research illuminated how grandmotherhood is regarded within the Chicano community and among older Chicanas. Hence grandmotherhood defined within this context warrants respect, under the condition that older women conform to the cultural expectation of caregiver. Thus grandmotherhood as defined contributes to a status of both power and powerlessness. The dichotomy of power/powerlessness is also illustrated in Espin's research on older Hispanic women (1992).

In Facio's research the element of powerlessness lies in the potential exploitation of older Chicanas as convenient caregivers or baby-sitters. Generally, grandmothering is a difficult task. However, of greater concern is the limited view of older women simply as caregivers. The process of establishing oneself as a cultural teacher involves retaining and capitalizing on respect granted to older women who conform to the caregiver role. The conditions under which older women attempt to capitalize on respect differ for widowed and married grandmothers.

Facio's research (1996) was conducted among 30 women in northern California; 26 were widowed grandmothers, 2 were married grandmothers, and 2 had never had children. For the widowed grandmother to retain respect, she must remain single and refrain from seeking male companionship. The widowed grandmother is expected to respect the memory of her past marriage by remaining widowed and conforming to a traditional role of caregiver. Older widowed grandmothers are discouraged from seeking male companionship. This proscription ultimately controls their sexuality, whether in fact they seek companionship. Thus, *la abuela*, like most aged persons, is considered asexual. Even though companionship among older people may not necessarily be sexual, older Chicanas do have a sense of sexuality. Cultural expectations, ageism, and patriarchy define and subsequently influence the expression of older Chicana sexuality.

An older widowed grandmother who challenges this expectation risks being judged as a "bad" woman or *una mujer sin verguenza*. The dichotomy of the "good" versus "bad" woman serves to ensure that aged widowed grandmothers will commit themselves to cultural expectations of caregiving. If widowed grandmothers do not concede to this cultural expectation, they risk losing the respect needed to establish themselves as cultural teachers.

According to Espin (1992), "The honor of Latin families is strongly tied to the sexual purity of women" (p. 142). The idea of the virgin/whore dichotomy stems from Catholicism. Again, according to Espin, "The Virgin Mary, who was a virgin and a mother, but never a sexual being, is considered an important role model for Hispanic women" (p. 142). Young women are encouraged to remain virgins until marriage, and older women are encouraged to be celibate after marriage. Thus the implication is that women should engage in sex only to procreate and should shun sexual pleasure.

Married grandmothers are not bound by the restriction. It is assumed that they will not seek male companionship. Therefore, their aspirations as cultural teachers should not be hindered. However, they are still expected to conform to the traditional caregiving role.

With respect to the two surrogate grandmothers who are childless women, one woman was a surrogate grandmother to her goddaughter's children. The other woman married late in life and did not have any children of her own. She too acted as a surrogate ''grandmother'' to her younger sibling's children. Given that they were widows, they also were discouraged from seeking male companionship. These women were expected to retain a sense of respect among their immediate families and the larger Chicano community by remaining single.

Older women's children, and the community in general, tend to regard Chicana grandmothers as ready, willing, and able to provide child care. It is important to clarify that caregiving carries no guarantee of respect. Being caregivers does not necessarily earn women the respect they need to become cultural teachers. If an aged grandmother does seek male companionship, she may not be granted the respect needed to become a cultural teacher. However, having male companionship in no way bars her children and, in some cases, grandchildren from seeking her services as a caregiver. Grandmothering is viewed as culturally valid. Seeking male companionship is culturally disrespectful.

In Facio's research (1996) one respondent, Antonia, had been living alone for nearly twenty years. Because of the expectations that are held about older Chicano women, Antonia had difficulty addressing the issue of companionship during the interview. She began by rationalizing why some older women may seek companionship. She stated that many women have had ''hard lives.'' By this she meant that many women were physically, emotionally, and/or psychologically abused in their marriages. According to Antonia, once these women become widows, they now ''feel free'' and are anxious to have a ''good'' relationship with someone. Second, she adopted the Chicano community's cultural norms by adamantly telling Facio not to repeat the story of her friend Carmen. The following is Antonia's account of Carmen's experience:

I haven't seen, but I have heard that a lot of men treat their wives really bad. When they die, well, a woman feels free. So they're anxious to marry whoever not thinking that it might not be good, they just think it'll be better, but sometimes the second is worse than the first. That's what I've heard (long pause) . . . that's what's happening with my friend, Carmen. Don't say anything! There's a man who's courting her, but don't you say anything to anyone! (Facio, 1996, p. 96)

Concepcion Villegas had been widowed for fourteen years and lived alone. She addressed the expectations placed on the older Chicana widows, focusing in particular on how women who seek male companionship run the risk of being categorized as either good or bad. This categorization perpetuates a traditional relationship to the older woman's family. Concepcion said,

When I became a widow, if you talk to men, they think you are bad, that you talk to them and want them to have maybe an affair, become a sweetheart or whatever, and that's when I changed because I couldn't talk to my friends or to a man like friendly. (Facio, 1996, p. 96)

Mercedes had been widowed for ten years, and she too lived alone. Mercedes was the most comfortable and adamant in addressing the issue of companionship:

Well, there's a lot of women . . . well, when their husbands pass away they begin to have a lot of friends, both men and women, and they go out and all that. Sometimes that can be good, and other times it isn't when other people see you and they begin to talk. They'll say, "Look at the way she's acting now, before don't you remember what a saint! Now look what's happening, that woman's up to no good." That's the first thing that people say! They don't say, "She's trying to enjoy herself because she needs to get out, she needs to keep busy, she needs to keep preoccupied." They don't say that, they say just the opposite. (Facio, 1996, p. 96)

Finally, Maria shared her experiences of how the community and particularly her children reacted to her companionship. Maria Gonzales had been widowed for ten years and lived with her 30-year-old daughter.

There were many people who criticized me. And my children said I was too old to have a friend. Your kids think that once you're old, you're dead or something. They get very jealous. And the first thing they say is "what about my father?" Well, what about their father, he's dead, may he rest in peace, but I'm not! See, if you're a widow, they want you to stay home, be a good little grandma. Yes, we can go out, but don't uh . . . don't try to make friends with men. (Facio, 1996, p. 97)

Generally, members of the community, but particularly children of older Chicanas, hold strong objections to their mother's involvement with men. Some children threaten to withhold financial support. Others discontinue regular visits and phone calls. Still others display their discontent by playing on their mother's guilt for not respecting their father's memory.

Given the constraints imposed on the older Chicana's womanhood, how then do these women remain respected while challenging cultural expectations? As illustrated in the preceding discussion, Chicana grandmothers are altering the traditional role of caregiving. Chicana grandmothers will provide child care out of necessity but not for convenience's sake. This, in turn, grants them independence and leverage in defining their relationship to the family. Under these conditions, child-care services are viewed as an important form of mutual aid to the family. The attempt, on the part of older Chicanas, is to socially construct the caregiver role as an important form of familial support rather than a form of control. Nonetheless, their womanhood, with respect to grandmothering, continues to be defined within a traditional context.

The process of socially constructing Chicana old age also involves capitalizing on symbolic respect for the aged. Symbolic respect refers to acknowledgment of a specific age hierarchy, which is largely manifested through language. Younger generations are expected to acknowledge the presence of older Chicanos, not render them invisible. They are taught to respect the aged for their wisdom and knowledge, for their survival into old age.

Older Chicanas' quest to redefine their womanhood obviously depends on their relationship to their children. However, given the cultural prerequisite of respect for the aged, older Chicanas are placed in an advantageous situation. This enables them to maintain contact with their children and, most important, grandchildren and, for some, great-grandchildren. Such contact, whether through visits, social gatherings, or caregiving services, allows older Chicanas to establish themselves as cultural teachers and subsequently to redefine womanhood while maintaining positive familial relationships.

The challenge for married grandmothers, according to Facio, is to maintain positive familial relationships, thus capitalizing on symbolic respect for the aged. Widowed grandmothers who try to reconstruct old age may violate cultural norms related to female sexuality. For the remaining 28 widowed grandmothers, living alone, involvement with senior centers and/or the church, and friendship networks are additional resources that contribute to an identity independent from the family. As older Chicanas' involvement in such environments grows, they move from a dependent to an interdependent relationship with their families that provides them with more leverage in negotiating and resolving their womanhood.

As cultural teachers, older Chicanas want to socialize grandchildren and/or great-grandchildren with certain cultural values and traditions, particularly their behavior toward older people and the maintenance of Spanish. The preservation of music, food, and, for some, religion is viewed as equally important. Given their socioeconomic status, older Chicanas are placed in a position where they can leave a legacy of cultural rather than monetary value. For example, Mercedes said, "I would like for all my grandchildren to speak Spanish. I have some grandchildren who speak Spanish and others who don't. I'm not trying to take their English away because I know real well that they need it, that's how I feel. (Facio, 1996, p. 99)

CONCLUSION

The social construction of womanhood for older Chicanas involves reconceptualizing the traditional expectation of caregiving and the role of cultural teacher. In altering rather than dismantling the caregiving role, older Chicanas continue to define their womanhood within a traditional context. Generally, they continue to view themselves as grandmothers who are both caregivers and nurturers. Hence reconceptualization involves the way in which the caregiver role is regarded among the Chicano community. At present, cultural expectations and the conditions under which older Chicanas are pressured to conform as caregivers serve as mechanisms of social control. For older Chicanas, the caregiver role should be valued and respected as an important form of financial and social support.

As cultural teachers, older Chicanas are recognized as people of knowledge and wisdom. Most important, they act as carriers of the cultural legacy, thus playing an important part in preserving culture. Interestingly, in providing child care, older Chicanas are more likely than men to have contact with their families, allowing the role of cultural teacher to develop. This is not to say that one cannot establish oneself as a cultural teacher outside of a child-care context or that men cannot establish themselves as cultural teachers. The implication is that women have effectively used their limited resources in socially constructing their womanhood, namely, their family and their relationships to the family.

In moving toward definitions of womanhood among older Chicanas, the concept *abuela* or grandmother merits attention. The term *abuela* connotes a romanticized image of older Chicanas that only serves to disempower women within their families and among the community. It is interesting to note that when older Chicanas are discussed in the literature, they are almost always referred to as grandmothers. Thus the terms grandmother and older woman are synonymous.

For older Chicanas, grandmotherhood should be a status of respect, not only because of their age and their potential as caregivers. Grandmotherhood should bring recognition for their position in the family, their labor as caregivers and nurturers, and their contributions to familial support systems. Facio (1996) and to some extent Espin (1992) suggested that older Chicanas desire an age hierarchy that would recognize them not only as grandmothers, but also as cultural teachers and older women who are not necessarily asexual.

NOTES

1. See Maldonado (1975). Maldonado argued that social change is breaking down the supportive quality of the traditional family structure. Also see Wallace and Facio (1987). Torrez (1996) argued that industrialization and urbanization have contributed to the changing structure of the traditional Mexican-American extended family, resulting in the unavailability of family support services that older Mexican Americans/Chicanos expected in their old age. Therefore, Torrez concluded, "Mexican American elderly need programs to provide them with services that the traditional extended family social support system may have previously provided" (p. 93).

2. Older Chicanos/Chicanas would probably refrain from using the term *Chicano* as a means of self-identity. Rather, they seem to prefer *Mexicano* or *Mexican*. Other acceptable terms are *Mexican American* or *Spanish-speaking* (Facio, 1996, p. 9).

3. Research on Chicano aging has focused primarily on the interrelationship of aging and the concept of familism. This approach has been widely accepted and is a primary guiding concept in Chicano aging studies. With few exceptions, Chicano aging research is grounded in an analysis of families as the driving force behind the relationship of the elderly to the larger society. Also, research guided by this concept assumes that most elderly are active exclusively within a family context.

REFERENCES

Alford, R. R., & Friedland, R. (1985). *Powers of theory*. New York: Cambridge University Press.

Almaguer, T. (1975). Class, race, and Chicano oppression. *Socialist Revolution, 5,* 71–99.

Alvirez, D., Bean, F. D., & Williams, D. (1981). The Mexican American family. In C. H. Mindel & R. W. Habenstein (Eds.,), *Ethnic families in America* (pp. 269–292). New York: Elsevier.

Barrera, M. (1979). *Race and class in the Southwest*. Notre Dame, IN: University of Notre Dame Press.

Bastida, E. (1984). Age and gender linked norms among older Hispanic women. In Robert Anson (Ed.), *The Hispanic older woman*. Washington, DC: National Hispanic Council on Aging.

Boone, M. S. (1980). The uses of traditional concepts in the development of new urban roles: Cuban women in the United States. In E. Bourguignon (Ed.), *A world of women*. New York: Praeger.

Boswell, T. D., & Curtis, J. R. (1984). *The Cuban-American experience*. Totowa, NJ: Rowman & Allenheld.

Coles, R. (1989). *The old one of New Mexico*. Albuquerque: University of New Mexico Press.

Cuellar, J. (1978). Senior citizens club: The older Mexican-American in the voluntary association. In B. Myerhoff & A. Simic (Eds.), *Life's career—aging* (pp. 207–230). Beverly Hills, CA: Sage Publications.

Elsasser, N., MacKenzie, K., & Tixier y Vigil, Y. (1980). *Las mujeres: Conversations from a Hispanic community*. Old Westbury, NY: Feminist Press.

Espin, O. M. (1992). Cultural and historical influences on sexuality in Hispanic/Latin women: Implications for psychotherapy. In M. L. Andersen & P. H. Collins (Eds.), *Race, class, and gender: An anthology* (pp. 141–146). Belmont, CA: Wadsworth.

Facio, E. (1996). *Understanding older Chicanas: Sociological and policy perspectives*. Thousand Oaks, CA: Sage Publications.

Fitzpatrick, J. P. (1971). *Puerto Rican Americans*. Englewood Cliffs, NJ: Prentice-Hall.

Lacayo, C. (1982, Spring). Triple jeopardy: Underserved Hispanic elders. *Generations,* p. 25.

Maldonado, D. (1975). The Chicano aged. *Social Work, 20,* 213–216.

———. (1979). Aging in the Chicano context. In D. E. Gelfand & A. J. Kutzik (Eds.), *Ethnicity and aging* (pp. 175–183). New York: Springer.

Markides, K. S., Boldt, J. S., & Ray, L. A. (1986). Sources of helping and intergenerational solidity: A three-generations study of Mexican Americans. *Journal of Gerontology, 41,* 506–511.

Minkler, M., & Estes, C. L. (1991). *Critical perspectives on aging: The political and moral economy of growing old*. Amityville, NY: Baywood.

Mirande, A., & Enriquez, E. (Eds.). (1979). *La Chicana: The Mexican American woman*. Chicago: University of Chicago Press.

Perez, L. (1986). Immigrant economic adjustment and family organization: The Cuban experience. *International Migration Review, 20,* 4–20.

Sanchez-Ayendez, M. (1986). Puerto Rican elderly women: Shared meanings and informal support networks. In J. B. Cole (Ed.), *All American women: Lines that divide, ties that bind* (pp. 172–186). New York: Free Press.

Schmidt, A., & Padilla, A. M. (1983). Grandparent-grandchild interaction in a Mexican American group. *Hispanic Journal of Behavioral Sciences, 5,* 181–198.

Segura, D. (1986). *Chicanas and Mexican immigrant women in the labor market: A study of occupational mobility and stratification.* Unpublished doctoral dissertation, University of California, Berkeley.

Sotomayor, M. (1973). *A study of Chicano grandparents in an urban barrio.* Unpublished doctoral dissertation, University of Denver School of Social Work.

———. (Ed.). (1995). *In triple jeopardy: Aged Hispanic women: Insights and experiences.* Washington, DC: National Hispanic Council on Aging.

de la Torre, A. & Pesquera, B. (Eds.). (1993). *Building with our hands: New directions in Chicana studies.* Berkeley: University of California Press.

Torrez, D. J. (1996). Independent living among Mexican American elderly: The need for social services support. In Roberto M. DeAnda (Ed.), *Chicanas and Chicanos in Contemporary Society.* Needham Heights, MA: Allyn & Bacon.

Velez, C. G. (1978). Youth and aging in central Mexico: One day in the life of four families of migrants. In B. Myerhoff & A. Simic (Eds.), *Life's career—aging* (pp. 107–162). Beverly Hills, CA: Sage Publications.

Wallace, S. P., & Facio, E. (1987). Moving beyond familism: Potential contributions of gerontological theory to studies of Chicano/Latino aging. In J. F. Gubrium & K. Charmaz (Eds.), *Aging, self, and community: A collection of readings* (pp. 207–224). Greenwich, CT: JAI Press.

Zepeda, M. (1979). Las abuelitas. *Agenda, 9,* 10–13.

Twenty-Two

Rural Older Women

VIRA R. KIVETT

Rural older women form a varied group from small towns, open country, and farms. The ever-changing rural context contributes to this diversity. Despite differences, many rural older women share a common heritage passed to them by earlier generations of women living off of the land (Kivett, 1990). Vestiges of this heritage still may be seen in their courage, optimism, efficiency, imagination, skill, common sense, and determinism (Stratton, 1981). The qualities of self-reliance, mutual support, and rurality, while positive forces, have helped to keep many rural women isolated and underserved (Carlton-LaNey, 1992). The purpose of this chapter is to profile contemporary rural older women according to their general status, roles, life outcomes, and needs as observed through the empirical literature.

A substantial number of studies were conducted on older women during the past two decades (see Coyle, 1989; Krout, 1986; and Wilkinson, 1982, for annotated bibliographies of this research). Approaches have been of two types (Mokuau & Browne, 1994). The first approach has placed considerable emphasis on the oppression of women, particularly of minorities, by ageism, classism, and racism. The second has placed emphasis upon their strengths and adaptive life patterns. Little research has specifically addressed women in rural areas. The lack of attention given to rural older women is primarily related to their historical lack of power, status, and visibility (Cool & McCabe, 1983). Rural older women are of particular interest because of their higher rates of poverty, poorer housing, and lesser access to medical and social services than corresponding urban older women (Bastida, 1984; Carlton-LaNey, 1992; Kivett & Schwenk, 1994).

Table 22.1

Population Profile of Rural Older Women According to Proportion in Rural
Population, Ethnic Status, and Male/Female Ratios

Profile Variable	Total Rural 65+ N	%[a]	Total Rural Women 65+ N	%[b]	Rural Males per 100 Rural Females
Totals	7,673,277	24.6	4,287,697	55.9	79
Age Groups					
65-69	2,587,975		1,352,440	52.3	91
70-74	2,011,190		1,086,588	54.0	85
75-79	1,494,962		846,492	56.6	77
80-84	911,386		551,799	60.5	65
85+	660,375		446,413	67.6	48
Ethnic Status					
White	7,162,085		3,994,413	55.8	79
Black	408,324		239,053	58.5	71
Hispanic	94,836		48,659	51.3	95
Native Americans	54,628		30,263	55.4	81
Asian-Pacific	22,965		11,582	50.4	98

Note: Totals vary in accordance with census figures.
[a]Percentage of the total population 65 years or older.
[b]Percentage of the rural population 65 years or older.
Source: U.S. Bureau of the Census. (1992). *1990 Census of Population: General Population Characteristics* (1990, CP-1-1). Washington, DC: U.S. Government Printing Office.

THE PREVALENCE AND LOCATION OF RURAL OLDER WOMEN

Rural refers to areas ranging from 50,000 or more persons to 2,500 persons
or less. The greatest socioeconomic and related differences from those of the
general population of older adults are found in areas of 2,500 population or less
(U.S. Bureau of the Census, 1992).

Approximately 4 million women 65 years or older live in areas of 2,500
population or less (table 22.1). They comprise approximately 56 percent of the
rural population 65 years or older. Relatively few older minorities are located
in rural areas. Considerable variation is found among rural minority older
women in terms of acculturation, educational level, level of income, family
structure, and worldviews (Kivett, 1993a). The ratio of older rural males to
females varies considerably according to ethnic group (table 22.1), an observation important to a number of economic and social outcomes of rural women.

RESEARCH APPROACHES IN THE STUDY OF RURAL OLDER
WOMEN

Despite a paucity of literature on rural older women, research approaches
have varied. Research designs have included cross-sectional (Dorfman & Mof-

fett, 1987; Kivett, 1993b; Krout, 1988), longitudinal (Blackburn, Greenberg, & Boss, 1987; McCulloch, 1991; Kivett & McCulloch, 1989; Wallace & O'Hara, 1992), and ethnographic or qualitative types (Carlton-LaNey, 1992; Shenk, 1987; Weinert & Long, 1987). Studies have seldom examined the process in the life outcomes of rural older women, but rather have considered the predictors and correlates of outcomes. Moreover, rural older women generally have been treated as an independent variable rather than as a major unit of analysis. As a result, issues of gender frequently are compounded with other structural variables such as education, race, and income.

THEORETICAL PERSPECTIVES

Few studies of older women have been theoretically based. Although a number of theoretical perspectives may be applied to studies of older women, none of the major psychological perspectives (mechanistic, organismic, and dialectic) or sociological perspectives (normative and interpretive) were designed to address processes and outcomes among women (Gee & Kimball, 1987). There would seem to be some support for a dialectic perspective. The proclivity of rural older women to act upon and react to social issues affecting the institutions and values important to rural life strongly supports a dialectic approach.

Occasionally, midrange theories such as activity, disengagement, and continuity theories have been used to explain social outcomes in the rural elderly (Dorfman, Kohout, & Heckert, 1985). Similarly, the theory of intergenerational solidarity has also served as a basis for studies on rural older adults (Atkinson, Kivett, & Campbell, 1986). Emerging perspectives such as those of feminists, many of which are based upon the premises of gender and power, not age, may have special application to rural older women. For example, more traditional or provincial views of rural women suggest lower status and power among rural women than among those in urban areas.

RESEARCH FINDINGS ON RURAL OLDER WOMEN

A general lack of research on rural older women requires that extrapolations of research findings on the general population of older women or rural older adults frequently be made to this important group.

GENERAL STATUS

Physical Well-being

Data on a rural health disadvantage are equivocal depending upon the health measure (Kivett & McCulloch, 1989; Krout, 1986). Furthermore, health issues among older women vary significantly according to age group and ethnic and socioeconomic background (U.S. Department of Health and Human Services,

1985). Data have shown that rural older women are more likely to report poor health, 25 percent, than the general population of older adults, 10 percent (McCulloch, 1991; U.S. Department of Health and Human Services, 1985). Limited information shows no differences in health dependency between rural older men and women. Krout (1986) found that health dependency among the rural elderly, professional health care, and related in-home health care services did not differ according to gender. Older rural women have a higher probability of surviving to very old age than older rural men (McCulloch & Kivett, 1995). The probability of surviving to a very old age for both rural men and women is more dependent upon their early life achievement, for example, education, than upon later-life events such as health.

Longitudinal data have shown that rural older women who survived to very old age had few increases in the number of physical ailments over a ten-year prior period (McCulloch, 1991). Considerable change occurred, however, in the extent to which their physical conditions affected their daily activities. Physical problems in the order of their prevalence were arthritis, 77 percent; hypertension, 48 percent; circulatory problems, 45 percent; and diabetes, 9 percent. Primary causes of death of nonsurvivors over the ten-year period were cerebrovascular disease, 22 percent; ischemic heart disease, 18 percent; and congestive heart failure, 13 percent. With regard to health management, the majority of rural older women, both survivors and nonsurvivors, visited a doctor for checkups when ill and took prescription medications. McCulloch concluded that the health problems and primary causes of death among this group of women were consistent with national findings on the general population of older adults.

The health problems of rural older black women differ sharply from those of other racial groups because of their physical environment, income, work, and health conditions (Carlton-LaNey, 1992). Strong concern has been expressed regarding the health status and outcomes of rural older black women. Studies have found that the range of health behaviors of rural older black women is enmeshed in the sociocultural fabric of the rural community. Findings suggest the importance of understanding the health behaviors of rural older ethnic women within their sociocultural milieu.

Many health practices are indigenous to the prescribed beliefs and practices of rural elderly people. These include ignoring or forgetting existing physical conditions until they become disabling, praying and living by religious principles, and using home remedies and self-medication. These health behaviors are congruent with the value system of independence and self-reliance found in the rural community. Data show that rural older adults in general acknowledge illness only to the extent that it interferes with the ability to function or "to work" (Weinert & Long, 1987).

A number of health issues remain unaddressed among rural older women. Little is known of the incidence of drug interactions due to multiple medications, drug reactions, and the use of over-the-counter medications. There appear to be no alcohol or drug-abuse disorders unique to older women (U.S. Department of Health and Human Services, 1985). Rowe (1992) found no drinking-related problems among a sample of rural women in Nebraska aged 80 to 98 who lived alone.

Psychological Well-being

The overall life satisfaction of rural older women has been found to be primarily a function of health, perceived adequacy of income, frequency of aid from relatives, quality of relationship with a confidant, and income. Dorfman, Mertens, and Lemke (1990), using results from a national retirement survey, found that the life satisfaction of rural older women increased with good health, actual and perceived adequacy of income, more frequent aid from relatives, and a good relationship with a confidant. Whether the retirement event had been immediate or gradual, voluntary or mandated, was not related to overall life satisfaction.

Dorfman et al. (1990) also examined retirement satisfaction among rural older women. Women who were more likely to have higher overall satisfaction with retirement than other women were healthier, had increased their number of voluntary memberships since retirement, had a high-quality relationship with a confidant, had encountered only small cutbacks in spending since retirement, and perceived their income as adequate. Rural older women having higher overall retirement satisfaction also had held more prestigious occupations and were younger than women who perceived less satisfaction.

Kivett and McCulloch (1989) found that rural older adults who survived to very old ages, most of whom were women, had relatively high morale. Predictors of the mental health status of rural older adults have been examined. Longitudinal data on rural older adults have shown perceived adequacy of income and adequacy of hearing to be the most consistent predictors of morale over time (Kivett & McCulloch, 1989). There is little evidence of gender differences in psychological well-being. Revicki and Mitchell (1990), in a study of 210 rural elderly, found that rural older women showed no higher levels of psychological distress or emotional distress or lower levels of life satisfaction than corresponding men. Similarly, Kivett (1979) found that gender did not discriminate levels of loneliness among rural older men and women. Scheidt and Windley (1983), however, found that more factors explained the psychological outcomes of rural older women than those of rural men. Longitudinal data on depressive symptomatology in the rural elderly have shown a gender crossover in level of depression, with level of depression increasing more rapidly for men than for women after age 85 (Wallace & O'Hara, 1992). Little is known of the frequency of dementia or specific areas of mental health problems among rural older women.

Social Characteristics

The social characteristics of rural older women vary according to a number of factors, which include marital status, education and work status, and social roles.

Marital status. Research on representative groups of the rural elderly shows that the majority of persons 65 years or older, 51 percent, are married, 39 percent are widowed, 7 percent never married, and 3 percent are divorced or separated (Kivett & Scott, 1979). The percentage of married rural older women is seen to decrease to 38 percent by age 75 or older (Kivett & Suggs, 1986). As a result, widowhood in old age is primarily an issue of older women.

Research on rural older adults shows marital status to be significantly associated with a number of life outcomes: residence, morale, and life satisfaction (Kivett & Scott, 1979) and economic well-being (Kivett & Schwenk, 1994). Married rural older adults are more likely than the nonmarried to live with another person and to have higher morale and life satisfaction. Research on widowhood has shown a high level of adjustment among rural widows at both six and twelve months after the death of a spouse (Blackburn et al., 1987). The results suggest that rural widows generally adjust to their new status and develop a positive and satisfying life within a relatively short period. Shenk (1987), in her in-depth study of rural older women, found that most of the women had adjusted well to enormous challenges and changes during widowhood, serious illnesses, and other crises. Others have reported that older women are better equipped to handle physical and social losses than men. This advantage is related to their superior ability to develop and sustain intimate relationships (Barer, 1994).

The acceptance of life changes, regret, and remorse appear to be functions of earlier personality and reaction styles. Successful coping mechanisms contributing to early adjustment in rural older widows have been found to be primarily functions of becoming independent and being enmeshed in the family: doing things with children, "showing strength in grief," becoming independent, trying to maintain family stability, and investing in children (Blackburn et al., 1987).

Education and work status. The educational level of some current groups of rural older adults, between six and seven years (Kivett & Suggs, 1986), is lower than that of the general population of older adults, approximately ten years (Schick, 1986). Older women's educational levels are found to be slightly higher than those of men. The majority of rural older women have worked both in the home and for remuneration (Jensen, 1981). For many, especially farm women, homemaking duties did not preclude intense involvement in farm work (Carlton-LaNey, 1992). The extent to which rural older women identify with the retirement role is not clear. Similarly, little is known about how retirement issues are perceived and addressed by them.

Social roles. Sex-role socialization has been found to benefit women's adjustment to old age through role continuity in late-life activities and relationships

(Barer, 1994). The social lives of rural older women traditionally have centered around the roles of wife, family member, worker, friend, leisure user, and community helper (Kivett, 1990). The wife role is the major family role of most rural women, with some women maintaining that status into very old age. Kinship and family membership are seen by feminists as the keys to understanding rural older women (Fink, 1986). Rural older women rate their feelings of closeness to kin as higher and report more value consensus with them than men (Dorfman & Mertens, 1990).

Studies have investigated the nature of the marital roles of rural older adults. Rural husbands' and wives' roles have tended to be traditional (Scanzoni & Arnett, 1987); however, household role segregation is seen to decrease significantly following retirement (Dorfman & Heckert, 1988). Age also has been found to level gender-role differences in the later years of marriage. With age, there is an egalitarian shift, more power is assumed by rural older women (Cool & McCabe, 1983), and there is more joint decision making among couples (Heckert & Dorfman, 1988).

Family roles, including that of wife, have been the primary roles open to most rural older women. Shenk (1987), in a qualitative study of older women, found that they described their family as the most important aspect of their lives. Several family roles performed by rural older women ground them to the social structure, in particular, the roles of mother and grandmother. Rural older women show high levels of affect for children and grandchildren (feelings of closeness and perceptions of getting along) (Powers & Kivett, 1992). The parent role appears to be a more salient role for rural older women than for men, as seen through assistance received from children and association with them (Atkinson et al., 1986; Powers & Kivett, 1992).

A family role of increasing interest is that of grandmother. Kivett (1993b) found that the grandmother role was more salient among rural black grandmothers than among white grandmothers, as seen through higher levels of exchanges with grandchildren. No racial differences were found in norms of grandfilial expectations, feelings of affect, or consensus with grandchildren when adjusted for grandmothers' income, number of grandchildren, and proximity to the grandmother.

The sibling role is thought to take on added significance in the later years among rural adults (McGhee, 1985; Suggs & Kivett, 1987). Availability of a sister has been found to increase the life satisfaction of rural older women. Despite this observation, research shows that rural older adults are not enmeshed in an emotionally supportive network of sibling relations, especially rural older men (McGhee, 1985; Suggs & Kivett, 1987).

Friend and neighbor roles of rural older women have been addressed infrequently. Limited data show that rural elderly women distinguish between neighbors and friends (Shenk, 1987). In contrast to friends, relationships with neighbors are described as casual, rather than intimate. Friends and neighbors may serve an important confidant function as well as that of an emergency resource. Longitudinal data on a representative group of rural older adults, most of whom were women, showed that the majority of older adults visited neighbors and friends at least once a month into very old age (Kivett & Suggs, 1986).

The leisure roles of rural older women have been investigated (Dorfman et al., 1990). Women satisfied with their retirement activities are more likely than others to have increased their number of voluntary activities following retirement. Other research on rural older adults showed that at least 60 percent of adults 74 years of age or older perceived having one-half day or more of discretionary time (Kivett & Suggs, 1986). Favorite pastimes in the order of their preference were television, church activities, having family over, having friends over, reading, and sitting and thinking.

Other research indicates the important role of the telephone in the social network of rural older adults. Kivett and McCulloch (1989) found that approximately 50 percent of their rural older panel (mean age, 84 years) had telephone conversations once or more a day with a friend, neighbor, or family member. Similarly, Rowe (1992), in a study of 100 single women ranging in age from 80 to 98, found that 75 percent talked daily on the telephone to others. No rural/urban differences were found.

Economic Well-being

Older women comprise 71 percent of the aged poor (U.S. Bureau of the Census, 1989). Few studies have examined the economic well-being of rural older women. Recent analyses of data from the 1990 Consumer Expenditure Survey showed significant differences in the economic well-being (annualized expenditures) of rural and urban older women (Kivett & Schwenk, 1994). Rural older women had significantly lower economic well-being than their urban counterparts regardless of race or marital status. Cross-sectional and longitudinal data on rural older adults have shown that approximately 80 to 84 percent receive Social Security benefits, a proportion similar to that of the general population of older adults (Kivett & Suggs, 1986).

Housing

Data show that according to most indicators of housing quality, the rural elderly live in lower-quality housing than either urban elderly or younger persons (Lee, 1986). Approximately 42 percent of women 65 years or older live alone (Golant, 1992). This percentage increases to over 50 percent among women over the age of 75. These figures may be slightly lower among rural older women because of the relatively higher male/female ratio than in urban areas. Nonetheless, very old rural women are significantly more likely to live alone than corresponding men (McCulloch & Kivett, 1995). The majority of rural older adults, 67 percent, own their home with no mortgage (Kivett & McCulloch, 1989). Considerable stability in housing is observed, with less than

2 percent of rural adults 65 years or older having plans to relocate (Colsher & Wallace, 1990). Rural older women are found to relocate more frequently than men. The chances for relocation also increase among those 84 years or older, persons living alone, and those with lower incomes and educational levels. Higher levels of depressive symptoms have been found to be associated with intent to move (Colsher & Wallace, 1990). Satisfaction with dwelling features has been found to be one of the most important predictors of mental health status among rural older women (Scheidt & Windley, 1983).

SUPPORTS

The supports of rural older women vary in accordance with their diversity. As with other groups, supports generally can be categorized as informal or formal in type.

Informal Supports

Major informal supports in rural areas are family, friends, neighbors, and other unrelated individuals such as those through affiliations with church and rural organizations. Most rural older adults receive in-home care exclusively from family members, friends, and neighbors (Newhouse & McAuley, 1987; Kivett & McCulloch, 1989). This observation increases with the impairment of the older adults (Coward, Cutler, & Mullens, 1990).

Although there is some disagreement in the literature as to a rural advantage in informal supports (Krout, 1988), there is evidence that the rural elderly are neither abandoned nor neglected in retirement, instead being well integrated into the kin network (Dorfman & Mertens, 1990). A female advantage has been found. Rural older women are both the recipients of assistance and "kinkeepers" more frequently than rural older men. No gender differences, however, are found in the frequency of in-home care from informal supports (Kivett, 1985; Newhouse & McAuley, 1987).

Women's relationships and social supports traditionally have been a strength and a key survival strategy in adversity (Mokuau & Browne, 1994). The support system of rural older women has been found to be flexible and amenable to adjustment to the loss of relationships through death or separation (Shenk, 1987). Its effectiveness is not based upon size of network but, rather, its flexibility and the availability of backup supports. Choices of support are determined by the nature of the specific relationships a woman has with her family, friends, and neighbors.

Most rural elderly have at least one child within thirty minutes of their residence (Dorfman & Mertens, 1990; Powers & Kivett, 1992). Only low to moderate amounts of assistance are exchanged, however (Powers & Kivett, 1992). Rural older adults have moderately high expectations for assistance from children, especially in illness and in visitation. Rural elderly women are found to receive more assistance from children than men, with the mother-daughter tie being more significant than the mother-son tie. Assistance from children may not always predict positive outcomes for the older adult. Dorfman and Mertens (1990), for example, found a negative relationship between the amount of assistance rural older women received from children and overall retirement satisfaction.

The majority of rural elderly have been found to have at least one sibling within sixty minutes' proximity (Dorfman & Mertens, 1990; Powers & Kivett, 1992). Powers and Kivett (1992) found that rural older adults held average and similar expectations of assistance from grandchildren and siblings. The amount of assistance from siblings, albeit only modest amounts, was found to increase with expectations for help. The amount of assistance rural older adults received from a sibling or a grandchild was mainly a function of proximity. Powers and Kivett found that rural older women were more likely than rural older men to receive assistance from a sibling-in-law.

Data are equivocal on rural/urban differences in availability of and assistance from family in later life. Scott and Roberto (1987) found relatively few rural/urban differences in the types of help received when proximity, gender, and marital status were controlled.

Friends and neighbors are potential sources of support to rural older women. Scott and Roberto (1987) observed that rural widows were more actively engaged in exchanges with friend networks than urban widows. Friends benefited older married women and widows most often through comfort. Other areas in order of their frequency for both married and widowed women included assistance when ill, transportation, and financial aid. Support from friends has been linked to the life satisfaction of rural older women. Dorfman and Moffett (1987) found that certainty of aid from friends was a significant predictor of life satisfaction among elderly rural married women. Furthermore, the maintenance of preretirement friendships and frequency of visits with friends were important to the satisfaction of widowed women.

The black church has been found to function as a "family surrogate" for childless married couples and unmarried persons, filling both social and emotional needs (Taylor & Chatters, 1988). "Para-kin" or "fictive kin" also are important components of the black family and support network (Johnson & Barer, 1990).

Formal Supports

Rural older women have been found to prefer a formal rather than an informal system of care for ongoing assistance with personal care (Shenk, 1987). Shenk found that rural older women used service providers to fill the gaps in their informal support system. Most existing models of service delivery in rural areas have been found to be largely unacceptable to rural older women (Shenk, 1987). Shenk found that in contrast to the preferences of rural elderly women, most delivery services are too all-encompassing, contribute to a feeling of loss of control through drawing women into a larger system of formal care, frequently carry a welfare stigma, and often are staffed by "outsiders" to the rural community. Shenk concluded that formal systems of support will work in the best interest of rural older women if they are based on clear understandings of the rural character, have a minimum of structure, and complement the informal system in maintaining the elderly in their homes.

CONCLUSIONS AND SUGGESTED RESEARCH

Information on rural older women is sparse. When studied, they are most frequently observed as an independent variable influencing aging outcomes. The paucity of data available show them to be a heterogeneous group. Because of their higher survival rates, most of the issues of aging, such as economic, health, and psychological outcomes, are primarily their issues rather than those of men.

The rich rural heritage of rural older women can be seen in their strong sense of independence and drive to remain in control of their lives for as long as possible. While they are open to assistance from sources outside of the informal network, their rural worldviews strongly condition the extent to which they accept nontraditional sources of assistance. Consequently, few existing service models have been applicable. A contributing factor to the lack of response to their needs is their largely "hidden" status and lack of power.

Major issues affecting older women in rural areas include economic well-being, health, isolation through migration of families, and transportation. Issues of increasing importance include crime, locating and linking to available services, and culturally sensitive programming.

Future cohorts of rural older women will become increasingly heterogeneous with regard to ethnicity, socioeconomic characteristics, marital status, family forms, and views toward assistance. Future cohorts of rural older women, too, will serve in more self-advocacy roles. They will acquire more power through their political actions and economic independence.

A number of research needs are indicated through a review of the literature on rural older women. More information is needed on the applicability of various theoretical perspectives to the life outcomes of rural older women. More longitudinal studies are needed to observe the relationship of a number of life processes and life outcomes. Multivariate studies are needed that control for confounding factors such as socioeconomic characteristics, ethnicity, and region. Additional comparative research is needed on similarities and differences between rural and urban groups. Research, too, is needed on both between- and within-group differences among important subgroups of rural older women. More data are needed on the factors related to rural older women's utilization of services.

In summary, migration, acculturation to urban views and lifestyles, and technological and related changes will continually modify the profile and subsequent needs of rural older women. Implicit to these modifications is the importance of addressing the ever-changing needs of this important group.

REFERENCES

Atkinson, Maxine P., Kivett, Vira R., & Campbell, Richard T. (1986). Intergenerational solidarity: An examination of a theoretical model. *Journal of Gerontology, 41*(3), 408–416.

Barer, Barbara M. (1994). Men and women aging differently. *International Journal of Aging and Human Development, 38*(1), 29–40.

Bastida, Elena. (1984). Some critical issues affecting older women in rural areas. In E. Bastida (Ed.), *Convergence in aging: Older women: Current issues and problems* (pp. 99–104). Kansas City, KS: Mid-America Conference on Aging.

Blackburn, James A., Greenberg, Jan S., & Boss, Pauline G. (1987). Coping with normative stress from loss and change: A longitudinal study of rural widows. *Journal of Gerontological Social Work, 2*(1&2), 59–70.

Carlton-LaNey, I. (1992). Elderly black farm women: A population at risk. *Social Work, 37*(6), 517–523.

Colsher, P. L., & Wallace, R. B. (1990). Health and social antecedents of relocation in rural elderly persons. *Journal of Gerontology: Social Sciences, 45*(1), S32–S38.

Cool, L., & McCabe, J. (1983). The "scheming hag" and the "dear old thing": The anthropology of aging women. In J. Sokolovsky (Ed.), *Growing old in different societies: Cross-cultural perspectives* (pp. 56–71). Belmont, CA: Wadsworth Publishing Company.

Coward, Raymond T., Cutler, Stephen J., & Mullens, Russell A. (1990). Residential differences in the composition of helping networks of impaired elders. *Family Relations, 39*, 44–50.

Coyle, Jean M. (1989). *Women and aging: A selected, annotated bibliography.* Westport, CT: Greenwood Press.

Dorfman, Lorraine T., & Heckert, D. Alex. (1988). Egalitarianism in retired rural couples: Household tasks, decision making, and leisure activities. *Family Relations, 37*, 73–78.

Dorfman, Lorraine T., Kohout, Frank J., & Heckert, D. Alex. (1985). Retirement satisfaction in the rural elderly. *Research on Aging, 7*(4), 577–599.

Dorfman, Lorraine T., & Mertens, Carol E. (1990). Kinship relations in retired rural men and women. *Family Relations, 39*, 166–173.

Dorfman, Lorraine T., Mertens, Carol E., & Lemke, Jon H. (1990). *Informal social networks and retirement satisfaction in the rural elderly.* Paper presented at the 43rd Annual Scientific Meeting of the Gerontological Society of America, Boston.

Dorfman, Lorraine T., & Moffett, M. M. (1987). Retirement satisfaction in married and widowed rural women. *Gerontologist, 27*(2), 215–221.

Fink, D. (1986). *Open country, Iowa: Rural women, tradition, and change.* Albany: State University of New York Press.

Gee, E. M., & Kimball, M. M. (1987). *Women and aging.* Toronto, Canada: Butterworths.

Golant, Stephen M. (1992). *Housing America's elderly: Many possibilities/few choices.* Newbury Park, CA: Sage Publications.

Heckert, D. Alex, & Dorfman, Lorraine T. (1988). Egalitarianism in retired rural couples:

Household tasks, decision making, and leisure activities. In Ramona Marotz-Baden, Charles B. Hennon, & Timothy H. Brubaker (Eds.), *Families in rural America: Stress, adaptation, and revitalization.* St. Paul, MN: National Council on Family Relations.

Jensen, J. M. (1981). *With these hands: Women working on the land.* Old Westbury, NY: Feminist Press.

Johnson, Colleen L., & Barer, Barbara M. (1990). Families and networks among older inner-city blacks. *Gerontologist, 30*(6), 726–733.

Kivett, Vira R. (1979). Discriminators of loneliness among the rural elderly: Implications for intervention. *Gerontologist, 19*(1), 108–115.

———. (1985). Consanguinity and kin level: Their importance to the helping networks of older adults. *Journal of Gerontology, 40,* 228–234.

———. (1990). Older rural women: Mythical, forbearing, and unsung. *Journal of Rural Community Psychology, 11,* 83–101.

———. (1993a). Informal supports among older minorities. In C. N. Bull (Ed.). *Aging in rural America* (pp. 204–215). Newbury Park, CA: Sage Publications.

———. (1993b). Racial comparisons of the grandmother role: Implications for strengthening the family support system of older black women. *Family Relations, 42,* 165–172.

Kivett, Vira R., & McCulloch, B. Jan. (1989). *Support networks of the very-old: Caregivers and carereceivers (Caswell III).* Final Report to the AARP Andrus Foundation. Greensboro, NC: Family Research Center, School of Human Environmental Sciences, University of North Carolina at Greensboro.

Kivett, Vira R., & Schwenk, Frankie N. (1994). The consumer expenditures of elderly women: Racial, marital, and rural/urban impacts. *Journal of Family and Economic Issues, 15,* 261–277.

Kivett, Vira R., & Scott, Jean P. (1979). *The rural by-passed elderly: Perspectives on status and needs.* Technical Bulletin No. 260. Greensboro, NC: North Carolina Agricultural Research Service, University of North Carolina at Greensboro.

Kivett, Vira R., & Suggs, Patricia K. (1986). *Caswell revisited: A ten year follow-up on the rural by-passed elderly.* Final Report to the AARP Andrus Foundation. Greensboro, NC: Family Research Center, School of Home Economics, University of North Carolina at Greensboro.

Krout, John A. (1986). *The aged in rural America.* Westport, CT: Greenwood Press.

———. (1988). Rural versus urban differences in elderly parents' contact with their children. *Gerontologist, 28,* 198–203.

Lee, Gary R. (1986). Rural issues in elderly housing. In R. J. Newcomer, M. Powell Lawton, & T. O. Byerts (Eds.). *Housing an aging society: Issues, alternatives, and policy* (pp. 33–41). New York: Van Nostrand Reinhold.

McCulloch, B. Jan. (1991). Health and health maintenance profiles of older rural women, 1976–1986. In A. Bushy (Ed.), *Rural Nursing* (Vol. 1, pp. 281–296). Newbury Park, CA: Sage Publications.

McCulloch, B. Jan, & Kivett, Vira R. (1995). Characteristics of and survivorship among the very old. *Family Relations, 44,* 87–94.

McGhee, Jerrie L. (1985). The effects of siblings on the life satisfaction of the rural elderly. *Journal of Marriage and the Family, 47,* 85–91.

Mokauu, Noreen, & Browne, Colette. (1994). Life themes of Native Hawaiian female elders: Resources for cultural preservation. *Social Work, 39*(1), 43–49.

Newhouse, Janette K., & McAuley, William J. (1987). Use of informal in-home care by rural elders. *Family Relations, 36*, 456–460.

Powers, Edward A., & Kivett, Vira R. (1992). Kin expectations and kin support among older rural adults. *Rural Sociology, 57*(2), 194–213.

Revicki, Dennis A., & Mitchell, Jim P. (1990). Strain, social support, and mental health in rural elderly individuals. *Journal of Gerontology, 46*(6), S267–S274.

Rowe, G. P. (1992). Successful aging of women over 80 living alone. *Research News, 6*(1), 2–3. Lincoln: College of Home Economics, University of Nebraska–Lincoln.

Scanzoni, John, & Arnett, Cynthia. (1987). Policy implications derived from a study of rural and urban marriages. *Family Relations, 36*, 430–436.

Scheidt, Rick J., & Windley, Paul G. (1983). The mental health of small-town rural elderly residents: An expanded ecological model. *Journal of Gerontology, 38*(4), 472–479.

Schick, F. L. (Ed.). (1986). *Statistical handbook on aging Americans*. Phoenix, AZ: Oryx Press.

Scott, Jean P., & Roberto, Karen A. (1987). Informal supports of older adults: A rural-urban comparision. *Family Relations, 36*, 444–449.

Shenk, Dena. (1987). *Someone to lend a helping hand: The lives of rural older women in central Minnesota*. St. Cloud, MN: St. Cloud University.

Stratton, J. L. (1981). *Pioneer women*. New York: Simon & Schuster.

Suggs, Patricia K., & Kivett, Vira R. (1987). Rural/urban elderly and their siblings: Their value consensus. *International Journal of Aging and Human Development, 24*(2), 149–159.

Taylor, Robert J., & Chatters, Linda M. (1988). Church members as a source of informal social support. *Review of Religious Research, 30*(2), 193–203.

U.S. Bureau of the Census. (1989). *Poverty in the United States, 1987*. Current Population Reports, Series P-60, No. 163. Washington, DC: U.S. Government Printing Office.

———. (1992). *1990 Census of the Population: General Population Characteristics* (1990, CP-1-1). Washington, DC: U.S. Government Printing Office.

U.S. Department of Health and Human Services. (1985). *Women's health: Report of the Public Health Service Task Force on Women's Health Issues* (Vol. 2). DHHS Publication No. (PHS)85–50206. Washington, DC: U.S. Public Health Service.

Wallace, J., & O'Hara, M. W. (1992). Increases in depressive symptomatology in the rural elderly: Results from a cross-sectional and longitudinal study. *Journal of Abnormal Psychology, 101*, 398–404.

Weinert, Clarann, & Long, Kathleen A. (1987). Understanding the health care needs of rural families. *Family Relations, 36*, 450–455.

Wilkinson, C. W. (1982). *Aging in rural America: A comprehensive annotated bibliography, 1975–1981*. Morgantown: West Virginia University Gerontology Center, University of West Virginia.

Part V

Relationships

Twenty-Three

Family Relationships of Midlife and Older Women

JEAN PEARSON SCOTT

Family relationships have provided a central source of identity and of inter- and intragenerational support for midlife and older women. Women have been called the "kinkeepers" of families, an apt description due to their key roles and functions in families and their enduring family bonds. Yet dramatic demographic and technological changes have altered the pattern and functioning of family relationships of midlife and older women.

Twentieth-century declines in mortality rates and altered fertility patterns have reshaped women's family-life experiences. Greater life expectancies for both men and women have contributed to more golden wedding anniversaries, a longer postparental period, and a lengthier retirement stage for married couples. Women hold a seven-year advantage in life expectancy over men that results in increasing numbers of older women relative to men with each succeeding cohort. Consequently, a disproportionate number of elderly widows and greater numbers of older women who are heads of household and living alone are present in the population relative to men. In short, family members of mid- and later life, particularly women, have potentially more time to be involved with their kin although they may not live in a family setting.

Furthermore, changes in attitudes regarding women's roles in the labor force, greater access to and equality in higher education, use of birth control, greater acceptance of divorce, and renegotiation of roles within the family are important changes affecting family relationships and greatly differentiating women of pre–, young, and older baby-boom cohorts. These changes evolved out of the social and political turbulence of the 1960s and 1970s: the women's movement, the sexual revolution, the Vietnam War, the popularity of the counterculture and the drug culture, and the civil rights movement. Research with these cohorts will no doubt reveal distinctive changes in family relationships.

Indeed, midlife baby boomers have experienced family life in significantly different ways than their mothers who are now in their 60s and 70s. Baby-boom women were the first generation to use the birth-control pill and to delay marriage and childbearing. They have experienced divorce in significant numbers and were the first cohort to view singlehood and cohabiting relationships as legitimate and acceptable lifestyles (Jacobson, 1995). Furthermore, rapid social changes have created different experiences between the youngest cohort of midlife women (ages 35–40) and the oldest cohort of midlife women (ages 40–48). The younger midlife cohort has experienced fewer limitations with regard to sexuality, education, and career choices in comparison to older counterparts. They, more than older cohorts, have delayed marriage and childbearing (Jacobson, 1995). Sociocultural and demographic changes have altered family life, and theoretical views for explaining the gendered nature of family relationships are evolving as well. Not only has the sociocultural context for study of women's family relationships changed, but theoretical views of gendered behavior have undergone change as well.

THEORETICAL BACKGROUND

Theories of socialization and sex roles have predominated as conceptual explanations of women's attitudes and behaviors within the family. Traditional social scientific views have considered gender as a set of social roles learned as a product of socialization that began at birth and continued throughout life. Socialization processes were responsible for gender-typed learning of "appropriate" male and female behavior. The learning of one's appropriate gendered roles was accompanied by a dichotomization of "his" and "hers," the "public" and "private" spheres, and "instrumental" versus "expressive" functions. Thus wives did "wives' " work and husbands did "husbands' " work. Wives were involved in the making of a home; husbands were involved outside the home. Thus women have been viewed as the central, most salient actors in the family sphere (Ferree, 1990).

A more recent conceptual framework evolving out of feminist thought argues for a rethinking of how persons assume certain positions and behaviors. While traditional sex-role theories assume certain structures and behaviors, gender theory analyzes how certain gendered social constructions developed. The gender model views gender as an element of social relationships that is based on perceived differences between the sexes and is indicative of power. Thus gendered behaviors, from a gender-model perspective, are derived from the processes of categorization and stratification according to gender (Ferree, 1990).

Additionally, the gender model challenges the old view of family separateness and solidarity (Ferree, 1990). For example, rather than viewing the family as a social sphere where different norms operate and women play a major complementary role vis-à-vis the work sphere, families are viewed as operating according to the same kinds of power agendas as the social structure in which they are embedded. Indeed, a fundamental assumption of feminist thought is that values, norms, and power hierarchies that operate in the larger context affect families as well. This position contrasts with the idea that the family is a safe haven or refuge from the world, and, as such, women are treated differently and accorded a status that is different from that of other arenas of life (Ferree, 1990).

From a gender-theory perspective, families are not unified wholes that act as a common actor. To the contrary, families are viewed as having multiple actors whose needs and interests are negotiated or resolved through overt and covert conflict. The fundamental conflicts of power via gender and generation must be considered in a realistic understanding of the family (Ferree, 1990).

Among several identified shortcomings of the sex-role ideology is a dysfunctional view of families as being the primary source of early sex-role socialization and devaluation of women. By tying gendered behavior to the larger structural organization of society as gender theory does, the family is not separated from the same politics that operate in the larger sphere, and power can be exposed. Therefore, the gender-role model places the family within the larger historical and social context (Ferree, 1990). Although gender theory offers a potentially heuristic view of gendered behavior in families, it is too early to evaluate its impact on the study of women and family relationships. The following sections dealing with topical areas of family relations document the limited use of theoretical perspectives. Family development and sex-role socialization theories are frequently used, as are midrange theories such as equity.

MARRIAGE

For the majority of midlife and older women, the role of wife was or remains a central feature of family life for much of adult life. Marital status, however, shifts considerably by gender and with advancing age. For the older population as a whole, for example, 74% of men are married, compared to 40% of women. These figures mask significant age differentials. For those aged 65–74, approximately 80% of men and 53.2% of women are married, yet for Caucasian elderly 85 years of age or older, 49% of men and 10.3% of women are still married (U.S. Bureau of the Census, 1992). African-American men and women aged 65 to 74 are significantly less likely to be married than Caucasians.

Studies of mid- and later-life marriage must be interpreted with certain methodological caveats. First, samples of older married spouses are biased because of selective attrition factors including divorce or separation and death of partners. These events do not occur randomly, and so the study population is presumed to be healthier, better off on socioeconomic indicators, and represented by disproportionately happier marriages than the original pool of newlywed couples. The highly personal nature of marriage and taboos about discussing marital behavior outside the marriage also may bias the sample.

A second issue is that of time and the potential confounding of marital duration with stage in the family career, cohort effects, and other influences. Cross-sectional studies offer an assessment of marriage at one point in time, and when marriages of different lengths are compared, it is not possible to know if differences observed are due to true change in marital duration or to many other plausible reasons, such as cohort or family stage. Nevertheless, a growing body of literature has examined marital characteristics and satisfaction of long-term married couples.

On the whole, marriage is very satisfying for the majority of long-term married couples. Studies of couples married 50 years or more consistently report high marital satisfaction (Brubaker, 1985). When differences in self-reports occur, however, wives' scores are slightly lower than husbands' scores (Brubaker, 1985). In Lauer, Lauer, and Kerr's study (1990) of 100 couples married over 45 years, there was much similarity in the reasons given by both partners for successful marriages. The most frequent reasons given included liking one's mate as an enjoyable person and friend, being committed to the relationship and to the institution of marriage, humor, and agreement on aims and goals.

Marital satisfaction in later life is particularly important to women's morale. Lee (1978) found that marital satisfaction was important to morale of both older husbands and wives, but that the effect was much greater for wives. This suggests that for women the quality of the marital bond has an impact on their overall mental well-being. There is consistent evidence that women's physical as well as mental health is influenced by the marriage. In a study of long-term marriages middle-aged and older women reported more physical, psychological, and functional health problems, and these problems were closely tied to satisfaction with the marriage (Levenson, Carstensen, & Gottman, 1993). Only in dissatisfied marriages did wives report more problems than husbands. These findings are consistent with other data suggesting that marriage benefits the physical and psychological health of men more than women (Levenson et al., 1993; Steil, 1984). In another series of experiments, data supported the hypothesis that men's experience of negative affect was correlated with their level of physiological arousal, whereas women's experience of negative affect was not correlated with their level of arousal (Levensen, Carstensen, & Gottman, 1994). This gender difference may explain why men tend to withdraw from conflictive marital interactions as a means of reducing negative affect or physical arousal. Women, in contrast, are less likely to withdraw and more likely to remain engaged to seek resolution, particularly if they are less aware of negative affect when physiologically aroused. Because men will disengage as a way of lowering negative affect and physiological arousal, their health is not associated with marital satisfaction. For women, the link of health and marital happiness suggests that their tendency to remain engaged in a conflict and less sensitivity to their state of arousal have adverse effects on health. Further, Levenson et al. (1994) reasoned that women feel greater distress over the long term from marital problems and feel more responsibility for resolving problems than husbands, and these feelings take a physical and emotional toll over time.

Equity theorists have argued that perceptions of equity or fairness in a marriage are associated with the affective mood of the relationship. That is, spouses who perceive that they get out of the relationship pretty much what they contribute to it will feel fairly treated and contented. Overbenefited spouses may feel guilty that they do not reciprocate what they perceive as the greater contributions of the spouse. Underbenefiters may feel angry that their contributions to the marriage are greater than their spouses' contributions. These predictions were supported in a study of 400 women, aged 52–92, where the subjects were asked to assess retrospectively the equity of their marital relationship (Traupmann & Hatfield, 1983). The most prevalent pattern for the women as a whole was one of perceived overbenefit in the early years, a perceived slight underbenefit in the middle years, and a shift to perceived equity in the later years (70s and 80s). Reasons for older women's perception of equity in their marriages could be due to real changes precipitated by retirement or by a sense of good fortune to still have a spouse (Traupmann & Hatfield, 1983).

Equity, however, is a prevalent pattern for more specific aspects of the marital relationship. When 412 married respondents aged 50 years or older were asked specifically about support that was exchanged in the relationship, women perceived less social support within marriage than men (Depner & Ingersoll-Dayton, 1985). With regard to perceived love, a sample of 240 women ranging in age from 50 to 82 felt that they were loved more passionately by their partners than they loved them in return. Companionate love, however, was perceived by the wives as an equitable exchange (Hatfield, Traupmann, & Sprecher, 1984). Perhaps perceived inequities cancel out when more global evaluations of the relationship are requested.

Changes in marital dynamics as a result of the decision to retire are not adequately researched. The literature suggests that women have greater difficulty adjusting to retirement and that their decision to retire themselves is often prompted by family responsibilities (retirement of spouse, caregiving) rather than by a desire on their part (Szinovacz, 1987). Retired women reported significantly more negative life events prior to retirement than did male retirees, and life events after retirement more negatively affected recently retired women's adjustment in comparison to men's (Szinovacz & Washo, 1992). For retired couples, having both spouses in the home all day calls for reconsideration of how time is spent, of priority given to activities, and of territorial issues. Despite greater time for sharing household tasks, wives in dual-retired relationships reported few changes in the division of household tasks (Brubaker & Hennon, 1982; Keating & Cole, 1980; Szinovacz, 1980).

Presently, studies are equivocal with respect to the effects of retirement on marriage. Gilford's (1984) data indicated that older couples between the ages of 63 and 69 experienced a "honeymoon" phase shortly after retirement; however, no relationship between retirement variables and marital satisfaction was found by Lee and Shehan (1989). One exception was a small negative relationship between husband's retirement and employed wife's marital satisfaction (Lee & Shehan, 1989). Researchers have noted the value of examining the timing of retirement and the retirement status of both marital partners as factors affecting retirement and marital satisfaction (Brubaker, 1990; Szinovacz, 1987). These studies suggest that women retiring from the work force may have greater difficulties adjusting to retirement than women who worked at home.

A major thrust of the literature on marriage has focused on the question of marital satisfaction over the life course. Are couples happier at different points along the marital life cycle? Three patterns have been reported in the literature: one of continuous decline, a second pattern of relative stability into the later years, and the third of a U-shaped curve consisting of a drop in satisfaction after the honeymoon period and lower satisfaction in the middle years followed by higher satisfaction in the retirement years (Brubaker, 1990). Data from cross-sectional studies of marital satisfaction suggest a curvilinear pattern of satisfaction with a diminution of satisfaction in the child-rearing and launching years (Anderson, Russell, & Schumm, 1983; Rollins & Cannon, 1974; Rollins & Feldman, 1970). Levenson et al.'s (1993) comparison of middle-aged and older couples' marriages indicated less potential for conflict and greater potential for pleasure in several areas (including children) for the older couples.

Longitudinal studies of marital satisfaction have found more evidence of stability when couples were studied prospectively and a slight curvilinear pattern, compatible with cross-sectional data, when couples were asked to report retrospectively on their relationship (Vaillant & Vaillant, 1993). In the Vaillant and Vaillant study, 268 men who were Harvard sophomores between 1938 and 1942, the original subjects from the Study of Adult Development, were studied along with their marital partners into their later years. Despite a higher-than-average educational level for this cohort, the majority of the wives (60%) described themselves as home-centered wives engaged in traditional activities. Prospective data indicated similarity in husband and wife scores on marital adjustment until the 31+-year period, where wives were significantly lower on their reported marital adjustment than husbands. The source of the difference was the wives' more negative judgment about the relative difficulty of resolving disagreements with their husbands. Spouses did not differ in their perceptions of stability of the marriage or sexual satisfaction. Retrospective assessments of their marriage produced a slight curvilinear pattern, with both husbands and wives rating the middle years (approximately 20 years' duration) lower than at other times and wives reporting significantly less marital enjoyment overall than husbands. Vaillant and Vaillant concluded, however, that the U-curve patterns of marital adjustment may be an artifact of retrospective and cross-sectional research. Further research using more sophisticated designs that include both husbands and wives and utilizing more representative samples is needed before the issue will be settled. Many of the cross-sectional studies have asked married women only about their marriages, whereas the Vaillant and Vaillant study included the reports of husbands and wives.

Several explanations have been offered for the observed reduction in marital satisfaction at midlife: the presence of children, multiple role strains, midlife developmental issues, and combinations of these factors that are explained as "family stage." Not all of these reasons have found support. Family stage has not proved to be influential when other variables including length of marriage and presence of children were controlled (Anderson et al., 1983). For those studies that observed increases in marital satisfaction in the later years, several reasons, such as freedom from child-rearing responsibilities and enjoyment of retirement, may explain the high satisfaction of older couples.

Changes in health status of either partner or of aged parents can have a significant effect on the dynamics of a marriage. Spouses are the first persons that older adults turn to for support. Demographic trends and the tendency of men to marry younger women predispose wives to more opportunity for caregiving than their male counterparts. Wives often provide care for mothers-in-law, especially when daughters are not available to provide care. Nowhere is the gendered nature of caregiving more pronounced than in comparing the patterns of care provided by adult daughters and sons. Studies examining gendered caregiving patterns document the greater burden experienced by wives in comparison to husbands. Wives were more likely to carry out more personal care tasks, whereas husbands were more likely to hire outside help or receive the help of kin (Johnson, 1985). Despite the stress of caregiving, most marriages maintain their positive levels of adjustment (Brubaker, 1990).

Marriage serves as a major source of intimacy and support for midlife and older women. However, gender differences with respect to social support suggest that marriage provides a greater source of social emotional support for husbands than for wives. A consistent body of empirical literature demonstrates that older women have a greater number of persons in their social support networks and that they rely on spouses for support to a significantly lower degree than older men. Men tend to rely exclusively on their wives for social support (Antonucci & Akiyama, 1987). With respect to material, practical, and personal help, a comparison of wives and widows aged 60 and over ($N = 106$) revealed significant differences in the help given to friend and kin networks according to marital status. Marriage served to "privatize" the helping networks of older wives by reducing their help to friends and increasing their help to kin in comparison to help provided by widows (Gallagher & Gerstel, 1993). Although wives gave significantly more help to other family members than did widows, most of the difference could be explained by the additional material resources of older wives.

DIVORCE

Between 1975 and 1985 the proportion of divorces involving women over 40 ranged from a low of 19% in 1980 to a high of 23% in 1985 (Uhlenberg, Cooney, & Boyd, 1990). Most of these divorces were to women between the ages of 40 and 60, as no more than 2% of all divorces involved women over age 60. Uhlenberg et al.'s analysis of current and projected divorce patterns suggests a marked increase in the number of future elderly women who will be divorced. For example, for the birth cohort of women born between 1955 and 1959, fewer than half will be in first marriages by age 50. Indeed, nearly a fifth of this baby-boom cohort will be divorced. Thus the divorce experiences of current and future cohorts of midlife and older women will be quite diverse. It is true also that rates of divorce are higher among ethnic minority elderly than for the population as a whole, especially for older African-American females (Hooyman & Kiyak, 1993).

The current cohorts of older women were socialized at a time when divorce was stigmatized by most social institutions. For these women, the occurrence of divorce carried an added burden of social stigma. Midlife women, on the other hand, were on the leading edge of much societal change regarding divorce precipitated by a dramatic rise in divorce rates in the 1960s and 1970s. Even with greater social acceptance of divorce, the dissolution process entails grief work, resolving feelings of anger, fear, and rejection, and redefinition of one's self as a single person. Family and other social ties are altered as well. Though we know little about later-life divorce, it is clear from existing studies that termination of a long-term marriage is a complex and multifaceted process (Brubaker, 1985).

Who initiates the divorce? In Hagestad and Symer's (1982) study of divorced men and women between 41 and 60 years of age, women were more likely to recognize problems and to initiate the transition to divorce sooner. Likewise, divorced women with marriages of 30–50 years reported that they were initiators of the divorce process (Weingarten, 1988). They complained of their partner's lack of emotional and instrumental support and that retirement for their former husbands had resulted in identity loss and a desire for more hedonistic values, for example, second adolescence. Other marital problems cited included spousal infidelity, the emptiness of the relationship after launching children, and greater acceptability of divorce.

In contrast, several researchers found no clear gender differences in initiator status across age groups, but when duration of marriage was controlled, a trend of husband-initiated divorce emerged for older relationships. Gander's (1991, 1992) predominantly female sample of both young ($N = 206$) and older ($N = 111$) divorced persons had no significant gender differences regarding who initiated the divorce. Yet the persons over age 50 were surprised by the divorce, for which they reported having no forewarning. The older divorced group who had been married an average of 30 years more often reported "no choice" in the divorce process. The most frequently cited reason for divorce among both older men and women was "grew apart/incompatible." Older women frequently mentioned the irresponsibility of the former spouse, although older men did not, and older women cited communication problems, cruelty, and infidelity as reasons for divorce more frequently than older men (Gander, 1992). The sample was obtained from public divorce records in Salt Lake County, and more than half of the sample were members of the Mormon church.

Members of Cain's (1988) sample of 30 women divorced after the age of 60 after at least 30 years of marriage were opposed to and surprised by the divorce initiated by their husbands. However, one-third of the women reported that the marriage had been turbulent with such problems as infidelity, alcoholism, and tyrannically controlling husbands. They attributed the divorce to their husband's desire to recapture youth or blamed themselves for "lacking the allure of youth." These studies suggest that divorce in later life occurs for marriages that have a history of marital turbulence or apathy.

Long-standing marital unhappiness as a reason for divorce in mid- and later life is corroborated by findings in Deckert and Langelier's study (1978) of Canadians married 20 years or longer. The decision to divorce was made over a period of time (2 years or more) by the majority of the sample. Multiple reasons for the divorce, including adultery, sexual problems, in-law problems, alcoholism, and mental cruelty were cited. In addition, 75% of the respondents reported long-term marital unhappiness.

How do women adjust to divorce? Studies that have examined the economic well-being of midlife and older women show a bleak situation for most women. Divorced women experience financial setbacks that place them in a disadvantaged position relative to divorced men and other marital groups (Hennon, 1983; Uhlenberg et al., 1990). The effects of limited financial resources are reflected in the smaller proportion of middle-aged and older divorced women relative to married and widowed women who were living independently, owned their own homes, and were not employed (Uhlenberg et al., 1990). Thus divorce has stronger socioeconomic consequences for older women than widowhood.

Divorce of midlife children, particularly daughters, may have serious consequences for the family support systems of older women. Next to spouses, adult daughters are most frequently relied on for support by the older generation. If adult daughters are experiencing their own problems due to divorce, they will be unable to provide the support that a frail mother would require. Divorce in both generations may severely curtail support that female kinkeepers normally provide.

With regard to social supports, older divorced women appear to turn more readily to their support networks during the process of divorce and to report greater happiness and adjustment in comparison to divorced men (Hammond & Muller, 1992). Keith (1986) found that older divorced women, in comparison to their male counterparts, had greater interaction with family and friends and continued family contacts to a greater extent after divorce. Hayes and Anderson's (1993) sample of 338 recently divorced women 40 to 75 years of age cited several positive events since the divorce, including a majority who reported positive feelings about self, valuing their privacy and independence, making new friends, feeling a sense of achievement, and feeling free to be themselves.

REMARRIAGE

Remarriage after a divorce or death of a spouse is an option for midlife and older women. However, demographic trends and the social norm of women marrying older men work against the likelihood of remarriage for women as compared to men. For divorced women aged 45–64, only 29 of 10,000 remarried during 1985, and only 5 of 10,000 divorced women over the age of 65 remarried (U.S. Bureau of the Census, 1992). Also, a preference for remarriage is not as strong for women. In one study of divorced women, those who had divorced between the ages of 40 and 44 (29%) preferred their freedom over remarriage. This figure rose to 41% for women divorced between the ages of 45 and 49 and to 46% for women 50–59 years of age (Hayes & Anderson, 1993). With respect to widowed women, remarriage rates also remain low. On average, less than 1 out of 10 baby-boom women who are currently married are estimated to remarry after the death of a spouse (U.S. Bureau of the Census, 1992).

In a qualitative study of 35 persons aged 60 or over who were dating, women more than men reported increased prestige and sense of identity as a result of dating (Bulcroft & O'Conner, 1986). Dating men, on the other hand, cited the need for intimacy and self-disclosure. This study indicates that women and men are motivated by different needs in the decision to date.

McKain's (1972) study of 100 remarried couples concluded that the majority (75%) were highly successful. Five reasons contributing to marital success were that the partners had known each other well, had approval of family and friends, adjusted well to age-related changes, set up a new home, and had adequate income. Vinick (1978) interviewed 24 older remarried couples, of which the majority reported being highly satisfied. Men appeared to "need" remarriage more, as they reported having a more difficult time adjusting to the death of their first spouse and generally took the initiative in the new relationship.

There is much additional research needed on the complexities of remarriage. Brubaker (1990) noted that former intimate relationships may serve as a referent for new relationships and thus influence adjustment of the new marriage.

GRANDMOTHERS

Women become grandmothers involuntarily and may add this role as early as the 30s or as late as the 70s. The timing of grandparenthood has received attention in the literature. For some women, the grandparent role is a mixed blessing because while it means a new set of potentially rewarding role relationships, it may also be a reminder of one's own aging. Studies, for example, of African-American grandmothers suggest that women who become grandmothers at a young age (25–38 years, mean age of 32) experienced more discomfort with the role of grandparenting than did those who became grandparents at a more normative time (42–57 years) (Burton & Bengtson, 1985; Hagestad

& Burton, 1986). Young grandmothers felt greater discomfort because of associating the grandparent role with "old."

Grandparents have been described as the "family watchdogs" because of their function as a safety net for young families (Troll, 1983). Grandmothers are frequently relied upon for baby-sitting, advice, help in time of emergencies, emotional support, financial assistance, and the maintenance of family rituals and traditions (Troll, 1983; Wentowski, 1985). The grandparent role serves to give midlife and older women a meaningful role in the family, satisfaction in leaving a legacy and seeing the family line continued, and opportunity to indulge and enjoy grandchildren (Kivnick, 1982).

Grandparents play an expanded role in families experiencing divorce. Furthermore, the legal right of grandparents to visitation with their grandchildren is now recognized under most state laws. Contact with grandchildren, however, is often mediated by the middle generation and dependent on which parent receives custody. Maternal grandparents may have greater contact with their grandchildren because mothers more often receive custody (Matthews & Sprey, 1984). Proximity to grandchildren is a primary determinant of contact patterns with or without divorce (Gladstone, 1988).

The growing trend of grandparents parenting their grandchildren has received limited study. It is estimated that 3.3 million children live with grandparents, a 44% increase since 1980. A greater proportion of African-American children live with grandparents than do other groups; however, the largest rate of increase has occurred among white children. Jendrek's (1994) study of 114 primarily white grandmothers who provided regular care to their grandchildren showed three distinct types of care arrangements: custodial grandparents, living with grandparents, and day-care grandparents. Data on the three types of care arrangements reveal that grandmothers are more likely to parent a daughter's child than a son's. Most day-care (85.7%) and custodial (61.8%) grandparents said that they offered to provide care, but more of the living-with grandparents said that someone else had made the suggestion or that it was assumed that they would provide care. The decision to provide care was often described by grandmothers as a nondecision: the result of an impulse to care. That is, grandmothers reported an automatic, do what you have to do attitude about providing care (Jendrek, 1994). Black grandmothers parenting children of their drug-addicted children faced multiple stressors that exacted a toll on their financial, physical, and emotional well-being (Burton, 1992).

Consistent with other data revealing the stronger ties of female kin, maternal grandmothers are closer to their grandchildren than are paternal grandparents (Matthews & Sprey, 1984). Fischer's (1981) data suggest that the bonds of mothers and adult daughters are strengthened by the birth of a child because of the common interest in parenting (Sprey & Matthews, 1982). Likewise, grandchildren report the greatest closeness to maternal grandmothers. Thompson and Walker (1987) examined the mediating effect of mothers on the relationships of grandmothers and their granddaughters. The grandmothers' rating of the relationship with their college-aged daughters was largely undifferentiated from their feelings about their relationships with their daughters. Granddaughters' feelings of closeness, on the other hand, were associated with their direct contact with their grandmothers, by feelings toward grandmother mediated by their mothers, and by a spillover of feelings for their own mothers (Thompson & Walker, 1987).

The grandparenting role may create new tensions, particularly if the expectations of grandmothers and their adult children and in-laws differ. Tension between adult daughters and grandmothers was identified in a study of Italian-American families where the immigrant grandmothers desired greater freedom from family responsibilities and daughters expected more traditional role behaviors from their elderly mothers (Cohler & Grunebaum, 1981). Baby-boom grandmothers may lead an active lifestyle outside the home that does not allow for extensive investments of time in the grandparent role (Grambs, 1989). Further research will be needed to understand the variety of styles and meanings that succeeding cohorts will use in defining the grandmother role.

SISTERS AND THEIR SIBLINGS

The majority of midlife and older women have siblings. Baby-boom women may have more siblings than children due to their lower fertility patterns compared to those of their mothers. Siblings have a unique relationship that sets them apart from other kin: the long duration of the relationship, a common family history, shared memories, and being an age peer. These features are potentially important for provision of social emotional support to one another in old age.

Structural features of sibling relationships show a predominance of female involvement. Connidis (1989) found that sister-sister dyads in a Canadian sample lived in greater proximity to one another and had greater face-to-face contact than other dyads. Earlier international research documented that with one exception (Yugoslavia), older women had greater face-to-face contact with siblings than older men in Western industrialized nations, Eastern Europe, and Israel (Shanas, 1973). Shanas attributed this gender difference to marital status, which predisposed a greater number of older women to being widowed and in need of support from extended kin.

The earliest studies of sibling relationships have observed the close bonds of sisters (Adams, 1968; Cicirelli, 1977). Early and more recent studies have documented the strong bond of sister-sister dyads, followed by mixed-gender and brother-brother dyads. With the exception of Scott (1983), sisters are consistently rated as the most intimate of sibling dyads. Among five sibling typologies, those with the more intense positive qualities (intimate and congenial types) were associated with the presence of a sister, whereas brother-brother dyads were disproportionately represented in the apathetic and hostile types (Gold, 1989). Scott (1990) found similar results, with gender composition of the dyad significantly associated with sibling type. Sister-sister dyads more frequently fell in the intimate typology.

Despite the strong positive bonds of sisters, evidence of conflict in the sister-sister relationship also appears. Using projective techniques, Bedford (1989) found that female siblings were higher on conflict themes in discussing relationships with sisters than were men talking about brothers. Similarly, Lowenthal, Thurnher, and Chiriboga (1975) found that women who felt closest to sisters were also highest on conflict. Sisters in Cicirelli's (1977) study were stimulated and challenged in their social roles. These findings suggest a greater intensity and involvement between sisters than between brothers.

Other studies suggest that sisters have more intimate relationships with their siblings regardless of gender. In an Australian sample women aged 60–64 and women aged 75 or over were more likely to report a sibling as a confidant than were men (Kendig, Coles, Pittelkow, & Wilson, 1988). For the middle group (65–74 years of age), having a sister emerged as a salient factor in confiding in a sibling.

There is a small body of literature suggesting that certain features of the sister relationship are related to one's mental health. In McGhee's (1985) study, having a proximate sister enhanced life satisfaction for older rural women and approached significance for older rural men. Marital status of the sister dyad was important to the positive affect of recent widows (O'Bryant, 1988). Having a married sister nearby and having contact with her were significant predictors of positive affect.

Female siblings are important in the provision of instrumental support to siblings (O'Bryant, 1988). Seeing an unmarried sister was most predictive of recent widows' receipt of sibling support, followed by frequency of phone contact with a married brother, having a married sister nearby, having an unmarried sister nearby, and having an adult child nearby. Also, not having an adult child nearby was predictive of more sibling support.

In summary, older women appear more involved and invested than males in sibling relationships, particularly those with a sister. Although gender plays a role in shaping the sibling relationship of later life, other factors, including marital status and proximity, are important to understanding the relationship quality and interaction of siblings. As with other family relationships, more theoretical attention to gender differences is needed. Examination of sibling relationships over time, from midlife to old age, is needed.

SUMMARY AND DIRECTIVES FOR FUTURE RESEARCH

After a review of the literature on family relationships of midlife and older women, several recommendations for future research can be offered. A future need is more research that is grounded in theory. Presently there are no dominant theories that guide our understanding of family relationships of midlife and older women. Studies that have used mini- or midrange theories to understand specific topic areas represent an initial step toward greater theoretical understanding of mid- and later-life families and of how gender influences family experiences. Ferree (1990), for example, criticized sex role socialization theories as inadequate to explain fully how gender influences family relationships. She argued that gender-role theory offers a more heuristic approach that has yet to be widely used in the study of family relationships (Ferree, 1990).

Though not always explicit, family development perspectives have been used in much of the literature. Women's lives have been closely intertwined with socially expected family roles of wife, mother, and grandparent. Recent reworking of family-development theory that better accounts for individual and family change and "offtime" patterns offer potentially fruitful approaches to the study of women's family careers (Klein & White, 1996; Rodgers & White, 1993). Today, some women remain single by choice, are childless by choice, make early commitments to careers, divorce, or go back to school. With an emphasis on the individual level of analysis rather than the family, life-course analysis offers a contextual perspective to study individual life trajectories. The timing, sequencing, and meaning of events is analyzed by considering one's place in the social structure (gender, race/ethnicity, socioeconomic status) and the effects of personal biography and historical period (Stoller & Gibson, 1994). These theoretical perspectives hold promise for the systematic study of women's lives.

Brubaker (1990) recommended more studies that examine gender differences in family relations. Greater effort to understand how men and women of mid- and later life experience family transitions and relationships differently will be important as new cohorts reach mid- and later life. Furthermore, we must move beyond a focus on identifying differences to an examination of how differences are constructed and what the ramifications are for women's lives. Additionally, more qualitative research and process research are needed to examine processes of retirement decision making, divorce, remarriage, and mid- and later-life marital communication.

Methodological improvements are needed, including more representative samples (broader representation of social class, race/ethnicity, and region); sequential designs that allow the differentiation of cohort, age, and period effects; and the simultaneous assessment of family relationships and broader contextual (work, health care services) variables. As researchers noted in their reports, the differentiation and study of cohort influences will be critical to an understanding of the family experiences of women of the depression era and early and late baby-boom cohorts. The combination of the effects of significant sociohistorical influences, age, and cohort differences on women's lives over the last decades presents a rare opportunity to examine disruptions and continuities in family relationships.

REFERENCES

Adams, B. N. (1968). *Kinship in an urban setting.* Chicago: Markham.

Anderson, S. A., Russell, C. S., & Schumm, W. R. (1983). Perceived marital quality and family life-cycle categories: A further analysis. *Journal of Marriage and the Family, 45,* 127–139.

Antonucci, T., & Akiyama, H. (1987). An examination of sex differences in social support among older men and women. *Sex Roles, 17,* 737–749.

Bedford, V. H. (1989). Sibling research in historical perspective: The discovery of a forgotten relationship. *American Behavioral Scientist, 33,* 6–18.

Brubaker, T. (1985). *Later life families.* Newbury Park, CA: Sage.

———. (1990). Families in later life. *Journal of Marriage and the Family, 52,* 959–981.

Brubaker, T., & Hennon, C. (1982). Responsibility for household tasks: Comparing dual-earner and dual-retired marriages. In M. Szinovacz (Ed.), *Women's retirement: Policy implications of recent research* (pp. 205–219). Beverly Hills, CA: Sage.

Bulcroft, K., & O'Conner, M. (1986). The importance of dating relationships on quality of life for older persons. *Family Relations, 35,* 397–401.

Burton, L. M. (1992). Black grandparents rearing children of drug-addicted parents: Stressors, outcomes, and social service needs. *Gerontologist, 32,* 744–751.

Burton, L. M., & Bengtson, V. (1985). Black grandmothers: Issues of timing and continuity of roles. In V. Bengtson & J. F. Robertson (Eds.), *Grandparenthood.* Beverly Hills, CA: Sage.

Cain, B. S. (1988). Divorce among elderly women: A growing social phenomenon. *Social Casework: The Journal of Contemporary Social Work, 69,* 563–568.

Cicirelli, V. G. (1977). Relationship of siblings to the elderly person's feelings and concerns. *Journal of Gerontology, 32,* 317–322.

Cohler, B. J., & Grunebaum, H. U. (1981). *Mothers, grandmothers, and daughters.* New York: Wiley.

Connidis, I. (1989). Siblings as friends in later life. *American Behavioral Scientist, 33,* 81–93.

Deckert, P., & Langelier, R. (1978). The late-divorce phenomenon: The causes and impact of ending 20-year-old or longer marriages. *Journal of Divorce, 1,* 381–389.

Depner, C. E., & Ingersoll-Dayton, B. (1985). Conjugal social support: Patterns in later life. *Journal of Gerontology, 40,* 761–766.

Ferree, M. M. (1990). Beyond separate spheres: Feminism and family research. *Journal of Marriage and the Family, 52,* 866–884.

Fischer, L. R. (1981). Transitions in the mother-daughter relationship. *Journal of Marriage and the Family, 43,* 613–622.

Gallagher, S., & Gerstel, N. (1993). Kinkeeping and friend keeping among older women: The effect of marriage. *Gerontologist, 33,* 675–681.

Gander, A. (1991). After the divorce: Familial factors that predict well-being for older and younger persons. *Journal of Divorce and Remarriage, 15,* 175–192.

———. (1992). Reasons for divorce: Age and gender differences. *Women and Aging, 4,* 47–60.

Gilford, R. (1984). Contrasts in marital satisfaction throughout old age: An exchange theory analysis. *Journal of Gerontology, 39,* 325–333.

Gladstone, J. (1988). Perceived changes in grandmother-grandchild relations following a child's separation or divorce. *Gerontologist, 28,* 66–72.

Gold, D. (1989). Generational solidarity: Conceptual antecedents and consequences. *American Behavioral Scientist, 33,* 19–32.

Grambs, J. D. (1989). *Women over forty: Visions and realities* (Rev. ed.). New York: Springer.

Hagestad, G., & Burton, L. (1986). Grandparenthood, life context, and family development. *American Behavioral Scientist, 29,* 471–484.

Hagestad, G., & Symer, M. (1982). Dissolving long-term relationships: Patterns of divorcing in middle age. In S. Duck (Ed.), *Personal relationships: Vol. 4, Dissolving personal relationships.* New York: Academic Press.

Hammond, R. J., & Muller, G. (1992). The late-life divorced: Another look. *Journal of Divorce and Remarriage, 17,* 135–150.

Hatfield, E., Traupmann, J., & Sprecher, S. (1984). Older women's perceptions of their intimate relationships. *Journal of Social and Clinical Psychology, 2,* 108–124.

Hayes, C. L., & Anderson, D. (1993). Psycho-social and economic adjustment of midlife women after divorce: A national study. *Journal of Women and Aging, 4,* 83–99.

Hennon, C. (1983). Divorce and the elderly: A neglected area of research. In T. Brubaker (Ed.), *Family relationships in later life* (pp. 149–172). Beverly Hills, CA: Sage.

Hooyman, N., & Kiyak, H. A. (1993). *Social gerontology: A multidisciplinary perspective.* (3rd ed.). Needham Heights, MA: Allyn & Bacon.

Jacobson, J. M. (1995). *Midlife women: Contemporary issues.* Boston: Jones & Bartlett.

Jendrek, M. P. (1994). Grandparents who parent their grandchildren: Circumstances and decisions. *Gerontologist, 34,* 206–216.

Johnson, C. L. (1985). Impact of illness on late-life marriages. *Journal of Marriage and the Family, 47,* 165–172.

Keating, N., & Cole, P. (1980). What do I do with him 24 hours a day? *Gerontologist, 20,* 84–89.

Keith, P. M. (1986). The social context and resources of the unmarried in old age. *International Journal of Aging and Human Development, 23,* 81–96.

Kendig, H. L., Coles, R., Pittelkow, Y., & Wilson, S. (1988). Confidants and family structure in old age. *Journals of Gerontology, 43,* S31–S40.

Kivnick, H. (1982). Grandparenthood: An overview of meaning and mental health. *Gerontologist, 22,* 59–66.

Klein, D., & White, J. M. (1996). *Family theories: An introduction.* Thousand Oaks, CA: Sage.

Lauer, R., Lauer, J. & Kerr, S. T. (1990). The long-term marriage: Perceptions of stability and satisfaction. *International Journal of Aging and Human Development, 31,* 189–195.

Lee, G. R. (1978). Marriage and morale in later life. *Journal of Marriage and the Family, 40,* 131–139.

Lee, G. R., & Shehan, C. (1989). Retirement and marital satisfaction. *Journals of Gerontology, 44,* S226–S230.

Levenson, R. W., Carstensen, L. L., & Gottman, J. M. (1993). Long-term marriage: Age, gender, and satisfaction. *Psychology and Aging, 8,* 301–313.

———. (1994). The influence of age and gender on affect, physiology, and their interrelations: A study of long-term marriage. *Journal of Personality and Social Psychology, 67,* 56–68.

Lowenthal, M. F., Thurnher, M., & Chiriboga, D. (1975). *Four stages of life.* San Francisco: Jossey-Bass.

McGhee, J. L. (1985). The effects of siblings on the life satisfaction of the rural elderly. *Journal of Marriage and the Family, 47,* 85–91.

McKain, W. C. (1972). A new look at older marriages. *Family Coordinator, 21,* 61–69.

Matthews, S., & Sprey, J. (1984). The impact of divorce on grandparenthood: An exploratory study. *Gerontologist, 24,* 41–47.

O'Bryant, S. (1988). Sibling support and older widows' well-being. *Journal of Marriage and the Family, 50,* 173–183.

Rodgers, R. H., & White, J. M. (1993). Family development theory. In P. Boss, W. Doherty, R. LaRossa, W. Schumm, & S. Steinmetz (Eds.), *Sourcebook of family theories and methods: A contextual approach* (pp. 225–254). New York: Plenum.

Rollins, B. C., & Cannon, K. L. (1974). Marital satisfaction over the family life cycle: A reevaluation. *Journal of Marriage and the Family, 36,* 271–282.

Rollins, B. C., & Feldman, H. (1970). Marital satisfaction over the family life cycle. *Journal of Marriage and the Family, 32,* 20–28.

Scott, J. P. (1983). Siblings and other kin. In T. H. Brubaker (Ed.), *Family relationships in later life* (pp. 47–62). Beverly Hills, CA: Sage.

————. (1990). Sibling interaction in later life. In T. Brubaker (Ed.), *Families in later life* (pp. 86–99). Newbury Park, CA: Sage.

Shanas, E. (1973). Family-kin networks and aging in cross-cultural perspective. *Journal of Marriage and the Family, 35,* 505–511.

Sprey, J., & Matthews, S. H. (1982). Contemporary grandparenthood: A systemic transition. *Annals of the American Academy of Political and Social Science, 464,* 91–103.

Steil, J. M. (1984). Marital relationships and mental health: The psychic cost of inequality. In J. Freeman (Ed.), *Women: A feminist perspective,* 3rd ed. (pp. 113–123). Palo Alto, CA: Mayfield Press.

Stoller, E., & Gibson, R. (1994). *Worlds of difference: Inequality in the aging experience.* Thousand Oaks, CA: Pine Forge.

Szinovacz, M. (1980). Female retirement: Effects on spousal roles and marital adjustment. *Journal of Family Issues, 3,* 423–438.

————. (1987). Preferred retirement timing and retirement satisfaction in women. *International Journal of Aging and Human Development, 24,* 301–317.

Szinovacz, M., & Washo, C. (1992). Gender differences in exposure to life events and adaptation to retirement. *Journal of Gerontology, 47,* S191–S196.

Thompson, L., & Walker, A. (1987). Mothers as mediators of intimacy between grandmothers and their young adult granddaughters. *Family Relations, 36,* 72–77.

Traupmann, J., & Hatfield, E. (1983). How important is marital fairness over the lifespan? *International Journal of Aging and Human Development, 17,* 89–101.

Troll, L. (1983). Grandparents: The family watchdogs. In T. H. Brubaker (Ed.), *Family relationships in later life* (pp. 63–74). Beverly Hills, CA: Sage.

Uhlenberg, P., Cooney, T., & Boyd, R. (1990). Divorce for women after midlife. *Journal of Gerontology, 45,* S3–S11.

U.S. Bureau of the Census. (1992). *Sixty-five plus in America.* Current Population Reports, Special Studies, P23–178. Washington, DC: U.S. Government Printing Office.

Vaillant, C., & Vaillant, G. (1993). Is the U-curve of marital satisfaction an illusion? A 40-year study of marriage. *Journal of Marriage and the Family, 55*, 230–239.

Vinick, B. (1978). Remarriage in old age. *Family Coordinator, 27*, 359–363.

Weingarten, H. R. (1988). Late life divorce and the life review. *Journal of Gerontological Social Work, 12*, 83–97.

Weishaus, S., & Field, D. (1988). A half-century of marriage: Continuity or change? *Journal of Marriage and the Family, 50*, 763–774.

Wentowski, G. (1985). Older women's perceptions of great grandparenthood: A research note. *Gerontologist, 25*, 593–596.

Wyse, L. (1981). *Funny you don't look like a grandmother.* New York: Crown.

Twenty-Four

Single Women in Later Life

RICHARD L. NEWTSON AND PAT M. KEITH

Perhaps because marriage and parenthood have been normative for most older persons, scholars often have neglected those who remain unmarried throughout the life course. Yet, given the primacy of marriage as a focus for social relationships, it is perhaps surprising that persons who have never had this support have been studied infrequently. Combining the widowed, divorced, separated, or never-married in one group, as is commonly done, may blur subtle and not-so-obscure differences.

Marriage alters the life course of any individual and reshapes thoughts, values, and dependencies. Because they have chosen the marital relationship, it would be more appropriate to identify widowed, divorced, or separated women as formerly married, while leaving the classification of single to those women who have never entered a marital relationship. Macklin (1987) noted that because of the "tremendous heterogeneity among singles, resulting from such factors as reason for singlehood, age, social class, and living arrangement, it is relatively useless to refer to singles as a global category. . . . it is important to distinguish between the never-married and the once married, the widowed and divorced." Unfortunately, the scarcity of large diverse samples will contribute to the continued categorization as "single" or "unmarried" of all of those not in a marital relationship. This limits what we know and teach about older ever-single persons. A recent text on aging, for example, contains two brief paragraphs on "never-married older people" (Hooyman & Kiyak, 1993).

Words used to describe the single suggest attitudes toward them. "Old maid," "spinster," and other terms are often used to connote singleness among older women. Just as old maid and spinster are derogatory terms to label singlehood as atypical and deviant, so the term "never-married" indicates a lack. The absence of a marital relationship for women should not imply a void, lessened status, or lowered expectations. More appropriate and less biased terms may be used, such as ever-single or lifelong single. Being ever-single or a lifelong single means never having been in a marital relationship, but it does not necessarily connote a lack of desire to be or to have been married. Others have proposed typologies that take into account the context in which persons make decisions about marriage and the extent to which they are voluntary, involuntary, temporary, or permanent (Stein, 1978). The issue of chance and choice relative to the ever-single status is beyond the scope of this chapter. We use ever-single, lifelong single, and single interchangeably.

Shostak (1987) observed that over the life course singleness may be easier and smoother for men than for women despite the greater happiness of the latter in their 20s. He described the decline of the "social life options" of women over age 30 and their increased discontent. "Never-married middle-aged women may begin to doubt their own sex appeal, personal worth, and capacity to be happier than a grim 'spinsterhood' will permit when faced with the media image of married women: happy, sexy, and desirable" (Shostak, 1987, p. 358). Single men and married women have been primary referents against which stereotypes of lifelong singleness among women have been evaluated. Freedman observed that in contrast to never-married women, men are not seen as "pathetic, lonely creatures; they are not dried-up spinsters; indeed, there is no comparable word for men" (cited in Shostak, 1987, p. 358). Consequently, it is not surprising that a recent text on aging concluded that "the traditional stereotype of the elderly spinster is that of a lonesome, egocentric, neurotic, irresponsible, or immoral deviant" (Aiken, 1995, p. 217). Aiken observed that this is not an accurate characterization of older lifelong singles today. Shostak acknowledged that the new social and cultural climate with more assertive females may alter perceptions and promote greater gender equity in well-being of singles. To substantiate his view, however, Aiken (1995) used data from a 1975 study of 22 never-married persons, from which he concluded that they were more independent and competent than their elder peers who had made other choices. But conceptions of singleness among the general population that might serve as estimates of current thinking or counter widely held stereotypes are less often studied. Taking into account devaluation of both age and nonmarriage, O'Brien (1991) asked whether single older women are "subject to some of the common stereotypes of old age in addition to those associated with being never married."

The stigma attached to being ever-single is still present in American society. Yankelovich (1981) reported that in the late 1950s about 80 percent of the general public still held negative images of the unmarried; by 1978 this had dropped to approximately 25 percent. While attitudes have changed somewhat in recent decades, there is still a bias and ignorance about the elderly who have not married. For instance, when Allen (1989) asked her sample of widowed respondents about ever-single females, the majority responded by saying that they did not know any ever-single women. Whether they knew any singles or not, as a group they held very stereotypical views of ever-single females, regarding them as "old maids or bereft of family" (Allen, 1989, p. 125). Most of Allen's sample had been involved in providing assistance to their family of orientation earlier in their lives. The widowed, however, still regarded the assistance and duration of the assistance provided by the ever-single as deviant. Marriage and motherhood were the two careers regarded as normal by Allen's sample. Singleness as a life choice is not seen as a viable alternative by many; in the mid-1980s about 4 percent expressed it as a preference (Thornton, 1989).

TRENDS IN SINGLENESS IN LATER LIFE

Ever-single women in later life (age 65 or over) make up about 5 percent of the population, with the majority of these women living in urban rather than rural areas. Between 1970 and 1992, for example, the proportion of single women aged 65 or over declined from 7.7 to 4.9 (Bureau of the Census, 1995). In contrast to the United States, twice the proportion of elderly women in England and Wales have never married (10 percent) (Arber & Ginn, 1992). This seems to be consistent with findings of Van Solinge (1994), who reported that in 1950 the percentage of ever-single elderly women varied from 10.5 percent in France to 22 percent in Scotland; by 1960, in most European countries, this proportion had shrunk to about 10 percent.

Research indicates that the percentage of ever-single older women increases somewhat with advancing age (Barresi & Hunt, 1990). The percentage of ever-single older women increases from 4.9 percent for women between the ages of 55 and 64 and 4.4 percent for those between 65 and 74 to 5.4 percent for women 75 years or older (Bureau of the Census, 1995). The increase in the percentage of ever-single women with advancing age is a trend among white, Asian/Pacific Islander, and Hispanic women; however, for blacks, American Indians, and Eskimos, the reverse is true, although the pattern is most evident for elderly black women.

There is some debate as to whether or not the number of ever-single older women will continue to increase. Some researchers believe that the number of ever-single females peaked in the late 1970s, and therefore there will be lower numbers of these older women in the next several decades; others speculate that the number of singles may increase in the near future (Bumpass, Sweet, & Cherlin, 1991).

HEALTH OF THE EVER-SINGLE

Much of the literature on marital status among the aged has focused on health (Keith, 1989). In this section we present research that focuses on the health and disability of ever-single aged females. Generally, married elderly are reported to have better health and fewer disabilities than the unmarried as a group, although some studies have found that lifelong singles, especially women, approach the reported levels of good health for married spouses. But what is the health status for the almost half of all elderly who are not married? What are the differences in health and disability of the divorced, widowed, or ever-single?

In an investigation of the unmarried aged, Verbrugge (1979) found that separated and divorced persons were the least healthy, followed by widowed persons; the most healthy were the ever-single. Loss of a spouse (i.e., divorced, separated, or widowed status) is associated with poorer health over time. This is also consistent with work done by Fenwick and Barresi (1981), who found that widows, divorcées, or those older women who had separated were in poorer health than were the married or ever-single. Using longitudinal data from the Retirement History Study, Stull and Scarisbrick-Hauser (1989) found that ever-single men and women were in no poorer health than the other groups and were not at a higher risk of needing care. When asked about their satisfaction with the way they were living at that time, the ever-single were the most satisfied of the unmarried.

Over a ten-year period, ever-single aged women reported significantly fewer handicaps and disabilities than did the widowed or divorced (Keith, 1989). Health limitations on the ability to work were investigated. At the beginning and end of a decade widowed and divorced women were more likely to report a greater number of limitations affecting work or housework than did the ever-single. The ever-single tended to rate their own health more highly than did widowed or divorced females. In fact, Fenwick and Barresi (1981) reported that widowhood is associated with an immediate decrease in perceived health status. In addition to rating their own health more positively, ever-single older women tended to have more stable health over a ten-year period than did the divorced or widowed. Across several indices, ever-single women had fewer health limitations, whereas the divorced and widowed had more comparable health assessments.

Because good health is so closely linked to enjoyment of life and because chronic diseases increase with age, health-seeking behavior is crucial to the well-being of the aged. The decision to see a doctor or obtain needed treatment may be a factor in prevention, cure, or management of health difficulties. There are differences by marital status in decisions to seek care that may account for some of the variations in health noted earlier. Ever-single older females more often sought health care than widowed or divorced women at both the beginning and end of a ten-year period (Keith, 1989).

Barriers to accessing health care also may vary by marital status. When health care was postponed by aged women, the ever-single, for example, were less likely to name financial reasons for delaying care than were widowed or divorced women. In contrast, ever-single women cited emotional reasons for their delay in attending to health care needs significantly more often than the widowed or divorced. It is likely that financial concerns had a substantially greater impact on the decisions of the widowed and divorced to seek health care than they did for the ever-single.

Relationships between mental health and marital status among the unmarried are similar to those for physical health. Gove (1979) found that divorced or separated elderly women had the highest rates of mental illness. Hoeffer (1987) explained the association by suggesting that these women had inadequate support networks and that the quality of the support network was more important than quantity. This may help explain why Fenwick and Barresi (1981) reported that both widowhood and marital separation are associated with higher suicide rates among the elderly. The ever-single aged woman tends to have larger and more developed social support networks than some of the previously married, and this has a direct effect on mental health. The social support networks of ever-single aged women are described in more detail in the next section.

In summary, among the unmarried, those who have never married seem to have the best health and fewest health limitations or disabilities, followed by the widowed and divorced/separated (Cramer, 1993). Health conditions usually are implicated in admissions to long-term-care facilities, and differences by marital status in these living arrangements are discussed in another section.

SUPPORT SYSTEMS OF THE AGED EVER-SINGLE

The family life of ever-single aged persons revolves around parents, siblings, nieces and nephews, and friends; they are not bound by nuclear units (Brubaker, 1985). Older ever-single females may live with or are expected to care for aging parents; in fact, Brubaker wrote that in Amish and Mennonite families an unmarried daughter is expected to provide such care. This pattern is found in many other cultures of the world as well. For instance, in Asian cultures unmarried women are still expected to provide care to family members. Even within our own not-so-distant American past, unmarried daughters were expected to provide care for aging parents or the family of orientation (Allen, 1989).

Ward (1979) suggested that families are more important to the ever-single because of the shrinkage in their social support systems as they age. It is thought that for ever-single women, family relationships are very important; they likely have had more intensive relationships with their elderly parents, siblings, and more distant kin (i.e., aunts, uncles, nieces, nephews) (Bengtson, Rosenthal, & Burton, 1990). As core family members die, there is a natural decline in available providers of emotional support. Filling the void may be left to so-called fictive kin, people who may mean a great deal to the aged ever-single and also may be counted on for assistance. Brubaker (1985) alluded to the importance of "fictive kin" to elderly ever-single women and their importance as providers of social support.

When the ever-single reach later life, they seem to have less familial instrumental support than do the married or those with children (Johnson & Catalano, 1981). Aged parents, who probably long held a significant place in the social support network of their ever-single daughters, are likely deceased or dependent themselves. Siblings may be the next viable source of social support, and, in fact, sibling support to unmarried aged women is well documented in the literature (Cicirelli, 1981).

In their study of aged unmarried women, Goldberg, Kantrow, Kremen, and Lauter (1986) found that ever-single women named about the same number of close relatives as did the widowed, but both the ever-single and widowed named significantly more close relationships with relatives than did the divorced or separated. Of the close relationships with relatives identified by their respondents, intimate relationships with siblings were the most often named by elderly spouseless and childless women. In fact, Goldberg et al. (1986) reported that widows and ever-single elderly women were about equally likely to have a close sibling relationship, whereas the divorced and/or separated least often maintained an intimate relationship with a sibling. The role of siblings may be compromised. Siblings, who themselves are of comparable age and health, are likely either to need assistance themselves or are trying to meet the demands of their spouses, children, or other family members; there may be little time to help ever-single brothers and sisters.

Other than family members, to whom do ever-single aged women turn for help and support? Goldberg et al. (1986) found that in their sample of unmarried elderly women, both the ever-single and widowed women were similar in their use of informal support, while the divorced or separated tended to rely more on formal supports. Their findings certainly suggest the importance of the informal support system to ever-single aged women. Friends comprise a very crucial part of the informal social support system. Many single aged have social networks that include persons to whom they are psychologically close (Rubinstein, 1987). Babchuk (1978) observed that the ever-single had fewer primary and confidant kin, but they had more primary or confidant friends than the previously married. Stull and Scarisbrick-Hauser (1989) found that the ever-single are more likely than the married to get together with friends (not neighbors). Highlighting the importance of friends, Lee (1985) found that friends are associated more with well-being than are kin and that ever-single women had more friendship ties than the previously married. Lee, however, reported that the association between friendship and sibling ties and marital status was mediated by social class and income; poorer ever-single aged women had the fewest ties with siblings and friends.

Another way to conceptualize the importance of both friends and kin is to consider work by Gupta and Korte (1994). Using a nonrandom sample of unmarried elderly (i.e., widowed, divorced/separated, and ever-single), Gupta and Korte found that having a peer group is equal in importance to having a confidant, since these roles are usually performed by different persons and serve different functions. The authors concluded by suggesting that what is really necessary for well-being in later life is diversity in social relationships. Here, ever-single aged women may have the advantage in that they have greater friendship ties, friends who are more likely to be both primary and confidants. The ever-single usually have not centralized their social support systems around one or two people as have the married. Many studies clearly indicate that a spouse is the preferred provider of most types of informal social support, followed by adult children (Newtson & Hoyt, 1994; Cantor, 1979; Litwak, 1985). The effect of this dependency may be a weak or less effective informal social support system for the formerly married at a time when it is needed the most.

The negative outcomes of kinship patterns of singles can be compensated for somewhat by other attributes. Lifelong singlehood is likely to have resulted in "qualities of independence, self-reliance, and habituation to living alone" (Johnson & Catalano, 1981). Ever-singles have spent a lifetime developing friendship ties, are more likely to have friends who are both primary and confidants, and maintain ties with "fictive kin" (Brubaker, 1985). In addition, the ever-single do not experience the dramatic and powerful effects of divorce or widowhood.

EDUCATION AND INCOME

Previous research has found that older ever-single women tend to be more highly educated and more likely to have professional careers than the elderly women in the other marital statuses (Carter & Glick, 1976; Havens, 1973). Keith (1989) found that ever-single aged females had higher incomes than the divorced or widowed. Among female-headed households in later life, ever-single women were the least likely to be below the poverty line compared with widowed, divorced, or separated women. Divorced and widowed females were more economically disadvantaged than were ever-single women. The formerly married may have fared less well financially because they held lower-level jobs throughout their work lives and/or had more discontinuous work histories than their ever-single counterparts.

Differential occupational placement by marital status is reflected in access to pension income as well, with single women more often receiving a pension than the divorced or separated (Arber & Ginn, 1992). Single women have a higher pension income than the widowed, divorced, or separated. Because widows benefit from their former husband's earnings, they receive higher pension income than other previously married women (Arber & Ginn, 1992).

Uhlenberg and Myers (1981), however, reported that there was no significant difference in satisfaction with their current financial situation between widows and the ever-single. Divorced or separated aged women, however, reported the greatest dissatisfaction with their financial circumstances.

Income adequacy is an especially important factor in well-being and satisfaction with life and/or retirement (Palmore, Burchett, Fillenbaum, George, & Wallman, 1985). To the extent that education and occupational status are linked to financial well-being, ever-single aged women should fare better than most previously married women.

LIVING ARRANGEMENTS

Living arrangements of the unmarried aged are varied, and findings about differences among these marital statuses seem somewhat inconsistent and probably reflect the samples on which they are based, especially in regard to age and place in the family life cycle of respondents. In an examination of the living arrangements of the elderly, Harris and Associates (1987) found that fully 8 percent of its sample who reported living alone were ever-single (men and women), whereas 9 percent of those who lived with children or others were ever-single (men and women). In a national longitudinal study widowed and divorced women were slightly more likely than the formerly married to be heads of households but living with others at the beginning of a decade compared to the ever-single (Keith, 1989). Earlier in their lives the formerly married may have had children or grandchildren living with them. By the close of the decade, however, the ever-single were more likely to be heads of households and living with others. This latter finding seems to be consistent with previous work (Goldberg et al., 1986; Mutchler, 1990). Goldberg et al., for instance, found that about half of their sample of ever-single elderly women shared a home with at least one other person, compared to 25 percent of the widowed and 14 percent of the divorced/separated.

Stull and Scarisbrick-Hauser (1989) also noted that the ever-single elderly, compared to other unmarried persons, are much more likely to have siblings or other relatives living with them. However, ever-single persons are not any more likely than the separated or divorced to live with their parents (Stull and Scarisbrick-Hauser, 1989). The ever-single may care for other dependent relatives after the death or incapacity of their own parents.

Finally, in an investigation of rural and urban differences, Barresi and Hunt (1990) observed that in each age category (i.e., young-old, middle-old, and old-old) there are substantially more ever-single females in urban than in rural areas. This seems to be consistent with work by Van Solinge (1994), who reported that in the Netherlands ever-single women tend to live more in urban areas and are better educated.

The probability of institutional residence is closely associated with marital status (Arber & Ginn, 1992). Married persons in both Great Britain and the United States are less likely to receive residential care than are the unmarried. For example, ever-single British women in their 70s are eight times more likely to reside in an institution than their married counterparts (Arber & Ginn, 1992). Twenty percent of ever-single persons in the United States aged 75 or over were institutionalized, compared with 14 percent of the previously married and 4 percent of the married (Dolinksy & Rosenwaike, 1988).

In a longitudinal study of living arrangements, including living alone, living with others, and institutionalization, Worobey and Angel (1990) concluded that never having been married increases dependency. These graphic differences by marital status are thought to reflect the informal care given by spouses to their partners and by children to the widowed. Arber and Ginn (1992) observed that those ''closest'' to marriage and children are less likely to reside in a residential facility during the course of their lives. Not surprisingly, the absence of a spouse or child, followed by greater age or disability, is the strongest predictor of institutional care for older persons in the United States (Dolinsky & Rosenwaike, 1988). Regardless of race, lifelong singles and those with disabilities have a higher probability of being in an institution even when demographic, economic, and health characteristics are controlled (Burr, 1990).

The effect of race on other living arrangements was considerable. Black women more often headed complex households and less often lived alone or lived as a nonhead of a household. Nonheads of households tend to be less healthy and to have fewer financial resources, including lower incomes (Mutchler, 1990). Women with higher incomes more often head their own households, whether or not others live with them.

Even so, Stull and Scarisbrick-Hauser (1989) argued that the ever-single, because of their greater social connectedness, may represent fewer demands on long-term care in the future. Offering evidence from the National Nursing Home Survey to support their claim, they noted that 64 percent of new admissions to nursing homes are widowed elderly, 16 percent are married, and less than 14 percent are ever-single. As further evidence, Cohen, Tell, and Wallack (1986) pointed out that the never-married live in larger-size households than the formerly married and that through age 80 widowhood had a greater effect on entry into a nursing home than being ever-single. That larger percentages of admittances to nursing homes are widowed or married women reflects their greater proportions in the older population. Even so, a higher percentage of ever-single women than the formerly married aged 65 or over reside in congregate facilities.

The financial resources of the ever-single also may figure in the type of institutional care they can afford. The pension-income advantage of lifelong single women is found only among those in nonmanual occupations (Arber & Ginn, 1992). Furthermore, earlier in their lives, low-income ever-single women may have been less able to afford preventive care, which may enhance their chances for later residential care.

RETIREMENT

For many, retirement is one of the most significant events associated with later life. The effects of retirement are many and are long-lasting. For employed men and women, and even for spouses not employed outside the home, retirement necessitates a reevaluation of roles, finances, values, goals, and relationships with family members and others. Retirement affects the well-being, roles, and relationships of spouses with their newly retired partners as well as those without spouses.

The unmarried have been found to derive more of their social validity from work than their married peers (Veroff, Douvan, & Kulka, 1981; Birnbaum,

1975). Atchley (1975) noted that ever-single women had a stronger work orientation than the previously married. If, in fact, single women derive greater fulfillment from work and have stronger work ethics, it is little surprise that Ward (1979) found that retirement had a more negative effect on the happiness of the ever-single than it did on the previously married. The salience of employment to lifelong single women is juxtaposed to Allen's (1989) finding that these women sometimes interrupted or delayed paid work opportunities to remain at home to care for aging parents. Consequently, there are sometimes family effects on the career patterns of the ever-single that are not limited only to the married or formerly married.

The passage of time may have a positive effect on retirement satisfaction for older ever-single women. For instance, at the beginning of a decade widowed and ever-single women had quite similar views of retirement; by the end of the decade, however, ever-single women clearly had more positive views of retirement than did the widowed or divorced (Keith, 1989). Ever-single women who have had consistent work histories are better able to plan for retirement and ensure a more positive financial situation in retirement than the previously married.

Among unmarried women the ever-single were least likely to expect financial problems in their retirement and, in fact, had expectations comparable to those of men. Perhaps reflecting their more negative expectations, a greater proportion of previously married women than singles did not plan to retire.

Ever-single females do not find retirement a less desirable time of life than being employed. Ever-single women likely will experience career fatigue similar to that of men, resulting from their continuous work histories, and will likewise welcome retirement as do most men. Also, as noted earlier, ever-single women enjoyed better financial circumstances than previously married women. Those who are responsible for preretirement programs may want to give special attention to previously married women, who are likely to be less prepared and to appreciate retirement less than are other groups.

LIFE SATISFACTION AND HAPPINESS

What are the consequences of marital status for satisfaction and happiness in later life? The common conception is that being married increases life satisfaction and happiness at any point in the lifespan. Although this chapter does not address the entire lifespan, evidence suggests that in later life the married may not manifest substantially greater happiness and satisfaction than some of the unmarried. Ward (1979) reported that in earlier years the ever-single are happier, but in later years they are less happy than married persons. Ward, however, did not consider women separately. Work by Gubrium (1975), in which he found that older ever-singles and married persons had similar levels of life satisfaction, suggested that ever-single women may be at least as happy as the married.

What is known about the satisfaction and happiness of older single women?

First, research suggests that ever-single aged women are happier than ever-single older men (Keith, 1989). Furthermore, ever-single older women expressed greater happiness over time than previously married women. This finding from longitudinal data is supported by Gee and Kimball (1987), who reported higher life satisfaction for the ever-single women than for the previously married. One reason that ever-single aged women seem to be happier may have to do with their outlook on life. Hoeffer (1987) reported that ever-single women had a more positive outlook on life than widows, the divorced, or the separated.

Although ever-single aged women were more likely to be happy and satisfied with their lives, Allen (1989) found that the ever-single, who thought that they had led uneventful lives, had diverse experiences similar to those of the previously married. The ever-single did not appreciate the "fullness" of their lives as much as the previously married.

In an investigation of isolation as a source of unhappiness and discontent, the majority of ever-single women were "satisfied affiliated," which was about the same as for widows but more than for divorced women (Keith, 1989). In other words, the majority of the aged ever-single women were satisfied and had a high degree of contact with others. Of those women who were identified as satisfied and isolated, ever-single aged women were twice as often contented and isolated as were divorced women.

Essex and Nam (1987), who observed that single women were less lonely than the formerly married, also found that contact with others had a differential impact among the unmarried. The relationship of single women with their closest family member or with their closest friend had little effect on the frequency of their loneliness (Essex and Nam, 1987). In contrast, formerly married persons were lonely more frequently if they did not see their closest family member or if they were distressed by inequity in relationships with their most intimate friends and family members.

Consequently, Essex and Nam concluded that there were variations in sources of loneliness by marital status that revealed a complex pattern in which ever-single women were significantly different from their married and formerly married peers. Although ever-single women may be less vulnerable to loneliness, perhaps because of self-reliance, low need for contact, and independence, deteriorating health threatens these lifelong behavior patterns. In contrast, stressful intimate relationships more often fostered loneliness among the formerly married, but health status rather than limited interpersonal ties directly affected loneliness of the ever-single.

In addition to giving views of their satisfaction, happiness, and loneliness, single women also have described their regrets. For some unmarried women, the choices leading to the absence of children and their irrevocability in late life result in feelings of regret (Alexander, Rubinstein, Goodman, & Luborsky, 1992). A common pattern is for the intensity of regret to increase with age. The lack of generational continuity, feelings of marginality, and nontraditional gender identity are central to regrets about not having children. "These women's regrets were shaped and formed in the context of a culture that defines womanhood predominantly through childbearing and that forces women to evaluate themselves continually against the pressure of this cultural prescription'' (Alexander et al., 1992, p. 626). In addition to this prescription, the ever-single in this generation of older women must evaluate in their life reviews and reflections the atypicality of nonmarriage as well.

Yet on many indicators aged ever-single women seem at least as happy as married men and women, and happier than the widowed, divorced, or separated. They are not dissatisfied with their lives, nor are the majority isolated; if they are isolated, they are not necessarily displeased with their lives. The aged ever-single probably are more likely to view their lives as less eventful compared to those of the married in a society in which marriage is seen as more fulfilling. As Gubrium (1975) suggested twenty years ago, being ever-single and old does not necessarily lead to dissatisfaction with life.

CONCLUSIONS

When Allen (1989) asked whether or not the ever-single had regrets about their decision to remain single, the majority either had no regrets or regretted only not having children. When the previously married were asked if they had regrets, the majority had none. O'Brien also observed from her qualitative study that single women had not found their marital status a disadvantage, but some expressed regret at not having children. It would seem that for the most part, life-course decisions that lead to either marriage or singlehood, and the lack of regret expressed by the majority, suggest that there is little dissonance in later years over this important life choice. Despite the stereotypes and misconceptions of elderly ever-single women, their ever-single status places them at no more risk than formerly married peers with one exception, that of a greater likelihood of institutional placement resulting from a disability. In fact, the majority of research seems to suggest that in many ways ever-single older women may actually be slightly better off than the widowed, divorced, or separated. Clearly, they have a more diverse social support system (which is linked to well-being), made up of a greater number of friends, whom they see more often, than previously married older women. While there is less familial support in later life for these women, older ever-single women have about as many close relationships with relatives as do the widowed and significantly more than the divorced or separated are able to maintain. A close relationship with a sibling is most often noted.

Sisters and other female relatives contribute the most assistance to ever-single women (Coward, Horne, and Dwyer, 1992). The psychological ''costs'' of informal assistance for older recipients, however, need further attention among the ever-single (Mutchler and Bullers, 1994). There also may be considerable strain for sisters who believe they should provide care to an ever-single sibling but are unable to do so because of physical health or other circumstances.

Greater dependence on hired help by ever-single women (Coward, Horne, and Dwyer, 1992) may be the result of their higher incomes and occupational status. Indices of social class need to be taken into account more often in future research on social ties and well being of the ever-single.

Several other questions remain unanswered. For those ever-single women with chronic disabilities who live with others, either as heads or nonheads of households, do their living arrangements help delay institutionalization? We know little about the supportive functions of other householders for older ever-singles.

There is clear evidence that even today ever-single women are stereotyped, if their existence is even known or understood (Allen, 1989). How do married or formerly married persons interact with singles in the varied social situations (i.e., community and senior functions, volunteer work) that are common to the groups in later life? It may be a mistake to assume that all the damage done by societal misconceptions and prejudices are experienced earlier in life. Age does not necessarily mean greater empathy or even acceptance of a "deviant" lifestyle. Further research also is warranted on differences in rural and urban friendship patterns of singles. In rural areas where ever-single peers are fewer social ties may be harder to maintain.

In summary, when compared to the formerly married, older ever-single women rate their own health the highest, report fewer disabilities, and are more likely to seek health care. They are at less risk of mental illness and impoverishment. The advantages that ever-single women manifest in late life may be an indicator of their hardiness in spite of having occupied an atypical marital status. For most ever-single aged women, later life need not be a time of greater anxiety.

REFERENCES

Aiken, L. (1995). *Aging*. Thousand Oaks, CA: Sage.

Alexander, B., Rubinstein, R., Goodman, M., & Luborsky, M. (1992). A path not taken: A cultural analysis of regrets and childlessness in the lives of older women. *Gerontologist, 32*(5), 618–626.

Allen, K. (1989). *Single women/family ties: Life histories of older women*. Newbury Park, CA: Sage.

Arber, S., & Ginn, J. (1992). *Gender and later life*. Newbury Park, CA: Sage.

Atchley, R. (1975). Dimensions of widowhood in later life. *Gerontologist, 15*(1), 176–178.

Babchuk, N. (1978). Aging and primary relations. *International Journal of Aging and Human Development, 9*, 137–151.

Barresi, C., & Hunt, K. (1990). The unmarried elderly: Age, sex, and ethnicity. In T. Brubaker (Ed.), *Family relationships in later life*. Newbury Park, CA: Sage.

Bengston, V., Rosenthal, C., & Burton, L. (1990). Families and aging: Diversity and heterogeneity. In R. Binstock & L. George (Eds.), *Handbook of aging and the social sciences*. (3rd ed.). San Diego, CA: Academic Press.

Birnbaum, J. (1975). Life patterns and self-esteem in gifted family-oriented and career-committed women. In M. Mednick, S. Tangri, & L. Hoffman (Eds.), *Women and achievement: Social and motivational analyses*. New York: Halsted.

Braito, R., & Anderson, D. (1983). The ever-single elderly woman. In E. Markson (Ed.), *Older women: Issues and prospects*. Lexington, MA: Lexington Books.

Brubaker, T. (1985). *Later life families*. Newbury Park, CA: Sage.

Bumpass, L., Sweet, J. & Cherlin, A. (1991). The role of cohabitation in declining rates of marriage. *Journal of Marriage and the Family, 53*, 913–927.

Bureau of the Census (1995). *Statistical Abstract of the United States, 1994*. Washington, DC: U.S. Government Printing Office.

Burr, J. (1990). Race/sex comparisons of elderly living arrangements. *Research on Aging, 12*(4), 507–530.

Cantor, M. (1979). Neighbors and friends: An overlooked resource in the informal support system. *Research on Aging, 1*(4), 434–463.

Carter, H., & Glick, P. (1976). *Marriage and divorce: A social and economic study*. (Rev. ed.). Cambridge, MA: Harvard University Press.

Cicirelli, V. (1981). *Helping elderly parents: The role of adult children*. Boston: Auburn House.

Cohen, M., Tell, E., & Wallack, S. (1986). Client related risk factors of nursing home entry among elderly adults. *Journal of Gerontology, 41*, 785–792.

Coward, R., Horne, C., & Dwyer, J. (1992). Demographic perspectives on gender and family caregiving. In J. Dwyer and R. Coward (Eds.), *Gender, families, and elder care*. Newbury Park, CA: Sage.

Cramer, D. (1993). Living alone, marital status, gender, and health. *Journal of Community and Applied Social Psychology, 3*, 1–15.

Dolinsky, A., & Rosenwaike, I. (1988). The role of demographic factors in the institutionalization of the elderly. *Research on Aging, 10*, 235–257.

Essex, M., & Nam, S. (1987). Marital status and loneliness among older women: The differential importance of close family and friends. *Journal of Marriage and the Family, 49*, 93–106.

Fenwick, R., & Barresi, C. (1981). Health consequences of marital-status change among the elderly: A comparison of cross-sectional and longitudinal analyses. *Journal of Health and Social Behavior, 22*, 106–116.

Gee, E., & Kimball, M. (1987). *Women and aging*. Toronto: Butterworths.

Glick, P. (1979). The future marital status and living arrangements of the elderly. *Gerontologist, 19*, 301–309.

Goldberg, G., Kantrow, R., Kremen, E., & Lauter, L. (1986, March/April). Spouseless, childless elderly women and their social supports. *Social Work*, pp. 104–112.

Gove, W. (1979). Sex, marital status, and psychiatric treatment: A research note. *Social Forces, 58*, 89–93.

Gubrium, J. (1975). Being single in old age. *International Journal of Aging and Human Development, 6*, 29–41.

Gupta, V., & Korte, C. (1994). The effects of a confidant and a peer group on the well-being of single elders. *International Journal of Aging and Human Development, 39*(4), 293–302.

Harris, L., & Associates Inc. (1987). *Problems facing elderly Americans living alone*. New York: AARP, National Gerontology Resource Center.

Havens, E. (1973). Women, work, and wedlock: A note on female marital patterns in the United States. *American Journal of Sociology, 78*, 975–981.

Hoeffer, B. (1987). Predictors of life outlook of older single women. *Research in Nursing and Health, 10*, 111–117.

Hooyman, N., & Kiyak, H. (1992). *Social gerontology.* (3rd ed.). Needham Heights, MA: Allyn & Bacon.

Johnson, C., & Catalano, D. (1981). Childless elderly and their family supports. *Gerontologist, 21*, 610–618.

Keith, P. (1989). *The unmarried in later life.* New York: Praeger.

Lee, G. (1985). Kinship and social support of the elderly: The case of the United States. *Aging and Society, 5*, 19–38.

Litwak, E. (1985). *Helping the elderly: The complementary roles of informal networks and formal systems.* New York: Guilford Press.

Macklin, E. (1987). Nontraditional family forms. In M. Sussman & S. Steinmetz (Eds.), *Handbook of marriage and the family.* New York: Plenum Press.

Mutchler, J. (1990). Household composition among the nonmarried elderly: A comparison of black and white women. *Research on Aging, 12*(4), 487–506.

Mutchler, J., & Bullers, S. (1994). Gender differences in formal care use in later life. *Research on Aging, 16*(3), 235–250.

Newtson, R., & Hoyt, D. (1994). The provision of sibling support in later life. Unpublished manuscript, Iowa State University, Ames.

O'Brien, M. (1991). Never married older women: The life experience. *Social Indicators Research, 24*, 301–315.

Palmore, E., Burchett, B., Fillenbaum, G., George, L., & Wallman, L. (1985). *Retirement: Causes and consequences.* New York: Springer.

Rubinstein, R. (1987). Never married elderly as a social type: Re-evaluating some images. *Gerontologist, 27*(1), 108–113.

Shostak, A. (1987). Singlehood. In M. Sussman & S. Steinmetz (Eds.), *Handbook of marriage and the family.* New York: Plenum Press.

Stein, P. (1978). The lifestyles and life chances of the never-married. *Marriage and Family Review, 1*, 1–11.

Stull, D., & Scarisbrick-Hauser, A. (1989). Never-married elderly: A reassessment with implications for long-term care policy. *Research on Aging, 11*(1), 124–139.

Thornton, A. (1989). Changing attitudes toward family issues in the United States. *Journal of Marriage and the Family, 51*, 873–893.

Uhlenberg, P., & Myers, M. (1981). Divorce and the elderly. *Gerontologist, 21*(3), 276–282.

Van Solinge, H. (1994). Living arrangements of non-married elderly people in the Netherlands in 1990. *Aging and Society, 14*, 219–236.

Verbrugge, L. (1979). Marital status and health. *Journal of Marriage and the Family, 41*, 267–285.

Veroff, J., Douvan, E., & Kulka, R. (1981). *The inner American.* New York: Basic Books.

Ward, R. (1979). The never married in later life. *Journal of Gerontology, 34*(6), 861–869.

Worobey, J., & Angel, R. (1990). Functional capacity and living arrangements of unmarried elderly persons. *Journal of Gerontology, 45*, S95–S101.

Yankelovich, D. (1981, April). New rules in American life: Searching for self-fulfillment in a world turned upside down. *Psychology Today*, pp. 35–91.

Twenty-Five

Friendship Patterns among Older Women

REBECCA G. ADAMS

Gerontologists have focused more attention on friendship than other researchers have. This is probably due to the centrality of the study of friendship to activity and disengagement theories, which preoccupied social gerontologists for decades, and because of the more recent interest in friends as a source of informal support for older adults (Adams, 1989).

Unlike researchers in many subfields of social science, researchers interested in older adult friendship have focused on women to the almost complete exclusion of men. This is partly because women compose more of the older population than men do, partly because early work suggested that friendship was more central to the lives of women than to the lives of men (Hess, 1972), and partly because more female than male scholars seem to be interested in friendship.

Given the plethora of studies on older adult women's friendships, we should know more about them than we do. The problem is that these studies of women's friendships are often descriptive and gender biased, using a women's perspective rather than a gender-informed one. A women's perspective emphasizes what Wright (1982) called the face-to-face aspects of friendship (personalism and interpersonal sensitivity), while a men's perspective emphasizes the side-by-side aspects (instrumentality and activity-centeredness). A gender-informed approach incorporates the perspectives of both genders. The gender biases of friendship researchers are reflected in the questions they ask about friendship and in the way they operationalize concepts. Female researchers have been more likely than male researchers to examine qualitative content or process (e.g., closeness, confiding, supportiveness), to ask nonglobal questions (as opposed to questions

A version of this chapter was presented at the Annual Meetings of the Southern Sociological Society, Raleigh, NC, April 8, 1994.

asking the respondent to summarize across friends), and to include the dyad as the unit of analysis (rather than focusing on friendships in general). This gender bias thus means that we know only part of the story about older women's friendships.

In addition to studies focused exclusively on older women, other scholars have examined friendship in populations including both genders. The contribution of these studies including both genders to our understanding of older women's friendships, however, is limited for two reasons. First, a surprising number of these studies do not include examinations of the effects of gender, but only analyses in which older women and older men are combined (Blieszner & Adams, 1992).

Second, when researchers do study gender differences and operationalize friendship in a way that encompasses the perspectives of both genders, they usually do not develop a theoretical explanation for why gender might have an effect (Adams & Blieszner, 1994; Blieszner & Adams, 1992). They typically add the variable ''sex'' to a set of independent variables predicting friendship patterns without discussing it conceptually and without including independent measures of gender as psychological disposition and as social structural position. This is unfortunate, because it is quite different, for example, to attribute the greater intimacy of women's friendships to their superior psychological capacity for such relationships rather than to their better opportunities to pursue them.

In order to understand older women's friendships, it is necessary to study the effects of gender among older adults, as well as to study the interactive effects of age and gender across the life course. Unfortunately, the limitations of the literature examining the effects of age on friendship mirror those of the literature examining the effects of gender on it. Researchers have conducted very few studies of friendships across the life course; what we know about older-adult friendship comes almost entirely from studies exclusively focused on that age group. When researchers do study friendships among adults of various ages, they either fail to examine age differences or they use the variable ''age'' as a proxy measure for both stage of life course and stage of development without distinguishing between these two aspects of aging. For example, Weiss and Lowenthal (1975) found that older adults tended to have more complex and multidimensional friendships than middle-aged or younger ones. They interpreted these results in light of differing age-related psychological needs and social norms, though they did not measure these needs or normative effects separately.

Studying the effects of age on friendship is further complicated by a need to separate out the effects of aging (growing older), period (time of measurement), and cohort (the interaction of age and period). To accomplish this, a theoretical rationale for setting one of these three effects to zero is needed, or at least a cross-sequential study design in which longitudinal studies of several cohorts are conducted (see Maddox & Campbell, 1985, for a general discussion of this methodological dilemma). There have been virtually no longitudinal studies of older-adult friend relationships (see Adams, 1987; Hatch & Bulcroft, 1992; and Shea, Thompson, & Blieszner, 1988, for exceptions) and no longitudinal studies including more than one cohort.

In addition to the problems already outlined, our knowledge of older women's friendships is further limited by problems characteristic of friendship research in general. On the one hand, there is a lack of studies using representative samples and samples of general populations (Adams, 1989). This has limited our ability to make generalizations and to identify sources of variation. On the other hand, though friendship researchers have tended to study special populations or friendships in specific contexts, they have not identified how the characteristics of the special populations or contexts affect friendship. Replications of both types of studies—the general and the specific—appear to be nonexistent.

Given these serious conceptual and methodological limitations of the literature bearing on older women's friendships, it is difficult to summarize the relevant findings. Although we know more about older women's friendships than about older men's friendships, much remains to be learned (see Adams, 1994, for a discussion of the research findings about older men's friendships that parallels this one). The rest of this chapter summarizes what can be culled from friendship research focused exclusively on older women and from research including gender comparisons, using a framework Adams and Blieszner (1994) developed for this type of analysis.

AN INTEGRATIVE CONCEPTUAL FRAMEWORK

The framework posits that the social structural and psychological aspects of individual characteristics (such as age, sex, race, and class) operate together to shape behavioral motifs (the constellation of both the routine and unpredictable aspects of an individual's daily activities), which, in turn, influence friendship patterns (see figure 25.1). Friendship patterns are comprised of dyadic and network structure and phases and the interactive processes connecting them. Internal structure consists of the degree of homogeneity, solidarity, and hierarchy between the members of friendship pairs and among friendship network members and the size, density, and configuration of the network. Phases reflect the developmental status of the friendship or the network, the formation, maintenance, and dissolution of friendship dyads and of clusters of friends within networks. Interactive processes denote the overt behavioral events and the covert cognitive and affective responses that occur when people interact (Kelley et al., 1983).

The elements of this integrative framework and the relationships among them vary by structural and cultural context. Structural and cultural contexts, in turn, vary by their remoteness from the individual and, therefore, from the immediate social environment in which friendships are formed and maintained (e.g., church, apartment building, senior center, volunteer organization) to the com-

Figure 25.1
Integrative Conceptual Framework for Friendship Research

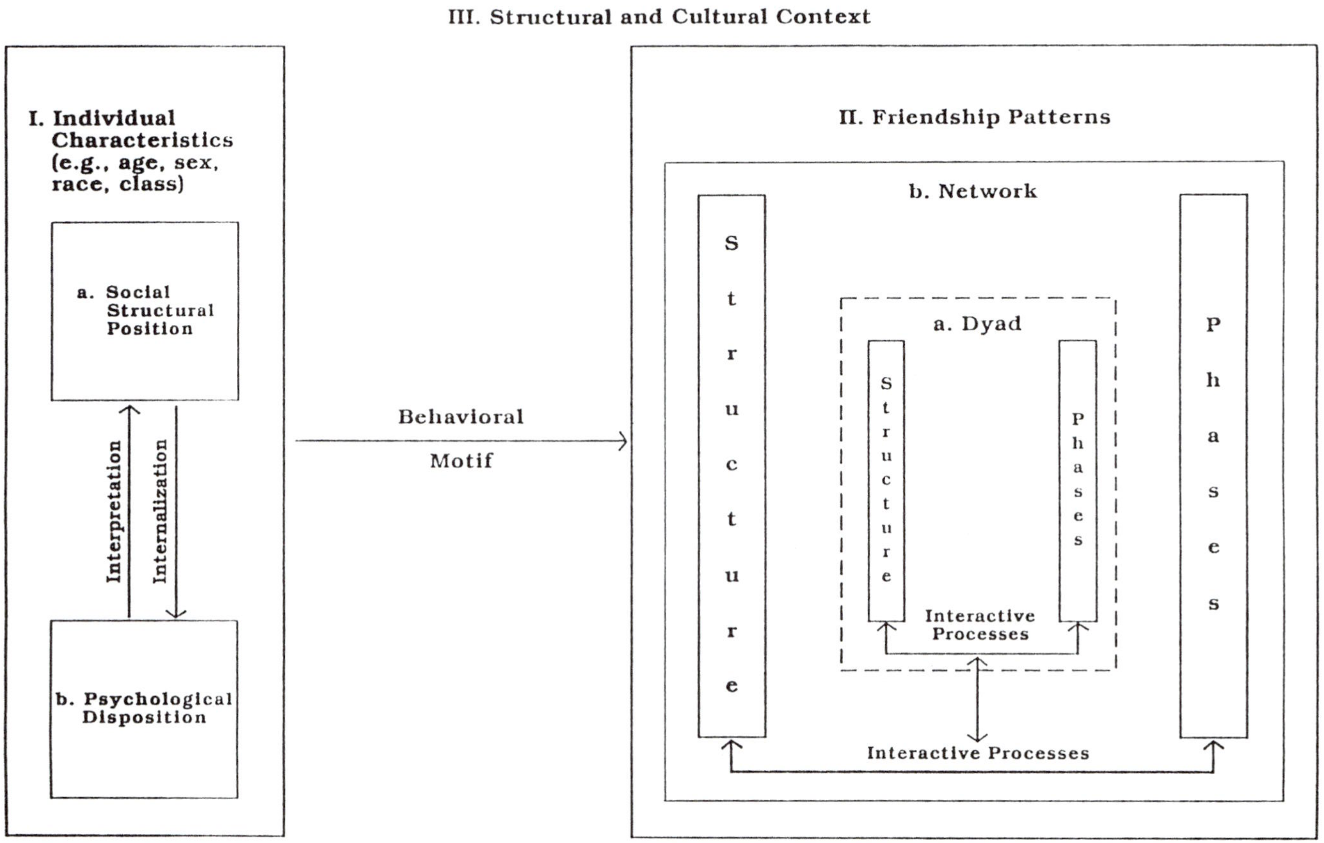

munity (e.g., ethnic and race subcultures, neighborhoods) and finally to the larger social system (e.g., nations, historical time periods).

It is perhaps easier to see how the framework would work differently in different immediate social environments than in different communities or societies. For example, compare the effects of social status on friendship among older people who have relocated to a nursing home and among those who are still living independently. Nursing homes are equalizers. Upon entering a nursing home, residents often shed their social identities—the material reminders of their past statuses are often left in storage. Status differences are thus much more salient in shaping the friendships of those fortunate enough to age in place.

FRIENDSHIP PATTERNS OF OLDER WOMEN

Using this integrative framework to organize what we know about older women's friendships immediately makes several substantive gaps in the literature apparent. Researchers have not studied the following aspects of older women's friendship patterns at all: network solidarity, dyadic and network hierarchy, multiplexity, maintenance, and dissolution. In addition, they have not examined many of the interactive processes characteristic of personal relationships. As mentioned in the introduction, though studies have been conducted in a variety of contexts and of different populations, systematic analyses of the effect of the characteristics of contexts or populations are not possible, because the researchers usually did not identify these characteristics.

In the following two sections the findings bearing on the internal structure, processes, and phases of older women's friendships are summarized in sequence, without systematic discussions of their relationship to one another and of contextual and population effects. The results of studies involving four types of samples are included in this synthesis: (1) those comparing women and men across stages of the life course, (2) those comparing older women and men, (3) one including women at various stages of the life course, and (4) those including only older women. See table 25.1 for a list and description of the studies that are summarized in the following sections.

Internal Structure

Size. The findings on the size of older women's friendship networks are inconsistent across studies, because the populations and the measures used to assess size differed. For example, in my study (Adams, 1987) of elderly female residents of a middle-class Chicago suburb, respondents listed an average of 10 friends. Three years later they listed an average of 12.2 friends. In a sample of widows, only 60% of whom were 65 years old or older, Lopata (1979) reported an average of only 1.25 friends per widow. Older women in a midwestern city reported an average of 5.6 close friends (Babchuk & Anderson, 1989).

Several studies of more or less general populations examined the difference between size of older women's and older men's friendship networks. Weiss and Lowenthal (1975) found that at all stages of life, women reported about 1 more friend than men did. Fischer and Oliker (1983) found that while there were no gender differences in number of friends among young adults and middle-aged parents, among middle-aged childless people and among the elderly women reported more friendships than men did. In contrast, in their study of older adults in 64 small towns in Missouri, Pihlblad and Adams (1972) found that older women had fewer friends than older men.

Other studies of more specific populations also included measures of size of network. In the context of a nursing home, Retsinas and Garrity (1985) found no gender differences among the older residents in number of friendships. About a third of the residents were loners; the median number of friendships was 6; and the maximum number was also 6. Blindness, being mute, tenure in the nursing home, and lack of lucidity were negatively related to number of friendships.

Homogeneity. The two most frequently studied types of network homogeneity are gender and age homogeneity. Several studies of older women suggest that their networks are fairly homogeneous in terms of gender. Assessing older, midwestern, urban women, Babchuk and Anderson (1989) reported that only about one-fifth of the married or widowed women considered one or more males as friends. In my study of elderly female residents of a middle-class Chicago suburb (Adams, 1985), I reported a very similar proportion. Rubinstein and his colleagues (Rubinstein, Alexander, Goodman, & Luborsky, 1991) reported that very few of the never-married, childless women in their sample named a man as one of their very closest friends. It is quite clear that older women have more gender-homogeneous friendship networks than older men do (Dykstra, 1990; Litwak, 1989; Powers & Bultena, 1976; Usui, 1984).

Two studies suggested that older women and older men are equally likely to have age-homogeneous networks (Usui, 1984; Weiss & Lowenthal, 1975) and that older people tend to have less age-homogeneous networks than younger people. Weiss and Lowenthal (1975) reported that 85% of the friends of the preretired were approximately the same age as the respondent, in contrast to over 90% of the networks of those in each of the earlier stages of life. Usui (1984) found that age homogeneity decreased with age, probably due in part to the reduced availability of age peers.

Both Dykstra (1990), who studied Dutch elderly, and Usui (1984), who studied the elderly in Jefferson County, Kentucky, reported on types of homogeneity that other friendship researchers have not studied among the elderly. Dykstra (1990) reported that never-married and formerly married women had friendship networks characterized by higher marital-status homogeneity than their male counterparts. In contrast, Usui (1984) reported that older women had less marital-status homogeneity than older men did. He also reported no gender differences in education and race homogeneity.

Density. Network density is a measure of "the extent to which links which

Table 25.1
Studies Including Information on Older Women's Friendships

Study	Population	Sample Type	N
Gender & Life Course Comparisons			
Fischer & Oliker (1983)	Urban Northern California adults	Purposive	1,050
Fox, Gibbs, & Auerbach (1985)	Students in Liberal Arts classes	Availability	31
Weiss & Lowenthal (1975)	Families of HS students	Purposive	216
Gender Comparisons of Older Adults			
Albert & Moss (1990)	Older adults	Unknown	225
Antonucci & Akiyama (1987)	National, 50+, married with at least one child	Probability	214
Blau (1961)	2 NY State Health Districts	Unknown	500
Bryant & Rakowski (1992)	National, 70+	Probability	473
Connidis & Davies (1990)	London Canada, 65+	Probability	400
Dykstra (1990)	Dutch elderly, 65+	Probability	322
Eckert (1980)	SRO hotel occupants in California	Availability	43
Ferraro, Mutran, & Barresi (1984)	Census Survey of low income aged & disabled	Probability	3,683
Fisher, Reid, & Melendez (1989)	Members of Senior Center in Urban Area	Unknown	55
Hatch & Bulcroft (1992)	National, 60+ (time 1), 68+ (time 2)	Probability/Longitudinal	1,435
Husaini, Moore, Castor, Neser, Whitten-Stovall, Linn, & Griffin (1991)	Black elderly in Nashville, Tennessee	Probability	600
Johnson (1983)	Acute care hospital admissions in SF Bay Area	Saturation	167
Jones & Vaughan (1990)	Participants in community activities	Availability	76

Table 25.1 (Continued)

Litwak (1985)	65+ in NYC area & 2 Florida counties	Availability/Probability	1,818
Pihlblad & Adams (1972)	65+ in 64 small towns in Missouri	Probability	1,551
Powers & Bultena (1976)	60+ noninstitutionalized, in 5 Iowa counties	Unknown	269
Retsinas & Garrity (1985)	Nursing home residents, Pawtucket, Rhode Island	Unknown	145
Roberto & Scott (1986)	64+ in southwestern city	Probability	116
Rosow (1967)	Apartment residents, 62+, Cleveland, Ohio	Probability	1,200
Strain & Chappell (1982)	Homecare users & nonusers, 65+ in Winnipeg	Probability	800
Usui (1984)	60+ in Jefferson County, Kentucky	Probability	704
Stage of Life Course Comparisons of Women			
Goldman, Cooper, Ahern, & Corsini (1981)	Women, 12-65+, affluent New England suburb	Purposive	90
Older Women Only			
Adams (1983, 1985, 1985-86, 1986, 1987, 1988, 1993)	Unmarried elderly women in Chicago suburb	Purposive/Longitudinal	70/42
Babchuk & Anderson (1989)	65+, midwestern city, married & widowed	Probability	132
Blieszner (1993)	Senior center & community organization participants	Availability	192
Lopata (1979)	Social Security beneficiaries in Chicago	Probability	1,169
O'Brien (1991)	80+, never married women, Prince Edward Island	Purposive	15
Roberto & Scott (1984-85)	White, middle-class, urban women, 65+	Probability	150
Rook (1987)	Elderly widows in Los Angeles	Purposive	120
Rubinstein, Alexander, Goodman, & Luborsky (1991)	Never-married childless women	Purposive	31
Shea, Thompson, & Blieszner (1988)	Residents of new retirement community, 55+	Availability/Longitudinal	24
Wingrove & Slevin (1991)	Urban professional & managerial retirees, mid-Atlantic	Purposive	25

could exist among persons do in fact exist'' (Mitchell, 1969, p. 18) and is expressed in terms of a percentage of all possible friendship links actually named. Fox, Gibbs, and Auerbach (1985) reported that older women and young men were more likely than those in the other age and sex groups in their study to have dense networks. They attributed this commonality to their single status. The older women in their study took part in a "rich, group cultural life of theater and concert-going, museum visits and the like" (p. 499).

In my study of older women (Adams, 1983), I measured two types of density, acquaintanceship density (where a link was recorded if two of the respondent's friends knew one another) and friendship density (where a link was recorded if the respondent perceived two of her friends to be friends with one another). The average acquaintanceship density was 42.4%, and the average friendship density was 27.4%. Half of the women lived in age-segregated housing. The density of their networks was not significantly different from that of the networks of women residing in the community.

The predictors of density in the two types of setting were, however, different. Among the women in age-integrated settings, those with physically limiting conditions had low-density acquaintanceship and friendship networks. Among the women in age-segregated settings, physical condition was not related to either measure of density. This was because the women who lived in age-segregated settings listed many friends who lived in their building. Furthermore, in age-integrated settings both forms of density tended to be positively correlated with the use of various forms of transportation. Women who could travel away from home continued to participate in groups of friends, the members of which were friends with one another or at least knew one another. In contrast, in age-segregated settings the opposite relationship was found. Women who used various forms of transportation maintained ties with friends who lived elsewhere and thus were not part of the dense building networks on which their less mobile peers were dependent for friendship.

Solidarity. Solidarity is the horizontal dimension of internal structure, the degree of perceived closeness between dyad members. Solidarity is a fairly widely used measure of the strength of social ties and of lack of social distance (Marsden & Campbell, 1984).

Although it is quite clear that older women are more likely than older men to spend time with emotionally close friends (Fox et al., 1985; Powers & Bultena, 1976) and that older women consider a high percentage of their friends to be very close (Adams, 1985–86), researchers have not reported data on the relative solidarity of older men's and women's entire networks. In order to measure network solidarity, it is necessary to determine the degree of emotional closeness between the members of each pair in the respondent's network. Probably because this is a time-consuming task, researchers have typically not undertaken it.

Internal Processes

Cognitive. Cognitive processes reflect the internal thoughts that each partner has about herself or himself, the friend, and the friendship (Blieszner & Adams, 1992). Two of the cognitive processes involved in older women's friendships have been addressed—satisfaction with friendship and its definition or meaning.

Quite a bit of research has been focused on the friendship satisfaction of older women. O'Brien (1991) reported that even the never-married, octogenarian women she studied had satisfying friendships. Blieszner (1993) and I (Adams, 1983) both reported that among older women we each studied, closer relationships were more satisfying than casual ones. Furthermore, I found that the older Chicago-area women in my sample were most satisfied with relationships in which they either were underbenefited or overbenefited, apparently because these were their emotionally closest relationships. This suggests that the norm of reciprocity does not apply in close friendships. Roberto and Scott (1986) later reported findings to support this interpretation, but Rook (1987) reported that reciprocity of exchanges was positively related to friendship satisfaction.

Gender comparisons of friendship satisfaction have produced mixed results. Antonucci and Akiyama (1987) reported that among the married people with at least one child whom they studied, older women were more satisfied with their friendships than older men. In contrast, Jones and Vaughan (1990) reported no group differences in satisfaction with friends among the older married women, single women, and married men whom they studied. Roberto and Scott (1986) reported no overall gender differences in satisfaction with friends, but found that older women reported a lower level of satisfaction than did older men when overbenefited by their friends.

Other studies bearing on the cognitive processes of older women's friendships have addressed questions about the definition or meaning of friendship to those being studied. Fox et al. (1985) found that across all of the age groups they studied, women's and men's conceptions of friendship fell into expressive and instrumental categories, respectively. They also reported that the meaning of friendship deepened with age, but more so for men than for women.

Albert and Moss (1990) measured consensus on the attributes of closest friends and friends as a whole. Older women and men were equally likely to agree with others of their own sex and age. For older women, consensus about what is characteristic of a close friendship was lower than consensus about what is characteristic of a friend in general. For older men, the opposite was true. Across all marital-status categories, older women ranked "someone to pass the time with" as a less important quality of all friends than men did. They also ranked "someone to feel comfortable with" for closest friends and "someone to count on" for all friends more highly than older men did. Furthermore, Albert and Moss (1990) suggested that there are gender-linked differences in interpersonal culture. Consensus about close friendships appeared to matter more for older women than for older men. Consensus about all friendships was important for both older women and men, but for women deviation led to depression, while for men it led to lower personal mastery.

Weiss and Lowenthal (1975) listed six domains into which the descriptions of friendship their respondents gave fit—similarity, reciprocity, compatibility, structured dimensions, role model, and other. Women, across all stages of life, were more likely than men to mention reciprocity. Men, on the other hand, emphasized similarity more frequently than women. The oldest group of respondents gave the most complex descriptions.

This finding contrasts with that of Goldman, Cooper, Ahern, and Corsini (1981), who examined friendship expectations across the female life course. Their youngest (12–14 years old) and oldest (65 or more years old) respondents gave relatively shorter lists of expectations regarding friendship than those between them in age. The expectation most frequently mentioned by the oldest respondents was common interests and activities, followed by friend as giver, family commonalities, long-standing friendship, and admiration. The first two of these were important to women in all six age groups.

Affective. Only one article listed in table 25.1 addressed the topic of affective processes in older women's friendships. Affective processes encompass emotional reactions to friends and friendship. Empathy, affection, commitment, joy, and contentment are all positive or pleasurable emotions. Indifference, anger, hostility, and jealousy are examples of negative or unpleasant ones (Blieszner & Adams, 1992).

Fisher, Reid, and Melendez (1989) studied anger in friendships among older adults. They found that anger between age peers is related to envy and failure of friends to adapt successfully to the aging process. Although there were no gender differences in the tendency of older women and men to experience anger over unmet aging role expectations, this type of anger was more common among people in their 60s than among people in their 70s. Women were more likely than men to report envy in their friendships.

Behavioral. Behavioral processes are the action components of friendship. They include, for example, disclosure of thoughts and feelings, displays of affection, social support, resource exchange, cooperation, accommodation to a friend's desires, coordination, sharing activities, concealment, manipulation, conflict, and competition (Blieszner & Adams, 1992). Research on the behavioral aspects of older women's friendships includes discussions of what friends do when they are together and social support.

Oddly enough, we know very little about what older women do with their friends. In keeping with the tendency to see women's friendships as face-to-face rather than as side-by-side, researchers have focused the majority of their attention in this area on confiding and talking rather than on other activities. Not surprisingly, most of the literature shows that older women are more likely to confide in and talk to friends than older men are (Connidis & Davies, 1990; Fox et al., 1985; but see Strain & Chappell, 1982, and Husaini et al., 1991, for exceptions). Researchers who have asked their older respondents broader questions about what they do with their friends have often failed to report these findings in subsequent reports on their data or have grouped activities in ways that obscure details (e.g., see Dykstra, 1990). When I identified this gap in the literature, I reexamined my data on older Chicago-suburban women (Adams, 1993). They reported participating in the following activities with at least one friend, in order of decreasing occurrence: talking, eating meals, recreational activities, clubs, outings, cultural events, instrumental support, social gatherings, and exercise and sport.

Three studies describe the types of social support provided to older women by their friends. In her study of Chicago-area widows, Lopata (1979) found that they were unlikely to be involved in economic exchanges with their friends and that exchanges were most likely to involve transportation and shopping. My study (Adams, 1983, 1986) confirmed these findings, though I also found that friends were fairly likely to help during illness. My findings also suggested that friends help most often when it is convenient to give help and when the need for help is unpredictable.

Blieszner (1993) tested hypotheses regarding resource exchange among elderly women derived from the work of Foa and Foa (1974). She found that friends exchanged love, status, and information more frequently than services, goods, and money and that this pattern matched their expectations. These findings held for both close and casual friends, though giving love was more important in close friendships and giving status was more important in casual ones.

In another study focused on older women, Roberto and Scott (1984–85) found that widows received more help from friends than did married women. Furthermore, she reported that equitably benefited older women had a higher mean morale score than the overbenefited women.

Other studies of social support included gender comparisons. In their study of married older adults with at least one child, Antonucci and Akiyama (1987) reported no gender differences in the number of friends in the helping network. Ferraro, Mutran, and Barresi (1984) found that married women were less likely than their male counterparts to have friendship support, but that there was not a gender difference among the widowed. In his study of older single-room-occupant hotel dwellers, Eckert (1980) reported that women were more likely to be involved in supportive relationships than men. Similarly, Roberto and Scott (1986) reported that compared to older men, older women had more involvement in instrumental and expressive exchanges with friends.

Two studies compared the equity involved in the friendships of older men and women. Roberto and Scott (1986) reported that older women were less likely than older men to be involved in equitable friendships. In contrast, in their study of senior adults (married women, single women, and married men), Jones and Vaughan (1990) reported no group differences in equity or reciprocity. They did observe that most of the people in their sample were slightly over-benefiting from their friendships.

Litwak (1989) examined the effect of the gender composition of the friendship support network rather than the effect of the gender of the respondent. He reported that the amount of help older married women, older single women, and older single men received was not affected by the gender composition of their friendship network.

Proxy measures of interactive processes. My discussion of processes has thus far focused on specific thoughts, feelings, and actions that take place between and among friends. Other process variables have received research attention as well. These include measures of how often and how long interactive processes occur and the variety of interactive processes that take place. These variables are proxy measures of process in the sense that they reveal only that interaction takes place but not the nature of the processes involved (Adams & Blieszner, 1994; Blieszner & Adams, 1992). The underlying assumption of researchers who use these measures exclusively seems to be that a larger quantity and variety of processes are better than less (see, for example, Bryant & Rakowski, 1992, for an examination of the connection between frequency of visiting and talking with friends and risk of mortality). The literature on older women's friendships includes many studies on frequency of interaction and duration, but none on multiplexity.

Several studies examined gender effects on older people's frequency of interaction with friends. The researchers involved in three studies found that gender did not affect frequency of interaction (Husaini et al., 1991; Johnson, 1983; Retsinas & Garrity, 1985); those involved in three other studies reported that women talked to friends (Albert & Moss, 1990) and saw friends (Pihlblad & Adams, 1972; Rosow, 1967) more frequently than men did; and those involved in two studies reported that women had less frequent contact with friends than men, but that more of their contacts were with intimate friends (Hatch & Bulcroft, 1992; Powers & Bultena, 1976). These discrepant findings probably reflect differences in the populations studied and measures of frequency of interaction.

A few studies provided information on the connection between contact with friends and aging. Pihlblad and Adams (1972) found that frequency of visiting friends did not decline with length of widowhood for women, but did for men. In a cross-sectional study Blau (1961) reported that widowhood affected the social participation of both women and men more in their 60s (when widows and widowers are less common) than in their 70s. The impact of a loss of a spouse during the 60s was less for women than for men. Hatch and Bulcroft (1992) noted that withdrawal from the labor force attenuated gender differences in contact with friends. Wingrove and Slevin (1991) observed that among female retired professionals and managers weekly contact with friends was typical.

Several studies have addressed the duration of the friendships of older women. Weiss and Lowenthal (1975) reported that for both women and men, the older the person was, the longer was the duration of their friendships. Babchuk and Anderson (1989) emphasized the high degree of stability in the friendship networks of the older widows and married women they studied. About two-thirds of the widows relied on friends of long standing. One-fifth of the widows had established all of their friendships since their husbands' deaths, but these women had been widows for so long that even their friendships tended to be of long duration. The data for married women showed a similarly stable pattern. Fox et al. (1985) observed that women were better at retaining intimate friendships than men were and that women's longest-term friends were also their emotionally closest friends. My study (Adams, 1985–86) confirmed this latter finding and also showed that older women have less contact with their longest-term, emotionally closest friends than with their other friends because they are more likely to live far from them.

Phases

Two studies have examined the formation phase of older women's friendships, but none have explicitly studied friendship maintenance or dissolution. Babchuk and Anderson (1989) investigated the contexts in which older women were likely to establish ties. Their findings underscore the importance of proximity for friendship formation. In order of decreasing frequency, their respondents established friendships in their neighborhoods, at work, at church, and through voluntary organizations. Many of these associations were self-initiated, though neighbors and relatives (and sometimes friends) sometimes provided them with introductions. Although widows were more likely than married women to have established friendship ties through work, the differences between them in how and where they met others were minor.

Shea, Thompson, and Blieszner (1988) examined the friendships of older women when they had first moved into a newly constructed rural retirement community and then again four months later. They compared the changes in resource exchange in those friendships that had existed before relocation to those established afterwards. The long-standing friendships remained stable in resource exchanges and in affection, despite the relocation of the respondent. The new relationships, however, showed increases in frequency of resource exchange and in affection as the respondents and their friends moved from acquaintanceship to friendship.

CONCLUSIONS

Applying the integrative conceptual framework (Adams & Blieszner, 1994) to the research on older women's friendships reveals that not much is "known" about them. In part this is due to the conceptual and methodological limitations of previous studies. But, as mentioned previously, researchers have neglected some aspects of older women's friendships entirely. Other aspects have been adequately studied, but only once or twice, using different measures on different populations.

Consistent findings across two or more studies are rare enough that only a few scattered hypotheses can be generated. Compared to older men, older women (a) have friendship networks higher in gender homogeneity, (b) have friendship networks equal to theirs in age homogeneity, and (c) are more likely to be involved in supportive relationships. Among older women, (a) close relationships seem to be more satisfying than casual ones, (b) longest-term friendships appear to be the emotionally closest, and (c) friends are unlikely to be involved in economic exchanges. This is not much, but it is a start.

Researchers interested in contributing to our knowledge of older women's friendship patterns need to replicate previously conducted studies and to design new ones including questions on neglected topics. For example, those of us who do research on the role of friendship in the lives of older women assume that it is important to them. The research on the effects of friendship needs development, however. Although it is clear that among older women friendship activity and psychological well-being are correlated with one another (see Larson, 1978, for a review of this literature and many of the studies cited in this chapter for more up-to-date findings), it is not clear what the causal direction is. Most researchers assume that friendship activity affects psychological well-being, but the results of my longitudinal study suggested that either the reverse is true or it is a reciprocal relationship (Adams, 1988). In order for the direction of the relationship to be specified, longitudinal research, on larger samples than mine was, is needed. Friendship might also have effects on other aspects of older women's lives, such as their physical health, mortality (Bryant & Rakowski, 1992), values, attitudes, and behaviors. Friendship might also have broader social effects, such as maintaining class cultures, reinforcing the institution of marriage (O'Connor, 1992), creating environments conducive to successful aging, or mediating the stigma associated with being old. Researchers have just recently begun to consider these possibilities.

But merely asking unasked questions, such as those about the myriad possible effects of friendship, is not enough. These new studies should be designed to do one or more of the following: compare women and men across stages of the life course; separate out age, period, and cohort effects; distinguish between the sociological and psychological effects of age and gender; and identify other sources of variation in friendship patterns (especially class and ethnicity). Above all, researchers must continue to work toward the development of a gender-informed approach to the study of friendship, so that older women's friendships can be examined with a broader perspective. This is an ambitious agenda, but at least the necessary methodological and conceptual tools are now available to friendship researchers.

REFERENCES

Adams, Rebecca G. (1983). *Friendship and its role in the lives of elderly women.* Unpublished doctoral dissertation, University of Chicago.

————. (1985). People would talk: Normative barriers to cross-sex friendships for elderly women. *Gerontologist, 25,* 605–611.

————. (1985–86). Emotional closeness and physical distance between friends: Implications for elderly women living in age-segregated and age-integrated settings. *International Journal of Aging and Human Development, 22,* 55–75.

————. (1986). Friendship and aging. *Generations, 10,* 40–43.

————. (1987). Patterns of network change: A longitudinal study of friendships of elderly women. *Gerontologist, 27,* 222–227.

————. (1988). Which comes first: Poor psychological well-being or decreased friendship activity? *Activities, Adaptation, and Aging, 12,* 27–41.

————. (1989). Conceptual and methodological issues in studying friendships of older adults. In Rebecca G. Adams & Rosemary Blieszner (Eds.), *Older adult friendship: Structure and process* (pp. 17–41). Newbury Park, CA: Sage.

————. (1993). Activity as structure and process: Friendships of older adults. In John Kelly (Ed.), *Activity and aging.* Newbury Park, CA: Sage.

————. (1994). Older men's friendship patterns. In E. H. Thompson, Jr. (Ed.), *Older men's lives.* Newbury Park, CA: Sage.

Adams, Rebecca G., & Blieszner, Rosemary. (1994). An integrative conceptual framework for friendship research. *Journal of Social and Personal Relationships, 11*(2), 163–184.

Albert, Steven M., & Moss, Miriam. (1990). Consensus and the domain of personal relations among older adults. *Journal of Social and Personal Relationships, 7,* 353–369.

Antonucci, Tony C., & Akiyama, Hiroko. (1987). An examination of sex differences in social support among older men and women. *Sex Roles, 17,* 737–749.

Babchuk, Nicholas, & Anderson, Trudy B. (1989). Older widows and married women: Their intimates and confidants. *International Journal of Aging and Human Development, 28,* 21–35.

Blau, Zena S. (1961). Structural constraints on friendships in old age. *American Sociological Review, 26,* 429–439.

Blieszner, Rosemary. (1993). Resource exchange in the social networks of elderly women. In Uriel G. Foa, John M. Converse, Jr., Kjell Y. Tornblom, & Edna B. Foa (Eds.), *Resource theory: Explorations and applications.* San Diego: Academic Press.

Blieszner, Rosemary, and Adams, Rebecca G. (1992). *Adult friendship.* Newbury Park, CA: Sage.

Bryant, Sharon, & Rakowski, William. (1992). Predictors of mortality among elderly African-Americans. *Research on Aging, 14,* 50–67.

Connidis, Ingrid A., & Davies, Lorraine. (1990). Confidants and companions in later life. *Journals of Gerontology, 45,* S141–S149.

Dykstra, Pearl A. (1990). *Next of (non)kin.* Amsterdam: Swets & Zeitlinger.

Eckert, J. Kevin. (1980). *The unseen elderly: A study of marginally subsistent hotel dwellers.* San Diego: Campanile Press.

Ferraro, Kenneth F., Mutran, Elizabeth, & Barresi, Charles M. (1984). Widowhood, health, and friendship support in later life. *Journal of Health and Social Behavior, 25,* 245–259.

Fischer, Claude S., & Oliker, Stacey J. (1983). A research note on friendship, gender, and the life cycle. *Social Forces, 62,* 124–133.

Fisher, Celia B., Reid, James D., & Melendez, Marjorie. (1989). Conflict in families and friendships of later life. *Family Relations, 38*, 83–89.

Foa, Uriel G., & Foa, Edna B. (1974). *Societal structures of the mind.* Springfield, IL: Thomas.

Fox, Margery, Gibbs, Margaret, & Auerbach, Doris. (1985). Age and gender dimensions of friendship. *Psychology of Women Quarterly, 9*, 489–501.

Goldman, J. A., Cooper, P. E., Ahern, K., & Corsini, David. (1981). Continuities and discontinuities in the friendship descriptions of women at six stages in the life cycle. *Genetic Psychology Monographs, 103*, 153–167.

Hatch, Laurie R., & Bulcroft, Kris. (1992). Contact with friends in later life: Disentangling the effects of gender and marital status. *Journal of Marriage and the Family, 54*, 222–232.

Hess, Beth B. (1972). Friendship. In Matilda W. Riley, Marilyn Johnson, & Anne Foner (Eds.), *Aging and society* (Vol. 3, pp. 357–393). New York: Russell Sage.

Husaini, Bagar A., Moore, Stephen T., Castor, Robert S., Neser, William, Whitten-Stovall, Richard, Linn, J. Gary, & Griffin, Denise. (1991). Social density, stressors, and depression: Gender differences among the Black elderly. *Journals of Gerontology, 46*, P236–P242.

Johnson, Colleen L. (1983). Fairweather friends and rainy day kin. *Urban Anthropology, 12*, 103–123.

Jones, Diane C., & Vaughan, Kristen. (1990). Close friendships among senior adults. *Psychology and Aging, 5*, 451–457.

Kelley, Harold H., Berscheid, Ellen, Christensen, Andrew, Harvey, John H., Huston, Ted L., Levinger, George, McClintock, Evie, Peplau, Letitia A., & Peterson, Donald R. (1983). Analyzing close relationships. In Harold H. Kelley et al., *Close relationships* (pp. 20–67). New York: Freeman.

Larson, Reed. (1978). Thirty years of research on the subjective well-being of older Americans. *Journal of Gerontology, 33*, 109–125.

Litwak, Eugene. (1985). *Helping the elderly.* New York: Guilford Press.

———. (1989). Forms of friendships among older people in an industrial society. In Rebecca G. Adams & Rosemary Blieszner (Eds.), *Older adult friendship: Structure and process* (pp. 65–88). Newbury Park, CA: Sage.

Lopata, Helena Z. (1979). *Women as widows.* New York: Elsevier North Holland.

Maddox, George L., & Campbell, Richard T. (1985). Scope, concepts, and methods in the study of aging. In Robert H. Binstock & Ethel Shanas (Eds.), *Handbook of aging and the social sciences* (2nd ed., pp. 3–31). New York: Van Nostrand Reinhold.

Marsden, Peter, & Campbell, K. (1984). Measuring tie strength. *Social Forces, 63*, 482–501.

Mitchell, J. Clyde (1969). The concept and use of social networks. In J. Clyde Mitchell (Ed.), *Social networks in urban situations* (pp. 1–50). Manchester, England: Manchester University Press.

O'Brien, Mary. (1991). Never-married older women: The life experience. *Social Indicators Research, 24*, 301–315.

O'Connor, Patrica. (1992). *Friendships between women: A critical review.* New York: Guilford Press.

Pihlblad, C. Terrence, & Adams, David L. (1972). Widowhood, social participation, and life satisfaction. *Aging and Human Development, 3*, 323–330.

Powers, Edward A., & Bultena, Gordon L. (1976). Sex differences in intimate friendships of old age. *Journal of Marriage and the Family, 38*, 739–747.

Retsinas, Joan, & Garrity, Patricia. (1985). Nursing home friendships. *Gerontologist, 25*, 376–381.

Roberto, Karen A., & Scott, Jean P. (1984–85). Friendship patterns among older women. *International Journal of Aging and Human Development, 19*, 1–10.

———. (1986). Friendships of older men and women: Exchange patterns and satisfaction. *Psychology and Aging, 1*, 103–109.

Rook, Karen S. (1987). Reciprocity of social exchange and social satisfaction among older women. *Journal of Personality and Social Psychology, 52*, 145–154.

Rosow, Irving. (1967). *Social integration of the aged.* New York: Free Press.

Rubinstein, Robert L., Alexander, Baine B., Goodman, Marcene, & Luborsky, Mark. (1991). Key relationships of never married, childless older women: A cultural analysis. *Journal of Gerontology: Social Sciences, 46*, 270–277.

Shea, Laurie, Thompson, Linda, & Blieszner, Rosemary. (1988). Resources in older adults' old and new friendships. *Journal of Social and Personal Relationships, 5*, 83–96.

Strain, Laurel A., & Chappell, Neena L. (1982). Confidants: Do they make a difference in quality of life? *Research on Aging, 4*, 479–502.

Usui, Wayne M. (1984). Homogeneity of friendship networks of elderly blacks and whites. *Journal of Gerontology, 39*, 350–356.

Weiss, L., & Lowenthal, Marjorie F. (1975). Life-course perspectives on friendship. In Marjorie F. Lowenthal, Majda Thurnher, David Chiriboga, & Associates, *Four stages of life* (pp. 48–61). San Francisco: Jossey-Bass.

Wingrove, C. Ray, & Slevin, Kate F. (1991). A sample of professional and managerial women: Success in work and retirement. *Journal of Women and Aging, 3*, 95–117.

Wright, Paul H. (1982). Men's friendships, women's friendships, and the alleged inferiority of the latter. *Sex Roles, 8*, 1–20.

Twenty-Six

Older Women and Widowhood

JULIA E. BRADSHER

The death of a spouse or partner has been described as the most disruptive and difficult role transition that an individual confronts throughout the life course (Lopata, 1973, 1979, 1987). It involves the loss of a master status, that of spouse (George, 1981), bringing with it a number of changes and losses in economic status, social status, and, often, personal self-identity (Lopata, 1973, 1979, 1984). The widowhood event is not an uncommon life experience among persons who have lived to an old age, especially women. The purpose of this chapter is to review the research on widowhood, particularly as it relates to older women. The first section will review the demographic profile of widows in the United States. Second is a discussion of the widowhood event as a life-course event. In the third part of the chapter the impact of widowhood on older women is examined, focusing on the health, social, and economic impacts of widowhood. Also part of this discussion will be the mediators of the impact of widowhood. Fourth is a discussion of the social relationships of older women in the context of widowhood. Throughout the chapter an effort has been made to draw comparisons to other groups, such as widows compared to married women and widows compared to widowers. In most of the research cited the research was conducted with samples of women. In some cases research was comparative, and in many cases the research focused on the death of a spouse, with the majority of the sample being widows. The chapter ends with some suggestions for future research directions.

A DEMOGRAPHIC PROFILE OF WIDOWS IN THE UNITED STATES

Almost one-half of all older women are widows. That is, approximately 49 percent of women aged 65 or older, or about 8.4 million women, were widows in 1990 (U.S. Bureau of the Census, 1992). This compares to only about 14 percent of men, or about 1.8 million men, who were widowers in 1990.

The proportions of older women who are widowed is even more impressive when they are broken down by age groups. Of women between the ages of 45 and 54, 5.3 percent were widowed. For women aged 55–64, only 17.2 percent were widowed in 1990. Thirty-six percent of women between the ages of 65 and 74 were widowed in 1990. By the time a woman reaches the age of 75, the likelihood that she will be widowed increases dramatically. For women between the ages of 75 and 84, there was a three-in-five chance of widowhood (62 percent), and 79.8 percent of women aged 85 and over were widowed in 1990, a four-out-of-five chance of widowhood (U.S. Bureau of the Census, 1992).

Among proportions of widowhood by race, there are some notable differences between racial and ethnic groups. Hispanic women have the lowest proportion of widowhood among those aged 65 or older with 42.2 percent. Among white older women, 48.1 were widowed. Older black women have the largest proportion of widows with 53.7 percent (U.S. Bureau of the Census, 1992).

There are a number of explanations for the differences in proportions of widows to widowers in the United States and for the greater likelihood that minority women will be widowed. First, there are sex differences in mortality at every age. Women at any given age have lower mortality rates than men and, therefore, are more likely to survive husbands the same age than to be survived by their husbands. Second, women tend to marry men who are somewhat older than themselves, making it more likely for the women to survive and become widows. Third, widowers at any given age are much more likely to remarry than are widows the same age. Fourth, race differences in mortality and remarriage place older minority women, particularly blacks, at greater risk for widowhood (Matras, 1990). While these demographic differences are notable, it is the social context and social factors in interaction with the demographic factors that play a significant role in the impact of widowhood on women.

THE CONTEXT OF WIDOWHOOD IN AMERICAN SOCIETY

The context of widowhood in American society has been an important focus for one of the foremost researchers of widowhood, Helena Lopata (1979, 1980, 1987). Through her years of research on widowhood, she has identified many of the factors that make American society a unique historical, social, and cultural context for widowhood. First is the expectation that the modern American nuclear family is socially and economically independent. Women have ties to the broader kinship network, but they are, at most, loose ones. Of particular significance is the independence from the male family line, which is characteristic of more modern societies. The second factor is that wives, particularly those who are traditionally socialized, are economically dependent on their husbands' sources of income. However, this situation is beginning to change somewhat. The third factor identified by Lopata is that American society places high importance on marital relationships and on the development of strong mutual dependence between marital partners (Lopata, 1980). Thus the social context for women as they move into old age is that they are to be socially, emotionally, and economically dependent on their husbands. This is juxtaposed with the high probability that they will become widowed and lose the person upon whom they are socialized to be dependent. In order to accept this order of events, women are socialized to expect to become a widow as a normative part of their life course.

WIDOWHOOD AS A LIFE-COURSE EVENT

The widowhood event has been described as a normative part of the life course for the majority of women in American society. Neugarten (1968) introduced the concept of "on time" versus "off time" when describing the occurrence of a major life event in the life course. As individuals pass through major life transitions throughout the life course, there is a socially prescribed timetable for the ordering of these transitions. Most adults hold a particular set of anticipations of the normal and expected life course. If events occur "off time" and upset the sequence and rhythm of the life cycle, the event is likely to pose a greater challenge for the person to cope with that event. Thus, for women, the temporality of widowhood, that is, the age of a woman when her husband dies, and the timing in the life course can significantly affect its impact. The impact of widowhood is greater for younger widows than for older ones, and thus, the older a woman is when she becomes widowed, the more normative is the widowhood event (Morgan, 1976).

Some research has pointed out that the death of a spouse marks a normative status passage for most women. This is because widowhood is expected for most women, and many other women have experienced it or are in the same situation. Furthermore, some scholars of widowhood assert that there is an understood role for widows in America. On the contrary, other research has described the role of a widow as ambiguous, roleless, or role deprived. There are no clear expectations for behavior in the role of a widow, particularly younger widows (Lopata, 1973, 1987; Brock & O'Sullivan, 1985; Atchley, 1994). Regardless of whether or not becoming a widow is normative, immediately following the death of a spouse is the time at which the greatest social and emotional impact occurs.

Bereavement and Grief

Most bereavement and grief occur following the initial loss of a spouse. Lopata (1973) found that almost half (48 percent) of widows in her study reported that they had gotten over their husband's death within one year. Another 20 percent said that they had not gotten over it and had no expectation that they would get over it in the future. What is evident from the research on bereavement and grief is that there are a number of factors that influence the successful mastery of bereavement (Wortman & Silver, 1990). Some of these factors include the level of dependency in the relationship, circumstances surrounding the loss of the spouse, whether the death was unexpected and/or untimely, the existence of concurrent crises such as economic hardship, and the existence of a social support network (Wortman & Silver, 1990).

The negative effects of bereavement are usually seen more readily in the recently widowed, but this is not always the case. Some women grieve for many years (Parkes, 1973). Kelly (1991), in her ethnographic case study of an 83-year-old bereaved nursing-home resident, found a prolonged state of bereavement. The woman had continued to suffer profound grief over the loss of her husband even twelve years after his death. Based on her findings, Kelly (1991) identified a number of important factors that shape the bereavement experience of older women. These include the multiplicity of losses, the particular characteristics of the relationship between the bereaved and deceased spouses prior to death, and personal characteristics of the bereaved.

Role Transition from Married Woman to Widow

The largest portion of research on widowhood has focused on the personal and social consequences that accompany the changes from wife to widow. Lopata (1987) has stated that the transition of becoming and being a widow requires a social-psychological process of acquiring a different or separate identity that replaces the role of wife and being half of a couple. It is a process of renegotiating one's self-concept and identity, a process in which many contextual, social, and psychological factors play a significant role and in which there are multiple stages that a woman passes through.

Lopata (1973, 1979, 1987) has described the process that a woman goes through in transitioning from wife to widow. The first stage is the official recognition of the event. This is usually the initial mourning period and the time in which the funeral occurs. It is during this time that the "grief work" must begin. However, there is no societally instituted period of grief, and many widows are left in a somewhat undefined situation. While it is expected that a widow go through grief, the length of time she should go through it is unclear.

Grief work continues in the second stage of the process, and this is the period in which the woman may go through temporary disengagement from her usual social obligations. The transition from wife to widow also brings with it certain obligations. For example, in her study in Chicago, Lopata (1973) found that one of these obligations is the duty to preserve the social presence of the husband and to sanctify his personality.

The next part of the process the widow must go through is reengagement. It is during this time that the widow begins to look forward and to be involved in social relations again (Lopata, 1973). The reengagement may include some friendship networks that existed prior to the husband's death and may also include new ones. Following reengagement, the widow continues to deal with some of the problems of being a widow. Reengagement does not mean the end of the problems associated with widowhood, but rather is a period of coping and adjustment in widowhood that is influenced by a number of factors and is the topic of the next section.

IMPACT OF WIDOWHOOD

Becoming widowed can have profound effects on physical health, mental health, mortality, social situations, and economic status (Ferraro, 1989; Wortman & Silver, 1990; Umberson, Wortman, & Kessler, 1992; Dodge, 1995; Mc-Gloshen & O'Bryant, 1988). The consensus of the literature is that the physical and mental health impacts seem to lessen over time, with minimal effects in the long run (Ferraro, 1989). The impact of widowhood is affected by a number of factors such as age at widowhood, whether the event is "on time" or "off time," gender, social class, race/ethnicity, living environment, and health (Bengtson, Rosenthal, & Burton, 1990).

Physical Health Impact

Widowhood can have a tremendous impact on the health of older women (Ferraro, 1989; Bowling, 1987; Gass & Chang, 1989). Most studies of widowhood demonstrate some declines in health (Ferraro, 1989). However, the more important questions, according to Ferraro (1989), are when, how severely, and upon whom these effects are most likely to occur. The consensus of the research literature is that the negative health consequences of widowhood are most likely to occur immediately following the death of a spouse and that the extended effects of widowhood on health are minimal (Ferraro, 1989).

Osterweis, Solomon, and Green (1984) found that the death of a spouse leads to increased mortality risk, reduced immuno-competence, and increased morbidity for a variety of physical and psychological disorders. Stroebe and Stroebe (1987) found that the negative health effects of bereavement are greater for men than for women. They concluded that this is because the marital relationship is a more effective support system for men than for women, and thus men are more negatively affected by its loss. However, in another study Feinson (1986) found the opposite. In her review of mortality studies and studies of psychological distress, she concluded that there are no definitive studies showing that widowed women suffered less than widowed men.

In a more recent study Stevens (1995) found that there were no major gender differences in bereavement outcomes in the long run. However, most research has found that there are important mediating factors that are also associated with gender, including income, education, health, social networks, and relationships with children.

In addition to health consequences, widowhood may also impact the utilization of health care. Feld and George (1994) examined the effects of social resources before widowhood on changes in subsequent hospitalizations. They used hospitalizations as an indicator of serious health outcomes as a way of having a measure that was unlikely to be biased by a widowed person's emotional state. They found that widows' perceptions that they had inadequate social support from persons other than their spouse exacerbated the effects of bereavement on hospitalizations. In another study on widows and health care use, Wolinsky and Johnson (1993) looked at widowed persons aged 70 or older and found that widowhood was not related to any change of health status, but that being a widow increased the probability of nursing-home placement.

Mental and Emotional Health Impact

Loneliness is one of the serious problems associated with widowhood (Lopata, 1984). With loneliness of widowhood can come mental and emotional trauma that is part of the grief process. There have been some recent studies focused on mental and emotional outcomes associated with widowhood. Mendes de Leon, Kasl, and Jacobs (1994) examined depressive symptomatology during bereavement. They found that depression scores increased during the first year of bereavement, but returned to prewidowhood levels thereafter. They also found that depression scores remained elevated among young-old widows (65–74 years old) well after the first year of widowhood. They concluded that young-old widows are particularly at risk of developing chronic depressive symptomatology during bereavement.

In another study Umberson, Wortman, and Kessler (1992) examined long-term gender differences in vulnerability to depression among widows and widowers. They found that having ever been widowed was associated with current levels of depression and that the association was greater for men than for women. They stated that some of this difference was because men have been widowed for a shorter average period of time than women and the effects of widowhood appear to lessen over time. Widowhood was also associated with different types and amounts of life strain for men and women. Their results suggested that the primary mechanism linking widowhood and depression among women was financial strain. Among men, the critical mechanism was strain associated with household management.

Finally, McGloshen and O'Bryant (1988) examined the psychological well-being of older, recent widows. They found that higher levels of positive affect were associated with religious involvement, number of siblings, and support from children and families. Negative affect was more often associated with having experienced other deaths (in addition to the husband's), housing dissatisfaction, and a history of employment outside the home during marriage.

Economic and Social Impact

In addition to physical and mental health consequences of widowhood, there are also economic and social ones. Widows may experience significant disorganization in social networks and support systems (Lopata, 1979; Matras, 1990). The economic impact of widowhood can be particularly severe for women. Recent research has focused on the economic impact and some of its mediating factors.

Bound, Duncan, Laren, and Oleinick (1991) examined the links between poverty and widowhood. They found that widowhood reduces living standards by 18 percent, on average, and pushes 10 percent of women whose incomes were above the poverty line prior to widowhood into poverty after it. Economic status prior to widowhood was the strongest predictor of economic status during widowhood. Their results also demonstrated instability of family income during the widowing process.

In another study Dodge (1995) examined movements out of poverty for elderly widows. Using an event-history approach, Dodge found that living with a family member is a strong predictor for the transition out of poverty among poor elderly women. Among elderly widows who moved out of poverty with relatively large increases in income, those who exited poverty due to an increase in pension income or gifts increased their income significantly more than those who exited through other sources.

Widowhood also brings with it sometimes significant changes in social networks and social participation. Lopata (1979) has described the lack of community resources available to widows as they try to rebuild their lives and deal with their particular problems. Fry and Garvin (1987) have described a "culture of widows" that exists among women who age in place in a community with social stability and continuity. Most of the women in their study were middle class. The culture of widows they described was not a communitywide phenomenon but existed through informal networks that formed through more formalized networks such as organizations, clubs, or religious affiliations. They stated that the culture of widows is, for the most part, "a peer culture that is brought together through commonalties in gender, widowhood, and common experiences in the community." The findings of Fry and Garvin build on Lopata's earlier work on the transitions that women go through when they become widowed. As in Lopata's study, Fry and Garvin found that widows' peers were a major source of support as they go through transitions associated with widowhood.

Gallagher and Gerstel (1993) examined the effects of marriage and widowhood on older women's help to kin and friends. Married women in their study provided more help to kin than widows, but most of those differences were explained in terms of the greater material resources marriage provides. In contrast, even when other social characteristics are controlled, widows spend more time and give more practical help, in particular, to more friends than do wives. In two senses, then, marriage privatizes women's help to others—it provides them with both the resources and the opportunity to help those related, while it reduces both the breadth and intensity of help for those not related.

Pellman (1992) examined the degree to which widows were integrated in their community, the daily hassles and stress they may have experienced, and their social networks and support-seeking behavior. She found that widowhood, in and of itself, did not appear to be a predictor either of community integration or the lack of it or the experience of stress and hassles. Those who experienced hassles were not the same persons as those who experienced stress. She also found that those who sought social support did not seem most in need of it.

Van Den Hoonaard (1994) examined the relationships between the widowed and married members of a Florida retirement community. She found the existence of stigma associated with widowhood, which resulted in lower status than for married members. She also found that if widowed members of the community wanted to maintain relationships with married residents, certain norms required that the newly widowed person accept a marginalized social position. Otherwise, the newly widowed were obliged to establish a new set of friends and a new social network.

Another area of study concerning widowhood and its social impact is geographic mobility. While there has been some research in this area, it is somewhat limited. Nelson and Winter (1975) studied how moving becomes a part of a readjustment plan in the event of a major life disruption when this event is discussed in future hypothetical terms. They found that anticipated major life disruptions, such as the death of a spouse, tend to cause an increase in experienced physical dependence. Persons in their study said that they were more likely to consider making a residential move if their living environments were no longer suited to their relative dependence or independence as a result of widowhood. In a more recent study Bradsher, Longino, Jackson, and Zimmerman (1992) found that the interaction of declining health and becoming widowed increased the probability of a move for older men and women.

Mediators on the Impact of Widowhood

Gender is a differentiator in the experience of widowhood. Some studies indicate that widowers experience more negative health problems, greater social isolation, and more restricted social networks, have fewer emotional ties with families, and are less likely to have a confidant than are widows. Other studies have suggested no gender differences (Stevens, 1995).

Lopata (1973) described the importance of social class in mediating the impact of widowhood. Working-class women experience less disorganization in their lives immediately following the death of a spouse than do their middle-class peers. In the long run, however, middle-class women are advantaged in widowhood, for example, with respect to social integration.

Race and ethnicity are associated with the likelihood of becoming widowed as well as with living arrangements. Pelham and Clark (1987) found that white and black widows tend to live alone and Hispanic and Asian widows to live with others. Hispanic widows had the largest household size and number of children. It may be these differences that cause Hispanic widows to appear to have stronger and more active support systems than white widows.

In her study of widows in the Chicago area, Lopata (1979) examined the concept of "age as a resource" when looking at the impact of widowhood. She pointed out that the age at widowhood had a number of influences on the impact of widowhood. First, she found that age influenced the manner and degree of disorganization of prior social networks and support systems. She also found that age influenced the content of new networks and support systems that developed following the widowhood event. Palmore (1981) had similar findings in his three-decade study. He found that the widowhood event was more stressful in middle age than in old age. Furthermore, for those who had been caring for a spouse who had a chronic disability or terminal illness, the death of a spouse brought relief and improved adjustment.

Another important mediator on the impact of widowhood is social support. A support network that includes children, siblings, and other family members plays a critical role in the adjustment and well-being of widows, especially the recently widowed (O'Bryant, 1988; McGloshen & O'Bryant, 1988). In her study of older recent widows, O'Bryant (1988) found that interactions with married sisters were second only to health in predicting higher positive affect in older widows.

Waehrer and Crystal (1995) found that coresidence living improved well-being for both the widow and the other household participants in the majority of their sample. Among nonwhites, coresidence benefited the widow less and other members more than among whites. Similarly, Silverstein and Bengtson (1994) investigated whether social support from adult children improved the psychological well-being of elderly parents. They found that instrumental and expressive forms of social support were weakly related to change, over a three-year period, in positive and negative aspects of psychological well-being. They also found that both types of support moderated declines in well-being associated with poor health and widowhood.

In another study Silverstein (1995) examined stability and change in temporal distance between the elderly and their children. He found that declining health and widowhood increased the degree of noncoresident proximity and the likelihood of transition to coresidence.

COMPARISONS WITH WIDOWERS AND OTHER WOMEN

To conclude the chapter, it is important to discuss some of the research that has attempted to make some comparisons between widows and people in other similar situations, such as recent widowers or widows who remarried. It is through these comparisons that the impact of widowhood can be further assessed.

Smith, Zick, and Duncan (1991) examined remarriage among recent widows and widowers. For the men and women in their sample, remarriage was one of the most important determinants of physical and economic well-being among the widowed. They found strong age and duration dependence effects for middle-aged widows and widowers and for older widowers. Among middle-aged widows, blacks and those with dependent children in the home had lower rates of remarriage. Overall, they found that age and time since widowhood had the strongest and most consistent effects on remarriage rates for different widowed groups.

O'Bryant and Straw (1991) examined remarriage of widows who had been previously widowed or divorced and compared them to widows who had not had previous widowhood or divorce experiences. They found that while the groups did not differ on psychological well-being, both economic and environmental factors revealed significant group differences. Those widows with previous experience with either widowhood or divorce showed better adaptation and self-sufficiency than those without such experience.

RESEARCH NEEDS AND FUTURE RESEARCH DIRECTIONS

The research literature on older women as widows discussed in this chapter spans almost four decades. In spite of the richness of this research, much remains to be examined. Bleiszner (1993) has admonished us to examine widowhood from alternative perspectives, such as the socialist-feminist perspective. In an approach such as this, the research focus moves away from looking at the consequences of loss of a husband and the self-sufficiency of the widowed person and allows for the examination of issues such as past labor-market participation, gender-based power relationships at home, and other research areas.

The bulk of research on the impact of widowhood has focused on health and psychological impact of the widowhood event. There has been limited research that has focused on coping strategies and reliance of women who are widowed. There is also a need to further examine the long-range outcomes of women who become widowed. Another important area of research is the examination of bereavement and the loss of a partner in nontraditional relationships. Neither cohabiting heterosexual couples nor lesbian couples have had much research. As the construct of family changes in our society, so must the research that examines family experiences, such as widowhood.

REFERENCES

Atchley, R. (1994). *Social forces and aging.* (7th ed.). Belmont, CA: Wadsworth Publishing.

Bengtson, V. L., Rosenthal, C., & Burton, L. (1990). Families and aging: Diversity and heterogeneity. In R. H. Binstock and L. K. George (Eds.), *Handbook of aging and the social sciences* (3rd ed., pp. 263–287). San Diego, CA: Academic Press.

Bleiszner, R. (1993). A socialist-feminist perspective on widowhood. *Journal of Aging Studies, 7,* 171–182.

Bound, J., Duncan, G. J., Laren, D. S., & Oleinick, L. (1991). Poverty dynamics in widowhood. *Journal of Gerontology: Social Sciences, 46,* S115–S124.

Bowling, A. (1987). Mortality after bereavement: A review of the literature on survival periods and factors affecting survival. *Social Science and Medicine, 24,* 117–124.

Bradsher, J. E., Longino, C. F., Jackson, D. J., & Zimmerman, R. S. (1992). Geographic mobility among the recently widowed. *Journal of Gerontology: Social Sciences, 46,* S243–S248.

Brock, A. M., & O'Sullivan, P. (1985). From wife to widow: role transition in the elderly. *Journal of Psychosocial Nursing and Mental Health Services, 23,* 6–12.

Dodge, H. H. (1995). Movements out of poverty among elderly widows. *Journal of Gerontology: Social Sciences, 50,* S240–S249.

Feinson, M. J. (1986). Aging widows and widowers: Are there mental health differences? *International Journal of Aging and Human Development, 23,* 241–255.

Feld, S., & George, L. K. (1994). Moderating effects of prior social resources on the hospitalizations of elders who become widowed. *Journal of Aging and Health, 6,* 275–295.

Ferraro, K. F. (1989). Widowhood and health. In K. S. Markides & C. L. Cooper (Eds.), *Aging, Stress, and Health* (pp. 69–83). New York: John Wiley & Sons.

Fry, C. L., & Garvin, L. (1987). American afterlives: Widowhood in community context. In H. Lopata (Ed.), *Widows* (pp. 32–47). Durham, NC: Duke University Press.

Gallagher, S. K., & Gerstel, N. (1993). Kinkeeping and friend keeping among older women: The effect of marriage. *Gerontologist, 33,* 675–681.

Gass, K., & Chang, A. (1989). Appraisals of bereavement, coping, resources, and psychosocial health dysfunction in widows and widowers. *Nursing Research, 38,* 31–36.

George, L. K. (1981). *Role transitions in later life.* Monterey, CA: Brooks/Cole.

Kelly, B. (1991). Emily: A study of grief and bereavement. *Health Care for Women International, 12,* 137–147.

Lopata, H. (1973). *Widowhood in an American city.* Cambridge, MA: Schenkman.

———. (1979). *Women as widows: Support systems.* New York: Elsevier North Holland.

———. (1980). Widows and widowers. In H. Cox (Ed.), *Aging* (2nd ed.). Guilford, CT: Dushkin.

———. (1984). The widowed. In E. Palmore (Ed.), *Handbook on the aged in the United States* (pp. 109–124). Westport, CT: Greenwood Press.

———. (Ed.). (1987). *Widows.* Durham, NC: Duke University Press.

McGloshen, T. H., & O'Bryant, S. L. (1988). The psychological well-being of older, recent widows. *Psychology of Women Quarterly, 12,* 99–116.

Matras, J. (1990). Role transitions in middle and later life. In J. Matras, *Dependency, obligations, and entitlements* (pp. 230–258). Englewood Cliffs, NJ: Prentice-Hall.

Mendes de Leon, C. F., Kasl, S. V., & Jacobs, S. (1994). A prospective study of widowhood and changes in symptoms of depression in a community sample of the elderly. *Psychological Medicine, 24,* 613–624.

Morgan, L. A. (1976). A re-examination of widowhood and morale. *Journal of Gerontology, 31,* 687–695.

Nelson, L. M., & Winter, M. (1975). Life disruption, independence, satisfaction, and the consideration of moving. *Gerontologist, 15,* 160–164.

Neugarten, B. (Ed.). (1968). *Middle age and aging.* Chicago: University of Chicago Press.

O'Bryant, S. L. (1988). Self-differentiated assistance in older widows' support systems. *Sex Roles, 19,* 91–106.

O'Bryant, S. L., & Straw, L. B. (1991). Relationship of previous divorce and previous widowhood to older women's adjustment to recent widowhood. *Journal of Divorce and Remarriage, 15*, 49–67.

Osterweis, M., Solomon, F., & Green, M. (1984). *Bereavement: Reactions, consequences, and care.* Washington, DC: National Academy Press.

Palmore, E. B. (1981). *Social patterns in normal aging: Findings from the Duke longitudinal study.* Durham, NC: Duke University Press.

Parkes, C. M. (1973). Anticipatory grief and widowhood. *British Journal of Psychiatry, 122*(570), 615.

Pelham, A. O. & Clark, W. F. (1987). Widowhood among low-income racial and ethnic groups in California. In H. Lopata (Ed.), *Widows* (pp. 191–222). Durham, NC: Duke University Press.

Pellman, J. (1992). Widowhood in elderly women: Exploring its relationship to community integration, hassles, stress, social support, and social support seeking. *International Journal of Aging and Human Development, 35*, 254–264.

Silverstein, M. (1995). Stability and change in temporal distance between the elderly and their children. *Demography, 32*, 29–45.

Silverstein, M., & Bengtson, V. L. (1994). Does intergenerational social support influence the psychological well-being of elderly parents? The contingencies of declining health and widowhood. *Social Science and Medicine, 38*, 943–957.

Smith, K. R., Zick, C. D., & Duncan, G. J. (1991). Remarriage patterns among recent widows and widowers. *Demography, 28*, 361–374.

Stevens, N. (1995). Gender and adaptation to widowhood in later life. *Aging and Society, 15*, 37–58.

Stroebe, W., & Stroebe, M. S. (1987). *Bereavement and health: The psychological and physical consequences of partner loss.* Cambridge: Cambridge University Press.

Umberson, D., Wortman, C. B., & Kessler, R. C. (1992). Widowhood and depression: Explaining long-term gender differences in vulnerability. *Journal of Health and Social Behavior, 33*, 10–24.

U.S. Bureau of the Census. (1992). *Marital Status and Living Arrangements, March 1990.* Current Population Reports, Series P-20, No. 450. Washington, DC: U.S. Government Printing Office.

Van Den Hoonaard, D. K. (1994). Paradise Lost: Widowhood in a Florida retirement community. *Journal of Aging Studies, 8*, 121–132.

Waehrer, K., & Crystal, S. (1995). The impact of coresidence on economic well-being of elderly widows. *Journal of Gerontology: Social Sciences, 50*, S250–S258.

Wolinsky, F. D., & Johnson, R. J. (1993). Widowhood, health status, and the use of health services by older adults: A cross-sectional and prospective approach. *Journal of Gerontology: Social Sciences, 47*, S8–S16.

Wortman, C. B., & Silver, R. C. (1990). Successful mastery of bereavement and widowhood: A life-course perspective. In P. B. Baltes & M. M. Baltes (Eds.), *Successful aging: Perspectives from the behavioral sciences* (pp. 225–264). Cambridge: Cambridge University Press.

Twenty-Seven

Women and Caregivers for the Elderly

SALLY BOULD

It has long been recognized that the role of adult-child caregiver is typically the role of middle-aged daughters, not sons. Furthermore, the most common role of care recipient has become that of widowed elderly women. This is the result of women's traditional assignment as caregivers and the longer life expectancy, higher rates of disability, and lower remarriage rates for elderly women in comparison to men. While critics of the postindustrial family deplore the evidence that some families do not take care of their elderly, the reality is that these middle-aged daughters provide more elder care than earlier generations did. In fact, the burden of family care is much greater today because functionally disabled family members cannot engage in mutual aid or often cannot even provide for their own personal needs, for example, bathing, dressing, or getting out of the house. This leaves middle-aged daughters to provide the bulk of today's higher caregiving burdens. What motivates this care? This chapter argues that it is the emotional bond between elderly mothers and their middle-aged daughters.

Approaches to familial care are dominated by a belief system that claims that in some vague past, the exact historical context unspecified, families took better care of the elderly, providing economic and emotional security in sickness and in health. The "family bond" was "a reciprocal sense of commitment, sharing, cooperation, and intimacy" (Dizard & Gadlin, 1990, p. 6). According to Dizard and Gadlin (p. 38), this system of mutual aid began collapsing, and social policy sought to emphasize only the "self-sufficiency" of the nuclear family. The new emphasis on the nuclear family resulted, according to Dizard and Gadlin, and other commentators, in the family no longer providing care for elderly parents.

This chapter is a revision of a paper presented at the International Institute of Sociology Conference, Paris, June 1993.

THE MYTH OF A GOLDEN AGE OF ELDER CARE

The first problem with this "golden age" of family care is that there is little evidence in Northwest Europe or the United States that adult daughters or daughters-in-law ever provided extensive care to noncontributing elders until the first part of the twentieth century. The discussion concerning the collapse of mutual aid has focused on the process of industrialization and urbanization. Family sociologists of the 1940s, 1950s, and 1960s assumed that this system of mutual aid took place within preindustrial, extended-family households (Parsons, 1949; Goode, 1963). With the development of family history, beginning with Laslett (1971), it became apparent that the preindustrial, extended-family household typically involving an elderly parent was applicable to only a tiny proportion of families in England prior to the industrial revolution.

The familial group that did operate as a mutual-aid society including elderly parents was no doubt the Victorian upper-middle-class family of the late nineteenth century. The highest incidence of the extended family, according to U.S. and English data, was from 1850 to 1915 (Ruggles, 1987, p. 5, figure 1.1). Furthermore, evidence suggests that the family with the most resources, the family with servants, was the most likely to be extended. In Erie County, New York, in 1855, only 11% of families headed by unskilled workers were extended, compared to 34.8% of families with servants (see Ruggles, 1996, and Ruggles, 1987, p. 35, table 3.1; for Sweden see Tedebrand, 1996). By 1900 more unskilled families were extended (15%), but the proportion was still twice as high for the families with servants. The presence of servants allowed relief for adult daughters in dealing with problems of care for sick and disabled elders needing twelve- or even twenty-four-hour care. But a typical elder did not require such a high level of care.

Among elders who reported an occupation, the higher the status of the occupation, the more likely the elder was to coreside with adult children. Similarly, in 1910, elderly employers, the self-employed, and homeowners were more likely to reside with kin than male wage and salary workers (Ruggles, 1996). Elderly widows had often been provided for in the wills of their husbands so that the condition of the son's inheritance was providing a room, food, and care for his elderly mother (Haber, 1983). Thus care for an elderly woman was a result of her and her husband's financial success. This made the elderly woman a contributing member of the household. In the 1910s elders who coresided were least likely to be a burden to the family group.

THE POSTINDUSTRIAL FAMILY—A FAILURE TO CARE?

This situation in the 1910s contrasts dramatically with that of the 1980s. For elders in the 1980s, being disabled and/or poor was one of the best predictors of coresidence with an adult child or extended-family member. Today, the family is the key institution providing for the care of the functionally disabled elder, and, of course, within the family it is the middle-aged daughter who provides the hands-on care.

This increase in the burden of care has been the result of increased longevity of the elderly combined with increased life expectancy for those with disabilities. Medical advances have been instrumental in saving lives—for example, the elderly stroke victim. The family, specifically the middle-aged woman, is now called upon for the heavy care required by these survivors. Furthermore, the care often brings with it high medical costs as well as a disruption of the household's social and economic life. Because such lives were rarely extended in the past the way they are today, women seldom had to face these heavy care burdens in the past. For women with a surviving parent, the prevalence of caregiving increases steadily after age 45; at age 70 nearly half of all women with a surviving parent are involved with caregiving (Himes, 1994).

But what of public pensions? Have not these released adult children from caring for an elderly parent? Has not the state taken over the responsibility of providing a livelihood for the elderly (see Hareven & Adams, 1996)? While public pensions do factor into the calculation of the burden of care, these contributions do not make the burden of today's family care less than yesterday's family care.

Table 27.1 compares the hypothetical burden of elder care in the 1910s to the burden in the 1980s. This care is not exactly comparable because in 1910 about two-thirds of the elderly resided with kin, but less than one-fourth did so in 1980. However, many of the elders in 1910 were employers or self-employed, homeowners, or still economically active. For comparative purposes, the situation of an extended-family household near to the median family income in 1910 was one in which the elder did not provide any wage, salary, or unearned income to the household—or the house itself—while in 1980 the elder provided only the public pension check to the household. In 1910 the overall objective burden of caring for a noncontributing elderly parent or parent-in-law consisted of food, medical care, and household space. These items, in 1910, were relatively inexpensive for a median-income family and would not have represented an extraordinary burden on the family budget or greatly affected family activities or living standards. Furthermore, the cost of these factors could be balanced by the contribution of the widowed elderly mother in terms of household tasks such as baking and preserving. In about one-third of the cases it would be the widower who was living in his children's household. He would not be likely to contribute to the household management but would be able to take care of his own personal needs.

By 1980, however, the financial burden on the adult children could be very large. The vast majority of such care was provided by women aged 50 to 70 to elderly mothers. A woman's public pension was likely to be near the poverty line. If it was below the poverty line, it would not be supplemented by public assistance (SSI) because of the reduced SSI benefits available to elders living with their families. After payments for prescription medication, eyeglasses, and

Table 27.1
Objective Burden of Caring for an Elderly Parent in Child's Household (For households near the median family income where elder is not in the labor force)

	Elder's Contribution to Household		Elder's Cost to Household	
	Cash	In-Kind	Direct in order of importance	Indirect
1910	None	Limited, but likely to contribute to housekeeping or home management tasks.	1st Food 2nd Medical care 3rd Space	May require some extra housekeeping, so housewife may be less productive.
1980	Social Security	None. Elder is not likely to be physically or mentally able.	1st Drugs and medical care* 2nd Household space 3rd Food	Loss of caretaker's wages or housework.

*Medical costs not covered by Medicare.

other out-of-pocket medical costs, there was likely to be only a small amount (if any) left over to contribute to the family household. This small contribution might cover the costs of food, but not the cost of household space. Children in such a family might have to give up their own room in order to accommodate the elderly (Bould, Sanborn, & Reif, 1989). It was unlikely, then, that the widow's public pension would adequately pay for the direct costs of food, shelter, and medical care in her daughter's household.

An examination of indirect costs and contributions makes it clear that the objective burden of elder care today is even higher. This occurs primarily because the typical elder living with an adult child not only cannot contribute labor to the household economy, but also requires the labor of a caregiver. This can often mean the loss of the middle-aged daughter's wages, a loss of 30–40% of the family income. Even if the adult daughter is retired or a homemaker, there is still the indirect cost of the loss of her household labor.

The extension of life has meant a higher risk of disability and an increasing likelihood that physical or mental problems will require the help of another person (Bould et al., 1989). The adult children are often faced with the difficult choice of constant care at home or placement in a nursing home. Placement in a nursing home may relieve the adult children of the physical burden of care, but it often leaves a very heavy financial burden, as over half of all nursing-home costs are borne by the patient and the patient's family.

WHY FAMILIES CARE

The task of the remainder of this chapter is to understand why this radical change in familial caretaking took place between the 1910s and the 1980s. Why are families, typically middle-aged daughters, accepting these extraordinary burdens of care today? What factors influenced these women in their assumption of care burdens? How might the motivation of familial caregiving be explained?

For the period of early industrialization, the family household provided a system of mutual aid that included the elderly. The critical element of this mutual aid was that it was mutual—that is, reciprocal. Inclusion of the elder did not create a hardship for the middle-aged daughter or daughter-in-law. Initially, this pattern was found primarily among the upper middle class, for example, where the elder was the homeowner.

In the United States by 1915, however, there was evidence that family extension had become an economic strategy for working-class families also. As more working-class families included elders, these elders were contributing members to the family economy (Hareven, 1982). As industrialization progressed, working-class families found that including wage-earning kin was a viable survival strategy (Ruggles, 1987).

There is evidence that at about the same time as working-class families were taking in extended kin as a way of improving the families' economic situation, the upper-middle-class households were beginning to include noncontributing elders, providing care for elders who had no resources to contribute to the family enterprise. This new behavior of upper-middle-class families taking on the burden of care suggests that by the early twentieth century motivations other than mutual-aid strategies became important in determining who was included in a family household. Of course, an economic argument is still viable in that these families would be better able to afford the care of an elder. They had larger houses and servants to do much of the extra work, but these economic resources had not been provided to noncontributing elders in the mid-nineteenth century. What caused the change in behavior? This chapter will examine two noneconomic factors: the role of Victorian morality and the role of the Victorian emphasis upon nurturing the child.

The importance of family honor and morality was characteristic of the Victorian upper-middle-class families in England and the United States. Upholding family honor required assuming obligations for care of elders as well as other deserving kin (e.g., maiden aunts). Family "values," therefore, prompted a public display of inclusion of extended-family members. Nevertheless, this Victorian family was not obligated to care for all members, but only the morally deserving members. For deserving relatives, especially the elderly, the moral obligation to care was clear and enforced by informal social controls. Such informal controls were no doubt effective among this small circle of upper-middle-class families who feared public shame and dishonor (Berger & Berger, 1983). Newly arrived families with "new money" had to be especially careful that the family behavior met the high standards of Victorian morality.

The second noneconomic factor that strongly influenced elder care and, in particular, care for elderly mothers was the emotional bond between mother and child. The bonds of affection between mother and child were the result of the Victorian emphasis on mothers as the primary nurturers of young children. This new role for the mother was recognized in the legal system in the "tender years" doctrine, which changed the assumption of paternal custody by granting custody of the young child to the mother in cases of separation or divorce. Child-care manuals for the upper middle classes in the nineteenth century also emphasized the special quality of the mother-child bond (see Stone, 1990, pp. 170–171). It is this new emotional bonding between mother and child that can explain the primary motivations for the assumption of the caregiving burden by middle-aged daughters. This emotional bonding between mother and child, moreover, was no doubt enhanced by declining rates of infant mortality in this social class. Upper-middle-class mothers could emotionally invest in their children from birth with the expectation that the child would live into adulthood.

By 1915 in Erie County, New York, upper-middle-class families were almost twice as likely to include a nonworking extended-family member as to include an economically active extended-family member. Typically, the nonworking extended-family member included in the upper-middle-class family circle would have been an elderly mother; an elderly father of this social class would continue his working role, especially as a business owner or member of a board of directors. These data are one of the first indications of the pattern of extended families providing care for a family member who is not directly contributing to the economic basis of the family household.

EXTENDED FAMILIES IN THE WORKING CLASS

In 1915 the working class had not yet adopted an extended-family structure to care for economically dependent extended-family elders; for the working class, the extended-family structure was an economic survival strategy. Ruggles (1987, p. 45) concluded that "the 1915 pattern makes sense from an economic point of view: the people with the greatest economic need usually adopted an extended-family structure only when this did not involve an additional burden." The reversal of the extended-family strategy between 1910 and 1980 requires an explanation. Today, it is poor and working-class families that are most likely to include nonworking extended-family members, especially the elderly. In order to explain this reversal, it is first necessary to examine the situation of poor and working-class families during the early industrialization years of 1880–1910. During these years there was greater inequality of incomes, and the wages of unskilled workers were further below the median income than they are today. These families could not afford to keep a noncontributing elder. (For the poor elderly, there was the poorhouse.)

Noneconomic reasons probably also played a role in these decisions. First, there was no community of peers who would publicly shame the family for failing in its moral obligation to care. These working-class communities did not exclude families who made these difficult decisions. The second noneconomic factor was that these families were not child centered, and emotional bonds between the generations were likely to be weaker than among upper-middle-class households. In addition, infant mortality was still high, influencing a more limited emotional investment in the young child who might not live.

This pattern of working-class households being least likely to include an elderly member and upper-middle-class households being most likely to include an elderly member gradually diminished between 1880 and 1940 for the United States. The change during these years is probably largely due to changes in the noneconomic factors. The growing impact of the Victorian ideal middle-class family upon working-class family behavior and rapid declines in infant mortality rates were critical noneconomic factors. The Victorian ideal was powerful as the image of the ideal family. Working-class families, in particular, sought to emulate this family style (Berger & Berger, 1983).

The more important noneconomic factor, however, is the development of mother-child bonding patterns among the working class. Efforts such as those of the Charity Organization Society and the kindergarten movement sought to teach working-class and poor mothers new methods of child rearing. This new emphasis upon the importance of the bonding of mother and child found its expression in a radical shift in policy in dealing with the unwed mother and her child. In the United States prior to the 1920s it was recommended that she give up her child, but in the 1920s the emphasis was on the importance of mother-child bonding, thus enabling the mother to keep her child. Furthermore, efforts in public health and sanitation had greatly reduced infant mortality, so that working-class mothers could expect their children to live. These patterns, together with the rising life expectancy of the mothers, led to the inclusion of the elderly mother in the working-class household of her middle-aged daughter.

There is also no doubt that economic factors also played a role in enabling working-class families to take on care burdens of their economically dependent elders. While there was a gradual change from 1880 to 1940 in that working-class families became as likely as middle-class families to contain elderly parents, a dramatic change took place between 1940 and 1960. By 1960 poor and working-class families were most likely to have an elderly parent in their home (Ruggles, 1996). What explains this reversal? The noneconomic factors were already in place by the 1940s in terms of emotional bonds and moral obligation. The reversal is therefore most likely due to the growing availability of public pension benefits, which gradually expanded between 1940 and 1960 to cover most of the elderly population. Now the working-class families could include the elder precisely because the elder was contributing income to the household. The elder's retirement check became a significant contribution to the working-class family economy. At the same time, the pattern among better-off families became that of "intimacy at a distance" (Rosenmayr & Kockeis, 1963). Elderly widows with means chose to live close to, but not with, their adult children. This reflects the growing importance of the value of independence for women as well as men.

It is plausible, therefore, that the Social Security legislation of the 1930s in the United States, by providing Social Security payments to the elderly, has enabled poor and working-class families to develop mutual-aid strategies including members, especially elderly mothers, whom they otherwise could not have afforded. This evidence supports the position that Social Security payments have neither weakened families nor made families less responsible for their elderly members. These transfer payments have enabled families to provide care that in the past they could not have afforded.

While the economic argument for enabling working-class families to care is important, the noneconomic variables discussed earlier must be considered as key motivating factors. The nineteenth-century ideal of the Victorian family with its structure of moral obligations had trickled down to the working class. Similarly, the education and uplift movements, the new home economics, the emphasis on biological motherhood, and the kindergarten movement all resulted in a more child-centered family among the poor and the working class. The result of this was no doubt strong emotional bonding between mothers and children in these families as well as in middle-class families. Thus working-class families sought to fulfill moral obligations to extended-family members, especially elderly mothers, and they were often prompted to do so by the emotional bonds developed during childhood. This trend was enhanced by the fact that between 1940 and 1960 the death rates fell much more rapidly for women than for men. In addition, elderly women are more likely to be disabled than elderly men at advanced ages (Bould, Longino, and Worley, 1997). Therefore, the most likely elder to need care would be the mother, the parent most likely to have established emotional bonds with the child (Bould, 1993). If the demographic situation had been reversed, with elderly fathers more likely to be in need, the patterns of care might have been different. Freedman (1993) has found that mothers benefit from a three-month reduction in their nursing-home stay, but fathers' nursing-home stays are not affected by the presence of an adult child.

THE DECLINE OF MORAL OBLIGATIONS

In family care for dependent members from the 1940s to the 1990s, the primary motivational aspect to have changed is the role of moral obligations. In the 1950s many states had laws requiring care of elderly parents or a disabled spouse. In Delaware until 1990 the state required the child to pay for the care of an elderly parent who was a patient in the state mental hospital. In England there has been no legal requirement to care for elderly parents since 1948 (Finch, 1993, p. 6). These changes are part of an overall weakening of Victorian morality in public life. With regard to overall attitudes, a recent survey in Manchester, England, found that 57.7% agreed that "there are circumstances under which it is reasonable to refuse to provide personal help for a sick or elderly relative" (Finch, 1993, p. 201). In the case of a frail elderly person who can no longer live alone, 54.9% said that he/she should move into an old people's home, while only 27.4% said that he/she should "live with relatives" (p. 205). While this study, as well as studies in the United States, indicates a strong support for filial obligation (Brody, 1985; Shanas, 1979; Finley, Roberts, & Banahan, 1988), this is primarily in terms of contact or help. In terms of "unconditional" responsibility for care of elderly parents, the support is less (cf. Campbell & Brody, 1985; Logan & Spitze, 1993).

The research in the United States on the relation between emotional bonds and moral obligations has examined affection as a cause for filial obligation. There are two problems with this research. First, the emphasis is upon "affection" rather than emotional bonds (cf. Walker, Pratt, Shin, & Jones, 1990). The latter is a more complex emotional entanglement. Cicirelli (1993) used the term "filial attachment." The second is the assumption of cause and effect when affection is related to a sense of moral obligation (cf. Finley et al., 1988). This chapter assumes that these are independent dimensions in the motivation to care (cf. Guberman, Maheu, & Maillé, 1992).

Finley et al. (1988) explored the relationship between affection and filial obligation for an urban sample from Alabama. They found that affection was not related to filial obligation for sons and suggested that "the male's sense of obligation may be satisfied with little investment of his actual time" (p. 77) and therefore is not related to affection. The strong relationship between affection and filial obligation for adult daughters, however, reflects a greater commitment of time and energy. For fathers, adult daughters' filial obligation is lessened by role conflict and high educational attainment. An adult daughter must calculate the costs of caregiving for her father. Only the mother-daughter bond supersedes these calculations. Cicirelli (1993) in his study of mothers and caregiving daughters found no relationship between his measure of filial attachment (which is close to the concept of emotional bonds) and obligation. Attachment motives, however, decrease the subjective burdens of caregiving, while obligation increases this sense of burden. The results of these two studies indicate that the mother-daughter bond is critical to long-term caregiving by the daughter. Part of this emotional bonding, moreover, is likely to be related to the daughter's reporting a happy childhood.[1]

To what extent does her motivation to care supersede a calculation of the costs of caring, the costs of her time available to her own family as well as her individualistic pursuit of self-interest? The weakening of Victorian moral obligations and the greater emphasis placed upon individual self-interest have led rational-choice theorists to claim that the state must take over all family functions because an individualistic cost/benefit analysis will result in the elderly, and even children, being abandoned (Coleman, 1993). Coleman's analysis stressed individual economic strategies rather than family economic strategies and concluded that families will break up under individual strategies.

The economic costs and benefits of caring for an elderly widowed mother can be assessed in terms of factors such as inheritance, but this cost/benefit analysis is by no means the entire picture. Nor can this factor be analyzed independent of emotional bonds. Emotional bonds between parents and children, especially between mothers and daughters, are of critical importance in the choice of economic or caregiving strategies for the middle-aged daughters. Elderly fathers with weak or conflictual ties to their middle-aged daughters are not likely to receive from them the kind of care necessary to stay out of a nursing home. When there is strong emotional bonding between generations, however, middle-aged women may face acute economic dilemmas when caught between the economic needs for college costs of their children and their own retirement in contrast to the need of an elderly mother for full-time care.

CONCLUSION

The postindustrial family has been transformed by the extension of life. First is the dramatic reduction in exposure to premature death, especially in the first year of life. It is in this context that the strong emotional bonds between mother and infant can develop. Second, the increasing extension of life among those over 65, especially women, exposes the family to the long-term-care needs of elderly widows with mental or physical disabilities. The percentage of families who face these heavy care burdens has increased dramatically due to the increasing numbers of such individuals, especially elderly women, who need this type of care. Furthermore, in order to perform these caretaking tasks, the middle-aged daughter must often forego wage-earning activities.

The widespread belief that families today, and especially women, are less accepting of the burdens of familial care than in earlier times is not substantiated by the evidence. Nevertheless, this belief persists in some scholarly contexts as well as in the popular culture. It is particularly popular among policy makers who wish to reduce payments for Social Security, Medicare, and especially home health care under the assumption that families—read women—should do more. Nevertheless, the level of care needed for elders today is very high and long-term.

The evidence of Ruggles (1987, 1996) points to the fact that the extended family was the result of early industrialization and that it was an economic strategy that excluded those most in need—the sick, the disabled, and the elderly. This family did not provide a refuge in life crisis. Even for the elderly, who were often included, their inclusion was related to their having economic resources—a house, a job, or a business. Poor elders were less likely to be included in the protected family circle.

Today, the evidence suggests that the vast majority of the functionally disabled unmarried elders are cared for by the family, typically by middle-aged daughters. The evidence is overwhelming that the level of care needed is far more burdensome than that of providing a spare room and food for an able-bodied elder. Public pension payments and Medicare do not compensate for this burden of care, although they permit poor families to include nonworking members who can contribute a Social Security check to the household maintenance.

The provision of this heavy care has increased during the same time as the moral obligation to care has decreased. Families today are less likely to provide this care out of Victorian moral obligation. What can explain this care today is primarily the emotional bonds, especially between mother and daughter. Those who are not tied by emotional bonds, of course, are at greater risk of requiring care by the state. There is no longer a moral obligation to care for an elderly parent who was abusive or just cold and distant. Furthermore, the emotional bonds supersede the individualistic cultural milieu, a milieu that encourages self-fulfillment and discourages self-sacrifice (Bellah, Masden, Sullivan, Swidler, & Tipton, 1985). The emotional bonds, then, operate in a hostile cultural environment, an indication of the power of these bonds. Indeed, what is extraordinary is the extent of care that adult daughters provide their mothers. Instead of blaming families, policy makers should investigate how to enhance the emotional bonds that motivate these middle-aged women to provide this high level of care.

NOTE

1. The Japanese women respondents, especially the granddaughter generation, were significantly more likely than the U.S. respondents to disagree with this statement linking

a happy childhood with parent care. In Japan moral obligation is still the overriding factor (Campbell & Brody, 1985, p. 590).

REFERENCES

Bellah, R. N., Masden, R., Sullivan, W. M., Swidler, A., & Tipton, S. M. (1985). *Habits of the heart.* Berkeley: University of California Press.

Berger, B., & Berger, P. L. (1983). *The war over the family.* Garden City, NY: Doubleday.

Bould, S. (1993). Familial Caretaking. *Journal of Family Issues, 14,* 133–151.

Bould, S., Longino, Jr., C. F., & Worley, R. (1997). Oldest old women: Endangered by government cutbacks. *International Journal of Sociology and Social Policy, 20,* 142–156.

Bould, S., Sanborn, B., & Reif, L. (1989). *Eighty-five plus: The oldest old.* Belmont, CA: Wadsworth.

Brody, E. M. (1985). Parent care as a normative family stress. *Gerontologist, 25,* 19–29.

Campbell, R., & Brody, E. M. (1985). Women's changing roles and help to the elderly: Attitudes of women in the United States and Japan. *Gerontologist, 25,* 584–592.

Cicirelli, V. G. (1993). Attachment and obligation as daughters' motives for caregiving behavior and subsequent effect on subjective burden. *Psychology and Aging, 8,* 144–155.

Coleman, J. S. (1993). The rational reconstruction of society. *American Sociological Review, 58,* 1–15.

Dizard, J. E., & Gadlin, H. (1990). *The minimal family.* Amherst: University of Massachusetts Press.

Finch, J. (1993). *Negotiating family responsibilities.* New York: Tavistock/Routledge.

Finley, N. J., Roberts, M. D., & Banahan, B. E. (1988). Motivators and inhibitors of attitudes of filial obligation toward aging parents. *Gerontologist, 28,* 73–83.

Freedman, V. (1993, June). Kin and nursing home lengths of stay: A backward recurrence time approach. *Journal of Health and Social Behavior, 34,* 138–152.

Goode, W. J. (1963). *World revolution and family patterns.* New York: Free Press.

Guberman, N., Maheu, P., & Maillé C. (1992). Women as family caregivers: Why do they care? *Gerontologist, 32,* 607–617.

Haber, C. (1983). *Beyond sixty-five: The dilemma of old age in America's past.* Cambridge: Cambridge University Press.

Hareven, T. K. (1982). *Family time and industrial time.* New York: Cambridge University Press.

Hareven, T. K., & Adams, K. (1996). The generation in the middle: Cohort comparisons in assistance to aging parents in an American community. In T. K. Hareven (Ed.), *Aging and generational relations over the life course: A historical and cross-cultural perspective* (pp. 272–293). New York: Walter de Gruyter.

Himes, C. L. (1994). Parental caregiving by adult women: A demographic perspective. *Research on Aging, 16*(2), 191–211.

Laslett, P. (1971). *The world we have lost.* (2nd ed.). New York: Charles Scribner's Sons.

Logan, J. R., & Spitze, G. D. (1993, November). *Self-interest and altruism in intergenerational relations.* Paper presented at the 46th annual meeting of the Gerontological Society of America, New Orleans.

Parsons, T. (1949). The Social Structure of the Family. In R. N. Anshen (Ed.), *The family: Its function and destiny* (pp. 173–201). New York: Harper.

Rosenmayr, L., & Kockeis, E. (1963). Propositions for a sociological theory of aging and the family. *International Social Science Journal, 15*, 410–426.

Ruggles, S. (1987). *Prolonged connections.* Madison: University of Wisconsin Press.

———. (1996). Living arrangements of the elderly in America, 1880–1980. In T. K. Hareven (Ed.), *Aging and generational relations over the life course: A historical and cross-cultural perspective* (pp. 254–271). New York: Walter de Gruyter.

Shanas, E. (1979). Social myth as hypothesis: The case of the family relations of old people. *Gerontologist, 19*, 3–9.

Stone, L. (1990). *Road to divorce.* New York: Oxford University Press.

Tedebrand, L. (1996). Gender, rural-urban, and socio-economic differences in co-residence of the elderly with adult children. In T. K. Hareven (Ed.), *Aging and generational relations over the life course: A historical and cross-cultural perspective* (pp. 158–190). New York: Walter de Gruyter.

Walker, A. J., Pratt, C. C., Shin, H. Y., & Jones, L. L. (1990). Motives for parental caregiving and relationship quality. *Family Relationships, 39*, 51–56.

Twenty-Eight

Fathers, Daughters, and Caregiving: Perspectives from Psychoanalysis and Life-Course Social Science

BERTRAM J. COHLER

> Particularly lacking is information on daughter-father relationships during the father's middle years. . . . our knowledge of the relationships adult daughters have with their fathers during these years is quite limited. (Barnett, Kibria, Baruch, & Pleck, 1991, p. 30).

The relationship between older fathers and their adult daughters has been largely neglected in studies of intergenerational relations. From earliest childhood through the middle years and beyond, much of the focus of study of parents and their offspring has concerned the mother-daughter tie. At least in part, founded on the assumption of inevitable tension between mother and daughter competing for the father's attention, much of the study of parent-offspring ties has focused on the conflict between mother and daughter from earliest childhood through the adult years. Further, since women generally outlive their husbands, even within the family of later life, the focus of study within the family of adulthood remains with the study of middle-aged daughters and their older mothers. At the same time, fathers continue as critically important relatives for the lives of their daughters, yet the significance of this relationship has been overlooked in much of the study of intergenerational relations and in the study of the family of the adult years.

This chapter reviews what is known regarding the relationship between older fathers and their middle-aged and older daughters. A primary concern of this chapter is to heighten our awareness of this little-studied relationship within the family and to foster enhanced interest in the study of the continuing relationship between older fathers, particularly with the advent of widowhood, and their caregiving middle-aged daughters. This discussion is informed both by understanding of the nature of family ties within contemporary urban society founded in systematic study of the relationship between parents and offspring within the family of adulthood, and by psychodynamic perspectives focusing on the meaning of such cardinal family relationships as that between father and daughter.

Freud (1900, 1905) initially pointed to significant issues between parents and children leading to points of tension between the two generations. Flügel (1927), Benedek (1970), and Rapoport, Rapoport, and Strelitz (1977) have extended this initial psychoanalytic focus on family process to include study of the complex ties taking place among family members across the course of life. Parker's (1972) detailed report on the significance of intergenerational ties for caregiving, Hess and Handel's (1959) report on the "psychosocial interior" of the family, and Cohler and Grunebaum's (1981) study of the tie between adult women and their own mothers have further enriched our understanding of the many factors entering into provision of care across the course of life. This psychodynamic perspective enriches our understanding of the significance of these relationships within the family and provides some additional understanding regarding the paucity of study of the tie between fathers and their middle-aged and older daughters.

From the time of the classic Greek dramas of family life by Aeschylus and Sophocles (Datan, 1986, 1988) to Shakespeare's tragedy of King Lear and Breuer and Freud's (1893–95) sensitive portrayal of daughters caring for their infirm fathers within bourgeois Viennese families in the last years of the nineteenth century, the conflict inherent in this tie, particularly when the wife and mother is deceased, has rendered caregiving particularly problematic. While, as Low (1978) and Cohler (1987–88) both have shown, the relationship between women and their mothers appears to become less tense as there is increasing role complementarity between middle-aged daughters and their own older mothers, there is little parallel reduction in tension between middle-aged or older daughters and their much older fathers.

As women attain middle age, their role portfolio comes increasingly to resemble that of their own mothers. Generally, both generations have attained the status of no longer actively parenting their own offspring and have entered more completely into work or other activities outside the house. Each of these two generations may enjoy the status of grandparent. Finally, each of these generations may have experienced widowhood as well. However, the conflict between daughter and father so characteristic across the first half of life within the contemporary family is not as readily ameliorated by changes in the middle-aged daughter's role portfolio. While grandchildren may provide an opportunity for increased positive experiences for middle-aged and older women and their much older fathers, many older fathers, particularly those representing cohorts of men growing older and whose years of active parenting were prior to the historical period 1965–1975, may find it difficult to relate to young adult offspring and may be bothered by the interests and lifestyles of their grandchildren (Boxer, Cook, & Cohler, 1986). Across the course of life, fathers find it somewhat more difficult than mothers to accept changing social circumstances that are associated with generation or cohort changes in lifestyle and attitudes (Hagestad, 1981; Boxer et al., 1986).

CAREGIVING, GENDER, AND RELATIONSHIPS WITHIN THE FAMILY OF ADULTHOOD

Much of the focus in the study of the relationship between adult offspring and their older parents in our society focuses on issues of caregiving provided by middle-aged and even older offspring for their much older parents. While caregiving is not the only aspect of the relationship among middle-aged offspring and their own older parents, it is most often the focus of continuing contact between the generations and a source of both satisfaction for offspring in having realized their responsibility toward their own older parents and, at the same time, a source of role conflict and overload for the younger generation (Cohler, 1983). Indeed, as Coward, Horne, and Dwyer (1992) have observed, roughly four-fifths of all support for older adults in the contemporary community is provided by offspring. Barnett, Kibria, Baruch, and Pleck (1991) have observed that nearly half of persons in their 50s still had at least one living parent.

With the group of persons over age 85 being the most rapidly growing age group in contemporary society (Rosenwaike, 1985; Mancini & Blieszner, 1989) and with enhanced longevity, there has been increased study of the manner in which older parents are cared for by their offspring. Indeed, concern with provision of care, principally with the goal of fostering continued physical mobility and independent living of even much older parents, is among the most significant issues confronting the family of the adult years. While these issues become particularly complex when parents have moved to warmer climates such as Florida or Arizona, leaving offspring in the Northeast or Midwest to manage caregiving from afar, even when generations live close to each other, efforts to preserve the older parents' independence and morale may become a difficult task for offspring and one involving feelings of resentment as well as obligation and responsibility in providing this care.

Perspectives on Family Caregiving

Contemporary urban society is unique in the extent to which caregiving for older family members both is voluntary and also reflects shared commitment of family and community. Within traditional societies, where families live together over time and across generations, caregiving is a formally assigned task (Nydegger, Mitteness, & O'Neil, 1983). Questions such as the degree of role strain imposed on adult offspring caregiving for these elders are irrelevant among societies where such caretaking is intrinsic to family life. Even within our own society, aging is expected to bring with it the "right" to be dependent on others for at least some aspects of care (Blenkner, 1965; Brody, 1985).

Much older parents expect to be able to depend upon their offspring, who, in turn, are expected to provide this care. Ironically, while it is assumed that geographic mobility interferes with this goal, as Litwak (1960, 1965) has shown, generations within the family continue to live close together. Indeed, as Young and Geertz (1961) have shown in their classic paper, families in the San Francisco Bay area reported about the same geographic mobility as families in East London housing districts where the relationship between generations was particularly close (Young & Wilmott, 1957; Kerr, 1958). Supporting this view, an analysis of geographic mobility across the year March 1993–94 reported that while about 18% of the population under age 65 had moved in the past year, only about 3% of these moves had been out-of-state (Treas, 1995).

As adults live to older age, caregiving demands upon middle-aged offspring, particularly daughters, have become increasingly significant. Brody (1985) has highlighted the problems for middle-aged and older women of providing care for their own much older parents while, at the same time, still providing care for their own adult offspring. At no time in history have there been as many generations within the family alive at the same time as presently characterize intergenerational relations in our own society. It is common for the family to realize four or even five generations alive at the same time, with adolescents enjoying the companionship and stories of their own great-grandparents. At the same time, the very longevity characterizing life within contemporary society poses issues for caregiving younger relatives. Neugarten (1979) has written of the significance of the distinction between the young-old (roughly ages 65–75) and the old-old (above age 75). As she noted, chronic illness is common and to be expected among these oldest old. At the same time, more than half of these oldest old maintain independent households and seek personal independence, which is essential for continued morale and sense of well-being.

A major goal in providing care for these older adults is maintenance of personal independence. Even among the oldest old (those over age 85), more than three-quarters of women and virtually all older men live with their spouse or live alone (Treas, 1995). Less than 5% of elders live in institutional care, although half of all older women and about one-third of older men may spend some time in a skilled-nursing-care facility. The reality is that most such patients either recover within about six months and return to independent living or else die while in care. Lieberman and Tobin (1983) have documented the rapid decline that often accompanies transition to long-term care. Increased use of such formal community services as the Visiting Nurse Association or "meals-on-wheels" may be of assistance in maintaining independent living.

However, much of the burden, as well as the sense of satisfaction with caregiving, rests on middle-aged and older daughters caring for their often-infirm parents. Women typically marry men somewhat older than themselves; traditionally, women have lived to older ages than men (a difference of about eight years favoring women). Schoen and Weinick (1993) have shown that widowhood for women may extend to fifteen years or longer, as contrasted with about eight and one half years for men who are widowed. Figures calculated from the 1990 census (Treas, 1995) have shown that among persons over the age of 65, there were 60 men for every 100 women; by the age of 85 sex ratios become even more unbalanced, 39 men for every 100 women. Since, as Treas (1995) noted, mortality figures favor women over men at all ages, it is understandable that with the mother the parent most likely to live into oldest age, much of the focus in the caregiving literature would be on the mother-daughter tie.

It is generally acknowledged that women in our society continue to be socialized from earliest childhood into the roles of kinkeeper and mother and maintain a relational perspective regarding self and others that supports this role of kinkeeper (Kerr, 1958; Chodorow, 1978; Gilligan, 1983; Troll, 1987; Walker, 1992; Lee, 1992; Antonucci, 1994). At the same time, much of the discussion to date regarding relations between the generations has focused on the tension existing in our society between mother and daughter. This tension, explicitly recognized by Freud (1900) from the outset of his work, has continued to our own time, as reflected in the large number of popular books portraying the relationship of mothers and daughters from earliest childhood to oldest age. Although much of this literature focuses on the relationship between mothers and daughters across the daughter's childhood, adolescence, and young adulthood, it is well recognized that the significance of this tie continues on through oldest age. In part, the lifelong shared focus on relationship characteristic of woman's role as kinkeeper, together with the matrifocal tilt in our society (preference, when possible, live near the wife's parents), reinforces the intensity of this tie (Sweetser, 1963).

Based on the reality of the continuing tie between mothers and daughters, it is understandable that much of the literature regarding the relationship between middle-aged and older daughters and their much older mothers has been the focus of the most intense study in the literature on intergenerational relations across the second half of life. At the same time, there is a paucity of literature regarding the relationship of daughters and fathers within the family of the second half of life. In part, this greater emphasis upon the daughter and mother than the daughter and father relationship reflects the reality that as long as both parents are alive, it is the spouse who is the most important family caregiver. Issues in caregiving first emerge with the death of one parent.

It should be noted that there has been little study of relationships between middle-aged offspring and their older parents even across the years when parents are healthy and have little need for care. Further, while there are a number of reports regarding the relationship between middle-aged mothers and their own much older mothers (Low, 1978; Cohler & Grunebaum, 1981; Baruch & Barnett, 1983; Fischer, 1986; Troll, 1987), there has been much less study of the relationship between fathers and their sons or daughters within the family of adulthood. It should also be noted that while the relationship between mother and daughter is an important source of morale, among many older adults, relationships with friends are as important or even more important as a source of morale than relationships with offspring.

Within families where both parents are still alive, and particularly within those families in which the father is the sole surviving spouse, the question of the tie between the older father and middle-aged offspring becomes particularly significant. Widowed men are less able to look after themselves than widowed women; widowed fathers require greater attention and assistance than widowed mothers, and daughters (and daughters-in-law) become the expectable kinkeepers. Additional problems have been posed in caring for an older father when, as happens frequently within the contemporary family, parents may have been divorced; most often, the biological father remarries and experiences diminished contact with his own offspring. With the advent of widowhood, even if his first wife is still alive, the divorced, now-widowed father may find himself particularly alone, while his daughter may find it additionally difficult to provide care and assistance, recognizing the intensity of her own feelings regarding the earlier divorce and later difficulties in maintaining a relationship following the divorce.

Fathers, Daughters, and the Family of Later Life

The most significant caregiver within the family is the spouse, typically an older woman caring for her ill or infirm husband. Further, as Cohler, Groves, Borden, and Lazarus (1989) have noted, while wives generally tend to call upon other family caregivers as a source of additional assistance, husbands tend to rely more explicitly upon formal community services. Husbands caring for ill wives are generally better able than wives caring for ill husbands to recruit a larger number of other kindred, particularly women, to assist in caregiving. It is assumed that husbands are ill equipped to render care and that they require assistance in caregiving from other family members. However, Coward et al. (1992) noted that among much older women caring for infirm husbands, the daughter becomes an additional source of support and assistance. While sons play a more prominent role in providing care for their father than for their mother (as Gay [1988] has noted, Freud was an exceptionally devoted caregiver during his father's last illness), daughters still play the most prominent role in caregiving for each parent (Lee, 1992; Lee, Dwyer, & Coward, 1993).

The requirement for care most often becomes apparent with the advent of widowhood. Since women so often outlive their husbands, the surviving parent is most likely to be the mother, while the caregiver is most often likely to be the daughter or daughter-in-law. However, in those instances in which it is the father who is the surviving spouse, the daughter is again the most preferred caregiver, raising once again lifelong issues in the father-daughter relationship. While sons are more likely to be involved in the care of older fathers than in the care of older mothers, even when the surviving parent is a father, it is the daughter who is the most visible caregiver (Coward et al., 1992; Montgomery, 1992; Lee et al., 1993).

Sons are relied upon only in those instances in which there is no daughter available to be of assistance; sons are more likely than daughters to fulfill a significant part of their caregiving responsibility through reliance upon formal community resources and to focus on less personal aspects of caregiving such as home repair and paying bills (Montgomery, 1992). However, daughters who are single are also more likely than their married counterparts, often with children of their own, to have experience using formal community resources and to call upon these resources in the same manner as do sons (Cohler et al., 1989; Montgomery, 1992). The important factor appears to be less the gender of the caregiver than community participation—women with significant household responsibilities are less likely to work outside the home and are therefore less likely than their single counterparts to have acquaintance with community resources. Further, single women have learned to use these resources in the absence of informal, family caregiving.

Barnett et al. (1991) have noted the lack of attention given to the relationship between middle-aged and older women and their much older fathers. Indeed, there is so little literature on the father-daughter tie within the family of the second half of life that these authors were required to extrapolate from the literature on the mother-daughter tie in discussing issues of aging and caregiving among women and their fathers. As might be expected, Barnett et al. (1991) have found that the better the past relationship between women and their fathers, the better the present relationship. Indeed, caregiving relationships were overwhelmingly positive for both generations. Widowed fathers reported greater caregiving satisfaction from daughters who were married, while still-married fathers were particularly committed to their single middle-aged and older daughters.

Rubinstein (1986) and Barnett et al. (1991) have observed that the relationship of father and daughter assumes particular importance for each generation following the loss of the wife and mother. While the relationship of mother and daughter may be the most significant within the family of the second half of life, daughters are able to turn to their fathers for the support that they had previously received from their mothers. However, Mancini and Blieszner (1989) cautioned that the relationship between older parents and offspring is more complex than has been discussed in the literature. In the first place, as Lee had earlier noted, the most important source of morale for older parents is friends rather than offspring.

In the second place, the extent of the older parent's feelings of satisfaction with the parental role is associated with the extent of the satisfaction received from the continuing relationship between the generations. Further, offspring provision of support and assistance may make daily life more manageable for an older parent but may do little to reduce feelings of loneliness. Too often, studies assume that frequency of contact may be simply equated with quality of contact. Finally, more detailed study is required not only of the father-daughter relationship within the family of later life, but also of the manner in which offspring divide responsibilities as well as of the experience each offspring has of the caregiving process (Matthews, 1987; Matthews & Rosner, 1988).

Illustrative of this call for increased study of the experience of the daughter-father tie within the family of the second half of life is a report (Abel, 1992) of caregiving by a middle-aged daughter for her father in a midwestern rural community late in the nineteenth century. Abel located the diary of a middle-aged daughter caring for her widowed father over a period of several years. When her widowed 77-year-old father was no longer able to support himself through a meager living from the family farm, Emily, his oldest daughter, brought him into her household. Separated from her own husband and firmly committed to the economic success of her two young adult children, Emily struggled for several years to support her children and manage her father's increasing dependence while at the same time dealing with her depressed and irresponsible former husband.

Over the course of the middle years, Emily's life became ever more burdensome. Her children left home for responsible middle-class positions. At the same time, she found herself increasingly alienated from her next-younger sister, who constantly quarreled with her regarding the manner in which she was caring for their father. When the sister's farm failed, she sought financial support from the ever-prudent Emily. At the same time, Emily's brother was unable to make his own way in the world and lived "hand-to-mouth," while her other sister struggled in poverty on a farm that could hardly provide a living for her own family. Faced with the care of her older, widowed father, who was in failing health, Emily turned to her own daughter for help and assistance.

Even though Emily's brother, as the only son, had inherited the family farm, he made little contribution to his father's support. Her father, in turn, did little to intercede in increasingly bitter conflicts among his children. Abel (1992) suggested that Emily's father may have been so despondent over his own help-lessness that he had little energy available for mediating conflicts. It is not clear how the situation became so grave, but ultimately Emily's sisters and brother decided that she was unfit to care for their father. Emily was clearly bothered by her father's depression, his inability to provide for his own self-care, and his increased incompetence. She found it frightening that he was acting like a child and unable to care for himself with his former pride. As her father faltered, he expressed ever greater rancor against Emily, together with increasingly bitter resentment regarding her care of him. Believing that he could do better with another sibling, after a seven-month stay he was moved to the house of his next-oldest daughter. Exhausted by her struggle to care for her father, overwhelmed by the intensity of his needs, struggling with her own burdens, and feeling defeated in her effort to manage the family, Emily died of exhaustion four years later.

While Abel (1992) viewed Emily's struggles in terms of feminist issues, most relevant in this context is the picture that is provided of issues posed for middle-aged and older daughters in the care of their own much older, often-infirm fathers. The struggle between the siblings regarding provision of care and locus of responsibility for the several aspects of providing for their older, widowed father is one familiar in our own time as well. Experiencing her father fall down while doing the simplest chores, Emily clearly was troubled by these changes in her once-proud, competent, and effective father. She was ill prepared to see her father acting like a helpless child. These feelings were in addition to those posed in providing for her own children and in dealing with an unsupportive and abusive husband. For his part, although we have only the reports from Emily's diary, her father seems to have acted as did Lear in Shakespeare's drama. Her father became incessantly critical of the only sibling honest enough to say what she thought and determined enough to be of help in spite of her own personal struggles. Ultimately, the father had no place to go when all offspring refused further care.

PSYCHODYNAMICS OF THE ADULT DAUGHTER-FATHER RELATIONSHIP

Abel's (1992) diary of Emily and her struggle to provide care for her older father while at the same time dealing with tensions with her brother and sisters is among the few accounts in the literature on family and aging to portray the human experience of caring for an older, widowed father. It is significant that Abel selected a life story as the means for studying the meaning for each generation of caregiving. In order to understand the process of caregiving for older parents, it is essential to move beyond study of social structure and residential propinquity. As Abel's account shows, it is not only structural features, but also those related to the relationships among brothers and sisters, the relationship of each with older parents (Cicirelli, 1981), and aspects of the kinkeeper's own life history that are of particular importance in the decision to provide care for an older relative. Rubinstein's (1986) account shows the importance of studying meaning systems and life histories in understanding the significance of this decision. Life histories provide a unique opportunity for understanding the meanings that members of each generation provide regarding both tensions and sources of satisfaction inherent in family caregiving, from that for young children to that for much older parents.

The "Family Romance" and Caregiving within the Family of Later Life

If we are to understand the dynamics of the provision of care and to have a better understanding of the role of the family in providing care for older family members, it is important that we have a better understanding not only of just who in the family provides care, but of the meaning of this provision of care for each generation (Goldfarb, 1965; Cohler & Grunebaum, 1981). From the outset, psychoanalysis has been concerned with the meanings that are made regarding the experience of generation and family. Most often, psychoanalytic inquiry has focused primarily on the relationship between young adult offspring and their parents. Freud himself had great difficulty with aging, perhaps a reflection of earlier life experiences with an older governess who terrified him, and did not believe that psychoanalysis could profitably lead to personality change across the second half of life (Gay, 1988).

However, over the course of the past several decades, perhaps reflecting the aging of the larger society, psychoanalysis has begun to consider the position of the middle-aged and older offspring's experience of parents (King, 1980; Nemiroff & Colarusso, 1985) and has increasingly focused on the meaning for middle-aged daughters of the care that they are expected to provide for often much older parents and in-laws. (While continuing enactment of wishes stemming from the continuing nuclear conflict of early childhood is reflected in the transference of middle-aged and older offspring, as Nemiroff and Colarusso [1985] and Cohler and Galatzer-Levy [1990] have noted, additional enactments stemming from subsequent life experiences, together with efforts to seek the analyst's admiration and respect for caregiving activities, also play a significant role in the transference enactments of these middle-aged and older offspring.)

Freud was fascinated with the tragedy of Oedipus the King (Rudnytsky, 1987). Earlier in his career it was Oedipus's struggle with the riddle of nature that fascinated the young scientist Freud. However, after his father's death, the self-analysis he undertook in order to resolve feelings of grief and guilt, and his discovery of the son's ambivalence regarding his father, Freud turned increasingly to Oedipus as a metaphor for the study of intergenerational relations and of the psychological significance of caregiving. As Datan (1986, 1988) has noted, the classic Greek dramas of Aeschylus and Sophocles provide important understanding of the meaning of caregiving in ways that have survived for several thousand years. In particular, the tension between fathers and daughters and the father's destructive actions regarding the daughter have been documented from Aeschylus to Shakespeare.

In the classic Greek trilogies a common fate befalls the legacy of Pelops, both the House of Atreus in Aeschylus's drama and Laius and Oedipus in Sophocles' tragedy of Oedipus so important in Freud's study and in contemporary arts and letters. In the beginning Pelops had three sons, Atreus, Thyestes, and Chrysippus. One brother, Atreus, murdered all but one of his brother Thyestes' children and fed them to their unsuspecting father, who then put a curse on all the lineage of Pelops, which included not only Atreus and Thyestes, but also Chrysippus, homosexually assaulted and abducted by Laius, Oedipus's father, who was supposed to be teaching horsemanship to this son of a neighboring king.

In Aeschylus's tragic trilogy Clytemnestra waits with her lover Aegisthus, the sole surviving son who escaped the dreadful murder and unwitting cannibalism, for her husband Agamemnon to return from his victories in the Trojan War. Alas, in order to propitiate the gods, Agamemnon had sacrificed their daughter Iphigeneia and returns home with his own young mistress. Clytemnestra urges

Aegisthus to kill both her husband and his mistress. In this act of retribution, Aegisthus not only avenges the murder of his brothers, but also Agamemnon's murder of Iphigeneia. These killings by Aegisthus are avenged in the second of the dramas, in which Orestes avenges the murder of his father Agamemnon by the murder of his mother and her lover. In the third of the dramas of this trilogy, Orestes is pursued by the Furies, brought to trial, and ultimately acquitted by Apollo.

The third of the brothers, Chrysippus, raped as a young boy by Laius, a neighboring king recruited to teach horsemanship and later the father of Oedipus, brings the curse on the house of Pelops to Oedipus, whose father abandoned him as an infant in order to avoid the curse that his own son would slay him, and who, in adulthood, commits incest as well as the killing of his father and is subsequently banished from Thebes in the care of his middle-aged daughter Antigone. Significantly, the relationship between father and daughter comes full circle; Agamemnon murdered his daughter Iphigeneia as a sacrifice necessary to win the Trojan War, while Oedipus is cared for by his daughter Antigone (Grene [1991] indicates that it is not clear whether Antigone was the daughter of her father's first marriage to Jocasta or the second marriage to Euryganeia), who leads him blinded through his old age and into the sacred grove at Colonus, where, in the third act of the drama *Oedipus at Colonus*, Oedipus is finally able to die a hero recognized by his city, which had formerly rejected him.

While the tragedy of Oedipus, so central in understanding the family romance (Freud, 1909b) within the bourgeois family of Western Europe and the United States, is still relevant, the first play in the dramatic cycle, *Oedipus the King*, may be much less relevant than the two later plays in this group, *Oedipus at Colonus* and *Antigone*. Antigone was a devoted caregiver to her father and overcame her own complex feelings to lead her blind father through the wilderness, insure his death truly as a king, and then take her own life following criticism from the community for having so honored her father.

Ross (1990) has commented that it is striking that Freud should choose to construct a psychology focusing on sons and fathers (perhaps a consequence of the discoveries of his self-analysis following his father's death, which overshadowed his clinical experience with daughters over the preceding decade), particularly Oedipus the son, rather than on the daughters of tragedy, ranging from the sisters Iphigeneia and Elektra to the devoted and caring Cordelia, the youngest and only devoted daughter in Shakespeare's tragedy of King Lear. In each case, the mother died, leaving the care of the old and infirm father to a daughter able to overlook her father's earlier disregard of her in order to provide care.

Breuer and Freud (1893–95) focused very much on the issue of the adult daughter and her father. Many of the reports in *Studies in Hysteria* concern a daughter attempting to provide care for an ill, widowed father and the personal pain evoked by unrecognized wishes encountered by the caregiving daughter in the process of being the primary caregiver. However, the reality of contemporary family life requires that psychoanalysis focus not only on the "family romance" of the young child (Freud, 1909b), but also on the enactment anew of this family romance across the years of middle and later adulthood. It is particularly likely that daughters will be called upon to provide service and support for their older parents as prolongation of the lifespan requires offspring to provide at least some assistance for their much older parents in at least some necessary activities of daily life. Caregiving may evoke anew conflicts unresolved since early childhood regarding the girl's wish for an exclusive relationship with her father; this conflict may be a particular problem within those families in which the mother dies, leaving the daughter responsible for her father's care.

Daughters, Fathers, and Psychoanalysis

Freud (1900, 1909b, 1910) understood the conflict between offspring and parent primarily from the offspring's perspective. Freud maintained that daughters expressed in disguised form wishes first stimulated by the nuclear conflict of sexual wishes experienced across the years of early childhood regarding attraction to the parent of the opposite gender together with rivalry with the parent of the same gender. These wishes are unacceptable as contents of awareness because of a shared sanction regarding acknowledgment of sexual feelings toward parents. As a consequence, these wishes are maintained outside of awareness, returning as compromise formations, primarily as dreams or as psychological symptoms. After his own father's death in 1896, Freud entered a period of heightened self-scrutiny or self-analysis (Anzieu, 1986), in which he explored his own ambivalent experience of his father as both caregiver and rival.

While Freud's psychology of the nuclear wish has most often been applied in understanding offsprings' experience of their continuing relationship with their parents across the years of adulthood, the conflict that he portrayed regarding the "family romance" (Freud, 1905, 1909b) within the bourgeois family of the West may also be applicable in the study of the parents' experience first of caregiving for younger offspring and, subsequently, of relations with adult offspring. Missing in Freud's work, but clearly addressed in more recent clinical psychoanalytic inquiry (Nemiroff & Colarusso, 1985, 1990) is the meaning of caregiving for the older parent who must deal with feelings of inadequacy and shame when confronted by increasing limitations on mobility and even mental activity (Goldfarb, 1965; Cohler & Galatzer-Levy, 1990; Donow, 1990).

Freud's self-scrutiny, resulting in the discovery that he harbored feelings both of tenderness and concern and also of competition and resentment, added to his growing conviction that the important psychological issue across the course of life was that of the child's experience of wishes toward the parents, together with the manner in which these wishes stemming from early childhood were amplified in the recounted experience of the family of early childhood and were understood as unacceptable and maintained outside of awareness. These wishes continued to be coactive in the present and provided the foundation for understanding all subsequent ties, including the range of other ties in the adult's life and the continuing complex tie between adult offspring and their middle-aged and older parents.

Psychoanalysis offers a particularly significant psychology for understanding the middle-aged and older daughter's experience of providing care for older parents. Freud had an opportunity to observe the manner in which daughters experienced their relationship with their older fathers. Freud's observations (Breuer & Freud, 1893–95) suggested that the task of caregiving led to the evocation anew of sexual wishes first experienced during the years of early childhood and maintained out of awareness across the course of adult life. Caregiving for an older, now-widowed father provided renewed opportunity for the satisfaction of the nuclear wish of early childhood.

The hysterical neurosis for which his women patients sought relief represented a symbolic enactment of both wish and counterwish stimulated by the physical and psychological intensity of the process of providing care for a widowed older father. This focus on the meaning for the caregiver of aspects of the caregiving relationship is as important as the focus on social structural aspects of caregiving in understanding the totality of the caregiving situation. Indeed, at least a part of Emily's struggle in caring for her father, portrayed so clearly in Abel's (1992) review of Emily's diary, concerned the evocation anew of her previously un-acknowledged wishes regarding her father, the impact of the nuclear conflict played out anew with her brother and sisters, her father's own response to the intensity of the caregiving situation, and his struggle to come to terms both with these wishes and with his own experience of enhanced infirmity and loss of independence.

In these and other accounts that Breuer and Freud provided in *Studies in Hysteria* (1893–95), as in the much later report on the "homosexual woman" (Freud, 1920), Freud strikingly showed a clear association between the act of caregiving and the sexual wishes that this act evokes for the adult caregiving daughter. While there is clearly much more to the relationship between middle-aged women and their fathers than issues of sexuality, neglect of this and other issues of meaning in much of contemporary social science study of adult inter-generational relations leads to a neglect of important psychological issues that have a direct impact both on larger relationships within the family and on the course of caregiving itself.

Particularly in the case of Elizabeth von R (Breuer & Freud, 1893–95), Freud suggested that the impact of caring for her dying father led to a "retention hysteria" in which Elizabeth von R was not able to recognize her feelings of resentment stemming from exhaustion due to the demands placed upon her. Freud himself had been a devoted caregiver for his father, who died of cancer after a lingering illness (Anzieu, 1986). Both father and child, Freud had focused on his feelings as child caring for his father and had apparently not explored the impact of being a parent upon his experience of caregiving for his father.

Finally, and particularly relevant in this discussion of psychoanalytic perspectives on the middle-aged daughter's caregiving for her much older father, is recognition of Anna Freud's own complex relationship with her father. Her father analyzed her over a period of several years, claiming that no other analyst could do as competent a job of analyzing his daughter (Gay, 1988). Further, middle-aged daughter Anna Freud served as a particularly devoted caregiver across more than a decade during which Freud struggled with his own recurrent cancer while maintaining an active clinical practice and writing many major papers. Largely unaware of the conflict overpowering Europe, Freud remained in Vienna until 1938, when increased persecution forced him and his family to flee to London, where he died the following year. There is a wonderful picture in Young-Bruehl's (1988) biography of father and daughter leaving Vienna for France and freedom, their noses pressed to the train window as they watched the old world slip away from them while facing an uncertain future. (Freud's wife, Martha Bernays Freud, who survived him for more than a decade, is nowhere in the photograph.)

Anna had long since succeeded her mother as her father's intellectual caregiver. She was the devoted caregiver both for her father and his ideas. Gay (1988) noted that it was Anna who went in Freud's stead to the funeral of his own mother in 1930. Certainly, Anna became her father's confidante and the acknowledged guardian of psychoanalysis in the later years of her father's life and following his death. Indeed, Gay (1988) suggested that Freud may have even discouraged suitors in order to maintain the close working tie with his daughter. Just as Antigone led a blinded Oedipus out of Thebes and into exile, devoted caregiver Anna led an infirm Sigmund out of Vienna, into exile in London, and through the last months as he succumbed to his illness (Young-Bruehl, 1988).

Society, Psychodynamics, and Caregiving within the Family of Later Life

Freud's discussion of Elizabeth von R's experience of caring for her father during her father's last illness and Freud's own experience of caregiving both highlight the significance of caregiving for adult offspring. This is particularly an issue for adult women in our urban society, so often charged with the care of their own infirm parents and, most often, those of their husbands as well. Although the image has often been portrayed of ours as a society stressing personal autonomy and independence, the reality is that we live in families, and that lives are more interdependent than independent (Kohut, 1981a, 1981b; Cohler, 1983; Pruchno, Blow, & Smyer, 1984).

The reality that the mother-daughter relationship is the most significant of ties within the family (Chodorow, 1978; Troll, 1987; Lee, 1992), considered together with patterns of preadult socialization that lead women rather than men to become primary kinkeepers in bourgeois Western society, leads to a focus on women as primary caregivers for widowed, older parents. Further, the matrifocal tilt evident in American society insures that a daughter will be available to serve in the caregiving role. Finally, the reality that women outlive their husbands by more than a decade, through the years when they, too, may become infirm, additionally enhances the significance of the daughter as caregiver for an older, widowed mother. Recognizing the importance for family and society of this caregiving role, it is understandable that the tie between older fathers and their middle-aged and older daughters should be so little studied.

However, given the tensions inherent in cross-gender caregiving, it is worth noting that there is also a dearth of literature regarding the son-mother caregiving role. While sons and daughters alike feel uncomfortable providing physical care for their much older parents and experiencing a role reversal as parents become dependent upon offspring for such basic care as bathing, since daughters are more likely than sons to be in a position to provide bodily care not only for mothers but also for fathers, psychological issues evoking a sense of discomfort are particularly salient for them.

Within the modified extended family characteristic of contemporary society, in which adult offspring maintain frequent ties with their own older parents and feel that this is an appropriate obligation to assume, daughters bear a special burden. Komarovsky (1950, 1962), Kerr (1958), Firth, Hubert, and Forge (1970), Sweetser (1963), and others have pointed to the "matrifocal tilt" of contemporary society in which the wife and mother is the kinkeeper and care-giver for a complex set of relatives. Adult daughters first learn this kinkeeping role during early childhood and assume it as a part of the expectable obligations of adult life (Komarovsky, 1950; Chodorow, 1978). Further, adult daughters are also mothers and perhaps even grandmothers. Even as they provide care for older relatives, they may have significant responsibility for still-dependent off-spring. This position as caregiver for both parents and offspring has been well portrayed by Elaine Brody (1985, 1990) as the "generation in the middle."

Findings from the study of adult lives have highlighted both the satisfactions and problems realized from providing care for older parents (George, 1986; Cohler & Galatzer-Levy, 1990). Daughters comment on the satisfactions re-ceived from doing what they believe to be right. As one daughter observed about the process of caring for her father, who was showing signs of personality disorganization often accompanying midphase Alzheimer's disease: "I visit my Dad once a week in the nursing home. Sometimes it's hard.... I hate to see him like this, but he cared for us all our lives and it's only right that we should do the same for him. My mom (deceased three years ago) would have expected me to do that too." Living up to an ideal set for oneself is an important aspect of caregiving. While much has been written about the realistic burdens of care-giving for older parents, there has been much less attention to the satisfactions realized from satisfying one's own ego-ideal (Schafer, 1960; Kohut, 1977, 1978, 1981a, 1981b). Even in the instance in which this caregiver is responsible for the care of both older parents and still-dependent offspring, there is the sense of pleasure realized from living up to one's own expectations and standards.

The position of this woman, providing care for her own older father, is very much like that which Breuer and Freud (1893–95) described for Elizabeth von R in *Studies in Hysteria*. The contributions of psychology of the self, including emphasis upon satisfactions realized from living up to one's own goals and ideals, poses another perspective for understanding Elizabeth's caregiving. The woman caring for her older, widowed father is in much the same position as Elizabeth caring for her father. Indeed, findings from life-course social science, reporting on caregiving across the course of life, suggest that the impact of the family romance continues across time, through the adult years. Just like Elizabeth, the participant in this study of caregiving also realized the pleasure of finally being able to provide for her father in the manner of her mother. Psychoanalysis provides increased understanding of the many and complex factors entering into the daughter's experience of caregiving. To date, although this is a common circumstance, there has been little systematic, psychoanalytically informed study of the meaning of caregiving. Such study needs to be undertaken employing the several theoretical perspectives presently available for understanding the meaning for daughters of providing this care.

The relationship between older fathers and their middle-aged and older daughters may be the most complex and least well understood of all relationships within the family. From the time of the epic Greek tragedies to contemporary intergenerational study, much of the discussion has concerned the relationship of mothers and both daughters and sons, while neglecting that between fathers and daughters. Indeed, the most interesting aspect of the complex family drama portrayed by Aeschylus and Sophocles is less the incest between Oedipus and Jocasta than the complex tie between fathers and daughters within the houses of Pelops (Iphigeneia, Elektra), and Oedipus (Antigone). This important relationship within the family of adulthood is largely neglected in both literature and the contemporary social sciences. Perhaps this neglect may be attributed to the reality that the relationship between father and daughter may be potentially the most intense of all family relationships. The recent concern with the father's use of power in the enactment with the daughter of incestuous wishes (Herman, 1992; Terr, 1994) may reflect this continuing focus on the implicit sexuality so difficult to resolve in the father-daughter relationship and much less explicitly discussed than that of mother and son.

While much of Freud's early study of psychoanalysis focused on daughters and their experience of providing caregiving for their fathers, the significance of this clinical study was eclipsed by Freud's "discovery" of the son's ambivalence regarding his father in the aftermath of his own father's death. Freud invoked the analogy of King Oedipus as a theme of universal significance. With the cases of Little Hans and of the Rat-Man and the Wolf-Man, much of the focus in psychoanalysis shifted away from the study of daughters and fathers to that of sons and fathers. Subsequently, additional problems were introduced when Freud attempted to portray the little girl's sexual development as symmetrical to that of the little boy and focused on the problems posed by the lack of castration anxiety among women. It is in Freud's early cases that the dilemma of fathers and daughters may be best understood.

Freud's (1905) understanding of the complex tie between Dora and her father is in marked contrast with his preoccupation with the impact of anatomical differences upon the course of personality development (Freud, 1925, 1931). While Freud can be faulted in this case for the lack of attention paid to Dora's experience of Freud as the reenactment of her sentiments regarding her father, he paid careful attention in this case to the "family romance" that ultimately led Dora as a caregiver both for her father and for her own family to reenact her mother's "housewife psychosis," failing to provide for her husband and children in her preoccupation with her housework in the same manner as had been the pattern of her mother's care of her. The case of Elizabeth von R also provides evidence of the problems that may arise as adult daughters undertake the care of their own older fathers.

CONCLUSION

Clinical psychoanalytic study provides an important means for understanding the meaning for daughters of caring for their own older fathers within contemporary society. However, this study must be informed both by life-course social science and by contemporary perspectives within psychoanalysis and must recognize that caring for an older father is an adult experience, but one that evokes wishes and sentiments salient for both generations across the course of life. Detailed study of relations between middle-aged and older daughters and their much older fathers must focus not only on social structural aspects of the relation, but also on the meanings for each generation of aspects of caregiving.

It is important to understand the manner in which caregiving is provided in contemporary society; detailed study of relations among kindred is clearly requisite in order to undertake more detailed study of the experience for each generation of caregiving for older parents. Study to date has not only highlighted the importance of understanding the role of middle-aged and older adult daughters caring for their much older fathers, but also the dearth of previous study regarding this most important relationship within the family of later life. While it is most often the case that it is a widowed mother who requires caregiving, widowed fathers are particularly poorly equipped to manage life on their own and both are particularly in need of care and find it difficult to accept such care, which is experienced as a threat to their autonomy and which may also evoke uncomfortable incestuous wishes, against the awareness of which these men may try to protect themselves. Similar, potentially disruptive feelings that may evoke anew unresolved aspects of the nuclear conflict of earlier life may also be experienced by daughters, who also seek to protect themselves from awareness of these issues.

The factors leading to selection of a particular caregiver, the meaning for each generation of this caregiving, and the impact of this caregiving on aspects of the caregiver's relationships with her or his own sisters and brothers all represent important issues for future study. Clearly, detailed, systematic study of this neglected relationship within the family should be a priority in subsequent intergenerational inquiry. This study should take advantage of both social and psychoanalytic perspectives and rely upon life-history interviews and other personal documents in an effort to better understand the interplay between social structure and personal experience within the family of later adulthood.

REFERENCES

Abel, E. (1992). Parental dependence and filial responsibility in the nineteenth century: Hial Hawley and Emily Hawley Gillespie, 1884–1885. *Gerontologist, 32*, 519–526.

Aeschylus. (ca. 458 B.C./1953). *Aeschylus, I. The Oresteia (Agamemnon, The libation bearers, The Eumenides)* (R. Lattimore, Ed. and Trans.). Chicago: University of Chicago Press.

Antonucci, T. (1994). A life-span view of women's social relations. In B. Turner & L. Troll (Eds.), *Women growing older: Psychological perspectives* (pp. 239–269). Thousand Oaks, CA: Sage Publications.

Anzieu, D. (1986). *Freud's self-analysis* (P. Graham, Trans.). London: Hogarth Press.

Arling, G. (1976). The elderly widow and her family, neighbors, and friends. *Journal of Marriage and the Family, 38*, 757–768.

Barnett, R. (1988–89). On the relationship of adult daughters to their mothers. *Journal of Geriatric Psychiatry, 21*, 37–50.

Barnett, R., Kibria, N., Baruch, G., & Pleck, J. (1991). Adult daughter-parent relationships and their associations with daughters' subjective well-being and psychological distress. *Journal of Marriage and the Family, 53*, 29–42.

Baruch, G., & Barnett, R. (1983). Adult daughters' relationships with their mothers. *Journal of Marriage and the Family, 45*, 601–606.

Benedek, T. (1970). The family as a psychologic field. In E. J. Anthony & T. Benedek (Eds.), *Parenthood* (pp. 109–136). Boston: Little, Brown.

Blenkner, M. (1965). Social work and family relationships in later life, with some thoughts on filial maturity. In E. Shanas & G. Streib (Eds.), *Social structure and the family: Generational relations* (pp. 46–61). Englewood Cliffs, NJ: Prentice-Hall.

Boose, L. (1989). The father's house and the daughter in it: The structures of Western culture's daughter-father relationship. In L. Boose & B. Flowers (Eds.), *Daughters and fathers* (pp. 19–74). Baltimore, MD: Johns Hopkins University Press.

Boxer, A., Cook, J., & Cohler, B. (1986). Grandfathers, fathers, and sons: Intergenerational relations among men. In K. Pillemer & R. Wolf (Eds.), *Elder abuse: Conflict in the family* (pp. 93–122). Dover, MA: Auburn House.

Breuer, J., & Freud, S. (1893–95/1955) *Studies in Hysteria.* In J. Strachey (Ed. and Trans.), *The standard edition of the complete psychological works of Sigmund Freud* (Vol. 2, pp. 1–305). London: Hogarth Press.

Brody, E. (1985). Parent care as a normative family stress. *Gerontologist, 25*, 19–29.

———. (1990). *Women in the middle: Their parent-care years.* New York: Springer.

Chodorow, N. (1978). *The reproduction of mothering: Psychoanalysis and the sociology of gender.* Berkeley: University of California Press.

Cicirelli, V. (1981). *Helping elderly parents: The role of older children.* Dover, MA: Auburn House.

Cohler, B. (1983). Autonomy and interdependence in the family of adulthood: A psychological perspective. *Gerontologist, 23,* 33–39.

———. (1987–88). The adult daughter-mother relationship: Perspectives from life-course family study and psychoanalysis. *Journal of Geriatric Psychiatry, 21,* 51–72.

Cohler, B., & Galatzer-Levy, R. (1990). Self, meaning, and morale across the second half of life. In R. Nemiroff & C. Colarusso (Eds.), *New dimensions in adult development* (pp. 214–259). New York: Basic Books.

Cohler, B., Groves, L., Borden, W., & Lazarus, L. (1989). Caring for family members with Alzheimer's disease. In E. Light & B. Lebowitz (Eds.), *Alzheimer's disease, treatment, and family stress: Directions for research* (pp. 50–105). Washington, DC: U.S. Government Printing Office (ADM89–1569).

Cohler, B., & Grunebaum, H. (1981). *Mothers, grandmothers, and daughters: Personality and child care in three-generation families.* New York: John Wiley.

Coward, R., Horne, C., & Dwyer, J. (1992). Demographic perspectives on gender and family caregiving. In J. Dwyer & R. Coward (Eds.), *Gender, families, and elder care* (pp. 18–33). Newbury Park, CA: Sage Publications.

Datan, N. (1986). Oedipal conflict, platonic love: Centrifugal forces in intergenerational relations. In N. Datan, A. L. Greene, & H. W. Reese (Eds.), *Life-span developmental psychology: Intergenerational relations* (pp. 29–50). Hillsdale, NJ: Lawrence Erlbaum.

———. (1988). The Oedipus cycle: Developmental mythology, Greek tragedy, and the sociology of knowledge. *International Journal of Aging and Human Development, 27,* 1–10.

Donow, H. (1990). Two approaches to the care of an elder parent: A study of Robert Anderson's *I never sang for my father* and Sawako Ariyoshi's *Kokotsu no hito* [the twilight years]. *Gerontologist, 30,* 486–490.

Dwyer, J., & Coward, R. (1992). Gender and family care of the elderly: Research gaps and opportunities. In J. Dwyer & R. Coward (Eds.), *Gender, families, and elder care* (pp. 151–162). Newbury Park, CA: Sage Publications.

Firth, R., Hubert, J., & Forge, A. (1970). *Families and their relatives: Kinship in a middle-class sector of London.* New York: Humanities Press.

Fischer, L. (1986). *Linked lives: Adult daughters and their mothers.* New York: Harper and Row.

Flügel, J. C. (1927/1960). *The psycho-analytic study of the family.* London: The Hogarth Press and the Institute of Psychoanalysis.

Freud, S. (1985). *The complete letters of Sigmund Freud to Wilhelm Fliess: 1887–1904.* (J. M. Masson, Trans. and Ed.). Cambridge, MA: Harvard University Press.

———. (1900/1958). The interpretation of dreams. In J. Strachey (Ed. and Trans.), *The standard edition of the complete psychological works of Sigmund Freud* (Vols. 4–5). London: Hogarth Press.

———. (1905/1953). Fragment of an analysis of a case of hysteria. In J. Strachey (Ed. and Trans.), *The standard edition of the complete psychological works of Sigmund Freud* (Vol. 7, pp. 7–124). London: Hogarth Press.

———. (1909a/1955). Analysis of a phobia in a five-year-old boy. In J. Strachey (Ed.

and Trans.), *The standard edition of the complete psychological works of Sigmund Freud* (Vol. 10, pp. 5–147). London: Hogarth Press.

———. (1909b/1959). Family romances. In J. Strachey (Ed. and Trans.), *The standard edition of the complete psychological works of Sigmund Freud* (Vol. 9, pp. 235–244). London: Hogarth Press.

———. (1909c/1955). Notes upon a case of obsessional neurosis. In J. Strachey (Ed. and Trans.), *The standard edition of the complete psychological works of Sigmund Freud* (Vol. 10, pp. 158–250). London: Hogarth Press.

———. (1910/1957). Five lectures on psychoanalysis (the Clark lectures). In J. Strachey (Ed. and Trans.), *The standard edition of the complete psychological works of Sigmund Freud* (Vol. 11, pp. 9–58). London: Hogarth Press.

———. (1920/1955). The psychogenesis of a case of homosexuality in a woman. In J. Strachey (Ed. and Trans.), *The standard edition of the complete psychological works of Sigmund Freud* (Vol. 18, pp. 146–172). London: Hogarth Press.

———. (1925/1959). Some psychical consequences of the anatomical distinction between the sexes. In J. Strachey (Ed. and Trans.), *The standard edition of the complete psychological works of Sigmund Freud* (Vol. 20, pp. 173–179). London: Hogarth Press.

———. (1931/1961). Female sexuality. In J. Strachey (Ed. and Trans.), *The standard edition of the complete psychological works of Sigmund Freud* (Vol. 21, pp. 225–243). London: Hogarth Press.

Gay, P. (1988). *Freud: A life for our times.* New York: Norton.

George, L. (1986). Caregiver burden: Conflict between norms of reciprocity and solidarity. In K. Pillemer & R. Wolf (Eds.) *Elder abuse: Conflict in the family* (pp. 67–92). Dover, MA: Auburn House.

Gilligan, C. (1983). *In a different voice.* Cambridge, MA: Harvard University Press.

Goldfarb, A. (1965). Psychodynamics and the three generation family. In E. Shanas & G. Streib (Eds.), *Social structure and the family: Generational relations* (pp. 10–45). Englewood Cliffs, NJ: Prentice-Hall.

Grene, D. (1991). Introduction, "Theban Plays" by Sophocles. In D. Grene (Ed. and Trans.) *Sophocles, I* (pp. 1–8). Chicago: University of Chicago Press.

Hagestad, G. (1981). Problems and promises in the social psychology of intergenerational relations. In R. W. Fogel, E. Hatfield, S. Kiesler, & E. Shanas (Eds.), *Aging: Stability and change in the family* (pp. 11–46). New York: Academic Press.

———. (1990). Social perspectives on the life course. In R. Binstock & L. K. George (Eds.), *Handbook of aging and the social sciences* (3rd ed., pp. 151–168). New York: Academic Press.

Herman, J. (1992). *Trauma and recovery: The aftermath of violence from domestic abuse to political terror.* New York: Basic Books.

Hess, R., & Handel, G. (1959). *Family worlds.* Chicago: University of Chicago Press.

Kerr, M. (1958). *The people of Ship Street.* London: Routledge & Kegan Paul.

King, P. (1980). The life-cycle as indicated by the nature of the transference in the psychoanalysis of the middle-aged and elderly. *International Journal of Psychoanalysis, 61,* 153–160.

Kohut, H. (1977). *The restoration of the self.* New York: International Universities Press.

———. (1978/1985). Self psychology and the sciences of man. In C. Strozier (Ed.), (1985), *Self psychology and the humanities: Reflections on a new psychoanalytic approach by Heinz Kohut* (pp. 73–94). New York: Norton.

————. (1981a/1985). Idealization and cultural selfobjects. In C. Strozier (Ed.), (1985), *Self psychology and the humanities: Reflections on a new psychoanalytic approach by Heinz Kohut* (pp. 224–231). New York: Norton.

————. (1981b/1985). On the continuity of the self and cultural selfobjects. In C. Strozier (Ed.), (1985), *Self psychology and the humanities: Reflections on a new psychoanalytic approach by Heinz Kohut* (pp. 232–243). New York: Norton.

Komarovsky, M. (1950). Functional analysis of sex roles. *American Sociological Review, 15*, 508–516.

————. (1962). *Blue-collar marriage.* New York: Random House.

Lee, G. (1992). Gender differences in family caregiving: A fact in search of a theory. In J. Dwyer & R. Coward (Eds.), *Gender, families, and elder care* (pp. 120–131). Newbury Park, CA: Sage Publications.

Lee, G., Dwyer, J., & Coward, R. (1993). Gender differences in parent care: Demographic factors and same-gender preferences. *Journals of Gerontology, 48*, S9–S16.

Lieberman, M. & Tobin, S. (1983). *The experience of old age: Stress, coping, and survival.* New York: Basic Books.

Litwak, E. (1960). Geographic mobility and extended family cohesion. *American Sociological Review, 25*, 385–394.

————. (1965). Extended kin relations in an industrial democratic society. In E. Shanas & G. Streib (Eds.), *Social structure and the family: Generational relations* (pp. 290–325). Englewood Cliffs, NJ: Prentice-Hall.

Low, N. (1978). *The relationship of adult daughters to their mothers.* Paper presented at the Annual Meetings of the Massachusetts Psychological Association.

Mancini, J., & Blieszner, R. (1989). Aging parents and adult children: Research themes in intergenerational relations. *Journal of Marriage and the Family, 51*, 275–290.

Masson, J. (1984). *The assault on truth: Freud's suppression of the seduction theory.* New York: Farrar, Straus & Giroux.

Matthews, S. (1987). Provision of care to old parents: Division of responsibility among adult children. *Research on Aging, 9*, 45–60.

Matthews, S., & Rosner, T. (1988). Shared filial responsibility: The family as the primary caregiver. *Journal of Marriage and the Family, 50*, 185–195.

Montgomery, R. (1992). Gender differences in patterns of child-parent caregiving relationships. In J. Dwyer & R. Coward (Eds.), *Gender, families, and elder care* (pp. 65–83). Newbury Park, CA: Sage Publications.

Nemiroff, R., & Colarusso, C. (Eds.). (1985). *The race against time: Psychotherapy and psychoanalysis in the second half of life.* New York: Plenum Press.

————. (Eds.) (1990). *New dimensions in adult development.* New York: Basic Books.

Neugarten, B. (1979). Time, age, and the life-cycle. *American Journal of Psychiatry, 136*, 887–894.

Nydegger, C., Mitteness, L., & O'Neil, J. (1983). Experiencing social generations: Phenomenal dimensions. *Research on Aging, 5*, 527–546.

Parker, B. (1972). *A mingled yarn: Chronicle of a troubled family.* New Haven, CT: Yale University Press.

Pruchno, R., Blow, F., & Smyer, M. (1984). Life-events and interdependent lives. *Gerontologist, 27*, 31–41.

Rapoport, R., Rapoport, R., & Strelitz, Z. (1977). *Fathers, mothers, and others: Towards new alliances.* London: Routledge & Kegan Paul.

Rosenwaike, I. (1985). A demographic portrait of the oldest old. *Milbank Memorial Fund Quarterly, 63,* 187–205.

Ross, J. M. (1990). The eye of the beholder: On the developmental dialogue of fathers and daughters. In R. Nemiroff & C. Colarusso (Eds.), *New dimensions in adult development* (pp. 47–70). New York: Basic Books.

Rubinstein, R. (1986). *Singular paths: Old men living alone.* New York: Columbia University Press.

Rudnytsky, P. (1987). *Freud and Oedipus.* New York: Columbia University Press.

Schafer, R. (1960). The loving and beloved superego in Freud's structural theory. *Psychoanalytic Study of the Child, 15,* 163–188.

Schoen, R., & Weinick, R. (1993). The slowing metabolism of marriage: Figures from 1988 U.S. marital status life tables. *Demography, 30*(4), 737–746.

Shakespeare, W. (1605/1991). *King Lear.* London: J. M. Dent & Everyman Books.

Sophocles. (441–405 B.C./1991). *Sophocles, I* (2nd ed.) (*Oedipus the king, Oedipus at Colonus, Antigone*) (D. Grene, Ed. and Trans.). Chicago: University of Chicago Press.

Sweetser, D. (1963). Asymmetry in intergenerational family relationships. *Social Forces, 41,* 346–352.

Terr, L. (1994). *Unchained memories: True stories of traumatic memories, lost and found.* New York: Basic Books.

Townsend, A., Noelker, L., Deimling, G., & Bass, D. (1989). Longitudinal impact of interhousehold caregiving on adult children's mental health. *Psychology and Aging, 4,* 393–401.

Treas, J. (1995). Older Americans in the 1990s and beyond. *Population Bulletin, 50*(2), pps. 48.

Troll, L. (1987). Gender differences in cross-generation networks. *Sex Roles, 17,* 751–766.

Walker, A. (1992). Conceptual perspectives on gender and family caregiving. In J. Dwyer & R. Coward (Eds.), *Gender, families, and elder care* (pp. 34–48). Newbury Park, CA: Sage Publications.

Willbern, D. (1989). *Filia Oedipi*: Father and daughter in Freudian theory. In L. Boose & B. Flowers (Eds.), *Daughters and fathers* (pp. 75–96). Baltimore, MD: Johns Hopkins University Press.

Young, M., & Geertz, H. (1961). Old Age in London and San Francisco: Some families compared. *British Journal of Sociology, 12,* 124–141.

Young, M., & Wilmott, P. (1957). *Family and kinship in East London.* New York: Humanities Press.

Young-Bruehl, E. (1988). *Anna Freud: A biography.* New York: Summit.

Twenty-Nine

Conclusions and Research Implications

JEAN M. COYLE

There has been an increase in research on issues affecting midlife and older women in the past twenty years. However, it was not until 1978 that the Baltimore Longitudinal Study added women to its study of normal aging (Markson, 1983). In that same year the Gerontological Society of America emphasized older women at its annual meeting (Markson, 1983).

The authors in this volume—writing on diverse topics—have identified some of the essential areas on which research still is needed. In particular, among questions of great interest are those about midlife and older women in all racial/ethnic groups. Many groups have not been investigated at all, for example, some of the new immigrant groups, such as Vietnamese and other Asian groups. Others still have not been thoroughly examined. As noted by Yee, Ralston, and John, Blanchard, and Hennessy, there still exist rather sizeable gaps in knowledge about minority women, especially older women. How similar/different are these women to/from one another? How similar/different are they to/from men in their own groups and in other groups? Given differing life expectancies, do variances in lifespan development patterns exist? Especially given a new focus on preventive health care measures earlier in life, how and when might these be instituted for these groups of women?

While older women in these groups may face triple jeopardy at least, all midlife and older women in general continue to become the objects of sexist and ageist attitudes. Are women still perceived as "old" sooner than are their male age counterparts? Is women's aging still seen as a greater obstacle for them, for example, in terms of employment after age 40, than is men's aging? What approaches might American society adopt to instill positive gender and age perspectives in future generations? What educational techniques would be most effective in countering prevailing age and sex stereotypes? In short, how does American society instill new, positive images of women as they grow older?

What steps can society take to prevent an old age of impoverishment for women? As Betty Friedan indicated (as quoted by Rubin), there is a need to integrate economic policies with social concerns. For example, how does an early-retirement policy affect women, who actually live longer than men, meaning that more of women's lives may be spent in a non-income-producing retirement period? How would income parity throughout working life affect women as they age? In what ways might pension reform prevent poverty among older women?

Does age discrimination in the work force particularly affect women—for example, women reentering the work force at midlife? Rife asks whether there are particular job-search techniques that would be most effective for midlife women and what the long-term effects of unemployment are.

Carp reminds us of the continuing need to look at women and retirement, especially financial issues—Social Security, pension, and earnings equity. How to be inclusive of women in retirement-planning programs remains an issue.

Understanding and acknowledging the differences in health status among subgroups of older women is a priority concern, as indicated by Torrez. Further consideration is needed of the interfacing among biological, behavioral, and social factors impacting women's health. Sinnott and McCulloch have provided models to utilize in future study of human development and life satisfaction. Attention to suicidal behavior in older women is particularly needed, as noted by Osgood and Malkin. Looking at the "survivor" quality of old-old women may provide insight into preventive health measures that may be instituted for both women and men, especially as more women and men become centenarians.

With the dramatic changes occurring demographically and technologically, noted by Scott, how will family relationships for women change? How will changing definitions of "family" determine new relationship patterns? With increasing numbers of women working outside the home, how will caregiving of elders be affected? How will women in geographically isolated areas—rural America—change as the next century dawns? What housing options will be needed to meet new and different requirements of midlife and older women in the next decades? What is the spiritual life of midlife and older women like, and how does their spirituality change with the aging process?

These questions provide a very limited list of research issues for the future. Data resulting from answering these and a multitude of research questions about the lives of midlife and older women have definite policy implications. For example, if more women are working outside the home, what caregiving alternatives for elder care need to be provided? If women spend more of their lives in paid employment situations, what will be the effects on their retirement income and their retirement planning?

How can policy initiatives recognize the heterogeneity of older women? What will be the effect of positive stereotypes on policy development? Steinhauer and Auslander (1984) clearly stated essential policy objectives:

The tasks and responsibilities of policymakers and program designers are threefold: 1) to enhance public awareness of older women, 2) to stimulate and conduct research and disseminate findings, and 3) to develop support services and community resources designed to benefit older women. (Steinhauer and Auslander, 1984, p. 175)

Researchers and policy makers alike need to recognize the vital interfacing of current research and future policy and to work together to improve the lives of all women as they age. It is hoped that this book has provided an overview of important issues and has raised some key questions—and that another volume will begin to provide some of the crucial responses.

REFERENCES

Markson, E. (Ed.). (1983). *Older women*. Lexington, MA: Lexington Books.

Steinhauer, M., & Auslander, S. (1984). Policy directions and program design: Issues and implications in services for older women. In G. Lesnoff-Caravaglia (Ed.), *The world of the older woman: Conflicts and resolutions* (pp. 175–186). New York: Human Sciences Press.

Selected Bibliography

Apter, T. (1995). *Secret paths: Women in the new midlife*. New York: W. W. Norton.

Arber, S., & Ginn, J. (1991). *Gender and later life*. London/Newbury Park, CA: Sage Publications.

Backer, J. (1995). Perceived stressors of financially secure, community-residing older women. *Geriatric Nursing, 16*(4), 155–159.

Barnes, C., Given, B., & Given, C. (1995). Parent caregivers: A comparison of employed and not employed daughters. *Social Work, 40*(3), 375–381.

Barusch, A. (1994). *Older women in poverty*. New York: Springer Publishing Co.

Bird, C. (1995). *Lives of our own: Secrets of salty old women*. Boston: Houghton Mifflin.

Browne, C. (1995). Empowerment in social work practice with older women. *Social Work, 40*(3), 358–364.

Butler, R., Collins, K., Meier, D., Muller, C., & Pinn, V. (1995a). Older women's health: Clinical care in the postmenopausal years. *Geriatrics, 50*(6), 33–36+.

―――. (1995b). Older women's health: "Taking the pulse" reveals gender gap in medical care. *Geriatrics, 50*(5), 39–40+.

Butler, S., & DePoy, E. (1996). Rural elderly women's attitudes toward professional and governmental assistance. *Affilia, 11*(1), 76–94.

Campbell, J., & Huff, M. (1995). Sexuality in the older woman. *Gerontology and Geriatrics Education, 16*(1), 71–81.

Chevan, A. (1995). Holding on and letting go: Residential mobility during widowhood. *Research on Aging, 17*(3), 278–302.

Claridge, K., Rowell, R., Duffy, J., & Duffy, M. (1995). Gender differences in adjustment to nursing home care. *Journal of Gerontological Social Work, 24*(1–2), 155–168.

Coyle, J. (1989). *Women and aging: A selected, annotated bibliography*. Westport, CT: Greenwood Press.

Davis, N., Cole, E., & Rothblum, E., (Eds.). (1993). *Faces of women and aging*. New York: Haworth Press.

Dodge, H. (1996). *Poverty transitions among elderly widows.* New York: Garland Publishing.

Dorfman, L. (1995). Health, financial status, and social participation of retired rural men and women: Implications for educational intervention. *Educational Gerontology, 21*(7), 653–669.

Drebing, C., Gooden, W., Drebing, S., Van de Kemp, H., & Malony, H. (1995). The dream in midlife women: Its impact on mental health. *International Journal of Aging and Human Development, 40*(1), 73–87.

Ettner, S. (1995). The impact of "parent care" on female labor supply decisions. *Demography, 32*(1), 63–80.

Facio, E. (1996). *Understanding older Chicanas.* Thousand Oaks, CA: Sage Publications.

Fingerman, K. (1995). Aging mothers' and their adult daughters' perceptions of conflict behaviors. *Psychology and Aging, 10*(4), 639–649.

Fischer, K. (1995). *Autumn gospel: Women in the second half of life.* New York: Paulist Press.

Franks, M., & Stephens, M. (1996). Social support in the context of caregiving: Husbands' provision of support to wives involved in parent care. *Journal of Gerontology: Series B: Psychological Sciences and Social Sciences, 51B*(1), P43–P52.

Freysinger, V. (1995). The dialectics of leisure and development for women and men in mid-life: An interpretive study. *Journal of Leisure Research, 27*(1), 61–84.

Friedan, B. (1993). *The fountain of age.* New York: Simon & Schuster.

Grambs, J. (1989). *Women over forty: Visions and realities.* (Rev. ed.). New York: Springer Publishing Co.

Hammond, J. (1995). Multiple jeopardy or multiple resources? The intersection of age, race, living arrangements, and education level and the health of older women. *Journal of Women and Aging, 7*(3), 5–24.

Handa, V. L., Landerman, R., Hanlon, J., Harris, T., & Cohen, H. (1996). Do older women use estrogen replacement? Data from the Duke Established Populations for Epidemiologic Studies of the Elderly (EPESE). *Journal of the American Geriatrics Society, 44*(1), 1–6.

Hannon, K. (1995, September). Why the rules are different for women. *Working Woman,* pp. 20+.

Hershey, D. (1995). Influence of age and gender on estimates of long-term financial growth functions. *Aging and Cognition, 2*(3), 231–250.

Hibbard, J. (1995). Women's employment history and their post-retirement health and resources. *Journal of Women and Aging, 7*(3), 43–54.

Jacobs, R. (1993). *Be an outrageous older woman: A RASP.* (Rev. ed.). Manchester, CT: Knowledge, Ideas, & Trends.

Jacobson, J. (1995). *Midlife women: Contemporary issues.* Boston: Jones & Bartlett.

Jirovec, R., & Erich, J. (1995). Gray power or power outage? Political participation among very old women. *Journal of Women and Aging, 7*(1–2), 85–99.

Lanetto, S., Keminski, P., & Felicio, D. (1995). Typical and optimal aging in women and men: Is there a double standard? *International Journal of Aging & Human Development, 40*(3), 187–207.

Laws, G. (1995). Understanding ageism: Lessons from feminism and postmodernism. *Gerontologist, 35*(1), February, 112–118.

Levinson, D. (1996). *The seasons of a woman's life.* New York: Knopf.

Macdonald, B. (1991). *Look me in the eye: Old women, aging, and ageism.* (2nd expanded ed.). San Francisco: Spinsters Book Co.

Macunovich, D., Easterlin, R., Schaeffer, C., & Crimmins, E. (1995). Echoes of the baby boom and bust: Recent and prospective changes in living alone among elderly widows in the United States. *Demography, 32*(1), 17–28.

Melamed, E. (1983). *Mirror, mirror: The terror of not being young.* New York: Linden Press/Simon & Schuster.

Meyer, B., Russo, C., & Talbot, A. (1995). Discourse comprehension and problem solving: Decisions about the treatment of breast cancer by women across the life span. *Psychology and Aging, 10*(1), 84–103.

Minick, P., & Gueldner, S. (1995). Patterns of conflict and anger in women sixty years old or older: An interpretive study. *Journal of Women and Aging, 7*(1–2), 71–84.

Ozawa, M. (1995). The economic status of vulnerable older women. *Social Work, 40*(3), 323–331.

Perkins, K. (1995). Social [in]security: Retirement planning for women. *Journal of Women and Aging, 7*(1–2), 37–53.

Peterson, B., & Klohnen, E. (1995). Realization of generativity in two samples of women at midlife. *Psychology and Aging, 10*(1), 20–29.

Pogrebin, L. (1996). *Keeping time: Angst, body blues, and other obsessions.* Boston: Little, Brown.

Porcino, J. (1991). *Growing older, getting better.* New York: Continuum.

Quinn, P., & Walsh, S. (1995). Midlife women with disabilities: Another challenge for social workers. *Affilia, 10*(3), 235–254.

Rabey, L. (1995). *Coming of age.* Nashville: Thomas Nelson Publishers.

Richardson, V., & Kilty, K. (1995). Gender differences in mental health before and after retirement: A longitudinal analysis. *Journal of Women and Aging, 7*(1–2), 19–35.

Rife, J. (1995). Older unemployed women and job search activity: The role of social support. *Journal of Women and Aging, 7*(3), 55–68.

Rosenthal, E. (Ed.). (1990). *Women, aging, and ageism.* New York: Haworth Press.

Rountree, C. (1991). *Coming into our fullness: On women turning forty.* Freedom, CA: Crossing Press.

Seltzer, M., Greenberg, J., & Krause, M. (1995). A comparison of coping strategies of aging mothers of adults with mental illness or mental retardation. *Psychology and Aging, 10*(1), 64–75.

Sharpe, P., & Mezoff, J. (1995). Beliefs about diet and health: Qualitative interviews with low income older women in the rural South. *Journal of Women and Aging, 7*(1–2), 5–18.

Soehnel, S. (Ed.). (1995). *Women's solutions to problems of aging.* Oakland, CA: S. Soehnel.

Stephens, M., & Franks, M. (1995). Spillover between daughters' roles as caregiver and wife: Interference or enhancement? *Journals of Gerontology: Psychological Sciences and Social Sciences: Series B, 50B*(1), P9–P17.

Thone, R. (1992). *Women and aging: Celebrating ourselves.* New York: Haworth Press.

Turner, B., & Troll, L. (Eds.). (1994). *Women growing older: Psychological perspectives.* Thousand Oaks, CA: Sage Publications.

Waskel, S. (1995). Ranking of words chosen to describe older women in general and older female relatives. *Journal of Women and Aging, 7*(3), 93–104.

Weinrich, S., Coker, A., Weinrich, M., Eleazer, G., & Greene, F. (1995). Predictors of Pap smear screening in socioeconomically disadvantaged elderly women. *Journal of the American Geriatrics Society, 43*(3), 267–270.

Welsh, W., & Stewart, A. (1995). Relationships between women and their parents: Implications for midlife well-being. *Psychology and Aging, 10*(2), 181–190.

Index

About the Editor and Contributors

JEAN M. COYLE is President of Jean Coyle Associates, a gerontological consulting firm, of Alexandria, Virginia. Coyle has been a social gerontologist since 1976. She is the author of *Women and Aging* and *Families and Aging*, both published by Greenwood Press. She founded the first academic gerontology program in the state of Louisiana in 1976. She also has taught at universities in Indiana, Texas, Illinois, Washington, D.C., Virginia, New Mexico, and Kansas and has held tenured professorships at Eastern Illinois University in Charleston, Illinois, and at New Mexico State University in Las Cruces, New Mexico. She has been Secretary of the Association for Gerontology in Higher Education (1978–1980), National President of Sigma Phi Omega gerontology honor society (1992–1994), and a founder and President of the Southwest Society on Aging. She is a Fellow of the Gerontological Society of America.

REBECCA G. ADAMS is Associate Professor in the Department of Sociology at the University of North Carolina at Greensboro. She received her doctorate from the University of Chicago with an emphasis on the sociology of aging. Her major research interest is friendship patterns, especially as they are affected by geographic separation and by cultural and structural context. She is coeditor of *Older Adult Friendship: Structure and Process*, coauthor of *Adult Friendship*, and author of numerous articles. She is conducting two studies of friendships— one an examination of the cultural conventions and structural conditions affecting the development of friendships among members of a nonterritorial music subculture and the other a study of older adult friendship patterns and mental health.

PATRICE H. BLANCHARD received her M.S. in aging studies from the University of North Texas and is currently Economic Security Representative, Southwest Region, American Association of Retired Persons. She has previous experience in international business, marketing, and management of health care and nonprofit organizations. She is also a Research Scientist in the University of North Texas Minority Aging Research Institute and has research interests in applied gerontology, cultural diversity in aging services, and American Indian aging.

SALLY BOULD is Professor of Sociology at the University of Delaware. Her research on social policy issues has focused on family policy and poverty and the elderly. She has published research on the relationship between unemployment and early retirement and poverty. Her book *Eighty-five Plus* (co-authored with S. Sanborn and L. Reif) examines the issues of state and family responsibilities for the oldest old and caregiving and social support for the oldest old. Her doctorate is from Bryn Mawr College.

JULIA E. BRADSHER is a Research Scientist with the New England Research Institutes in Watertown, Massachusetts. She completed her doctoral work at the University of Miami, Coral Gables, Florida, and held a postdoctoral fellowship at the Institute for Health and Aging at the University of California in San Francisco. Her research focuses on aging, disability, and health policy, with particular interests in minorities and women. Currently, she is the project director for the Coordinating Center of the Study of Women's Health across the Nation, a longitudinal, multisite study of women in midlife.

FRANCES M. CARP received the doctorate in general psychology from Stanford University "with greatest distinction" and the diploma in clinical psychology from the American Board of Examiners in Professional Psychology. She is a member of Phi Beta Kappa and Sigma Xi, a Public Health Fellow, and a Fellow of the American Psychological Association, the Gerontological Society of America, and the Association for Personality Assessment.

BERTRAM J. COHLER is William Rainey Harper Professor of Social Sciences at the University of Chicago and Co-Director for the Social Sciences of the University of Chicago Center on Health, Aging, and Society.

EILEEN DEGES CURL is Assistant Professor of Nursing, Fort Hays State University, Hays, Kansas.

WINIFRED DOWLING has twenty years experience in the field of aging and voluntarism. She is Aging Services Administrator for the city of El Paso, Texas. She spent ten years in Washington, D.C., as a staff member of VISTA (Volunteers in Service to America), the Peace Corps, and ACTION, the federal volunteer agency. She is Past President of the National Association of Retired

Senior Volunteer Program (RSVP) Directors, is President-Elect of the Southwest Society on Aging, and is the founder of the first senior volunteer program in Mexico.

ELISA FACIO is a core faculty member in the Department of Ethnic Studies at the University of Colorado at Boulder, where she previously served as a faculty member in the Department of Sociology. Her areas of research include aging, health care policy, and Chicana feminist theory. She received her B.S. in sociology with honors from Santa Clara University and her M.A. and Ph.D. in sociology from the University of California at Berkeley. From 1988 to 1990 she was a National Institute on Aging Postdoctoral Fellow at the University of California at San Francisco under the direction of Carroll L. Estes. She has published articles on older Chicanas in the *Journal of Aging Studies, The Oxford Companion to Women's Writing in the United States*, and the edited anthologies *Race and Ethnicity in Research Methods* and *Building with Our Hands: New Directions in Chicana Studies*, and a book entitled *Understanding Older Chicanas*. She is currently working on an article, "Health Care Policy toward Chicanas: Assumptions, Values, and Implications of Medicaid," and on an edited anthology on Cuba, the latter a collaborative project among North American sociologists and political scientists and Cuban social scientists from the University of Havana, Cuba.

MARY GRIZZARD is an internationally known Latin Americanist with a specialty in cultural and political history. She was a tenured professor at the University of New Mexico for sixteen years and currently teaches at American University. She is the author of three books and has written sixteen chapters and forty-eight articles in juried publications. She has taught courses ranging from Latin American studies to art and architectural history.

CAROLE HABER is Chair of the Department of History and Professor of History at the University of North Carolina at Charlotte. She received her doctorate from the Department of American Civilization of the University of Pennsylvania. She is the author of *Beyond Sixty-five: The Dilemma of Old Age in America's Past* and, with Brian Gratton, *Old Age and the Search for Security.*

CATHERINE HAGAN HENNESSY is trained in anthropology and public health gerontology. She received her doctorate in public health from the University of California at Berkeley in 1990. Her major research interests are in the areas of long-term care, case-management practice, and the delivery of geriatric services to minority populations. Her current activities include several assessments of the long-term-care needs of American Indian elders.

ROBERT JOHN received his doctorate in sociology from the University of Kansas. He has long-standing research interests in applied aspects of American

Indian aging and has recently published a monograph written for the Indian Health Service entitled *American Indian and Alaska Native Elders: An Assessment of Their Current Status and Provision of Services.*

PAT M. KEITH is Professor of Sociology and Assistant Dean in the Graduate College at Iowa State University. Her recent research on guardianship was reported in *Older Wards and Their Guardians* (Praeger), coauthored with Robbyn Wacker.

VIRA R. KIVETT is an Excellence Professor in the Department of Human Development and Family Studies, School of Human Environmental Sciences, University of North Carolina at Greensboro. She has published extensively in the areas of family roles and relationships in later life, with particular emphasis on women, ethnicity, and the rural elderly.

CHARLES F. LONGINO, JR., Wake Forest Professor of Sociology and Public Health Sciences at Wake Forest University and the Bowman Gray School of Medicine, has led eight major investigations of older populations. He has authored or coauthored 13 books, monographs, and compendia, most recently *Retirement Migration in America, 1970–1990* (1995) and *The Old Age Challenge to the Biomedical Model: Paradigm Strain and Health Policy* (with John Murphy, 1995), and 116 other publications, nearly all on aging topics. He has taught the introductory sociology course every semester of the first twenty-five years of his academic career.

B. JAN McCULLOCH is Assistant Professor with a joint appointment in the Department of Family Studies, College of Human Environmental Sciences, and the Sanders-Brown Center on Aging, University of Kentucky. Her research interests include longitudinal investigations of well-being among older, rural adults, rural aging—especially gender differences in rural aging and home-based labor experiences among rural women—and methodological issues in aging research.

DEBRA McDONALD is a Nursing Instructor at Cloud County Community College. A long-term interest in promoting mental health in the elderly led to research on the phenomenon of reminiscence in elderly women. McDonald received B.S. and M.S. degrees in nursing from Fort Hays State University in Hays, Kansas.

MARJORIE J. MALKIN is Associate Professor, Department of Health Education and Recreation, Southern Illinois University at Carbondale.

ELIZABETH W. MARKSON received her B.A. from Bryn Mawr College in French literature and M.A. and Ph.D. degrees in sociology from Yale University.

She has a long-term interest in research on older women and is currently focusing on depictions of older women in film. She is associate director of the Gerontology Center and Project Director of a training grant in aging research at Boston University, where she is Professor of Socio-Medical Sciences and Community Medicine, Research Professor of Medicine, and Adjunct Professor of Sociology.

RICHARD L. NEWTSON is Assistant Professor at Eastern Oregon State College. He received a doctorate in sociology at Iowa State University in 1994. His recent research has been on sibling support in later life.

NANCY J. OSGOOD is a Professor in the Department of Gerontology, Virginia Commonwealth University and Medical College of Virginia.

ERDMAN B. PALMORE is Professor Emeritus of Medical Sociology at the Duke University Center for the Study of Aging and Human Development. He has done extensive research on ageism and has written a book called *Ageism: Negative and Positive*. He is also the author of fourteen other books, including *The Facts on Aging Quiz* and *Handbook on the Aged in the United States*.

BARBARA PAYNE-STANCIL is Professor Emerita of Sociology and Director of the Gerontology Center, Georgia State University, Atlanta. She is Chairperson of the Georgia Council on Aging and a member of the Georgia Board of Nursing Homes. Her major research and writings are in religion and spirituality.

PENNY A. RALSTON is Professor and Dean, College of Human Sciences, Florida State University, Tallahassee, Florida. She received her doctorate at the University of Illinois. She has published in the areas of community-based programs for older adults and nutrition and health promotion, with an emphasis on minority elderly. She is a Fellow in the Gerontological Society of America and has served on the Board of Directors for the Association for Gerontology in Higher Education and the Older Women's League. She is President-Elect of the American Association of Family and Consumer Sciences.

JOHN C. RIFE is Associate Professor of Social Work and Director of the bachelor of science in social work program at the University of North Carolina at Greensboro. He has completed research on older workers, their characteristics, and effective intervention strategies and has written *Employment of the Elderly: An Annotated Bibliography*, published in 1995 by Greenwood Press.

ROSE M. RUBIN is Professor and Chair of the Department of Economics at the University of Memphis. She has taught in the areas of the economics of health care and economics of social welfare. Her research has been focused on the economics of working wives and dual-earner families and on the economics of health care, with emphasis on health and aging.

JEAN PEARSON SCOTT is Associate Professor of Human Development and Family Studies at Texas Tech University. Her research interests focus mainly on family support networks of older adults. Recent articles have addressed family caregiving, sibling relationships, the oldest old, and rural aging.

SUSAN R. SHERMAN is Professor of Social Welfare, Rockefeller College of Public Affairs and Policy, Professor of Public Health, and Faculty Research Associate of the Ringel Institute of Gerontology at the State University of New York at Albany. She is Past President of the Association for Gerontology in Higher Education and of the New York State Society on Aging and is a Fellow of the Gerontological Society of America. Among her books are *Foster Families for Adults: A Community Alternative in Long-term Care* (with Evelyn Newman) and *The Environment for Aging: Interpersonal, Social, and Spatial Contexts* (with Russell Ward and Mark LaGory).

JAN D. SINNOTT is a Professor of Psychology at Towson State University, Baltimore, Maryland, where she also has a private practice. Her research in positive aspects of adult cognitive development, following from postdoctoral work at the National Institutes of Health, has led to several books, including *Reinventing the University* (with Lynn Johnson), *Interdisciplinary Handbook of Adult Lifespan Learning, Bridging Paradigms* (with John Cavanaugh), *Everyday Memory and Aging* (with Robin West), and *Sex Roles and Aging*. She is currently completing a volume on her theory of adult logical development.

DIANA J. TORREZ is an Assistant Professor at the University of North Texas. She is on leave (1994–1996) as a National Institute on Aging/Pew Postdoctoral Fellow and is engaged in research on access issues to home health and adult day care. Her publications include "Sudden Infant Death Syndrome and the Stress-Buffer Model of Social Support," *Clinical Sociology Review*, 1992; "Ethnicity, Gender, and Parental Grief: The Case of Sudden Infant Death Syndrome (SIDS)," *Latino Studies Journal*, 1994; and "Independent Living among Mexican American Elderly: The Need for Social Services Support," *Contemporary Chicanos: Explorations in Culture, Politics and Society*, 1995.

DARLENE YEE is a Professor of Gerontology in the College of Health and Human Services at San Francisco State University, where she is also Coordinator of the Long-Term Care Administration Program and Project Director of the Health, Mobility, and Safety Laboratory. Her current research interests focus on improving and maintaining health, mobility, and safety of older adults, as well as minority management-training issues in long-term-care administration.

ISBN 0-313-28857-7

HARDCOVER BAR CODE